Outcome-Based Massage™ *Putting Evidence into Practice*

THIRD EDITION

Carla-Krystin (ck) Andrade, PhD, PT

Associate Clinical Professor
Department of Physical Therapy and Rehabilitation Sciences, School of
    Medicine, University of California–San Francisco
University of California–San Francisco/San Francisco State University
    Graduate Program in Physical Therapy
Private Practice: Wellness Workshops/Stress Free Zone

Photographs by Marc Boulay, BFA, MA

 Wolters Kluwer | Lippincott Williams & Wilkins
Health

Philadelphia • Baltimore • New York • London
Buenos Aires • Hong Kong • Sydney • Tokyo

Acquisitions Editor: Emily J. Lupash
Product Manager: Linda G. Francis
Marketing Manager: Sarah Schuessler
Production Editor: Vanavan Jayaraman
Designer: Stephen Druding
Compositor: Integra Software Services Pvt. Ltd.

Third Edition

351 West Camden Street   Two Commerce Square
Baltimore, MD 21201   2001 Walnut Street
                                Philadelphia, PA 19103

Printed in China

9 8 7 6 5 4 3 2 1

Library of Congress Cataloging-in-Publication Data
Andrade, Carla-Krystin, 1962-
Outcome-based massage : putting evidence into practice/Carla-Krystin Andrade, PhD, PT, associate clinical professor, Department of Physical Therapy and Rehabilitation Sciences, School of Medicine, University of California-San Francisco, University of California-San Francisco/San Francisco State University Graduate Program in Physical Therapy; photographs by Marc Boulay, BFA, MA.—Third edition.
    pages cm
Includes bibliographical references and index.
  ISBN 978-1-4511-3033-1
  1. Massage. 2. Massage—Decision making. I. Title.
  RA780.5.A53 2014
  615.8'22—dc23

                                                        2012041542

DISCLAIMER

To purchase additional copies of this book, call our customer service department at **(800) 638-3030** or fax orders to **(301) 223-2320**. International customers should call **(301) 223-2300**.

Visit Lippincott Williams & Wilkins on the Internet: http://www.lww.com. Lippincott Williams & Wilkins customer service representatives are available from 8:30 am to 6:00 pm, EST.

A truly good book teaches me better than to read it. I must soon lay it down, and commence living on its hint. What I began by reading, I must finish by acting.

HENRY DAVID THOREAU

TO

Trish Dryden and Linda Francis

Words cannot begin to express my sincere gratitude for your words of wisdom, unflagging enthusiasm, and ongoing encouragement through two editions of Outcome-Based Massage™.

Contributors

Paul Clifford, BSc, RMT
Professor, Massage Therapy Program
School of Health and Wellness
Sir Sandford Fleming College
Peterborough, Ontario, Canada
(Coauthor, *Outcome-Based Massage* 1st and 2nd editions)

Bryan Ausinheiler, DPT, CPT
University of California–San Francisco/San Francisco State
    University Graduate Program in Physical Therapy
(Evidence research for Chapters 1 to 14)

Celia Bucci, MA, LMT
Clinical Massage Therapy
Chicago, Illinois
(Passive Movement Techniques for Chapter 11;
    Percussive Techniques for Chapter 12; Clinical Cases
    for Chapter 14; Quick Treatment Guides)

Trish Dryden, MEd, RMT
Associate Vice-President, Research and Corporate
    Planning
Centennial College
Toronto, Ontario, Canada
(Evidence for Massage for Chapter 3)

Pamela Fitch, BA, RMT
Professor, Massage Therapy Program
School of Health and Community Studies
Algonquin College
Ottawa, Ontario, Canada
(Interpersonal and Ethical Issues for Chapter 2; Quick
    Treatment Guides)

Jane Galvan, PT, MS, DPT, OCS
Assistant Clinical Professor
University of California–San Francisco/San Francisco State
    University Graduate Program in Physical Therapy
San Francisco, California
(Client Examination Techniques for Chapter 4; Quick
    Treatment Guides)

Jocelyn Granger, MT
Director
Ann Arbor Institute of Massage Therapy
Ann Arbor, Michigan
(Neuromuscular Techniques for Chapter 9; Connective
    Tissue Techniques for Chapter 10; Clinical Cases for
    Chapter 14)

Theresa Jaramillo, PT, DPT, MS
Assistant Clinical Professor and Academic Coordinator
    of Clinical Education
University of California–San Francisco/San Francisco State
    University Graduate Program in Physical Therapy
San Francisco, California
(Client Examination Techniques for Chapter 4, Quick
    Treatment Guides)

Alfonse T. Masi, MD, DrPH
Professor of Medicine and Epidemiology
University of Illinois College of Medicine at Peoria
Peoria, Illinois
(Scientific Basis of Soft-Tissue Examination for
    Chapter 4, Quick Treatment Guides)

Stacey Shipwright, BA, RMT
Research Analyst
Applied Research and Innovation Center
Centennial College
Toronto, Ontario, Canada
(Evidence for Massage for Chapter 3)

Paula Tanksley, BA, MPT
Private Practice, Tanksley Physical Therapy
Oakland, California
(Client Examination Techniques for Chapter 4)

Christine Zampach, DPT
University of California–San Francisco/San Francisco State
    University Graduate Program in Physical Therapy
San Francisco, California
(Pain Examination Techniques for Chapter 4)

Subject Matter Experts

Stephen Goring, BSc, MA, RMT
Private Practice
Toronto, Ontario, Canada
(Client's emotional response to massage treatment
    for Chapter 2)

Teresa Randall, MPT
Staff Physical Therapist
Alameda County Medical Center–Fairmont Campus
San Leandro, California
(Strategies to enhance client adherence for Chapter 2)

The author wishes to thank the following individuals who reviewed portions of the manuscript and provided constructive feedback or clinical expertise during critical stages of the development of the various editions of this text. Their thought-provoking comments prompted much discussion and helped refine the final content.

Lorraine Allen, DPT

Amanda Baskwill, RMT

Benjamin Boyd, MSPT

Bridget Bouyssounouse, BS, PT

Nancy Byl, PT, PhD, FAPTA

Nancy Mezick Cavender, MM, LMT, LNMT

Sandi Chan, BS, PT

Kevin K. Chui, PT, PhD, GCS

Tara Detwiler, Certified Advanced Rolfer

Deborah Edmondson, PT, EdD

Alexandra N. Fallot, BA, MPT

Paul Finch, PhD, MSc, DPodM

Meghan Gordineer, MPT

Betty Ann Harris, BSc, RMT

Susan Klingaman Estilaei, PT, DPT, OCS

Wendy Katzman, PT, DPTSc, OCS

Shawn Jarman, MPT

Lee Kalpin, RMT

Julianne Lepp, CNMT

Liz Lester, RMT

Everett L. Lohman, DSc, PT, OCS

Wendy Moore, BA, MSc, MD, FRCP(C)

Rosalyn Pitt, PT, EdD, SPE

Gaye Raymond, BS, MS, PT

Kenneth Resznyak, RMT

Rick Ritter, PT, DPT, OCS

Jarek Szymczak, RMT

Kimberly Topp, PT, PhD

Foreword

Nearly five years ago I was moved to write an enthusiastic foreword for the second edition of *Outcome-Based Massage*™. For a number of reasons, I felt that book was an invaluable, truly unmatched resource for both massage educators and clinicians. When I learned that the third edition was about to come out, I honestly wondered whether improvements could be made, and whether the world of massage had changed enough or produced enough new data to warrant a third edition. The answer is yes and yes.

Healthcare in North America is changing dramatically, with implications for the role of massage that make this rich text more important than ever. In addition, Dr. Andrade has made changes, including the very important addition of the Quick Treatment Guides, that render this work not only likely the best book on your shelf, but also something akin to a coach in your own office, guiding you step by step in the care of your patients. I recommend this improved text even to those who have already purchased the first two editions.

First, a few words on the changing nature of health care in North America and the role of massage within it. Opportunities are coming, but we must be ready. Nothing will be handed to us. That is the punch line. And I believe this book can help practitioners be ready.

Health care is changing because what ails us is changing. In the 21st century, we are not dying from the bubonic plague or any of its relatives. We are, increasingly and at great expense and suffering, dying from our own collective and individual bad habits. We are dying from chronic illnesses that result from stress, obesity, substance abuse, lack of good sleep, and physical inactivity. We are also experiencing unprecedented rates of chronic musculoskeletal pain. The Affordable Care Act of 2010, recognizing this situation, is changing the way health care is delivered in the United States. Some of these changes have already taken place in Canada and others likely will. I will only mention two here because they relate directly to the strengths of *Outcome-Based Massage*™: *Putting Evidence into Practice.*

- In 2014 a section of the Affordable Care Act (Section 2706) is slated to go into effect, which will make it illegal for an insurer or insurance company to discriminate against a health care provider who is practicing within his or her licensed scope of practice. While it may take some legal and political work to hold all insurers to this standard, I believe it is inevitable that this will come to pass and will open doors of reimbursement for clinicians who are ready. I emphasize "who are ready" because an insurer will not need to include *every* therapist in order to heed the law, just *some* therapists. Therapists who will be most ready are those who can develop and execute plausible, effective treatment plans that are in keeping with existing research literature. That is, therapists who understand how to go from *evidence* (which they know how to locate) to *practice,* which they know how to explain and execute.

- The Affordable Care Act mandated the creation of a Patient-Centered Outcomes Research Institute (PCORI) in recognition of the fact that traditional double-blind placebo-controlled randomized clinical trials don't answer all of our health care questions. PCORI will focus on issues that matter to clinicians and patients and will be conducting largely, though not exclusively, comparative effectiveness research. I think we can all see that when massage is being compared to other treatments, we want to make sure we are putting our best foot forward in our treatment. I believe this volume, like the previous editions of this text, will help us do that. In *Outcome-Based Massage*™: *Putting Evidence into Practice,* Andrade tackles the obstacles to integrating clinical decision-making and a focus on client outcomes within our massage treatment head on and provides us with practical solutions that we can all use.

For these reasons, I believe this third edition is particularly timely. It does, of course, offer us all the strengths that were apparent in the last two editions.

Earlier editions of *Outcome-Based Massage*^{TM} wiped away the excuses some clinicians have used to avoid staying abreast of the research literature and linking it to their daily practice. It also did away with the excuses of those who claim that their treatments are intuitive and therefore can't be planned or thought about. It erased the excuses of massage educators who emphasize technique and neglect teaching clinical reasoning and cultivating the mind of inquiry. Now, in place of our old excuses, Andrade and her multidisciplinary team of contributing authors have given us everything we need in the third edition of *Outcome-Based Massage*^{TM} to think intelligently about massage and apply the principles of *Outcome-Based Massage*^{TM} to our day-to-day treatment of patients with clinical conditions, as well as the wellness goals that will increasingly be recognized by insurers.

Personally, I was delighted to see that the third edition retains the key message of the earlier editions: *Intuition and compassion are not one end of a continuum with purposeful planning and delivery of theory-driven outcome-based treatment on the other end.* Rather than being at odds with one another, the heart and science of massage are two different and essential facets of good treatment. They are compatible, and their interplay is in fact the art of massage at its best. The structure of the book and each chapter reflect this philosophy beautifully by intertwining evidence and practice within the text and bringing the two together within the context of clinical practice in Clinical Cases.

This core message of "putting evidence into practice" is the springboard for the third edition. Andrade has surpassed all expectations by providing in this book the answers to our questions, spoken and unspoken, about how to do *Outcome-Based Massage*^{TM}. This book successfully achieves the right balance of theory and hands-on guidance for practitioners. The theory behind OBM is presented in clear prose with an emphasis on the concepts that are essential for clinical practice, as well as practical instruction on how to perform techniques. Additionally, the text takes on some often misunderstood concepts that form the scientific basis of soft tissue examination, such as resting muscle tension, and translates them into easy-to-grasp material that grounds it firmly in treatment applications.

The practical aspects of OBM are where this edition shines. Andrade and her contributors offer a comprehensive approach to assessment, treatment design, and treatment delivery that is meticulously explained in prose, pictures, charts, case studies, and video clips. The new Chapter 14, Practical Applications of OBM to Clinical Conditions and Wellness and the Quick Treatment Guides, picks up where the second edition left off by giving model examples, clinical cases, and guidelines for how to craft outcome-based treatments for clients with a wide variety of common clinical conditions and wellness goals. This content facilitates our transition from the more traditional approach of using standard massage regimens for patients with similar clinical conditions, to a clinical decision-making approach, to designing treatments that address each client's unique needs.

The authors also show us that, while treatments to enhance wellness may not look exactly like treatments to address impaired function, they can and should both be purposefully planned and outcome-oriented. Done well, they each rely upon careful observation, clinical reasoning, and clear goal setting. The goals are different, but the processes are the same. One of the gifts of this third edition of *Outcome-Based Massage*^{TM} is its direct attention to the similarities and differences in designing massage for both wellness and clinical conditions and extended content on wellness.

Andrade is an experienced and skilled educator. Learners of all types will find what is needed to give clients the best, which is, after all, what they deserve. The material in this book is as appropriate for advanced practitioners treating patients in a variety of settings and those responsible for setting the curriculum for our own continuing education as it is for the classroom student. This is a welcome resource for educators doing their best to teach skills (e.g., locating relevant research literature) and processes (e.g., clinical reasoning) that were not part of the curriculum when they were being trained. Our field is becoming more sophisticated, and this book helps us all keep pace with the changes.

There are important reasons for us as clinicians and as a profession to hone our skills of clinical reasoning and evidence-based practice. We don't do it to be trendy or to "succumb" to the medical paradigm. In applying the skills of treatment planning and evaluation presented in this text, the real wisdom of our profession, and of each of us, comes forward. The truth is that all good clinicians are alert observers with theories about how and why certain treatments work. One of our limitations as a profession has been that we have not encouraged ourselves, or one another, to articulate what we notice and what we think. The word intuition has too often been used in place of slowing down enough to notice and name the signals we are picking up from our clients—postural, palpatory, verbal bits of information that, combined with our past experience, lead us to choose the techniques, the pace, and the encouraging phrases of our treatments. *Outcome-Based Massage*^{TM} can teach us to name what we are noticing and organize it for the health and well-being of our clients. That is good massage.

It is also the basis of good research. Clinical reasoning and the researcher's mind of inquiry are intimately related, with overlapping skills used for somewhat different purposes. When, as clinicians, we articulate our observations and our theories about how massage works, we are able, as a profession, to identify the research agenda for our field. We can identify the unanswered questions coming from our clinical practice and encourage researchers to investigate these questions. Good practice and good research go hand in hand.

In fact, *Outcome-Based Massage*^{TM} should be essential reading for researchers of massage who are not practitioners.

It delineates the elements of the varied massage techniques in a way that will allow researchers to design more sophisticated protocols for clinical trials. It offers the best current thinking on the effects of specific techniques and mechanisms, both examined and unexamined. The technique-by-technique sections on how massage might work are invaluable.

This book is an important contribution to the field, a gift to anyone who cares about the development of therapeutic massage and its potential to help people.

Janet R. Kahn, PhD, NCBMT, LMT
Principal, Integrative Consulting
Executive Director, Integrated Healthcare
Policy Consortium
Member, Advisory Group on Prevention, Health
Promotion, and Integrative and Public Health

The field of massage has evolved considerably in recent years: our understanding of the potential effects of massage is deeper, our approach to evidence-based practice is more rigorous, and clinicians have recognized the importance of demonstrating and documenting the outcomes of their massage-based treatments. In keeping with these changes, *Outcome-Based Massage*™*: Putting Evidence into Practice* (3rd edition) shows students and practitioners how to integrate an Outcome-Based Massage™ (OBM) approach into their day-to-day clinical practice. The text gives them tools that they can use to increase client satisfaction and treatment effectiveness by designing and delivering treatments that explicitly address each client's unique needs and desired outcomes, instead of applying a standard treatment regimen to all clients who present with a given clinical condition.

This book is for healthcare students and professionals whose scope of practice permits them to perform massage techniques. We designed it so that entry-level students will find it to be an invaluable textbook and experienced practitioners will use it as an essential clinical reference. Consequently, a prior knowledge of massage is not needed in order to use this book effectively—simply a familiarity with basic scientific language and anatomy.

GOALS OF THE THIRD EDITION

In response to feedback from educators and clinicians, the third edition addresses the following goals:

■ *Emphasize the Practical Application of OBM Principles to Clinical Practice*

This edition of *Outcome-Based Massage*™ is even more "hands on" and practical than its predecessors. The first edition of *Outcome-Based Massage*™ was the first massage text to propose a systematic problem-solving approach in which clinicians design sequences of massage techniques to reflect a client's unique presenting issues and achieve specified treatment outcomes. Now that this approach is more widely accepted, the emphasis of this text shifts from the focus on "Why" and "What" of the earlier editions to a detailed discussion of "How," "When," and "With whom," as reflected in the Practice section of each chapter. This section gives instructions and clinical cases that show readers how to apply the concepts in their clinical practice.

■ *Demonstrate How to Plan and Progress Treatments Using OBM*

Students and practicing therapists who are new to OBM can benefit from guidelines on how to approach the care of a client who presents with a given clinical condition or wellness goals. To address this need, this book provides a variety of tools for learning how to apply the concepts of an Outcome-Based Massage™ approach to examination and treatment, including step-by-step guidelines, practice sequences, Clinical Cases, and the new, full-color Quick Treatment Guides for commonly treated clinical conditions, which appear as part of Chapter 14.

■ *Illustrate How to Integrate Evidence into OBM Treatment Planning and Delivery*

Evidence is a necessary component of the clinical care that we provide to our patients. Consequently, you will find sections in each chapter entitled "Evidence" that summarize the relevant current evidence, explain how to evaluate it and use it in practice, and reference the relevant research articles.

■ *Provide a Multidisciplinary Perspective on the Application of OBM*

For this edition, I have the privilege of including a stellar team of massage therapists, physical therapists, and physicians, who are practicing clinicians, authors, educators, and researchers. Their input complements my perspective as a physical therapist, clinician, researcher, and educator. In doing so, it introduces a broader, multidisciplinary view on how clinicians can use OBM in clinical practice and increases the relevance of this book to different healthcare professions.

■ *Retain the Best of the First and Second Editions*

This edition retains and updates all of the content on our unique integration of OBM clinical problem solving, manual skills, evidence-based practice, and interpersonal aspects of massage that readers found useful in the earlier editions.

WHAT'S NEW IN THE THIRD EDITION

The third edition goes beyond an update of the content of the second edition. No chapter goes untouched; every chapter of the book has been enhanced to make this edition of *Outcome-Based Massage*[TM] an even more effective textbook and clinical reference for student and practicing clinicians alike.

Structure

The approach of this text to teaching massage is based on the observation that practitioners need both clinical decision-making and manual skills, not merely a mechanical "laying on of hands," in order to use massage techniques effectively. Consequently, *Outcome-Based Massage*[TM]: *Putting Evidence into Practice* guides you through the steps of the OBM clinical decision-making process using the following framework.

Book Sections

Part I: Principles of Outcome-Based Massage[TM]

This section is concerned with the initial stages of clinical decision-making that form the foundation of clinical care. It provides a solid foundation of the essential concepts underlying Outcome-Based Massage[TM]; this foundation includes the definition of OBM, how to find and use evidence in practice, guidelines for effectively managing the ethical and interpersonal issues that arise in the therapeutic relationship, how to identify impairments and wellness issues through the client examination, and a step-by-step OBM clinical decision-making process for planning and progressing massage-based interventions that guides you from initial examination to discharge.

Part II: Application of Outcome-Based Massage[TM] to Clinical Conditions and Wellness

This section details how to apply all of the concepts of an Outcome-Based Massage[TM] approach to the examination and treatment of your patients including (a) discussions and examples of 68 outcomes and wellness goals that you can achieve using massage; (b) instructions on how to prepare yourself, your materials, and your client for treatment; (c) details of 17 commonly used massage techniques and instructions on how to perform them that are accompanied by photographs, palpation practice, and practice sequences; (d) guidelines on how to select massage techniques and develop sequences of massage techniques; (e) guidelines on how to plan and progress interventions to achieve treatment outcomes with massage; (f) an extensive set of Clinical Cases that illustrate the steps in developing OBM treatments for specific clinical conditions and wellness issues; and (g) the new, 1-page Quick Treatment Guides for 16 commonly treated clinical conditions and wellness issues that summarize the relevant anatomy, pathophysiology, examination techniques, outcomes, treatment techniques, and contraindications for treatment.

Chapter Sections

Objectives

Learning objectives for the chapter to focus you on the key concepts that will be covered within the chapter.

Evidence

This section (a) summarizes the relevant current evidence on the uses and physical and psychosocial effects of massage, examination techniques, and interpersonal and ethical issues in easy-to-understand terms and (b) uses it to explain how massage might work and how we might use it in practice. This edition also includes an updated comprehensive reference list of hundreds of research articles to support the evidence that we present, along with guidance on how to evaluate and understand this evidence.

Practice

This section provides detailed instructions, photographs, references for online videos, clinical cases, and practice sequences that show you how to use the concepts outlined in the chapter when you are examining and treating a client. This pertains to content on evidence-based practice, interpersonal and ethical aspects of massage, and therapist and patient preparation for treatment, as well as the material on client examination, treatment principles, and massage techniques.

Review

This section summarizes the key content of the chapter within the Takeaways and provides Critical Thinking Questions or OBM Clinical Decision-Making Exercises that you can use to facilitate your critical thinking about the information and test your grasp of the concepts.

Content

- **Chapter 1: Principles of Outcome-Based Massage™** provides an easier-to-digest definition of Outcome-Based Massage™ and its theoretical basis. This enables both students and practicing therapists to grasp the concepts of OBM more readily in preparation for later chapters.
- **Chapter 2: Interpersonal and Ethical Issues for Massage** includes new evidence and practical content on communication skills and strategies for the client interview.
- **Chapter 3: Evidence for Massage** highlights new evidence for the effects of massage, updates perspectives on levels of evidence, and introduces the concepts of whole systems massage and mixed methods research within the research on massage.
- **Chapter 4: Client Examination for Outcome-Based Massage™** has a new section entitled Scientific Basis of Soft-Tissue Examination that synthesizes relevant anatomy and current physiologic principles in its explanation of soft-tissue structure and function. It also has an extensive section on the examination of pain and new sections on how to perform palpation and commonly used client examination techniques.
- **Chapter 5: Outcome-Based Massage™ Clinical Decision-Making** now includes two levels of the systematic OBM clinical decision-making process for clinicians who are at different levels of mastery of the concepts of OBM. The basic, yet comprehensive, 9-step process is suitable for student and practicing clinicians who are new to the concepts of OBM. The detailed 27-step clinical decision-making process, which is accompanied by an extensive clinical case, facilitates clinicians' progress to a more advanced level of decision-making. This chapter now also shows the relationship among OBM clinical decision-making, evidence-based practice, and the therapeutic process.
- **Chapter 6: Preparation and Positioning for Outcome-Based Massage™** now adds Therapist's Preparation for Delivering Outcome-Based Massage™ Interventions, which describes the clinical frameworks that prepare clinicians for delivering OBM interventions: OBM's novel organization of massage technique, intelligent touch, and the intelligent practice of massage techniques. It also addresses the problem of clinician burnout by including a section on how to prevent burnout and suggested stress control strategies.
- **Chapters 7 to 12** on massage techniques have a new layout, and the organizational structure of these chapters will allow clinicians to follow the clearly written, updated, and illustrated instructions on how to perform massage techniques with greater ease. Revised Clinical Cases show how to use the massage techniques in the treatment of patients with clinical conditions.
- **Chapter 13: Sequencing Massage Techniques for Outcome-Based Massage™** extends the content on developing massage sequences for wellness massage, including practice sequences that are appropriate for wellness.
- The new **Chapter 14: Application of Outcome-Based Massage™ to Clinical Conditions and Wellness** outlines the outcomes that clinicians can achieve with massage, while showing clinicians how to plan and progress massage interventions that address client's impairments or wellness issues and achieve desired treatment outcomes. It also uses new clinical cases and OBM clinical decision-making exercises to illustrate how to apply OBM principles and techniques to the treatment of common clinical conditions and wellness issues. It reinforces the importance of the outcomes for massage by including up-to-date evidence for the latter.
- The new 4-color **Quick Treatment Guides**, which complement Chapter 14, were designed for treatment table-side use. They provide descriptions of anatomy and pathophysiology, key impairments or wellness goals, relevant examination techniques, massage treatment suggestions, complementary techniques, helpful hints, cautions and contraindications for 16 clinical conditions and wellness issues that the surveyed clinicians identified as those that they most often treat using massage techniques.
- Updated **Glossary** that reflects new terminology has been introduced in this edition.
- **References**: we strengthen the already impressive foundation of evidence with extended reference lists that include new evidence on massage techniques and highlight those references that are randomized clinical trials, systematic reviews, and meta-analyses.

HOW TO USE THIS BOOK

The content and features of this edition of *Outcome-Based Massage™* are intended to make it easier for you to learn how to integrate OBM clinical decision-making into your clinical practice as a means of increasing client satisfaction, enhancing your treatment effectiveness, and facilitating reimbursement for treatment. Whether you are a practicing clinician, student, or educator with patients who have clinical conditions or wellness goals, here are some guidelines for how to get the most out of this book.

Learning Objectives for This Book

When you use *Outcome-Based Massage™: Putting Evidence into Practice,* you will learn:

- A practical clinical decision-making process that you can use to examine clients, identify relevant impairments and wellness issues, determine appropriate outcomes, select massage and complementary techniques, design and progress interventions, and discharge clients
- When, why, how, and with whom to use massage techniques to achieve 68 different outcomes for wellness, the treatment of clinical conditions, and palliative care
- Guidance on how to prepare your clients and materials for massage
- Practical skills you need to perform neuromuscular, connective tissue, percussive, passive movement, superficial reflex, and superficial fluid massage techniques using correct manual technique
- How to complement massage with other techniques and homecare
- Therapist self-care and strategies to prevent overuse injuries and "burnout"
- How to successfully manage the unique interpersonal and ethical issues that accompany your use of massage techniques
- How to find, evaluate, understand, and apply the evidence for massage techniques

Structure

The book is divided into two parts: one focused on the principles of Outcome-Based Massage™ and the other on application of OBM to practice. The chapters are as follows:

Part I. Principles of Outcome-Based Massage™

Part II. Application of Outcome-Based Massage™ to Clinical Conditions and Wellness

Chapter Sections

There are four sections in each chapter that contain different types of information to enhance your understanding of the Outcome-Based Massage™ approach. You can use "Learning Objectives" to orient yourself to the key concepts in the chapter. Within the "Evidence" section, you will focus on the current evidence and theory to support practice. The "Practice" section is where you will find detailed instructions, photographs, references for on-line videos, clinical cases, and practice sequences that show you how to perform practical skills and apply theory to practice. Finally, you can enhance your understanding of the concepts within the chapter by using the material in the "Review" section.

Content

- **Content for a Broader Range of Healthcare Professions:** The content is intended to meet the needs of several healthcare professions that use massage such as physical therapy, massage therapy, occupational therapy, bodywork, chiropractic, athletic training, nursing and naturopathy. We now include content and a level of material that addresses licensure and credentialing requirements in massage for a broader range of healthcare professions. For example, we cover material that is relevant to (a) the National Certification Examination for Therapeutic Massage and Bodywork: pathology, therapeutic massage and bodywork assessment and application, professional standards, and ethics sections; and (b) the American Physical

Therapy Association Required Skills of Physical Therapy Graduates examination: evaluation, plan of care, body mechanics and positioning, interventions–manual therapy techniques, evidence-based practice, and professionalism sections.

- **Video Clips of Massage Techniques:** Almost 70 video clips that show how to perform many of the techniques and sequences illustrated by the photographs in the book are available online. These share the same labels as the photographs in the book and are cross-referenced within the text so that readers can use this material with ease.

- **Using Massage to Treat Patients with Clinical Conditions:** We show practitioners how to make the transition from the traditional approach of using standard massage sequences for clinical conditions to an outcome-based approach. In particular, we demonstrate how to identify the impairments associated with a client's clinical condition and create an intervention that treats those impairments and achieves specific treatment outcomes. We do so by discussing the clinical relevance, treatment considerations, guidelines for using massage techniques, and complementary modalities for 30 impairments related to common musculoskeletal, circulatory, respiratory, neurological, and psychoneuroimmunological conditions.

- **Using Massage to Treat Clients with Wellness Goals:** We describe the key differences between providing interventions for clients with clinical conditions and those who present for Wellness Massage in the absence of a clinical condition. We present a new, holistic model of wellness and demonstrate how to conduct a client examination and treatment planning to create effective massage interventions that achieve a client's wellness outcome. This provides practitioners with a more flexible alternative to using a standard "full-body wellness massage" sequence for their clients. We also provide step-by-step sample sequences that you can use for wellness interventions.

- **Sample Sequences of Massage Techniques:** As an adjunct to the principles of designing sequences, we provide step-by-step examples of short regional sequences, long regional sequences, general sequences, and full-body sequences for wellness and the treatment of impairments due to a variety of clinical conditions.

- **Physiological and Psychological Effects of Massage:** We offer more detailed discussions of the possible mechanisms for the physical and psychological effects of massage techniques in the How Techniques Might Work and Outcomes and Evidence sections for each of the techniques.

- **Comprehensive Overview of Client Examination Techniques:** This unique chapter synthesizes information on a wide range of clinical examination techniques that you can use to assess clients who present with a variety of impairments or wellness goals.

- **Expanded Instruction on How to Perform Massage Techniques:** We provide exemplary step-by-step instruction on manual technique and approximately 400 illustrations and photographs of massage techniques along with several components that will assist readers in learning manual techniques in, and beyond, the classroom. These include practice sequences for each technique, details of contraindications and cautions to using each technique, and details of how to use the techniques in treatment. We also discuss Eastern and European massage traditions.

- **Palpation Training:** We introduce the concept of "intelligent touch" and provide extensive instruction on how to use palpation for examination and treatment. Dozens of palpation exercises, which specifically relate to each technique, show you how to use palpation within the context of treatment.

- **Application of OBM to Practice:** The text contains examples of ways in which readers can apply the principles introduced in the chapter to real-life clinical situations such as Clinical Cases, Applications of OBM Cases, and Quick Treatment Guides.

- **Evidence-Based Practice:** We introduce the concepts of Evidence-Based Practice and the steps practitioners can use to find, understand, evaluate, and apply current evidence for massage techniques. We also provide an overview of the current state of research and theory on massage and a discussion of the issues related to creating a body of evidence for massage practice.

- **Putting Evidence into Practice:** We show practitioners how to integrate evidence into their daily clinical practice in several ways. Each chapter contains an "Evidence" section that summarizes key evidence. Furthermore, Chapters 7 to 12 contain "Examining the Evidence" sections for each category of techniques that demonstrate how to understand and apply evidence within daily practice. In addition, the "How Techniques Might Work" sections in Chapters 7 to 12 provide a summary of the current evidence that explains the possible therapeutic effects for each of the massage techniques.

- **Integrated Clinical Decision-Making and Documentation:** We demonstrate the OBM clinical decision-making process and relevant clinical documentation (using SOAP format) for the

Evaluative, Treatment, Treatment Planning, and Discharge phases of the clinical decision-making process using flowcharts and clinical cases.

- **Ethical and Interpersonal Issues in Massage:** The physical proximity of massage techniques often generates a heightened level of trust between the practitioner and the client. To address this, we have devoted an entire chapter to ethical and interpersonal issues. This includes details of the therapeutic relationship, a three-phase therapeutic process, an overview of therapists' and clients' rights, and several clinical scenarios to help practitioners understand these issues and the guidelines for practice.

- **Clinical Scope:** The scope of the book includes information on the treatment of clinical conditions, wellness, and palliative care that is relevant to clinicians who practice in a variety of settings.

- **Extended Glossary:** We have enlarged the glossary to include a larger number of massage-related terms and modalities.

- **References:** We provide an extensive reference list of research articles and other references on massage within two lists: References, which may be found at the end of the book (divided by chapter), and Further Reading, which may be found online at http://thePoint.lww.com/Andrade3e.

Key Features

The following features enhance the instruction in the text and help readers navigate.

Outcome-Based Massage^{TM} logo that appears on the front cover appears at the beginning of each chapter to orient the reader to which component of OBM the information in the chapter covers.

Key Points call out supplementary content that is of interest to the reader.

Examining the Evidence analyzes a research article on a massage technique discussed in the chapter.

Practice Sequence is massage sequence that you can use to practice a specific massage technique.

Online Videos demonstrate many of the techniques presented in the text; these are indicated with the icon <online>.

Takeaways summarize the key concepts in the chapter.

Clinical Case features a brief clinical case that illustrates how to use OBM to treat a patient with a given clinical condition or wellness issue.

Application of Outcome-Based Massage^{TM} (Chapter 14 only) is a longer clinical case that includes an OBM Clinical Decision-Making exercise and a sample treatment plan.

Critical Thinking Questions at the end of each chapter invite students to engage more deeply with the material for better understanding.

Quick Treatment Guide is a 1-page guide on how to use OBM for a specific clinical condition that includes anatomy, examination, and treatment information (these can be found in pages A432–A447).

*Randomized Controlled Trial, *†Systematic Review or Meta-Analysis*: These labels are used in the reference lists at the end of the book to identify the **Level of Evidence (Sackett)** of a given research article.

RESOURCES FOR LEARNING AND TEACHING

Hands-On Treatment References

This edition includes several features and sections that can serve as easy-to-use references for daily patient care.

- The 1-page Quick Treatment Guides summarize the relevant anatomy, pathophysiology, examination techniques, outcomes, treatment techniques, contraindications, and helpful hints for the treatment for 16 commonly treated clinical conditions.

- Chapters 7 to 12 on massage techniques include a "Practice" section for each massage technique that contains step-by-step instructions for therapist positioning and how to perform manual techniques accompanied by photographs, guidelines for what to palpate and observe, what to communicate to clients, cautions and contraindications, and how to use each technique in treatment.

- Chapter 13: Sequencing Massage Techniques for Outcome-Based Massage^{TM} contains a "Practice" section that gives guidelines for designing and performing regional and full-body sequences of massage techniques that you can use to achieve a variety of treatment outcomes for clients with clinical conditions and wellness issues.

- Chapter 14: Application of Outcome-Based Massage^{TM} to Clinical Conditions and Wellness includes 10 detailed Clinical Cases in the "Practice" section that illustrate how to apply OBM to common clinical conditions (acute, chronic, and palliative) and wellness issues. This complements the detailed guidelines on how to plan and progress interventions to achieve outcomes for patients with musculoskeletal, cardiopulmonary, neurologic, psychoneuroimmunological, and multisystem (including pain) clinical conditions and wellness issues.

Online Resources

This edition of *Outcome-Based Massage*™ provides a wealth of information on the theory and manual technique of massage for students, educators, and clinicians at all levels. We also provide several online instructional aids to simplify the process of using *Outcome-Based Massage*™ as the primary text or an adjunct to your program.

- PowerPoint presentations synthesize the key information from each chapter, which you can use within lectures or as handouts
- The Instructor's Guide is a flexible resource that provides recommendations and ideas for effective presentation of each objective listed in the book, no matter the length and focus of a particular class.
- The Test Generator contains numerous questions on the content
- The Image Bank includes all of the art that appears in the text, including the extensive set of manual technique photographs.
- The video clips of manual techniques are organized in alphabetical order and listed by chapter.
- Student Resource Center gives students access to the videos as well.

A Note on Language

This text addresses the needs of a variety of different healthcare practitioners. For the sake of simplicity, we use the terms *practitioner*, *therapist*, and *clinician* interchangeably to refer to the individual who is providing care. Furthermore, practitioners will be treating clients or patients depending on their practice setting. Consequently, we use the terms client and patient interchangeably, to refer to the individual who is receiving care.

Contact Dr. Andrade

In essence, the third edition is a judicious balance of what worked in the first editions and new material that will enable readers to make OBM an integral part of daily practice. I trust that *Outcome-Based Massage*™ (3rd edition) will be a book that you will read and then act on.

I welcome your questions, comments, and suggestions. Please feel free to contact me at askdrck@stressfreezone.com or on Facebook at CK Andrade or Carla-Krystin Andrade.

Acknowledgments

Each edition is a chance to try something new, and this edition was no exception. Frankly, this new edition could not have happened without Trish Dryden, Celia Bucci, Pamela Fitch, Jocelyn Granger, Stacey Shipwright, Jane Galvan, Theresa Jaramillo, Bryan Ausinheiler, Alfonse Masi, and Christine Zampach, our contributors; Linda Francis, our Product Manager; and Emily Lupash, our Acquisitions Editor, who embraced the idea of this interdisciplinary collaboration and took a leap of faith with me. Their generosity with their time and considerable expertise, their patience, and their excitement about the project were heartwarming and humbling—I could fill a book with the millions of ways in which I would like to thank them. A new look for the interior was part of the new concept for the book and I am grateful to Steven Druding (design) and Vanavan Jayaraman (production) for their visually engaging design and layout. Michael Connors, Manual A. Domenech, Deborah Edmonson, Robin Helton, Beth McNeill, Jeff Moggach, Lou Peters, Diane H. Pitts, Jessica Rogers, Edith Smith, and James Kevin Tenpenny gave valuable input during reviews. And Sarah Schuessler contributed her marketing know-how to the project.

The strength of this edition rests on the foundation of the prior editions. For this I owe a debt of gratitude to Paul Clifford for the years that we spent brainstorming new approaches, honing the concept of Outcome-Based Massage™, and writing the first two editions together. In that vein, I would like to add a note of thanks to our contributors from the early editions, Trish Dryden, Pamela Fitch, Paula Tanksley, Teresa Randall, and Stephen Goring, and the reviewers for their wonderful additions to those texts. In addition, I would like to acknowledge other key people whose guidance and assistance shaped the early editions: Peter Darcy, Peter Sabatini, John Goucher, and Margaret Biblis on the editorial side; Freddie Patane and Mark Flanders for their video expertise; Marc Boulay for his outstanding photographs; and Chanelle Andrade, Christopher Alger, Tricia Bachman, Joanne Baker, Dan Boon, Paul Bucciero, Brian Burgess, Melissa Cole, D!ONNE (Francis), Etienne Harris, Lee Kalpin, Rahima Kassam, Michael Kitney, Amy Knapp, Chris Lemieux, Frank Marincola, Colin Outram, Shahnaz Suteria, Jarek Szymczak, and Jane Wellwood, our models for photographs and videos.

And in the midst of all of the book production craziness, my special treat for this edition was to be able to share my work in progress and my downtime with my son Alan, who was a newborn for the first edition (my, how the years have flown!). Thanks for helping me keep things in perspective.

Contents

PART

I

Principles of Outcome-Based Massage™

OVERVIEW OF CHAPTERS IN PART I

Chapter 1: Principles of Outcome-Based Massage™

Therapists can use Outcome-Based Massage™ to achieve client-specific outcomes for medical massage, wellness massage, and whole systems massage treatments. To prepare them for doing so, this chapter explains the principles of Outcome-Based Massage™, the concept of outcomes, and relevant outcomes for medical massage, wellness massage, and whole systems massage.

Chapter 2: Interpersonal and Ethical Issues for Massage

Since interpersonal issues are often more subtle and less easily addressed than direct mechanical problems, this chapter provides clear explanations of the therapeutic relationship, the therapeutic process, and problems that may arise in the therapeutic relationship. It also outlines concrete strategies for ethical decision-making and enhancing the therapeutic relationship in typical "in the moment" clinical situations.

Chapter 3: Evidence for Massage

This chapter addresses questions such as: "What is good evidence?" and "What constitutes best evidence when making clinical decisions?" It also describes how evidence helps therapists to serve their clients better. Finally, it introduces concepts related to the steps of finding, understanding, critically evaluating, and applying best evidence to clinical practice.

Chapter 4: Client Examination for Outcome-Based Massage™

This chapter reviews selected issues for therapists to consider when conducting a client examination prior to using massage techniques. These topics include the focus of an examination for the use of massage techniques, body structures and functions that are relevant to massage, client reports that arise during the course of history-taking that can suggest soft tissue dysfunction, and the use of palpation and nonpalpatory examination techniques.

Chapter 5: Outcome-Based Massage™ Clinical Decision-Making

This chapter discusses Outcome-Based Massage™ clinical decision-making over four phases: the evaluation phase, the treatment planning phase, the treatment phase, and the discharge phase. It provides guidelines for therapists to use to enhance the appropriateness and adequacy of the client examinations, plans of care, and interventions they plan and provide. In addition, it shows the relationship between Outcome-Based Massage™ clinical decision-making and evidence-based practice and the therapeutic relationship.

Principles of Outcome-Based Massage™

OBJECTIVES

After studying this chapter, you will have the information that you need to do the following:

1. Describe the goals and components of Outcome-Based Massage™.
2. Describe the relationship between Outcome-Based Massage™ clinical decision-making, evidence-based practice, and the therapeutic relationship.
3. Identify the components of the structure, process, and outcomes of clinical care.
4. Describe and distinguish among outcomes for medical massage, wellness massage, and whole systems massage.
5. Identify when it is appropriate to establish different types of outcomes for clients.

Therapists can use Outcome-Based Massage™ (OBM) to achieve client-specific outcomes for medical massage, wellness massage, and whole systems massage treatments. To prepare them for doing so, this chapter explains the principles of Outcome-Based Massage™, the concept of outcomes, and relevant outcomes for medical massage, wellness massage, and whole systems massage.

Evidence

OUTCOME-BASED MASSAGE™: AN OVERVIEW

Outcome-Based Massage™ (OBM) is a systematic treatment approach in which therapists provide massage interventions with the goal of achieving specified **outcomes** that are tailored to address each client's unique needs, presenting issues, and preferences. Outcome-Based Massage™ has three key components: **Outcome-Based Massage™ clinical decision-making**, **evidence-based practice**, and the **therapeutic relationship** (Figure 1-1). Outcome-Based Massage™ clinical decision-making is a systematic process in which the therapist and client work together to (a) identify the

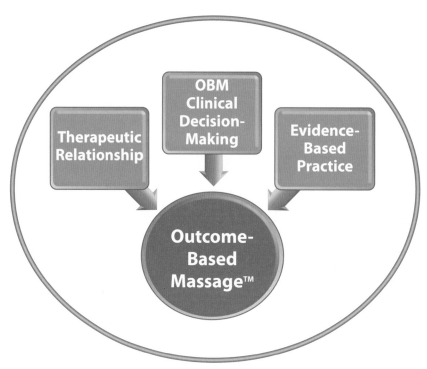

FIGURE 1-1 Components of Outcome-Based Massage™.

client's issues and the desired outcomes based on those issues and (b) develop and implement a treatment plan to achieve those outcomes. Evidence-based practice[1] provides therapists with a framework for using the evidence to guide the client evaluation, treatment planning, and treatment in Outcome-Based Massage™. Finally, therapists practice Outcome-Based Massage™ within a collaborative, client-centered therapeutic relationship that respects the ethical, sociocultural, and interpersonal aspects of the therapist–client interactions.

Outcome-Based Massage™ has several key features, some of which are outlined in Key Points 1-1. In particular, Outcome-Based Massage™ is distinguished from other treatment approaches because it delivers interventions that are focused on achieving outcomes that reflect each client's unique clinical presentation. It recognizes, for example, that two clients with the same clinical condition may present with different impairments and, consequently, have different desired outcomes that require a different treatment approach.

OUTCOMES FOR MASSAGE

The **outcomes of care** are the results of the care that the therapist delivered to the client within a given clinical setting. In the case of massage, outcomes can be the results

of a single **intervention** using massage techniques or of all of the interventions in the **plan of care** as a whole.[2] There are a multitude of ways to measure these outcomes. Administrators may be more concerned with cost-effectiveness, the efficiency

---

Key Points: 1-1

Features of Outcome-Based Massage™

- Uses the systematic Outcome-Based Massage™ clinical decision-making process for identifying each client's unique presenting impairments or wellness goals, defining treatment outcomes, and planning and delivering treatment

- Based on wellness models and models of functioning, disability, and health

- Classifies massage techniques on the basis of the tissue layer they treat and the outcomes they achieve

- Uses massage and other treatment techniques to achieve specific treatment outcomes

- Selects massage and other treatment techniques based on the evidence for their effects

- Modifies and progresses interventions based on the results of ongoing client reexamination

- Addresses the client's interpersonal and ethical needs

- Modifies interventions to address the client's interpersonal and physical needs

- Integrates massage techniques into interventions using effective practical skills of care, and client satisfaction. Therapists, on the other hand, may look at the short-term and long-term effects of care on the client's body structures and function, levels of activity and participation, or overall wellness. Clients, in turn, bring their own perspective on the relevant effects of care on their clinical condition, function, overall wellness, or **quality of life**.

There are several basic assumptions related to the use of outcomes within Outcome-Based Massage™.[3] First of all, massage techniques have a variety of possible outcomes, but not all of these outcomes are relevant for a given client or situation. Second, therapists can use massage to produce a variety of distinct outcomes related to impairments and wellness goals. The third assumption is that therapists can structure the massage treatment to produce some outcomes and not others. The fourth is that therapists can measure the client's progress toward the achievement of the desired outcomes. Finally, outcomes can encompass (a) client-centered outcomes based on the client's physical, psychological, social, and spiritual needs[4] and (b) broader whole systems–oriented outcomes that consider the therapeutic environment and the therapist–client interaction.[5]

Based on these assumptions, a therapist needs to use three steps to determine the appropriate treatment outcomes for a given client. First, the therapist must understand the potential **therapeutic effects** of massage and the evidence for those effects. The therapist must then identify which of the client's body structures and functions or aspects of activity or participation level can be treated appropriately with massage techniques. This commonly goes hand in hand with the final step of determining whether the therapist is treating the client using an approach of **medical massage**, **wellness massage**, or **whole systems massage**.

Therapeutic Effects of Massage

A massage technique can produce multiple therapeutic effects. These may occur locally, only on the site of manipulation, or generally throughout the client's body. The majority of the therapeutic effects of massage techniques fall into six categories: mechanical, physiologic, psychological, reflex, psychoneuroimmunological, and "energetic" (Table 1-1).[6-12] Mechanical effects result from the therapist physically moving the tissues by compression, tension (stretch), shearing, bending, or twisting. In the case of reflex effects, the client's nervous system mediates therapeutic changes. Physiologic effects involve a change in biochemical processes in the client's body. Psychological effects, on the other hand, occur in the client's mind, emotions, or behavior. Psychoneuroimmunological effects are those effects in which changes in hormone levels or immune function accompany changes in a client's feeling

Table 1-1 General Therapeutic Effects of Massage Techniques[6-11]

Effect[a]	Description	Example Outcome
Mechanical[b]	■ Effects are caused by physically moving the tissues by compression, tension (stretch), shearing, bending, or twisting	■ Increased lymphatic return ■ Mobilized bronchial secretions
Reflex[b]	■ Functional change is mediated by the nervous system	■ Sedation or arousal ■ Facilitation of skeletal muscle contraction
Physiologic[b]	■ Involves a change in biochemical body processes	■ Improved modeling of connective tissue ■ Reduced muscle spasm
Psychological	■ Effect occurs in the mind, emotions, or behavior	■ Improved social interaction ■ Improved physical self-image
Psychoneuroimmunological	■ Altered feeling state is accompanied by changes in hormone levels or immune function; this term emphasizes that "mere" feeling states like relaxation represent complex multisystem phenomena	■ Decreased anxiety and cortisol levels ■ Improved T-cell function
Energetic	■ Direct effects on the client's biomagnetic field and possible secondary effects on client's body structures and functions	■ Improved biomagnetic field pattern ■ Improved energy flow

[a]Any given massage technique produces multiple effects, and outcomes are usually achieved through several mechanisms operating simultaneously.
[b]Effects may be local, occurring only on the site of manipulation, or general, occurring throughout the body.

state. In this case, the term psychoneuroimmunological emphasizes that feeling states, such as relaxation, actually represent complex multisystem phenomena. Finally, energetic effects are direct effects on the client's biomagnetic field and possible secondary effects on the client's body structures and functions.

Impairments and Outcomes for Medical Massage

In medical massage, therapists use massage to help clients with clinical conditions return to an optimal state of **health**.[3,13,14] The **International Classification of Functioning, Disability and Health** (ICF)[15,16] is a commonly used model for explaining the dimensions of health. The ICF model represents the individual at three levels: **body structures and functions**, **activity**, and **participation** (Figure 1-2). Body structures are the various anatomical structures and systems of the body, and body functions are the physiologic functions of those anatomical systems (Table 1-2 and Key Points 1-2). Activity capacity is the individual's execution of a task or action in an ideal situation (Table 1-3). Finally, participation refers to the individual's involvement in a life situation or the ability to execute a task within his environment (Table 1-3). The individual's clinical condition, a disease or disorder, affects all three levels of his functioning concurrently. At the same time, the individual's **personal factors** and **environmental factors**, termed here as **contextual factors**, are all exerting an effect on the individual's body structures and functions, activity, and participation.

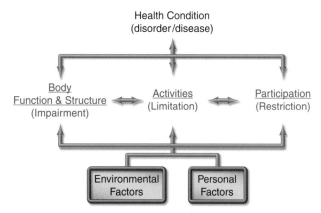

FIGURE 1-2 The International Classification of Functioning, Disability and Health. Reprinted from World Health Organization. *Towards a Common Language for Functioning, Disability and Health: ICF: The International Classification of Functioning, Disability and Health*. Geneva, Switzerland: World Health Organization; 2002, with permission from the World Health Organization.

Table 1-2	Summary of Body Structures and Functions from the ICF[15,16]
Body Structure	**Body Function**
Nervous system: brain, spinal cord, and peripheral nerves	■ Consciousness ■ Orientation (time, place, person) ■ Intellect ■ Energy and drive functions ■ Sleep ■ Attention ■ Memory ■ Emotional functions ■ Perceptual functions ■ Higher level cognitive functions ■ Language ■ Pain
Eye, ear, and related structures	■ Seeing ■ Hearing ■ Vestibular (including balance functions)
Structures involved in voice and speech: nose, mouth, pharynx, and larynx	■ Vocalization ■ Articulation ■ Rhythm and tempo functions
Cardiovascular, hematologic, immunologic, and respiratory systems	■ Heart functions ■ Blood pressure ■ Hematologic (blood) functions ■ Immunologic (allergies, hypersensitivity) functions ■ Respiration
Digestive, metabolic, and endocrine systems	■ Digestive functions ■ Defecation ■ Weight maintenance ■ Endocrine gland functions (hormonal changes)
Genitourinary and reproductive systems	■ Urination functions ■ Sexual functions
Neuromusculoskeletal structures related to movement: head and neck region, shoulder region, upper extremity (arm, hand), pelvis, lower extremity (leg, foot), trunk, and spine	■ Mobility of joint ■ Muscle power ■ Muscle tone ■ Involuntary movements
Skin and related structures (skin glands, nails, hair)	■ Protective functions ■ Repair functions ■ Sensation

Examples of Neuromuscular and Movement-Related Body Functions

Key Points: 1-2

Functions of the joints and bones

- Mobility of joint: Functions of the range and ease of movement of a joint
- Stability of joint: Functions of the maintenance of structural integrity of the joints
- Mobility of bone: Functions of the range and ease of movement of the scapula, pelvis, and carpal and tarsal bones

Muscle functions

- Muscle power: Functions related to the force generated by the contraction of a muscle or muscle groups
- Muscle tone: Functions related to the tension present in the resting muscles and the resistance offered when trying to move the muscles passively
- Muscle endurance: Functions related to sustaining muscle contraction for the required period of time

Clients who seek treatment for clinical conditions present with impairments in body structures or functions. An impairment can be any loss or abnormality of the client's body structures or functions that occur as a result of the pathophysiology of a clinical condition. Unlike pathophysiology, which occurs at the level of the cell, impairments and their effects are usually visible and/or palpable. For example, adhesions, elevated resting muscle tension, postural adaptive shortening, edema, anxiety, and depression are all impairments. Furthermore, each clinical condition has a characteristic set of potential impairments.[17] For example, the impairments associated with fibromyalgia may include muscle pain, muscle tenderness, elevated resting muscle tension, tender points, anxiety, disturbed sleep, and altered body image. An outcome for a client with a clinical condition is, therefore, a desired change in a specific impairment in body structure or function that stems from that client's clinical condition. Different clients with the same clinical condition can, however, present with different combinations of the characteristic impairments and, consequently, can require different outcomes and different treatment regimens. Consequently, the therapist's final step is to determine which outcomes are relevant for the client's needs and the intent of the intervention.

Relevant Massage Outcomes for Impairments

In the case of an intervention for the treatment of clinical conditions, the therapist will have a list of impairments

Table 1-3	**Activity and Participation Domains from the ICF[15,16]**
Learning and Applying Knowledge	**Mobility**
■ Watching	■ Lifting and carrying objects
■ Listening	■ Fine hand use (picking up, grasping)
■ Learning to read	■ Walking
■ Learning to write	■ Moving around using equipment (wheelchair, skates, etc.)
■ Learning to calculate (arithmetic)	■ Using transportation (car, bus, train, plane, etc.)
■ Solving problems	■ Driving (riding bicycle or motorbike, driving car, etc.)
General Tasks and Demands	**Self-Care**
■ Undertaking a single task	■ Washing oneself (bathing, drying, washing hands, etc.)
■ Undertaking multiple tasks	■ Caring for body parts (brushing teeth, shaving, grooming, etc.)
Communication	■ Toileting
■ Communicating with—receiving—spoken messages	■ Dressing
■ Communicating with—receiving—nonverbal messages	■ Eating
■ Speaking	■ Drinking
■ Producing nonverbal messages	■ Looking after one's health
■ Conversation	

(Continued)

Table 1-3	**Activity and Participation Domains from the ICF[15,16]** (*Continued*)

Domestic Life

■ Acquisition of goods and services (shopping, etc.)

■ Preparation of meals (cooking, etc.)

■ Doing housework (cleaning house, washing dishes, laundry, ironing, etc.)

■ Assisting others

Interpersonal Interactions and Relationships

■ Basic interpersonal interactions

■ Complex interpersonal interactions

■ Relating with strangers

■ Formal relationships

■ Informal social relationships

■ Family relationships

■ Intimate relationships

Major Life Areas

■ Informal education

■ School education

■ Higher education

■ Remunerative employment

■ Basic economic transactions

■ Economic self-sufficiency

Community, Social, and Civic Life

■ Community life

■ Recreation and leisure

■ Religion and spirituality

■ Human rights

■ Political life and citizenship

---

in body structures and functions and outcomes that revolve around the treatment of impairments, **recovery**, and the **prevention** of secondary impairments.[6,18] This list of impairments and associated outcomes may contain outcomes that cannot be achieved directly through the use of massage techniques. Consequently, the therapist needs to select those impairments that are amenable to treatment with massage techniques prior to finalizing the list of desired treatment outcomes. Recent work on summarizing the effects of massage concluded that reduction of anxiety and reduction of musculoskeletal pain, including low back pain, are among the most established outcomes for massage.[3,9] Nevertheless, massage can have other important physiologic and psychological outcomes such as positive effects on mood, stress reduction, reduction of lymphedema and impairments in patients with cancer, and improved oxytocin levels, immune function, sleep, and airway clearance. Table 1-4 provides a list of the impairments in body structures and functions that massage techniques can address and some of the associated outcomes that therapists can attain through the use of these techniques.

Relevant Functional Outcomes

Therapists must also bear in mind that a client's clinical condition can also have an effect on activity level or participation level. Although massage interventions will not address those directly, the therapist is also wise to consider the changes in the client's levels of activity and participation expected from a treatment approach. These are functional outcomes (Table 1-5) that provide meaningful changes for the client and justification for reimbursement for services.[18]

Outcomes for Wellness Massage

Health-care professionals now define **wellness** as encompassing both a balance of "mind, body, and spirit" and individuals' self-perception of their well-being, which is distinct from their state of "health."[19,20] In other words, a person can consider himself as having a high level of wellness, even though he has a clinical condition that leaves him with suboptimal health in one or more of the domains of health. For example, people who are living with chronic illnesses, disabilities, or clinical conditions associated with age are still capable of experiencing high levels of wellness.

It is a common misconception that wellness massage does not require a sound foundation of clinical reasoning and a systematic outcome-based approach to intervention. Therapists working in the area of wellness are better able to help their clients achieve optimal wellness when they provide massage interventions that are directed at achieving outcomes for wellness, rather than "back rubs." Clear definitions and models of wellness, such as the **Wellness Interactions Model (WIM)**, can provide the foundation for the effective use of massage to achieve wellness outcomes.

Table 1-4	Impairments in Body Structures and Functions Amenable to Treatment with Massage and Related Outcomes

Impairments	*Outcome*
Musculoskeletal	
■ Adhesions/scarring	■ Increased tissue mobility
	■ Decreased scarring
■ Impaired connective tissue integrity	■ Separation and lengthening of fascia
■ Fascial restrictions	■ Promotion of dense connective tissue remodeling
■ Abnormal connective tissue density	■ Increased connective tissue mobility
■ Decreased mobility of skin, superficial and deep fascia	
■ Impaired joint integrity	■ Decreased signs of inflammation of joint capsule, tendons, or ligaments
■ Inflammation of joint capsule or ligaments	■ Decreased capsular and ligament restrictions
■ Restrictions of joint capsule and ligaments	■ Increased joint mobility
	■ Increased joint integrity
■ Impaired joint mobility	■ Increased joint mobility
■ Decreased voluntary range of motion	■ Increased voluntary range of motion
■ Impaired muscle integrity	■ Increased muscle extensibility
■ Decreased muscle extensibility	■ Decreased signs of inflammation and promotion of healing of tendons
■ Muscle strains and tears	■ Decreased signs of inflammation and promotion of healing of muscle
■ Tendinopathies	■ Decreased trigger point activity
■ Trigger points	■ Increased joint mobility
■ Impaired muscle performance (strength, power, endurance)	■ Enhanced muscle performance secondary to the enhancement of muscle extensibility, reduction of pain, reduction of muscle spasm, enhancement of joint mobility, normalization of joint integrity, reduction of trigger point activity, etc.
	■ Balance of agonist/antagonist muscle function
■ Abnormal resting muscle tension	■ Decreased muscle spasm
■ Muscle spasm	■ Normalized resting muscle tension
	■ Increased joint mobility
■ Postural malalignment	■ Normalized postural alignment
	■ Increased postural awareness
■ Impaired sensation (secondary to entrapment neuropathy, nerve root compression)	■ Normalized sensation (secondary to the reduction of nerve and nerve root compression due to fascial restrictions and trigger points)
Psychoneuroimmunologic	
■ Stress	■ Systemic sedation
	■ Increased perceived relaxation
	■ Decreased levels of cortisol, epinephrine, and norepinephrine
Multisystem	
■ Pain	■ Pain reduction through primary treatment of dysfunction, e.g., active trigger points
	■ Counterirritant analgesia
	■ Systemic sedation resulting in decreased perception of pain

(Continued)

Table 1-4	Impairments in Body Structures and Functions Amenable to Treatment with Massage and Related Outcomes (*Continued*)

Impairments	*Outcome*
■ Swelling: edema, joint effusion, lymphedema	■ Increased lymphatic return ■ Increased venous return ■ Decreased joint effusion ■ Decreased edema ■ Increased joint integrity ■ Increased joint mobility
Cardiopulmonary	
■ Impaired airway	■ Increased respiration/gaseous exchange ■ Increased airway clearance/mobilization of secretions ■ Decreased dyspnea
■ Dyspnea	■ Decreased dyspnea due to increased airway clearance ■ Decreased dyspnea due to increased perceived relaxation
■ Impaired rib cage mobility (other than bony abnormality)	■ Increased rib cage mobility ■ Increased muscle extensibility ■ Increased ventilation
Neurological	
■ Abnormal neuromuscular tone: spasticity, rigidity, clonus	■ Normalized neuromuscular tone ■ Alteration of movement responses through proprioceptive and exteroceptive stimulation techniques ■ Balance of agonist/antagonist muscle function

Table 1-5	Sample Functional Outcomes

Activities of Daily Living	**General Outcomes**
■ Increased ability to perform grooming tasks, such as bathing and dressing ■ Increased ability to perform work-related tasks, such as lifting and keyboarding ■ Increased ability to perform leisure tasks ■ Increased ability to perform transfers, such as sit to stand ■ Increased ability to perform bed mobility tasks, such as rolling from side to side or scooting ■ Increased ability to perform gait and locomotion tasks ■ Increased ability to perform functional mobility tasks, such as toilet and bath transfers ■ Increased ability to perform cooking tasks ■ Improved quality or quantity of movement during functional activity ■ Improved safety during functional activity ■ Decreased level of supervision required for task performance ■ Increased tolerance for positions and activities	■ Improved self-management of condition ■ Decreased risk of recurrence of condition ■ Improved decision-making regarding health issues ■ Reduced utilization and cost of health-care services ■ Decreased need for adaptive, assistive, supportive, protective, or orthotic equipment or devices ■ Ability to recognize and seek intervention for a recurrence of the clinical condition ■ Decreased intensity of care required

Adapted with permission from American Physical Therapy Association. *Guide to Physical Therapist Practice*. 2nd ed. Alexandria, VA: American Physical Therapy Association; 1999.

FIGURE 1-3 The Wellness Interactions Model.

The Wellness Interactions Model created for Outcome-Based Massage™ is based on the ICF.[15] It does not have a continuum or progression through varying levels of disease and health to wellness like Travis' original Wellness Model.[20,21] Instead, it shows an ongoing interaction between a person, wellness, and his environment (Figure 1-3). In this model, an individual's level of wellness can affect any aspect of the person at any point in life, and vice versa. In the WIM, a person has multiple dimensions: **spirit**, brain and body structures and function, activity capacity, ability to participate in society, and **wellness behaviors**. Here, body structures and functions, activity capacity, and ability to participate in society are the same as in the ICF. In the case of wellness, however, the relevant body structures and functions are those that are free of impairments—grade 0. Spirit, a concept that is not part of traditional models of health, refers to that part of a person's nonphysical being that embodies his or her drive to transcend the physical world.[19,22,23] Wellness behaviors are personal factors that play a central role in wellness, such as self-nurturance, healthy lifestyles, readiness for change, and perceived health.[6,24,25] Finally, the WIM highlights the importance of **environmental factors**: facilitators and barriers to wellness that individuals encounter in their social setting. The environmental factors that can affect wellness are many and varied and can include social attitudes, available wellness services, education, and the individual's financial status.[15]

Relevant Massage Outcomes for Wellness

In wellness massage, the client does not present with impairments in body structures and function that are secondary to a clinical condition. Instead, the client has several body structures and functions that they wish to enhance as the focus of a wellness intervention. The therapist will examine these structures and functions to ensure that they are free of impairments prior to embarking on a wellness intervention that targets these areas. In the absence of impairments that stem from a clinical condition, the therapist will have a list of relevant impairment-free body structures and functions and associated outcomes for wellness, which are directed at optimizing them.[4] Outcomes for wellness focus, therefore, on the client's desired wellness goals. Relevant outcomes for wellness goals can include optimized functioning of any body part or body system, prevention of injury, improved body awareness, enhanced mental focus, enhanced ability to deal with stress, self-nurturing, and others noted in Table 1-6.[3,12] A common misconception is that massage treatments for increased muscle tension, anxiety, stress-related problems, and depression are wellness massage. Clients with these conditions are in fact presenting with impairments in a variety of body functions including mental functions, psychological functions, and immunologic functions. By definition, therefore, this treatment of stress-related disorders, anxiety, and other similar conditions is the treatment of impairments, whereas stress management interventions that prevent impairments and optimize function are wellness interventions.

Wellness Outcomes in the Presence of a Clinical Condition

The Wellness Interactions Model addresses the fact that individuals with clinical conditions can also have body structures and functions that are unaffected by the clinical condition and free of impairments and, therefore, are appropriate for wellness interventions. For example, a client with a hamstring strain still has other body structures

Table 1-6   Domains, Definitions, and Sample Outcomes for Wellness and Whole Systems

Domain	Definition	Sample Outcomes
Physical	Related to the body	■ Increased energy ■ Improved sleep ■ Enhanced postural awareness ■ Improved functional status ■ Enhanced immune function
Social	Related to the life and relations of humans in their community	■ Improved social functioning ■ Increased social support ■ Improved family relationships
Psychological	Related to the mind, emotions, or other mental phenomena	■ Increased general well-being ■ Positive mood ■ Increased relaxation ■ Improved coping skills
Spiritual	Related to the spirit or soul, as distinguished from the physical self	■ Enhanced spiritual well-being ■ Improved mindfulness
Health-related quality of life	Related to ability to function in and derive satisfaction from a variety of roles in the presence of impaired health status	■ Improved quality of life ■ Improved functional status
Holistic	Related to outcomes on a global level	■ Enhanced well-being ■ Improved wellness ■ Increased life satisfaction
Context	The set of circumstances encompassing the intervention or healing experience, such as the client–provider relationship	■ Increased empathy ■ Increased positive attitudes to therapy ■ Increased trust in health-care provider
Process	Related to the process of healing and personal transformation, such as learning	■ Enhanced capacity for transformation ■ Enhanced personal growth
Individualized	Important to, and as identified by, the individual client or research participant	■ Various

Adapted with permission from Dryden T, Moyer CA, eds. *Massage Therapy: Integrating Research and Practice*. Champaign, IL: Human Kinetics; 2012.

and functions for which the therapist can establish outcomes for wellness, despite the impairments and limitations in activity and participation that stem from the clinical condition.

Outcomes for Whole Systems Massage

The Whole Systems approach takes a broader view of the client within the therapeutic environment and therapist–client relationship, rather than focusing on the client's clinical condition or wellness goals alone.[3,5] Looking at outcomes from this perspective will consider the clients' experiences of massage, psychosocial effects of the therapeutic environment, clients' expectations of the therapist, and even the therapists' perspective. Within the realm of the clients' experiences of massage, for example, we see that clients report that massage contributes to improved body image, self-image, social identity, confidence, perceived relaxation, perceived well-being, and ability to cope with stress.[26-30] Furthermore, massage also helps clients connect mind and body and leaves them feeling good and feeling cared for. Clients also have characteristics that they report desiring in a Massage Therapy experience: personal time, a competent therapist, trust, holism/empowerment, effective touch, and relaxation.[31] Finally, from the therapists' perspective, the evidence has given us some insight into the positive and negative personal and professional experiences that influence an individual's professional choices.[32] Table 1-6 notes possible domains and outcomes for whole systems excerpted from the IN-CAM database.[4]

THE CLINICAL CONTEXT FOR OUTCOMES

As noted earlier in this chapter, a treatment **outcome** is a result that a therapist obtains through delivering a treatment to a client. Outcomes are one of the three components of clinical care defined by Donabedian.[2] The other two components, which are equally important, are the structure and process of clinical care (Figure 1-4). This chapter examines outcomes in the context of the structure, process, and outcomes of clinical care as a whole, to enable therapists to use and interpret outcomes more effectively within massage treatments.

The Structure of Care for Massage

According to Donabedian,[2] the **structure of care** refers to the human, physical, and financial resources available for

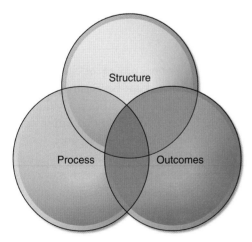

FIGURE 1-4 Components of clinical care. Adapted from Donabedian A. Evaluating the quality of medical care. *Milbank Q.* 1966;3:166-206, with permission of *Milbank Quarterly.*

delivering care. This includes the staff, the clinical environment, the organization's financing, and other resources.

Human Resources

- Organization of staff
- Number and distribution of staff
- Qualifications and training of staff

Physical and Financial Resources

- Size of facility
- Geographical location of facility
- Organization of facility
- Equipment available
- Formal financing

Often, despite the therapist's best intentions, the structure in which she provides care has an impact on her approach to treatment. Consider the situation of the therapist treating the client with carpal tunnel syndrome in a busy outpatient setting with restrictions on reimbursement for services, 20-minute treatment sessions, and a high proportion of aides assisting with treatment delivery. This setting presents different constraints and benefits than those that the therapist would encounter in an on-site occupational injury center with 45-minute treatment sessions, few adjunct personnel, and a flexible reimbursement structure. A therapist treating clients with industrial injuries in the busy outpatient setting is less likely to have time for extensive use of hands-on massage techniques, and will have a greater component of education in self-care, than the therapist treating the client in the on-site occupational rehabilitation setting. For this reason, therapists need to be aware of the context in which they treat their clients, even though this will not be an explicit component of treatment planning.

The Process of Care for Massage

The **process of care** is the manner in which the therapist delivers care.[2] It refers to how the activities between the therapist and the client take place. There are two aspects to the process of care: the technical aspects of how the therapist provides care and the interpersonal aspects of the client–therapist interaction. The importance of the process of care cannot be emphasized enough. Therapists need to understand the process by which they deliver care to their clients in order to improve their interventions. This understanding can also enable them to identify if they can improve the outcomes they achieve by changing the process of care—the manner in which they deliver care.

Technical Aspects of the Process of Care

Technical aspects of care include a range of issues related to the mechanics of delivering care such as

- Utilization patterns
- Appropriateness of referrals
- Completeness of diagnosis
- Appropriateness of examinations and evaluations performed by therapists
- Adequacy of interventions selected and provided by therapists
- Relevance of treatment goals set by therapists
- Patterns of treatment by therapists

Of these technical aspects of care, the appropriateness and adequacy of the examination performed, the therapist's evaluation of the client's presenting problems, the intervention plan outlined, and the interventions selected and provided by the therapist are the most relevant to the practicing therapist.[2] Examination, evaluation, treatment planning, and intervention are interdependent processes within the clinical decision-making process. For example, a therapist's failure to adequately evaluate the relevant impairments related to the client's clinical condition will lead to an intervention that does not effectively address the client's impairments. As a result, it is less likely that the client's functional limitations that result from these impairments will improve with treatment. In the case of a client with carpal tunnel syndrome, if the therapist evaluated only strength, and paresthesia, the intervention she provided would fail to address the pain that could be limiting the client's ability to perform functional activities and contributing to his other symptoms. As later sections will discuss, a therapist can use regular reexamination of the client's status to monitor the adequacy of the interventions he is providing. This will provide the therapist with several opportunities for refining the intervention and for enhancing the technical process of care delivery.

Interpersonal Aspects of the Process of Care

Three components make up the interpersonal aspects of the delivery of care: the client, the therapist, and the interaction between the two, which is often referred to as the **therapeutic relationship**.[2]

The Client

At the heart of clinical care lies the client and all of the things that he brings into treatment, such as physical and psychological characteristics, family history, lifestyle, work and home environment, and belief systems. In addition, the client enters treatment with expectations for treatment and outcomes that will affect the treatment process, whether or not the therapist inquires about these expectations. The International Classification of Functioning, Disability and Health (ICF) provides us with a framework for understanding the client who receives massage interventions for medical massage. The Wellness Interactions Model (WIM), on the other hand, explains different aspects of the client who receives wellness massage.

The Therapist

The therapist's interpersonal manner is the second component and includes aspects such as her interpersonal skills, her skill as an educator, and her ability to engage and motivate clients. A therapist's primary purpose is not merely to implement treatment plans. In reality, the therapist's ability to engage, educate, motivate, and support the client throughout the treatment process is as important as her technical skill.

The Client–Therapist Interaction

The interaction between the client and the therapist is the third component. The quality of this interaction can shape the level of client adherence, client motivation, and, in many ways, the outcomes of the plan of care. Therefore, the therapist is wise to engage the client in the therapeutic process, to solicit and respect the client's input on the plan of care and treatment outcomes, to consider the context in which the client lives and works, and to seek the client's feedback throughout the course of treatment. This is particularly true in the clinical use of massage techniques, because the use of touch can raise issues related to personal vulnerability, emotional responses to treatment, and the need to set appropriate boundaries between the client and the therapist.

Clinical Setting

Rarely is the interpersonal process of clinical care limited to the interactions that occur between the client and the therapist; typically, this process occurs within a specific clinical setting (Figure 1-5).[2] First, the clinical setting may include a variety of health-care professionals with whom both the therapist and the client may interact. In addition, the client has a social network of caregivers, relatives, and others who may participate in, or have an impact on, the process of clinical care. The complexity of the interactions will vary with the clinical setting, the client, and the client's presenting clinical condition. For example, a therapist who is treating a geriatric client with a stroke in a rehabilitation setting will have to manage numerous interactions over the course of treatment. These may include interactions

Social Context of Care

Health-Care Professionals

Client's Social Network

Clinician

Client

Client–Clinician Relationship

FIGURE 1-5 Social context of care. Adapted from Donabedian A. Evaluating the quality of medical care. *Milbank Q.* 1966;3:166-206, with permission of *Milbank Quarterly.*

with the client, the client's family, and the other members of the health-care team in the rehabilitation setting and possibly some community-based resources for the family. On the other hand, the therapist who is treating a client with carpal tunnel syndrome in the on-site occupational injury center will only have to interact with the client, the referring physician, and, perhaps, the client's supervisor.

The Outcomes of Care for Massage

Regardless of the type of outcome selected, the therapist needs to be cautious not to overemphasize outcomes and ignore the structure and process of care. In reality, a therapist needs to understand and evaluate the structure and process of care to determine why the intervention was successful or not. Furthermore, the danger always exists that a therapist may discard a potentially effective intervention because the outcomes achieved were poor, when in fact the problem lay in the manner in which the intervention was delivered (process of care). A holistic, client-centered intervention will, therefore, consider the structure, process, and outcomes of clinical care.

IN CONCLUSION

Outcome-Based Massage™ clinical decision-making, evidence-based practice, and the interpersonal and ethical issues in the therapeutic relationship combine to provide the theoretical framework for Outcome-Based Massage™ (OBM). One goal of Outcome-Based Massage™ is to identify and treat appropriate outcomes, which are the results that a therapist obtains through delivering a treatment to a client. In Outcome-Based Massage™, therapists evaluate a client's body structures and functions, levels of activity and participation, and contextual factors and use this information to define which body structures and functions need to be addressed in their interventions and set appropriate outcomes for treatment in collaboration with their clients. In addition, whenever relevant, they use findings on the client's limitations in activity and participation to define functional outcomes that they can reasonably expect to achieve through the intervention.

The types of outcomes set by the therapist will vary with the overall massage approach. First of all, in medical massage, therapists treat the impairments in the client's body structures and functions, which result from a clinical condition, as a means of enhancing the client's level of activity and participation and decreasing the client's impairments. Second, in wellness massage, therapists direct their interventions toward the client's body structures and functions that are free of impairments as a means of optimizing wellness. Finally, by contrast, whole systems massage considers the client within the therapeutic environment and therapist–client relationship, rather than focusing on the client's clinical condition or wellness goals alone. In all treatment approaches, therapists reevaluate the client's body structures and functions to refine their selection of treatment techniques from the taxonomy of six types of techniques. Finally, they reevaluate the client's body structures and functions and levels of activity and participation to determine when to terminate based on the client's achievement of identified outcomes.

Practice

Note: This section contains clinical cases and instructions that demonstrate how to use some of the principles of Outcome-Based Massage™ that were introduced in this chapter.

IMPAIRMENTS AND OUTCOMES FOR PATIENTS WITH CLINICAL CONDITIONS

Clinical Case 1-1: Impairments and Outcomes for a Patient with Postural Malalignment illustrates possible outcomes for a patient with a clinical condition. In this situation, the clinician is providing medical massage.

The patient has postural malalignment, which affects her body structures and functions, activity, and participation. The body structures involved are her lumbar spine and her abdominal, hip flexor, and erector spinae muscles. The associated impairments of these body structures are hyperlordosis of the lumbar spine and shortened musculature. The impairments in her body functions, such as pain and muscle weakness, are a consequence of her altered body structure. There are two key contextual factors affecting this patient. The personal factors are her dislike of exercise and her perceived decrease in her quality of life. The environmental barrier of a busy schedule of traveling results in increased exposure to activities that aggravate her pain and decreased time for exercise and treatment, which limit the level of function that she may be able to achieve. The result of the interaction among the body structures and functions, clinical condition, and contextual factors is that the patient has limitations in her capacity to perform work-related activities and leisure activities. Furthermore, she experiences restrictions in her participation in her life situation, namely a decreased ability to perform in and enjoy the activities of her social roles as a sales manager and a parent.

The problem list in Clinical Case 1-1 summarizes this patient's impairments and limitations that will form the basis for determining outcomes for her massage intervention. The clinician's final step is to determine which outcomes are relevant for the patient's needs and the intent of the intervention. Since this is an intervention for the treatment of a clinical condition, the clinician will have a list of impairments in body structures and functions and outcomes that revolve around the treatment of impairments, recovery, and the prevention of secondary impairments. Clinical Case 1-1 shows the patient's impairments in body structures and functions and some relevant outcomes.

This list of impairments and associated outcomes contains several outcomes that cannot be achieved directly through the use of massage techniques. Consequently, the clinician needs to select those impairments that are amenable to treatment with massage techniques prior to finalizing the list of desired treatment outcomes. Using Table 1-4 as a guideline will produce the list of impairments and outcomes for massage noted in Clinical Case 1-1. Based on this list of outcomes for massage, the clinician can select massage techniques whose therapeutic effects will achieve the desired outcomes. The chapters on massage techniques include tables that document possible outcomes for individual massage techniques to guide clinical decision-making.

Finally, the clinician also considers the changes in the patient's levels of activity and participation expected from a treatment approach. These are functional outcomes (Table 1-5) that provide meaningful changes for the patient and justification for reimbursement for services. Clinical Case 1-1 shows a sample of relevant functional outcomes for the patient with postural malalignment and muscular low back pain. Note that functional outcomes are an indirect result of the use of massage techniques, rather than outcomes that are specific to the individual massage techniques.

Clinical Case 1-1: *Impairments and Outcomes for a Patient with Postural Malalignment*

Note: This clinical case illustrates possible outcomes for a patient with a clinical condition (medical massage).

Patient Profile

A 50-year-old female who is employed as a sales manager has had a recent onset of low back pain following a busy period of traveling. She is overweight because her work and family schedule leave her little time for exercise. She has never been fond of exercising.

Clinical Findings

Presenting Issue

Postural malalignment (hyperlordosis) and muscular lumbosacral pain

Subjective Findings

- Aching in muscles across her lower back
- Pain increases with sitting, driving, and standing for >30 minutes
- Decreased ability to carry out her leisure activities of going to movies and bowling with her children
- Decreased ability to carry out her role as a sales manager who travels extensively by plane and car
- Demanding work schedule is necessary because she works partly on commission and has a busy territory

Objective Findings

- Hyperlordotic
- Tight erector spinae in lumbar region
- Erector spinae in lumbar region tender on palpation
- Tight iliopsoas muscles bilaterally
- Weak abdominal muscles—unable to perform >2 crunches

Impairments and Outcomes

Problem List

1. Impairments in body structure
   - Hyperlordotic
   - Tight erector spinae in lumbar region
   - Tight iliopsoas muscles bilaterally
   - Increased abdominal girth
2. Impairments in body function
   - Muscular pain in lumbar region
   - Weak abdominal muscles
3. Activity limitations
   - Decreased ability to carry out her role as a sales manager who travels extensively by plane and car
   - Decreased ability to carry out her leisure activities of going to movies and bowling with her children

4. Participation restrictions
   - Inability to perform job of sales manager
   - Inability to perform social role as a parent
5. Environmental factors
   - Demanding work schedule with a lot of traveling
6. Personal factors
   - Dislike of exercising
   - Perceived decreased quality of life and ability to function in and enjoy her social roles as sales manager and parent

Outcomes for Impairments

Impairments in Body Structures and Functions	Outcomes
■ Postural malalignment: hyperlordotic	■ Normalized lumbar spine posture ■ Improved postural awareness
■ Tight erector spinae muscles in lumbar region	■ Increased extensibility of erector spinae muscles ■ Decreased resting muscle tension in erector spinae muscles
■ Tight iliopsoas muscles bilaterally	■ Increased extensibility of iliopsoas muscles
■ Muscular pain in lumbar region	■ Decreased muscular pain in lumbar erector spinae muscles ■ Systemic sedation resulting in decreased perception of pain
■ Weak abdominal muscles	■ Increased functional strength of abdominal muscles; able to perform abdominal bracing during functional activities and maintain correct pelvic alignment
■ Imbalance of agonist–antagonist muscle function	■ Enhanced balance of agonist–antagonist muscle function

(Continued)

Functional Outcomes

Activity Limitations and Participation Restrictions

Activity limitations
- Decreased ability to carry out her role as a sales manager who travels extensively by plane and car
- Decreased ability to carry out her leisure activities of going to movies and bowling with her children

Participation restrictions
- Inability to perform job of sales manager
- Inability to perform social role as a parent

Outcomes

- Patient is able to sit for >30 minutes while traveling in a car or plane without complaints of pain
- Patient is able to walk carrying a briefcase >20 minutes without complaints of pain
- Patient is able to bowl for >30 minutes without complaints of pain
- Patient initiates functional activity readily without fear of pain

WELLNESS OUTCOMES

As noted earlier in this chapter, clinicians can identify wellness outcomes for patients who are free of impairments and for those who have impairments secondary to a clinical condition. Clinical Case 1-2: Wellness Outcomes for a Patient with Carpal Tunnel Syndrome illustrates the process of setting wellness outcomes for a patient who has a clinical condition.

Often in wellness massage, the patient does not present with a clinical condition. In the absence of impairments that stem from a clinical condition, the clinician will have a list of the patient's wellness goals and relevant body structures and functions. The clinician will examine these structures and functions to ensure that they are free of impairments and set wellness goals that are directed at optimizing the patient's body structures and functions.

Clinical Case 1-2 illustrates that individuals with clinical conditions can also have body structures and functions that are free of impairments and, therefore, appropriate for wellness interventions. In this situation, the clinician uses the same clinical decision-making process for setting these wellness outcomes as that for the patient who does not have a clinical condition. The 30-year-old with carpal tunnel syndrome in Clinical Case 1-2 still has body structures and functions for which the clinician can establish outcomes for wellness, despite the impairments and limitations in activity and participation that stem from his clinical condition. For example, his sleep pattern, energy levels, and resting tension in his shoulder and neck muscles are within normal limits. Consequently, he can have wellness goals for optimizing these body structures and functions, as illustrated in this clinical case.

Clinical Case 1-2: *Wellness Outcomes for a Patient with Carpal Tunnel Syndrome*

Note: This clinical case illustrates how to formulate wellness outcomes. The patient has a clinical condition and the clinician will deliver components of medical massage and wellness massage.

Patient Profile

A 30-year-old male, who is employed as a data entry clerk, has long-standing carpal tunnel syndrome on the right side as a result of long periods of keyboarding.

Clinical Findings

Clinical Condition and Pathophysiology

- Carpal tunnel syndrome
- Inflammation of the wrist and finger flexor tendons in the region of the carpal tunnel
- Inflammation results in pressure on the median nerve as it passes through the carpal tunnel

Subjective Findings

- Pain in fingers and hand
- Inability to perform customary job-related activities, especially typing, filing, and writing
- Inability to perform leisure activity of playing racquetball
- Inability to perform activities of daily living, especially grooming and household tasks that involve lifting
- Fear of experiencing pain during functional activity
- Inability to carry out social roles as a data entry clerk and a member of a racquetball club
- Limited health insurance to cover the cost of treatment for carpal tunnel syndrome

Impairments and Outcomes

Problem List

1. Impairments in body structure
   - Edema in the region of the carpal tunnel
   - Pressure on the median nerve
   - Decreased joint range of motion of wrist and fingers
2. Impairments in body function
   - Pain
   - Paresthesia
   - Decreased strength of hand and wrist muscles
3. Activity limitations
   - Inability to perform customary job-related activities, especially typing, filing, and writing
   - Inability to perform leisure activity of playing racquetball
   - Inability to perform activities of daily living, especially grooming and household tasks that involve lifting

4. Participation restrictions
   - Inability to perform job of data entry clerk
   - Inability to perform social role as a member of a racquetball club
5. Environmental factors
   - Limited health insurance
6. Personal factors
   - Fear of exacerbating pain limits initiation of functional activity
   - Perceived decreased ability to function in and enjoy his social roles of data entry clerk and member of a racquetball club

Patient's Wellness Goals

- Enhance sleep
- Increase level of relaxation of muscles
- Improved energy for activities

Wellness Outcomes

Relevant Body Structures	Relevant Body Functions
Structure of the nervous system - Brain	Mental functions - Energy and drive functions - Sleep
Structure of the respiratory system - Respiratory system	Function of the respiratory system - Respiration
Neuromusculoskeletal and movement-related structures - Head and neck region - Shoulder region	Neuromusculoskeletal and movement-related functions - Resting muscle tension

Body Structure or Function	Wellness Outcome
Brain	- Increased quality and quantity of sleep - Increased energy
Respiratory system	- Increased ventilation
Muscles of the head, neck, and shoulder region	- Normalized resting muscle tension

TAKEAWAYS

1. Outcome-Based Massage™ is a systematic treatment approach in which clinicians provide massage interventions with the goal of achieving specified outcomes that are tailored to address each patient's unique needs and presenting impairments or wellness goals.
2. Outcome-Based Massage™ has three key components: Outcome-Based Massage™ clinical decision-making, evidence-based practice, and the therapeutic relationship.
3. Outcomes are one of the three components of clinical care defined by Donabedian: structure, process, and outcomes.
4. The structure of care refers to the human, physical, and financial resources available for delivering care.
5. The process of care is the manner in which the clinician delivers care.

6. Massage techniques have a multitude of possible outcomes but not all of these outcomes are relevant for a given patient or situation.
7. Clinicians can use massage to produce a variety of distinct outcomes related to impairments and wellness goals.
8. An outcome for a patient with a clinical condition is a desired change in a specific impairment in body structure or function that stems from that patient's clinical condition.
9. Patients who present for wellness massage may not have clinical conditions and their associated impairments. Outcomes for wellness focus, therefore, on the patient's desired wellness goals for impairment-free body structures and functions.
10. Individuals with clinical conditions can also have body structures and functions that are free of impairments and, therefore, appropriate for wellness interventions.

Critical Thinking Questions

1. How is Outcome-Based Massage™ different from treating using a standard treatment protocol for all patients with the same clinical condition?
2. What are the situations in which a clinician would deliver different massage interventions to patients with the same clinical conditions?
3. What are the differences between the structure and the process of care?
4. What are the components of care that can affect the outcomes achieved by a clinician?
5. How can a clinician determine if a body structure or function is appropriate for a wellness intervention or for the treatment of a clinical condition?

6. What steps can a clinician take to ensure that he can achieve the outcomes he has established for his patient using a given set of massage techniques?
7. How will the list of clinical issues and associated outcomes differ if the clinician is planning an intervention for wellness versus an intervention for the treatment of clinical conditions?
8. What issues must clinicians consider when creating lists of outcomes for an intervention that will include massage techniques?
9. In which situations is it inappropriate to establish wellness outcomes for a patient?
10. What are functional outcomes and where do they fit into the process defining outcomes for massage?

References for Chapter 1 begin on p. 449.

CHAPTER 2

Interpersonal and Ethical Issues for Massage

OBJECTIVES	After studying this chapter, you will have the information that you need to do the following:

1. Describe the dimensions of the massage therapeutic relationship.
2. Explain the importance of client-centered care in massage therapy.
3. Outline key strategies for enhancing the massage therapeutic relationship.
4. Discuss strategies that support client adherence to the plan of care.
5. Explore the impact of personal history on client experiences of massage.

Therapists who use massage techniques are often not trained in psychotherapy. Yet, good hands-on therapy depends to a large degree on the therapist's ability to listen, observe, help clients be aware of changes, respond to discomfort, modify interventions according to client wishes, and reinforce the changes that clients make. Regardless of how well a therapist addresses impairments and functional limitations, the client may make little progress without participating in clinical decision-making. Ethical therapist behavior and clear communication are essential for a strong therapeutic alliance or relationship to develop. For teaching purposes, we often separate the clinical or technical aspects of care from the interpersonal interactions that occur between the therapist and client. In reality, the technical and interpersonal aspects of care are closely intertwined. Since interpersonal issues are often more subtle and less easily addressed than direct mechanical problems, this chapter will provide clear explanations of the therapeutic relationship, the therapeutic process, and problems that may arise in the therapeutic relationship. It will also outline concrete strategies for ethical decision-making and enhancing the therapeutic relationship in typical "in the moment" clinical situations when using Outcome-Based Massage™.

Evidence

At the heart of any treatment encounter is the therapeutic relationship between the practitioner and patient.

MITCHELL A, CORMACK M. *The Therapeutic Relationship in Complementary Health Care*. London: Churchill Livingstone; 1998:37.[1]

FOUNDATIONS OF THE THERAPEUTIC RELATIONSHIP

The Therapeutic Relationship

Donabedian's[2] model of clinical care (Figure 2-1) describes the interaction that occurs between the client and the therapist as a critical interpersonal component of the process of clinical care. This **therapeutic relationship** is a trust relationship, rather than a simple interaction between two people, because of the client's vulnerability and the therapist's responsibility not to exploit or harm the client through this vulnerability.[3] It is a rich and dynamic interaction in which a client's spoken and unspoken wishes interact with what the therapist perceives to be feasible, appropriate, and helpful. The therapeutic relationship provides a container for the hopes, expectations, and fears of the client. It provides a zone of safety for the client in which the client can stop, sense, reflect, and change with the help of the therapist.

A recent study suggests that despite whatever bodily changes a therapist hopes to achieve in a client's condition,

massage therapy clients actually seek significant interpersonal experiences, such as caring, connectedness, and compassion, in addition to therapist competence.[33,35] In addition, a meta-analysis of massage therapy research suggests that some of the positive responses to massage therapy may be attributable to the warmth and positive regard of the therapist toward the client and the development of an alliance between the therapist and the client, which are factors that are usually associated with psychotherapeutic interactions. According to Moyer et al.,[35] massage therapy may have more in common with psychotherapy than was previously considered. Such evidence puts considerable responsibility on the therapist to respond to clients in a supportive and compassionate way. Therapists must discern the most responsible and appropriate way of interacting with clients, a task that demands maturity, and understanding of the relationship that builds between client and therapist.

The therapist sets the tone of the therapeutic relationship based on her willingness to share information, support client goals, and empathize with the client's circumstances or condition.[2,3] Most importantly, the therapist must hold the best interests of the client above all other aspects of the interaction. Consequently, a healthy alliance between therapist and client depends on the therapist's awareness and acceptance of the client's needs (Key Points 2-1). If the therapist is skilled in observation, seeks clarification, and adapts the intervention to the client's abilities or tolerance, then therapeutic outcomes will most likely succeed.[3] If the therapist cannot read the client's desires, body language, and behavioral cues, then the client will not find the therapeutic relationship dependable. If this occurs, the client may feel unsafe and unable to trust the therapeutic process.

Client-Centered Care

Client-centered care is a philosophy of care that underlies the therapeutic relationship for Outcome-Based Massage™. This approach to care looks beyond the mere delivery of services to the client to include advocacy, empowerment, respect for the client's autonomy, and the client's participation in decision-making.[4] When a therapist commits to client-centered care, the client and therapist share the decision-making about how the

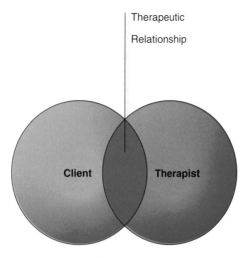

FIGURE 2-1 The therapeutic relationship.

<table>
<tr><td>

Key Points: 2-1

What Does a Client Need from a Therapeutic Relationship?

Safety
- Promotes trust and allows the client to explore sensation and make therapeutic change.

Predictability
- Reduces the need to adapt to a new situation.
- Further promotes trust in the therapeutic relationship.

Patience
- Gives the client permission to feel sensation and pain and to make therapeutic change.
- Compassion and empathy.
- Helps establish an alliance with the therapist that promotes desired outcomes.
- Clear consent negotiation.
- Involves client in making decisions about outcomes.

Clear and Explicit Interpersonal Process
- Underscores the integrity of the therapeutic process and the safety of the therapist.

Healthy Boundaries
- Contains and establishes the context for the therapeutic experience.
- Time to explore sensation.
- Teaches the client to be present in his or her body and aware of sensations and the willingness to change.

Responsible Closure
- Prepares the client to move from the therapeutic realm to the outside world.

</td></tr>
</table>

intervention will proceed. Other best practices for client-centered care can encompass recognizing that the clients are experts on their own lives, focusing on the client's goals, and providing timely, responsive, and consistent care.

The Therapeutic Contract

The therapeutic relationship provides the framework for negotiating the clinical care that the client will receive. The **therapeutic contract** is the form that this negotiation takes.[2,3] In the process of formulating this contract, the client brings his or her condition, wishes for treatment, and expectations for success to the therapist. The therapist sifts through all the information that can be gleaned from the client's story and an objective client examination

and then develops an intervention that she believes will help the client. Although it seems mechanical, the process of developing and working with a therapeutic contract can be complex. Sometimes this commitment seems simple and straightforward. At other times, therapists can forget or feel conflicted with their contractual responsibilities—a situation that puts their clients at risk for poor outcomes. In addition, while some aspects of the therapeutic contract are explicit, problems can arise, in part, because many aspects of the contract are unspoken.[5]

Rights and responsibilities are the cornerstone of the therapeutic contract. The client's rights and the therapist's responsibilities are the most commonly discussed. Nevertheless, the client also has responsibilities within the therapeutic contract and the therapist is not without rights.

Clients' Rights and Responsibilities

The client comes into the client–therapist relationship with rights that exist to protect her from victimization or harm by the therapist, as well as to ensure that she receives a high standard of care. The clients' rights summarized below revolve around issues of autonomy, privacy, information, confidentiality, and respect[6-14]:

- Accessible and impartial access to care.
- Autonomy: freedom of choice of therapist; right to participate in decision-making during treatment; right to refuse or leave treatment regardless of the therapist's opinion; right to a consultation with another therapist.
- Care in a safe health-care environment.
- Confidentiality: specifically, no disclosure of any information about the client without his or her written consent.
- Continuity of care.
- Dignity, including the right not to remain disrobed longer than necessary.
- Privacy, both visual and auditory; this includes not having to disclose any information that is not relevant to the care the client is receiving.
- Respect for client values and cultural beliefs.
- Right to be informed of his or her rights.
- Timely and accurate information on the status or background of the therapist providing care, the intervention provided, risks, side effects, alternatives, whether it is a research study, and post-discharge treatment needs.

However, the client is not without responsibility in the client–therapist interaction. As the clients' responsibilities outlined below suggest, the client must bear the responsibility of acting on his or her rights and must, in turn, treat the therapist with respect, as follows:

- Provide accurate information to the therapist.
- Accept the consequences of refusing care, altering care, or choosing an alternative option to care.
- Act with consideration and respect for therapists and others in that setting.
- Adhere to instructions provided by the therapist.
- Follow rules of conduct of the health-care setting.
- Assure that financial obligations to the therapist or facility are met.

Therapists' Rights and Responsibilities

The therapist bears the burden of responsibility in the client–therapist relationship because of the therapist's need to ensure that the power he or she holds in the relationship is not abused.[15] Not only do therapists have responsibilities to their clients (Key Points 2-2), but they also have responsibilities to the profession and society as a whole that are beyond the scope of this chapter. Consequently, therapists needs to seek out and understand the ethical code for their profession.

Unfortunately, therapists' rights are rarely discussed. It is important not to lose sight of the following therapists' rights:

- Ability to make independent clinical judgments.
- Freedom to decline to treat a client if it would compromise the therapist's ethics, dignity, or values.
- Right to work in an environment in which the therapist can practice without coercion, conflict of interest, or undue influence, including being pressured into over-utilization of services for the facility's financial gain.
- Right to be treated with respect and consideration by clients and colleagues.

Therapists are wise to familiarize themselves with their rights and ensure that they are being met in their practice settings.

Ethical Conduct within the Therapeutic Relationship

The need for a discussion of ethical decision-making and conduct stems from the difference in power between therapist and client.[15] In a therapeutic relationship, the client perceives the therapist as an authority figure with specific knowledge and influence. By consulting with the therapist, the client places a degree of trust in the competence and ability of the therapist to help. In

Key Points: 2-2

Therapists' Responsibilities to Clients

Ethical Guidelines for Client Interactions

- Demonstrate responsible caring and concern for the client.
- Do not guarantee a cure or misrepresent the potential effects of the intervention.
- Do not treat clients when under the influence of any substance that would impair the ability to treat safely.
- Listen to and respect client's values, beliefs, and needs.
- Maintain appropriate clinical boundaries and avoid sexual interaction of any sort with clients.
- Provide client-centered, preventative care.
- Provide the client with an opportunity to give voluntary and informed consent.
- Respond appropriately to client's emotional reaction to treatment.
- Use draping to maintain the client's privacy and appropriate clinical boundaries.

General Issues

- Act in the client's best interests.
- Act without conflict of interest.
- Assume responsibility for and provide appropriate examination, treatment, progression of care, and discharge planning.
- Communicate information on the client's care to the referring therapist (within restraints of maintaining confidentiality).
- Delegate care to and supervise adjunct staff or students appropriately and take responsibility for the care they provide.
- Document all of the client's findings accurately and appropriately.
- Ensure and maintain a high level of competence.
- Maintain confidentiality of records and information and obtain a signed release prior to disclosure.
- Do not refuse a client care on the basis of race, gender, culture, religion, sexual orientation, age, etc.
- Do not treat the client unless the client's clinical condition (prevention, curative, maintenance, and wellness) warrants it, thus avoiding the overutilization of services.
- Provide client-centered, preventative care.
- Provide services to meet the client's needs, rather than for financial gain.
- Provide the highest standard of care possible.
- Request consultation from other therapists as appropriate.
- Take responsibility for the care provided to a client.
- Transfer the client to another therapist, as appropriate, when the client–therapist relationship is ended or the client is discharged.
- Use sound judgment.
- Work within the scope of practice and refer to another therapist when the client's condition requires treatment that is beyond your legal scope of practice or level of competence.

manual therapies, the client may be partially or completely undressed, and the therapist may spend up to an hour touching the client's body. Under these circumstances, the client must trust that the therapist will not exploit her.

Ethical issues are not confined to any particular phase of the therapeutic process; instead, therapists must address these issues at all points during and beyond the therapeutic relationship. Both the client and the therapist have rights and responsibilities that result from their participation in the therapeutic relationship. The importance of these rights and responsibilities is underscored by the fact that health-care professions have a clearly articulated set of guidelines for ethical conduct in clinical practice to which they expect all members of their profession to adhere.[6-14] Professional ethical codes are sets of moral principles that promote commonly held values and beliefs that support technical standards of practice.[6-14] These codes of ethics provide a template for making clinical decisions that honor the clients' needs within a moral **framework** that is acceptable for therapists.

In order to respond appropriately to the needs of a client, a therapist must first understand the ethical framework that defines her professional behavior.[6-14] One of the first codes of ethics acknowledged in health care was *primum non nocere* or "first, do no harm." The therapist must first "do no harm." At first glance, this would mean no bruises, increased inflammation, or undue pain as a result of overly vigorous treatment. Clinical experience also suggests that the interaction between therapists and their clients is an aspect of client care that may cause significant concern or injury. Consequently, the therapist must ensure that all aspects of care that she provides promote positive outcomes.

Ethical decision-making requires that therapists consider the following factors when planning treatment.[6-14,16-18]

- What kind of intervention does this client really need?
- What are this client's expressed and unexpressed outcomes?
- How does the client's perception of the power imbalance between therapist and client affect outcomes?
- How comfortable is this client with authority?
- What information does this client need to know from the therapist in order to proceed?
- How comfortable is this client in this treatment room?
- What are the limits or boundaries to care in this circumstance?
- How far are you prepared to go in helping this client?

THE THERAPEUTIC PROCESS

The therapeutic process (Figure 2-2) outlines the interpersonal issues and phases in the therapeutic relationship that arise during the course of providing care to a client within an individual session or the overall episode of care. There is always a beginning, middle, and end to the therapeutic process.[15] If a therapist acknowledges where she and the client are in the therapeutic process, then she enhances the client's feelings of safety.[19] If therapists are unsure what phase is occurring, then the client may be vulnerable to therapist's miscommunication or assumption. This is particularly important when working with clients who have a history of trauma or other emotional challenges.

Beginning Phase: Building Trust

The first part of the therapeutic process establishes the norms of treatment and helps clarify the therapeutic relationship for the client.[1,3,15] When clients feel safe and comfortable, they are more likely to participate fully in the intervention. If clients appear unfamiliar with massage techniques, it is important to explain the approach to treatment and how the therapy works. Figure 2-3 outlines some steps that the therapist can follow within the building trust phase of the therapeutic process. Trust is an essential cornerstone of the therapeutic relationship, and it may only develop if the client feels safe. The following

FIGURE 2-2 The therapeutic process.

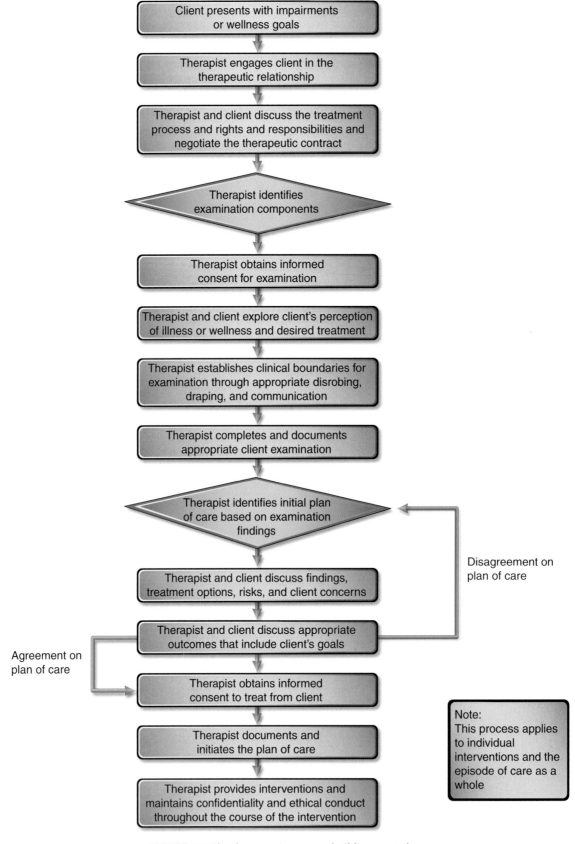

FIGURE 2-3 The therapeutic process: building trust phase.

are some basic actions that foster trust between the client and therapist.

- Create a clear and predictable framework:
  - Begin and end appointments on time.
  - Manage the time effectively during interventions.
  - Return phone calls promptly and demonstrate dependability.
- Respond to clients with honesty, integrity, compassion, and acceptance.
- Acknowledge when you do not have all the answers.
- Seek input on challenges or problems that are not easily solved.

Mid-phase: Exploring Sensations

Once the client feels confident in the therapeutic relationship, she may be ready to explore the physical sensations, conditions, or problems that led her to seek treatment using massage.[19] If a client feels emotionally vulnerable regarding the intimacy of touch, exploring her body's sensations in response to treatment may help her to change the attitudes toward touch. Exploring physical sensations may be painful, historically significant, pleasurable, or frightening for the client. Therefore, during this part of the therapeutic process, it is essential for the therapist to pay attention to the client's verbal and nonverbal cues so that the client does not progress beyond her level of comfort. If the pace of treatment supports the client's ability to process the sensations she experiences, then she may gain a better understanding of her body and her personal somatic history. Figure 2-4 outlines some steps that the therapist can follow within the Exploring Physical Sensations phase of the therapeutic process. Here are some actions that support the client's

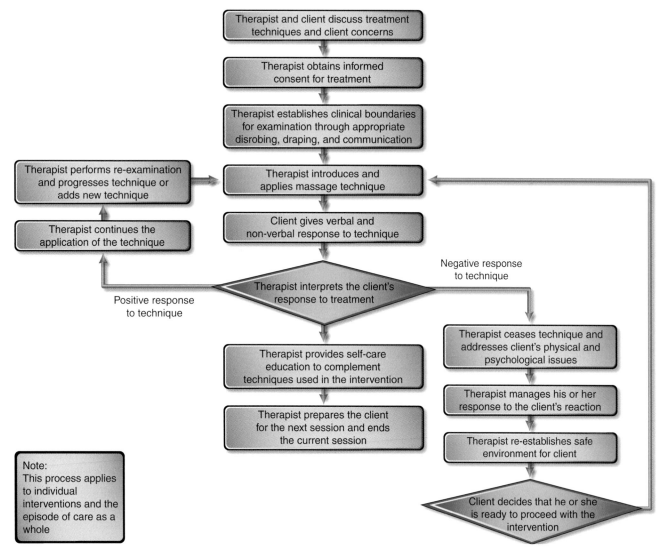

FIGURE 2-4 The therapeutic process: exploring physical sensations phase.

exploration of physical sensations and the therapeutic process as a whole:

- Adhere to guidelines for ethical conduct.
- Maintain clinical boundaries during the intervention through appropriate draping and communication with client.
- Use appropriate physical and psychological therapist self-care during the course of interventions.
- Use appropriate body mechanics and manual technique.
- Deliver interventions in a safe manner.
- Demonstrate responsible caring and concern for the client.
- Support client's willingness to explore sensations.
- Assist the client in deepening his or her relaxation and somatic awareness.
- Celebrate client successes and efforts to change.
- Actively listen and watch for cues throughout the intervention that require changing or adapting the course of the intervention.
- Respond appropriately to a client's emotional reaction to treatment.
- Facilitate client participation in and adherence to the intervention.
- Elicit client's ongoing feedback on progress with clinical outcomes.
- Provide the client with appropriate education.
- Encourage client self-care to help build independence.
- Delegate care to and supervise adjunct staff appropriately.
- Maintain updated documentation on the intervention provided and the client's response.
- Maintain communication with referring practitioner, as appropriate.

The therapeutic process is not linear; instead, it is a dynamic interaction in which the client can move back and forth among stages depending on her level of comfort, safety, and health.[1,3,15] At any time, it is possible for the client to lose focus and experience a need to rebuild trust with the therapist if she becomes distressed as a result of an increase in pain or a personal upset. If the therapist is fully aware of what is occurring at any given time and responds appropriately, then the client will feel safe. Furthermore, the therapeutic process can conclude naturally as the client becomes more independent and able to manage her condition.

Final Phase: Creating Healthy Closure

There comes a time in the therapeutic process when clients prepare to complete treatment and take on their own self-care.[1,3,15] This process is easier for some clients than for others. Clients who feel emotionally attached to therapists or appreciate their empathy and compassion may find it painful to leave the therapeutic relationship. Nevertheless, prolonging the therapy beyond its natural course is not helpful for either client or therapist. It is important for clients to understand at the outset of treatment that there is a natural point of closure that will come when they have achieved their outcomes and are ready for independent self-care. Like any good coach, the therapist can prepare her clients for the point of closure by encouraging independence and acknowledging their gains. Regularly re-examining and reviewing client gains can facilitate a positive closure. Figure 2-5 identifies a possible sequence of steps that therapists can use to promote healthy closure.

Therapists are human and may also feel attached to their clients.[1,3,15] It is very important at this stage that therapists not indulge themselves by encouraging clients to continue in a therapeutic relationship past a natural point of closure. This does not mean that clients cannot enter therapy again in the future to address another condition or part of their bodies with massage techniques. It does mean that each therapeutic process needs to have a natural beginning, middle, and ending; otherwise, one or both partners in the therapeutic relationship may find the therapeutic process stagnant.

Clients who have derived satisfaction from the therapist's use of massage techniques may wish to continue on a maintenance or preventative basis.[15] The therapist needs to negotiate this within the limits for intervention that are defined by her profession's scope of practice. Furthermore, it is often important for both parties to openly acknowledge a change in the therapeutic contract. Regardless of how closure occurs, the more open the discussion of the issues, the easier it will be for clients to explore different paths of healing and for therapists to let go and move on.

STRATEGIES FOR ENHANCING THE THERAPEUTIC RELATIONSHIP

Touch demands intimate human contact, interaction, and response.[15,20] The therapist's behavior in response to the client is every bit as important as the examination or massage techniques she uses. One may view the therapist as a "canvas" on which the client paints his or her therapeutic goals, hopes and fears, and abilities and limitations. How well the therapist responds to the client's wishes can

Therapist identifies client's
readiness for discharge

Therapist and client discuss
client's discharge needs

Therapist identifies initial
discharge plan based on clinical
findings and client needs

Therapist and client discuss
discharge goals and plan

Therapist identifies final
discharge plan

Therapist addresses client's
remaining clinical outcomes

Therapist completes discharge
arrangements

Therapist and client discuss
client's post-discharge concerns

Client participates in pre-discharge
education and preparation

Therapist facilitates appropriate
closure to client–
practitioner relationship

Therapist completes intervention

Therapist completes and
documents discharge examination
to confirm client status at discharge

Therapist arranges a follow-up
visit at an appropriate interval if
appropriate

Therapist transfers the client to
another practitioner or caregivers
for follow-up care if appropriate

Note:
This process applies
to individual
interventions and the
episode of care as a
whole

Therapist provides other
therapists or caregivers with
documentation on follow-up care

FIGURE 2-5 The therapeutic process: healthy closure phase.

influence the outcomes of the intervention. If a therapist believes that success depends wholly on the intervention she provides, then she may ignore one of the most fundamental aspects of manual therapies.

The manner in which a therapist supports the therapeutic relationship depends largely on her awareness of her morals, values, and beliefs regarding health, illness, and physical dysfunction, as well as the knowledge of the professional role and responsibilities.[15,18,21,22] In the same way that clients develop a frame of reference about touch and safety based on childhood experiences, therapist attitudes toward illness, health, and physical dysfunction shape their professional responses to clients' needs. When clients present with conditions that are puzzling and disturbing or remind the therapist of personal experiences, then it becomes more challenging for the therapist to remain present in the therapeutic relationship and accept the clients' needs. The strategies in this section will assist the therapist in supporting the therapeutic relationship with the client.

Obtain Informed Consent

Client-centered care supports the principle of **informed consent** by giving clients the information that they need in order to choose the type of intervention that will suit them best.[6-14] Before the therapist can examine the client or initiate the treatment plan, he requires the client's understanding and consent. Obtaining clear and informed consent for treatment from a client involves ensuring that the client understands the intent and direction of therapy. This process requires that the therapist explain exactly what he is going to do and how he will achieve the specified outcomes. It also requires that the client hears and understands the therapist's explanation, since clients who do not hear the explanation may agree without understanding what the therapist means.

Consent for Treatment

Consent for massage techniques can occur at three levels.[15] First, the client may agree "from the head," thinking to themselves, "This seems to make sense…." Second, if the client considers that the intent of the therapist is to help, the client may agree "from the heart" based on her emotional response to the therapist and the environment (for example, "I like Janey, she won't hurt me … I guess it's okay …"). Finally, in order for a client to agree "from the body," the client must feel safe and be prepared for the intervention. The acceptance of the intervention may take a while to register in the client's tissues. When the

intervention feels right to the client, the client's muscles will soften and release tension easily and the client will rest deeply, breathe slowly, and give control of the intervention over to the therapist.

Consent for Painful or Uncomfortable Procedures

Therapists who use massage techniques may need to cause the client temporary discomfort in order to give the client relief from pain, even as they maintain the client's overall comfort, safety, and trust.[15] In addition, although it appears paradoxical, clients who are in pain or uncomfortable with touch may seek a form of therapy that could be painful or intimate. This occurs because the prospect of a pleasurable sensation or relief from pain may be sufficient to entice the client to try an intervention that may be outside of her level of comfort with touch. In light of the pain and/or intimacy associated with massage techniques, the therapist must ensure that the client understands and accepts the responsibilities of the therapeutic relationship and the possible responses to treatment techniques before he proceeds with an intervention that the client may find uncomfortable.[6-14] Otherwise, if the client does not trust the therapist and the therapeutic relationship, she may mistakenly perceive that the therapist intends to inflict pain.

Consent for Intrusive Work

There are times during treatment using massage techniques that the therapist must place a finger or a hand in a sensitive location. Intra-oral work, massage on the attachments of the groin or psoas, or breast or abdominal massage may feel invasive to clients who are uncomfortable with the therapist touching them in these locations. In these situations, therapists must carefully negotiate with the client where and how deeply they touch them.[6-14] This clear and ongoing informed consent is particularly important when the client reports that she feels uncomfortable.

To obtain consent for intrusive work, the therapist must explain the procedure clearly, answer any questions, and ask for the client's permission to perform the techniques he deems appropriate.[6-14] Once the therapist has obtained permission, he must perform exactly the techniques that he said that he would perform. In addition, he must obtain client feedback about her comfort and response to those techniques. After he has completed the intervention, he must review what he did and must ask the client for any follow-up questions. This approach will communicate to the client that he is safe with the therapist and can trust the therapeutic process.

Communicate Clearly

Despite the therapist's efforts to achieve full informed consent prior to embarking on an intervention, the therapeutic contract may remain implicit or unspoken.[1-3,23] If a therapist does not communicate clearly, a client may misunderstand the intent of a particular intervention. If a therapist ignores the client's needs or insists on a particular form of treatment, then the client may feel hurt or traumatized by the experience. The responsibility for achieving the desired outcomes rests on the therapist's skill in reading and responding to the client's cues throughout the therapeutic process.

Interview with Care

Clients present with a variety of conditions, perspectives, and experience to therapists. Unfortunately, clients do not share complete personal histories with therapists for a variety of reasons.[5-14] This occurs during the clinical interview when either the details seem petty to the client or the client considers them far too significant to share with a stranger. Incomplete histories can lead to problems with treatment planning and the client's response to treatment. In addition, clients do not always articulate their expectations for treatment to therapists, although these are critical for a successful outcome.[5,6-14] Consequently, a therapist may not meet the client's expectations because the therapist is unaware that these unspoken wishes exist. Not fully appreciating the client's reason for seeking treatment using massage techniques can result in misunderstanding, confusion, and hurt. For these reasons, therapists must use active listening, observation, and full investigation of clients' reactions to gain a clear understanding of clients' problems, histories, and expectations for treatment.

Interviewing a client about personal and intimate health details takes time and skill. In order to understand the full case, a therapist must include adequate time on intake in order to explore the issues that arise. Clients may need reassurance that the time is well spent in order to feel permission to share their true desired goals and expectations of treatment.

Use Plain Language

Therapists who employ too technical language when explaining their approaches to treatment run the risk of alienating their clients through misunderstanding. Although it is important to be precise and accurate, using Latin terms or technical directions may be interpreted by the client incorrectly or as a way to suggest that the therapist wishes to be considered an expert. This puts the client in a "one-down" position from the therapist. Clients may feel too embarrassed to ask for clarification and accept an approach to treatment that is not comfortable. It is up to the therapist to ensure clients fully understand what is proposed and that means speaking in a language that is readily understood.

Ask Questions Effectively

Knowing how to ask questions effectively is an art that facilitates good therapeutic outcomes. Part of the challenge stems from realizing what information is necessary, what might be useful to know, and why specific information is sought. There are several specific types of questions that support good interviewing (Table 2-1). For example, open questions invite reflection and stimulate further discussion. They do not work especially well when therapists have limited time to discuss a problem or when seeking specific information. When clients are shy or unable to share details about their health, it may be helpful to "prompt" them. This shows clients that the therapist is interested in what the clients have to say and it engages and encourages the clients to continue with their story. Closed questions result in simple, straightforward answers. These questions fill in the blanks of the bigger clinical picture and are very useful when seeking details. If clients gives vague descriptions or has difficulty answering directly, therapists should clarify what is meant. Therapists clarify what is confusing and ask for more detail. Finally, how therapists employ "I," "we," and "you" ensures that the focus for the interview remains on the client's needs. "I" is used when a therapist describes her own perceptions or feelings. "We" is used when the therapist wants to include the client in decision-making. "You" is used to describe behaviors and is particularly effective in closed, specific questions.

Seek Information on Clients' Needs

Clear communication requires more than an ability to ask different types of questions. Therapists also need to put the information that they gather into context and avoid making assumptions about the client's needs or goals. When questions are too specific, clients may not feel that they have permission to tell the whole story. Seeking context for a client's condition gives therapists a broader picture

| Table 2-1 | Types of Questions |

Question Type	Example of Use of Question Type
Open questions: ■ Invite reflection and stimulate further discussion. These are used to learn more about a condition or attitude. There is no "right" answer.	Therapist: What brings you in for massage therapy today? (Open question) Client: I sprained my ankle last week.
Prompting: ■ Demonstrates interest and encourages the speaker to continue. This technique lets the speaker know that the listener is paying attention and wants to know more.	Therapist: Oh dear! Please tell me more. (Prompt) Client: Oh it's not too bad. I sprained it while playing soccer. We won the game though!
Clarification: ■ Restates what is heard and asks if this is correct or if there is another interpretation for the information given. ■ This essential interview technique helps the therapist clarify or understand more fully what the client means. It is especially helpful when therapists hear what sounds like contradictory information.	Therapist: Congratulations on the game! But I am confused. You told me you sprained your ankle but you just said that you are ok. So are you here for your ankle or do you want some other type of treatment? (Clarification) Client: Yes, I'm here for my sprained ankle. It's still swollen and it hurts.
Closed questions: ■ These questions have specific, black and white answers. They are used to get to the truth of the circumstance and result in simple, straightforward answers.	Therapist: Which ankle did you injure while playing soccer? (Closed question) Client: My right ankle. It's always been a bit weaker than my left.
Use of "I," "we," and "you" ■ "I" is used to describe feelings or perceptions. ■ "You" is used to describe specific behaviors. ■ "We" is used to encourage inclusion and helpful when summarizing an agreement.	Therapist: I think I understand now. You sprained your weak right ankle during the soccer game and now it is swollen. (I statement) Client: That's it exactly. Therapist: You are concerned that your ankle is still swollen and painful and are hoping that therapy can help decrease the pain and swelling. (You statement) Client: I guess that is so. Do you think that there is anything that you can do for my ankle? Therapist: We can complete your examination and identify the main problems with your ankle. Then we can discuss the different options for treatment. What are your thoughts on that? (We statement) Client: Works for me. When do we start?

Adapted from Fitch, P. *Talking Body Listening Hands*. Pearson. In press.

of why the client is seeking massage therapy. For example, if a client tells her therapist that she has headaches, it is essential to know whether the headaches derive from tension and life/work stress or whether they are related to hormonally induced migraines. In the first case, massage therapy can be very effective in alleviating the pain. In the second, massage therapy might make the migraine worse. In addition, when therapists assume what clients want from treatment, they may miss the most important

or essential reasons that clients have booked the session. Even if a client presents with a specific problem that can be helped by massage therapy, the principles of client-centered care require that the treatment reflects the client's desired goals and not the treatment that the therapist wishes to give. For example, if a client has just lost her best friend to cancer, then assuming that she wants a treatment for low back pain may ignore her need for nurturance and support during the time of grieving.

Use Self-Disclosure Carefully

As a rule of thumb, self-disclosure is only appropriate if the information that is shared contributes positively and relates directly to the client's case. An appropriate way of self-disclosing would affirm the client's experience, not take away from the client's story. For example: "Yes, I know how hard it is to park at the Institute. I have been there too." Not, "Oh I have been at the Institute many times before. I see Dr. Smith there. Do you know him?"

Pay Attention to Body Language

While there is considerable debate about the actual percentage of a person's message that is conveyed by verbal or non-verbal communication, there is agreement that non-verbal communication is an essential component. There are countless articles and textbooks on non-verbal communication. What follows are some basic suggestions to consider during communication with a client that therapists can modify to meet the different cultural and personal needs of each client. The therapist's position and posture can affect communication; therefore, the therapist needs to maintain a relaxed posture, face the client squarely, and lean slightly toward the client.[24-26] This position will also facilitate appropriate eye contact during therapist–client interactions. The distance between therapist and client is another important factor to consider. Hall[24] distinguished between intimate (6 to 18 in.), personal (1.5 to 4 ft), social (4 to 12 ft), and public (12 to 25 ft) distances, with social distance being appropriate for most therapist–client discussions. Finally, removing physical barriers between the therapist and client, such as furniture and equipment, will enhance the communication.

Ensure Privacy and Confidentiality

Therapists need to honor the clients' openness in disclosing personal information and allowing the therapist to touch their bodies by ensuring that they provide the client with privacy and confidentiality.

Maintain Privacy

Using appropriate draping to respect client privacy facilitates the sense of safety that the client feels and promotes a healthy therapeutic relationship.[6-14] At the same time, the therapist should accomplish draping with the least fuss possible. When therapists nervously spend extended periods of time attending to the draping or repeatedly tuck sheets in until the client feels overbound, they move the emphasis from the desired treatment outcomes to their concerns about exposing the client. This excessive concern may frighten clients into wondering what may happen next or annoy the client because it is taking time away from hands-on treatment.

Ensure Privacy for History Taking

Clients' words deserve as much privacy as their bodies, a fact that therapists often forget.[6-14] Conducting client interviews in open gyms and asking clients for feedback on their response to treatment in waiting rooms or hallways are among the ways in which therapists inadvertently violate clients' privacy. Clients differ in terms of what they consider to be sensitive topics. Consequently, therapists need to provide clients with as much privacy as possible within their clinical setting during history taking, feedback on response to treatment, and other discussions of client information. Doing so will include ensuring that sensitive discussions with clients do not occur in the presence of administrative staff, adjunct staff, or other clients.

Ensure that Client's Information Is Secure and Confidential

Finally, it is up to the therapist to ensure the security of the confidential information that the client has shared. Paper records should be secured and electronic records password protected and free from corruption. Therapists must seek the permission of the client prior to sharing any of their personal health history or information with another professional. Most jurisdictions require that the client sign a written authorization before this information may be shared. In jurisdictions where written authorization is not required, the client's record should indicate that the record-sharing was discussed and permission granted by the client.

In peer discussions about clients, it is essential that identifying information be omitted. Both parties should agree to keep the discussion confidential and only the aspects of the case that are of importance be shared with the peer. Peer discussions should not occur in public places, especially elevators, coffee shops, hallways, or bars.

Establish Health Therapeutic Boundaries

There are many obstacles to a successful therapeutic relationship. The client–therapist relationship is complicated by the imbalance of power from two sources.[16,17] The first is the therapist's presumed role of "healer" and his possession of information and skills that the client needs. The second is the client's vulnerability and dependence on the therapist. In addition, the use of massage techniques involves the therapist touching parts of the client's body that are often unclothed. How the client interprets and responds to this form of touch will depend on a variety of factors, such as culture, religion, gender, upbringing, and personal experiences of touch.[17,18] Finally, changing a person's body structure with massage techniques can evoke emotional responses or trigger tissue memories.[21,22,27-30] Clients' responses to touch can be exaggerated or negative if they are emotionally fragile or have had negative past experiences of touch.[15,19,20] Fortunately, there are a variety of strategies that therapists can use to overcome these obstacles and establish healthy therapeutic boundaries and a positive therapeutic relationship.

Recognize the Power Differential between Therapist and Client

The authority of the therapist creates a **power differential** between therapists and clients.[15,18] Clients are vulnerable, often fully or partially disrobed, and usually lying prone or supine. Therapists, on the other hand, are dressed and standing and hold the authority, knowledge, and responsibility for the intervention. Since clients may have little or no awareness of their own physical responses, therapists' professional experience puts clients at a considerable disadvantage. For these reasons, clients may interpret therapists' behavior as that of a friend, a parent, or an intimate partner if they do not understand the nature of the imbalance of power in the therapeutic relationship.

Because therapists are in a position of authority, clients' personal history with authority figures may also play into the therapeutic process.[15-18] Clients who are in the habit of agreeing with authority figures may agree with whatever therapists suggest during the course of treatment, regardless of whether they actually agree. It is, therefore, essential for therapists to acknowledge clients' susceptibility to suggestion and to clearly and unequivocally empower clients to ask questions, stop at any time, or change positions so that they remain safe, comfortable, and able to continue with treatment.[15] In addition, therapists must also ensure that they do not abuse the power they have within the therapeutic relationship by behaving inappropriately toward their clients.[15-18]

Understand Clients' Emotional Response to the Therapist

It is common for clients to project feelings from earlier relationships onto their therapists.[15-18] This occurs because it is human to interpret the present based on one's experience of the past. If the therapist reminds the client of an important person in her past, the client may relate to the therapist in the same way that she did in the relationship she remembers. This is called **transference**, and it forms an important component of the therapeutic process. Transference is particularly strong when a client receives touch from a person whom she perceives to have power and authority.

If the person the client remembers was a positive influence on her, like a coach or a teacher, then the client may be encouraged or motivated to do whatever the therapist asks and follow up with self-care strategies carefully. Unfortunately, it is also possible that the transference may stem from a historically negative relationship, and the client's transferred feelings may seem painful, unpredictable, confusing, and, at times, alarming for a therapist who does not recognize the possibility of transference.

Avoid Highly Emotional Responses to Clients

When the client is experiencing transference in his relationship with the therapist, the ability to succeed in treatment depends on how the therapist responds to his projected feelings. There are a variety of possible responses: the therapist may feel flattered by the client's intense positive regard, have an urge to challenge the client's misconceptions, accept the transference because it feels like the easiest course of action, or discharge the client out of alarm and confusion. If the therapist misinterprets or acts inappropriately toward a client's transference, she may ignore the articulated treatment outcomes or make it impossible to achieve them. This puts the client in the difficult situation of having his unconscious feelings for the therapist interrupt or jeopardize his therapeutic progress.

Countertransference occurs when a therapist allows his unresolved feelings and personal issues about people outside of the therapeutic relationship to influence his relationship with a client.[17,18] If a therapist is experiencing countertransference toward a client, then he may ignore the client's best interests and allow his own needs to direct the intervention. At the same time, the client in the therapeutic relationship is vulnerable to suggestion and may not realize the harm of the therapist's actions. In these circumstances, clients may feel confused or alarmed by the change in relationship and attention. To avoid the problems associated with transference and countertransference, the therapist needs to remain focused on the treatment goals and providing a healthy therapeutic relationship.

Prohibit Flirtatious, Seductive, or Sexualized Behavior

Flirtatious or seductive behavior on the part of the therapist or client abuses the therapeutic relationship and may seriously harm the client. It takes the focus away from the goals of treatment and increases the potential for transference or countertransference.[6-12,14,31,32] In addition, it may compound issues that arise because of the client's personal history of touch and attitudes about intimacy. Moreover, if the flirtatious behavior continues, it could result in negative and harmful consequences. For these reasons, therapists must avoid flirtatious and seductive behavior and politely discourage it in their clients.

When a therapist engages in sexualized contact with a client, he discards the purpose of the intervention, betrays the client's trust, and either minimizes or completely ignores the client's needs. Furthermore, it is unethical and abusive for therapists to engage in personal or sexualized contact with clients because of the power imbalance between therapists and their clients. In addition, therapists must not sexualize massage techniques because the degree of intimacy inherent in hands-on work, coupled with the authority of their position, makes clients vulnerable to suggestion. When a therapist acts on his fantasies about a client, he has abused the client.[6-12,14,31,32] Some jurisdictions consider comments of a sexual nature, in addition to sexualized touching and intercourse, to be sexual abuse.

Avoid Keeping Secrets about Treatment

It is important for therapists to ensure confidentiality in order for clients to trust the therapeutic process.[6-14,32-37] At the same time, it is essential that therapists refrain from asking their clients to keep secrets about the treatments that they receive.[18] All aspects of treatment and the therapist's comments should be explicit and clear. Asking a client to keep a secret about interventions confers a "special status" to the client that is linked to intimacy and promotes transference. This act also removes any freedom the client has to discuss, process, or question the therapeutic relationship and interventions with other clients or people.

Discourage Specialness

When the therapist treats a client in a special way or gives the impression that the care that the client receives

is different from or better than the norm, it enhances the potential for transference and **boundary violations**.[18] Therapists should, therefore, make a conscious effort to avoid behaviors that suggest that a particular client is special in some way. It is predictable that the therapist may find some clients more appealing than others. Acknowledging one's affection for a client is sometimes helpful in facilitating the therapeutic process. Conversely, telling the client repeatedly what a special person she is can only emphasize any existing transference or countertransference and may put the client at risk for abuse. Be sure that if you show affection for a client, then it is in the client's best interests for her to experience this affection.[18]

Maintain Clearly Defined Relationships

Dual relationships describe situations in which clients and therapists have more than one kind of relationship.[18,6-14,32-37] There are very good reasons why therapists are discouraged from engaging in dual relationships. Dual relationships challenge the objectivity of the therapist. They also put the therapist in an uncomfortable position of having to choose which relationship will define the therapeutic relationship. When a therapist is also a brother or sister or friend to a client, then the relationship that came first is likely to determine the therapist's behavior toward the client. For example, a therapist who is treating one of his parents will find it is difficult to remain objective because his parent–child relationship is the most dominant. Instead of the therapist feeling responsible to a client, the therapist may feel like a son or daughter to the client, with all the complications of long-standing family relationships attached to the situation. Dual relationships are not comfortable and can verge on being unethical if the therapist is asked to perform some task that compromises his professional responsibilities.

Maintain Physical Boundaries

As noted previously, the client–therapist relationship is complicated by the imbalance of power from the therapist's presumed role of "healer," the client's vulnerability and dependence on the therapist, and the use of massage techniques that involve the therapist touching parts of the client's body that are often unclothed.[15,19,20]

The proximity of the therapist's body to a client can convey strong, and possibly unintentional, messages, particularly if the therapist is attracted to the client.[17,18] Brushing the client's body with one's hips or abdomen may occur inadvertently during treatment. If, however, it appears to happen more frequently with one client than with others, there is a distinct possibility that countertransference is at play. In addition, the client may perceive the unintentional touch as an expression of intimacy, affection, or control. No matter how innocuous the therapist's unintentional touch is, there is a possibility that the client may interpret the message incorrectly. The following are some guidelines on the characteristics that people use to interpret touch[17,18]:

■ The part of the other person's body that touches the person
■ The part of the person's body that is touched
■ How long the touch lasts
■ How much pressure is used
■ Whether there is movement after contact is made
■ If anyone else is present to witness the touch
■ The relationship between the person performing the touch and the person receiving the touch
■ The verbal exchange that accompanies the touch
■ Other non-verbal behaviors that are present
■ Prior touch experiences

In addition, changing a person's body structure with massage techniques can evoke emotional responses or trigger tissue memories.[15,19,20] Clients' responses to touch can be exaggerated or negative if they are emotionally fragile or have had negative past experiences of touch.[15,19,20]

Extend Unconditional Positive Regard

Unconditional positive regard is one of the common factors that supports a therapeutic relationship.[18,15,19,20] When clients appear inhibited about their body size or appearance, it is not helpful for the therapist to make comments that underscore this discomfort. On the other hand, there are times when body size may contribute to pain, and a responsible therapist should find a tactful way of sharing this perspective so that the client is fully informed. Clients may tell personal stories or ask therapists for their opinion regarding relationships. Expressing opinions is not part of the professional scope of practice and may influence the client unduly. Offering unconditional positive regard while avoiding the provision of opinion is a skill that requires attention and care. Therapists may deflect client's requests for opinion by stating that they do not know the best answer for that individual. If the client is in need of support, the therapist may wish to provide the name of a psychotherapist, counselor, accountant, or lawyer, depending on the client's problem.

Enhance Client Adherence

The client's **adherence** to the plan of care is the final component of the interpersonal aspects of the process of clinical care addressed in this chapter. The literature defines adherence in a variety of ways.[38-56] Responsibility is placed on the client in the definition that adherence is the extent to which clients follow the instructions for care that they negotiate with their health-care providers. Adherence can also be viewed as being influenced by the therapist when it is defined as a positive behavior that occurs when a client is motivated by the therapist to adhere to the negotiated plan of care because of a perceived positive outcome or benefit. However it is defined, adherence to the prescribed plan of care is necessary for the attainment of positive outcomes. Several models attempt to identify the factors that influence clients' motivation and adherence. For example, Keller's ARCS[42] (attention, relevance, confidence, satisfaction) model suggests that clients' motivation to participate in health-care programs reflects several factors, including the extent to which therapists gain their attention, the relevance of the information to them, their confidence in their ability to perform the desired task, and their level of satisfaction with their performance. Based on research, various authors have suggested a variety of strategies for increasing clients' adherence to prescribed plans of care. These strategies revolve around the client's ability to understand the regimen and follow the directions that were provided, the type of instructions provided by the therapist, and the extent to which the therapist tailors the regimen to the client's needs. Some examples of these strategies include the following[38-56]:

■ Create a collaborative relationship between the client and the therapist.
■ Provide clients with information about their disease, the rationale and goals for treatment, and the benefits and risks of treatment.
■ Whenever possible, simplify and customize programs.
■ Prioritize activities and share this information with clients.
■ Evaluate clients' comprehension and ability to perform tasks at intervals.
■ Provide cues for remembering information.
■ Provide clients with strategies for self-monitoring of their programs.
■ Use behavioral contracts and positive reinforcement of clients' successes.
■ Involve clients' families and significant others in their care, as appropriate.

- Evaluate the level of client compliance at regular intervals during the episode of care.
- Discuss potential barriers to learning or adherence with the client and assist them in removing those barriers.
- Provide challenges and meaningful opportunities for clients to succeed.
- Keep the material you present to clients stimulating but not overstimulating.
- Use familiar concepts, concrete examples, and familiar language to increase clients' receptiveness to new information.
- Provide clients with ongoing opportunities to apply their newly learned skills.

Limit the Amount and Variety of Information

Unfortunately, the types of information that clients are least likely to remember are instructions and advice.[38-56] The more information a client receives, the more he is likely to forget. Clients generally remember what therapists tell them first and what they consider to be the most important. There is no correlation between the amount of information that is remembered and age or intelligence, although clients with more medical knowledge will recall more information. In addition, a myriad of factors can influence a clients' readiness to learn, such as their age, personality, health beliefs, knowledge about their conditions, understanding of the intents and benefits of treatment, and social factors. Furthermore, moderately anxious clients will recall more information than highly anxious clients or clients who are not anxious.

Make Instructions Clear

Adherence decreases when therapists give unclear instructions; conversely, specific advice may increase adherence.[38-56] For this reason, simple, direct, and repetitive instructions are most effective. For example, "You must do this exercise 10 times when you get out of bed every morning" will be recalled more readily than "Do this exercise several times each day." Furthermore, clients have difficulty complying when they are unclear why the various aspects of the regimen are important, even if the regimen is relatively simple. For example, the addition of the explanation "Putting ice on your ankle and elevating it by putting it up on a chair will help relieve the pain and swelling that you have in your ankle …" as a precursor to instructions for the application of ice may clarify for the client why it would be beneficial to adhere to those instructions.

Make Instructions Simple

Modification of the characteristics of the prescribed regimen can increase adherence.[38-56] Since adherence decreases with increasing duration of the episode of care and with increasing complexity of the intervention, therapists should simplify complex interventions by breaking the plan of care into sequential steps. Furthermore, clients are less likely to adhere to interventions that they perceive as intruding into their daily activities, and the simplest intervention that is compatible with the client's lifestyle is most effective. Consequently, therapists should also tailor self-care programs to clients' activities and lifestyles. Finally, clients respond positively when therapists appear to accept that problems arise in integrating a regimen into a client's lifestyle and are available to help the client make modifications.

Use Group Instruction if Possible

Clients place a high value on information, although therapists often underestimate the extent to which they do so.[38-56] Consequently, client education can become an intervention, not merely an adjunct to treatment. When a therapist is using client education as a primary intervention, small groups can be an effective approach. A small group format allows clients to hear information repeated several times and provides opportunities for reinforcing that knowledge. Other clients may ask questions that another client may be hesitant to ask either in a group setting or one-on-one with the therapist. Group participation may also contribute to a sense of community by allowing the client to be with others with similar conditions. Small group sessions can also facilitate the client's proficiency in specific skills that she requires for successful self-management of chronic conditions. If skill acquisition is the primary goal of a small group, then therapists should spend the majority of the time in the sessions on practice and the provision of feedback to the clients. In this context, breaking clients into pairs to practice skills and to develop action plans can be beneficial.

EMOTIONAL RESPONSES TO MASSAGE

Performing massage techniques on a client can evoke emotional responses for a variety of physiological and psychological reasons. Changing the structure of a client's tissues through massage may result in a tissue release and an accompanying emotional release. Clients may also experience an emotional response to being touched that can be either negative or positive, depending on their past experiences of touch. For this reason, therapists need to be aware of the possible causes and presentation of clients' emotional responses to massage and how to respond to these effectively.

Emotional Responses to Changes in Physical Structure

Reich, a student of Freud's, identified relationships between chronic muscular tension and psychological disorders.[21,30,57] He recognized that these patterns of muscular tension were not merely symptoms of his clients' neuroses but actually the means by which they avoided experiencing emotions related to childhood psychological traumas and maintained their psychological disorders. By incorporating bodywork into his psychoanalytic practice, he found that treating patterns of chronic muscular tension resulted in emotional and psychological responses that enabled his clients to become aware of the feelings that they were avoiding. Based on this observation, he formed a theory about the connection between the body and the emotions.

Reich proposed that the bodies of all living organisms vibrate or "pulsate" in an ongoing cycle of expansion and contraction.[21,30,57] During normal levels of nervous system activity, these "pulsations" are difficult to observe. The intensity of these "pulsations" will increase, however, with increases in the intensity of an individual's emotional response. For example, an individual will shake when she experiences intense excitement or fear or her chest will heave when she sobs. Furthermore, Reich theorized that people can learn to control their emotions by learning to control their physical reactions, or "pulsations," even when the reasons for avoiding these emotions are unconscious.

Essentially, individuals can control the "pulsations" in their bodies by tensing groups of opposing muscles around a specific skeletal structure that is related to the emotion that they are trying to control.[21,30,57] This controlled tensing of the muscles can be short term in nature or long term and habitual—not even relaxing in sleep. This muscle tension reduces the spontaneous movement in that part of the body and can result in that skeletal structure being generally held in a stiff and relatively fixed position known as "holding" or emotional structuring. Eventually, the posture of the entire body can reflect a psychological attitude. Not all muscle tension, however, is the result of an attempt to achieve emotional control. An individual's patterns of muscular tension may also be related to genetic predispositions, compensatory changes, injuries, and physical occupational stresses. Furthermore,

not only can psychological attitudes affect muscular tension, but the opposite may also be true.

Rolf, and others, maintained that a change in myofascial length or tension that changes the structure of an individual's body will shift the way he or she is in the world.[22,28,29] They believed that individuals become accustomed to a specific way of feeling their bodies and experiencing their usual physical sensations. In addition, during regular states of consciousness, individuals have their usual repertoire of emotional reactions with which they can identify. When the structure of their bodies is changed, they can experience new physical experiences—feelings of warmth and tingling or sensations in areas of which they were previously unaware. New thoughts and feelings, other than the ones that they normally recognize, can also accompany these changes in physical structure. These thoughts and feelings may be so subtle that they are difficult to recognize, such as a delicate feeling of openness or a momentary feeling of vulnerability. On the other hand, the change in their bodies' structure might evoke an emotional response that is so strong that it makes it difficult for them to function socially. Therapists should, therefore, recognize that the application of a massage technique always has the potential to evoke an emotional response that stems from a change in the structure of the client's body. They also need to distinguish between the emotional response to a release of the client's tissues and the usual emotional response to being touched.

Tissue Memory

Touch may trigger unexplained, odd, or unusual responses that appear to arise more from the client's history than from the actual therapeutic technique.[22,28,29] When clients have negative or traumatic personal histories, they may exhibit surprising or disturbing responses to the most benign touch. Without understanding the neurological underpinnings of trauma, therapists may be quite puzzled by the degree of **hyperarousal**, sensitivity, or **dissociation** that can occur with some clients.

It is important for therapists to recognize that **tissue memory** is encoded in the tissue of the body and not in the brain.[58] For example, if a person has a skiing accident that causes an anterior dislocation of the humerus, then each time the person's arm moves quickly into the same pattern as the dislocation, a memory of the injury will surface. This is a body memory or "kindling."[58] Tissue memory may not occur as a conscious, chronologic image of the experience but rather may be felt emotionally or somatically. Apprehension, nausea, anger, pain, or whatever describes the initial response to the injury may surface again when the therapist moves the client's humerus into a pattern that is reminiscent of the initial event.

When a therapist touches a client for the first time, it activates a cascade of neurological responses that help the client to interpret whether or not the touch is safe or threatening.[58] Textbooks on neurobiology describe this neurological response to touch in detail. It is essential for the therapist to respect the client's ability to receive touch when he is deciding on a treatment plan. If the client perceives the initial touch by the therapist as a threat, then the entire desired outcome for the intervention may be lost. Furthermore, it is unlikely that hands-on massage techniques will succeed until the client can receive touch without perceiving a threat. Therapists must also bear in mind that client vulnerability can increase the likelihood that a client who has negative history of touch will perceive therapeutic touch to be threatening.

Negative Past Experiences of Touch

If clients have experienced a painful or difficult past, traumatic injuries, abuse, or a fear of being touched, then they are particularly vulnerable to triggered responses to touch or potential misunderstanding regarding the intentions of the therapist. Clients who seem the most vulnerable or fragile in the therapeutic setting may have some or all of the following emotions, conditions, or behaviors:

- Emotionally vulnerable, distant, brittle, edgy, sad, distraught, guarded, or angry.
- Exhibit wide arcs and swings of emotion (sad, mad, and glad).
- Chronic pain, headaches, insomnia, hyperarousal, flattened affect, depression, and anxiety.
- Possible history of neglect, trauma, and abuse.
- Recently experienced deep grief, loss, or profound stress.
- Feel anxious with touch and intimacy.
- Have little or no frame of reference for positive and healthy touch or interpersonal relationships.
- May be distinctly prone to transference.
- Hyperaware of seductive or inappropriate behavior or may (mis)read a therapist's intentions. (Adapted from Fitch P. *Talking Body Listening Hands Workshops*, with permission from the author.)

How clients bonded with their parents and how they were touched as children create their frame of reference for interpreting the level of safety, pleasure, or fearfulness that accompanies touch experiences. A person who received hugs, love, and security while growing up is more likely to interpret touch in a positive and open way, without fearing

for her safety, because her first encounters with touch taught her that she is safe in the world.[15] Since only half to two-thirds of the general population fit into this category,[22] up to half of the people whom therapists encounter may have insecure touch histories. This half of the population may have childhood touch histories that are mixed with neglect, inconsistent caregiving, or frightening and disturbing circumstances that the therapist cannot ignore.[15,59]

If an individual's parents neglected or never touched her as a child, then the experience of massage techniques might seem bizarre or disturbing to her because she has no clear frame of reference for safe touch. On the other hand, if a client's caregiver was present and loving one day but unavailable or rejecting the next, then the client may need considerable reassurance and consistency from the therapist in order to trust the therapeutic process. Finally, if a client has experienced abusive touch, then a therapeutic environment that involves touch is unlikely to feel safe at all. Touch in this circumstance may remind clients of earlier negative and frightening encounters.[15] In all of these situations, the client may not be conscious or aware of the impact of her personal touch history. Reminders from earlier years may emerge as unwelcome sensations, sudden pain, emotional charge, or hypersensitivity, known as traumatic memory.[20]

In each of these circumstances, the client requires a feeling of safety within the therapeutic relationship.[7] Without this feeling of safety, the client cannot trust the process or the therapist. Furthermore, the client is unlikely to be able to relax and focus on the present instead. She will be drawn back into her unresolved past experiences of touch and may forget the present therapeutic intent.

Trauma and Anxiety

Some clients have experienced significant trauma that results in posttraumatic stress disorder.[19,60] The primary symptoms include hyperarousal, **hypersensitivity**, numbness to feelings or parts of the body, dissociation from the present, and an inability to relax. Key Points 2-3 lists some common symptoms to assist therapists in identifying these clients. These clients may find the treatment sessions anxiety provoking.

When faced with a threat, most people respond with a "flight or fight" reaction. On the other hand, when some people are faced with a threat and they cannot figure out how to respond, they will "freeze."[24] Fight, flight, or freeze responses relate to altered limbic pathways and disrupted homeostasis. The therapist may witness all three responses in his clients.

If a therapeutic encounter causes a client to react fearfully, then it may be very difficult for the client to

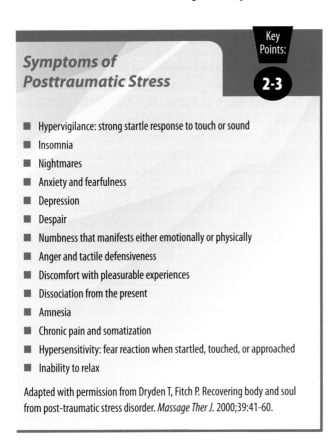

Key Points: 2-3

Symptoms of Posttraumatic Stress

■ Hypervigilance: strong startle response to touch or sound
■ Insomnia
■ Nightmares
■ Anxiety and fearfulness
■ Depression
■ Despair
■ Numbness that manifests either emotionally or physically
■ Anger and tactile defensiveness
■ Discomfort with pleasurable experiences
■ Dissociation from the present
■ Amnesia
■ Chronic pain and somatization
■ Hypersensitivity: fear reaction when startled, touched, or approached
■ Inability to relax

Adapted with permission from Dryden T, Fitch P. Recovering body and soul from post-traumatic stress disorder. *Massage Ther J.* 2000;39:41-60.

hear instructions, respond appropriately, remain present, or allow the intervention to proceed normally.[24] This occurs because the client is caught in a fight, flight, or freeze response. In an extreme case, the therapist's touch may recall painful personal history that can cause the client to dissociate or disconnect from the intervention, temporarily forget her surroundings, or temporarily lose touch with reality.

Addressing the Client's Emotional Response to Massage

Therapists are often unprepared for the client's emotional response to the application of massage techniques. The information in this chapter serves as an overview of some basic strategies for responding to the client. The therapist should ensure that she remains within the limits of her professional scope of practice and clinical training when addressing the client's emotional needs that arise during an intervention. In particular, the therapist should recognize when it is appropriate to refer the client to a physician or a health-care professional who can provide psychosocial care.

Recognize the Client's Emotional Process

Reichian theory suggests that levels of emotional release lie on a continuum from overt to subtle.[21,30,57] In this continuum, signs of overt emotional release are easily recognized, and those of subtle release are less easily recognized. The signs and sensations of the usual vibratory and spontaneous movement in the body that accompany a subtle emotional release in the body include an increase in the rate of breathing; gurgles in the throat and abdomen; swallowing; tearing; the production of sounds, such as sighing or moaning; spontaneous jerking of musculature; itches; sensations of heat and cold; and the movement of energy. These are usually simply signs and sensations of physical release or the movement from a tense state of sympathetic nervous system activation to a relaxed state of parasympathetic nervous system activation. When therapists use massage in a clinical setting, the occurrence of these signs and sensations in the client does not lead to anything other than a state of physical relaxation. By contrast, when the client's physical signs and sensations are accompanied by thoughts and beliefs that form an emotion, an emotional release occurs.

The client can also manifest the physical and behavioral signs of limiting or containing, rather than releasing, emotions.[21,30,57] These attempts to limit the vibratory or spontaneous movement in the body lead to reactions such as becoming still and silent, holding one's breath, a rigidity in the musculature, and focusing one's attention on an unrelated situation or distracting conversation. The individual will be able to maintain a distance from emotional content as long as these strategies are successful. The client's need to prevent emotional release can be in conflict with the massage-related treatment outcomes. For example, if a client needs to maintain a certain degree of muscular tension in order to limit the vibratory and spontaneous movement in his body, this may be in conflict with the goal of deep relaxation of his tense musculature. If the therapist is able to see the client's need to prevent emotional release and control his physical reactions as a reflection of fear of unresolved and difficult emotional terrain, then she may be better able to respect the need for these behaviors.

Accommodate Negative Experiences of Touch, Trauma, or Posttraumatic Stress Disorder

Clients can overcome the negative aspects of negative experiences of touch or trauma or the symptoms of posttraumatic stress disorder through a harmonious therapeutic process that has clear client–therapist boundaries.[19,33,34,36,37] First, the therapist must be able to read and respond to the client's reactions, proceed slowly and carefully with treatment, and modify interventions to prevent further hyperarousal and distress. In response, the client may experience increased comfort within the therapeutic relationship and may learn to accept, and even enjoy, touch and treatment using massage techniques. This can have physiological benefits for the client because the sense of safety and comfort that comes from being soothed can assist in shutting off the limbic response to stress (fight, flight, or freeze) and facilitate the relaxation or parasympathetic response. In this way, treatment using massage techniques can teach clients an alternative response to touch than a perceived threat. In addition, it can help them learn how to receive positive and healthy touch within a relationship that has clear boundaries.

Respond Appropriately to Emotional Release

The most appropriate response for a therapist without training in working with emotional and psychological issues is to provide an atmosphere in which the client feels comfortable and safe to express his emotions as they arise. This can be achieved by using the strategies outlined in the following sections.

Encourage the Client to Give Feedback

Therapists can facilitate open communication with the client by creating an open, accepting environment and encouraging the client to talk about what does not work for him during a session.[21,61-65] In addition, asking the client for his consent to treatment both before and during a session can reaffirm the right to refuse any aspect of the intervention and contribute to his sense of safety.

Respect the Client's Need to Avoid or Contain Emotions

There are times when the client needs to use strategies to avoid or contain emotions and the therapist finds that this need is in conflict with the goal of relaxation.[21,61-65] Paradoxically, acceptance of the client's need to avoid or contain his emotions can reduce the tension associated with his response and allow him to achieve a greater level of relaxation.

Containment

Unless the therapist has discussed a "contract" with the client that involves the exploration of his emotions, then she must simply deal with whatever arises when the client experiences an emotional release.[21,61-65] Although everyone has his or her own unique way of being with someone who is experiencing intense emotions, within the context of an intervention, this usually involves avoiding any actions that might intensify the client's emotional reaction. For example, engaging in the content of the emotion by asking the client questions can intensify his emotional reaction and lead to difficult interpersonal dynamics if the therapist's questions are not consistent with the client's emotional state and needs. In addition, moving to an area of the client's body where the emotional reaction is focused can also potentially intensify his emotional reaction. Although intensifying the client's emotional reaction may be desirable, asking for the client's consent before doing so allows him to control what he feels is appropriate for him and, in turn, helps contain the level of emotional reaction to what is suitable for the situation.

Manage Your Response to Clients' Emotional Expression

Being comfortable with clients' expressions of emotions is a skill that therapists develop with repeated exposure to clients' emotions.[21,61-65] It is important for the therapist to acquire this skill in preparation for a situation in which she encounters a client who starts to express his emotions. When a therapist exceeds her comfort level and pretends to be comfortable with her client's emotional expression, it can erode the client–therapist relationship for several reasons. The client may feel a lack of safety as a result of the therapist's falseness, or the therapist may feel that the client's emotional needs have gone beyond the proper boundaries of the client–therapist relationship.

Know One's Comfort Level with Clients' Emotional Responses

It is important for the therapist to learn the level of comfort with clients' emotions. When the therapist becomes aware that she has passed the acceptable comfort level, she must communicate to the client what level of emotions she can and cannot respond to within the session.[21,61-65] Communicating one's limits appropriately can result in the client feeling good about himself and understanding the limits for emotional expression and processing within a treatment session. This skill not only involves the therapist knowing ways of phrasing the appropriate information, but also requires that the therapist be aware of when she begins to feel discomfort so that she has time to communicate with the client in a calming and accepting manner. Appropriate communication can help avoid the interpersonal disconnection that can occur when the therapist suddenly feels overwhelmed and withdraws. This is important because these disconnections can leave the client feeling like there is something wrong about his emotions and can result in negative interpersonal dynamics between the client and therapist that are difficult to resolve.

Accept Clients' Emotional Expression

Ideally, the therapist will allow the client's emotions to arise with acceptance, rather than encouragement or discouragement. An excellent way to communicate this acceptance to the client is through "mirroring"[36] or feeding to the client an empathetic understanding or perception of his present emotional state through verbal statements or physical touch. These strategies include rephrasing or repeating the client's communications, applying massage movements that match the client's expression of his emotions, or respectfully stopping the treatment while the client expresses the emotional state. Regardless of the strategy the therapist uses, she needs to ensure that she matches the response to the state and level of intensity of the client's emotional expression, rather than engaging in the actual content of these emotions.[21,22,61-64] This becomes particularly important when the client is in the middle of an intense emotion because problems may arise when the therapist fails to match the client. For example, if the therapist noticeably lowers the intensity of her engagement when the client is increasing the intensity of emotions, then the client may feel that the emotional expression is not accepted. If, on the other hand, the therapist noticeably raises the intensity of her engagement beyond the intensity of the client's emotional expression, then the client may feel that he should be expressing something more than he is. With practice, it is possible for the therapist to develop a repertoire of phrases that she can use to ask the client what he needs in these situations. While both the timing and phrasing of these statements will improve with practice, it is important for the novice to attempt these communications, even if somewhat awkwardly, so that the client can have open communication with the therapist.

Emotions generally have an intensity that peaks and then passes, followed by a more reflective period.[21,27,61-64] A general rule of thumb is for therapists to provide clients with a "space" that is free from large amounts of verbal communication and difficult physical manipulations when they are in the intense phase of emotional expression.

Clients often appreciate the invitation, even if they choose not to accept it, to share their experience after the intensity of the emotions has passed. This sharing of emotions can help clients integrate their experiences in the presence of therapists' empathetic listening and monitoring.

Finally, therapists always need to be aware of the appropriate roles of the client–therapist relationship.[21,27,61-64] Although a small amount of sharing by the therapist may help reduce a client's sense of isolation, appropriate sharing is perhaps the most difficult art to master. The biggest danger faced by therapists is the subtle, or not so subtle, reversal of the client–therapist role. Because sharing by the therapist is not required for empathetic attunement, it is better to err on the side of caution and not share anything too personal. When therapists find that they have an emotional response to something that arises out of a clinical session, it is important for them to seek an appropriate means of dealing with those feelings such as talking with a supportive colleague, supervisor, or mentor.

IN CONCLUSION

The therapeutic relationship, a trust relationship, between the client and the therapist lies at the core of client-centered care for Outcome-Based Massage™. Within this relationship, the client and therapist negotiate a course of treatment that is called the therapeutic contract. The therapeutic process parallels the phases of the clinical decision-making process as the client and therapist move through the stages of building trust, exploring physical sensations, and healthy closure. The therapeutic process is complicated by a number of factors, including the client's vulnerability, because of the intimacy of touch, the therapist's authority and power in the therapeutic relationship, and the fact that clients do not always fully disclose their expectations and histories. Other client-related obstacles can be their negative experiences of touch, tissue memories, trauma, and anxiety. Strategies that therapists can use to enhance the therapeutic relationship include maintaining ethical conduct and addressing the client's emotional response to massage. Since both technical and interpersonal factors can have an impact on the outcomes of care that the client can achieve, therapists would be wise to attend to both of these aspects in the planning and delivery of care to their clients.

Practice

Note: This section contains instructions and clinical cases that demonstrate how to perform some of the approaches to addressing interpersonal and ethical issues that were introduced in this chapter.

Clinical Case 2-1: *Dealing with the Patient's Emotional Response to the Clinician*

Situation

A clinician is treating a patient for a hamstring strain that she sustained while playing badminton. During early sessions, the patient appeared shy and nervous. Over the course of the first four sessions, she began to trust the clinician's integrity and learned to relax into the massage techniques. Now, midway through the episode of care, the clinician has become alarmed because the patient told him that he is the first man who has ever made her feel so special.

The patient moans happily when the clinician applies massage techniques to her leg and shows signs of being attracted to him. As the intervention progresses, she expresses her attraction and appreciation for his therapy more openly.

The clinician knows that he does not intend to cross any professional boundaries, but he feels increasingly uncomfortable treating the patient and wishes that she would just go away.

Issues to Consider

1. What is going on here?
2. How would you describe the patient's behavior?
3. What can the clinician do or say to address the patient's behavior in an ethical manner?

It appears that the patient has transferred her feelings about men and intimacy to the clinician. Whatever her past experience with men, she enjoys the intimacy of the sessions. Consequently, she may be confusing therapeutic intimacy with the kind of closeness that one might have in a personal relationship.

The clinician is uncomfortable because he is receiving a type of attention that he does not want and does not intend to encourage. He does not appear to understand that her behavior has more to do with her past history with men than specifically with him.

Resolution

Baffled by the patient's behavior, the clinician discusses her case with a peer supervisor. He recognizes that the patient may continue to exhibit her attraction and appreciation for him unless he addresses her behavior directly. On the other hand, he also knows that this transference may gradually lessen, and she may be able to see him more clearly for the health-care professional that he is. The clinician decides, for the sake of future sessions, to gently and compassionately explain to the patient that he is pleased she finds the interventions beneficial but that his responsibility to her is strictly professional. Following his discussions with the patient, she gradually begins to respond to him in a more appropriate manner.

Clinical Case 2-2: *Unexpressed Expectations and Histories*

Situation

The patient was in a serious car accident over a year ago and her neck has never been the same. She has been seeing the clinician for more than 3 months. The patient has never had much luck with therapy because the clinicians always seemed to get frustrated with her and discharge her without really addressing her neck pain. She thinks that the present clinician is the first person who has really stuck by her. One day, she shyly admits to the clinician that she is the best thing that has happened to her since her car accident.

The clinician finds the patient's neck pain perplexing. She realizes that the car accident has caused some restriction and pain, but she cannot find any objective examination findings to corroborate the patient's subjective reports. The patient continues to report that her pain is constant, and she appears somewhat depressed. The clinician recognizes her discomfort, but she cannot understand why the patient continues to come for treatment when there does not seem to be any shift in her pain.

One day, the clinician discusses her "challenging patient" (without mentioning names) with an insurance adjuster who has been working with accident claims for years. The adjuster tells her that he has seen all this before. He suggests that the patient is just trying to get more treatment and tells her that the insurance industry calls this behavior malingering. He also suggests that the clinician should discharge the patient because she is just taking advantage of the system.

After her discussion with the adjuster, the clinician meets with the patient and informs her that she has done all that she can for her and that it is time for her discharge. Much to the clinician's surprise, the patient bursts into tears and becomes distraught. After calming her down, the clinician assures her that she does not have to leave therapy if she does not want to.

Issues to Consider

1. What just happened here?
2. Which aspect of the therapeutic process has the clinician negated?
3. What does the clinician need to do in order to re-establish the therapeutic relationship?
4. What actions of the patient have contributed to the current situation?
5. What else should the clinician address in the plan of care for her patient with chronic pain?

The clinician and the patient have been living in two different realities. Although the patient has not told the clinician about all the other clinicians, for the first time, she has begun to trust a therapeutic process. The clinician has been facilitating the patient's trust by simply bearing witness to her pain and treating her over the course of 3 months without questioning the need for discharge. When the clinician discussed her patient with the insurance adjuster, she heard an industry term "malingering" that made her doubt the patient's integrity. The clinician did not reflect further but simply acted on the adjuster's suggestion to discharge her patient on the basis of malingering.

The patient, having just begun to trust the therapeutic process, was dumbfounded when the clinician sought to discharge her. The distressing news removed the patient's fledging sense of safety, making it difficult, once again, for her to trust a clinician.

The clinician was not aware that the patient was still in the phase of building trust. She had been intuitively offering a safe environment in which the patient could experience her pain. When the clinician brought up the idea of discharge, the patient once again experienced the trauma of discharge and punishment for not getting better on a clinician's timetable.

Resolution

The clinician returned to the beginning of the therapeutic process with her patient by completing a full examination and negotiating a plan of care that clearly addresses her impairments and functional limitations. The patient, in turn, disclosed her full history of treatment and medical issues. Through these activities, both patient and clinician developed a greater understanding of the limits to care for the patient. In addition, the clinician involved other health-care professionals in her patient's care for additional physical testing and for psychosocial support, since she could not provide these within her treatment sessions.

At what point will the patient be ready for discharge? The clinician realized that she should have asked this question early in the intervention so that both parties could be prepared for and agree on the point of closure. To remedy this oversight, they set mutually agreed upon times for re-examination as a team so that they knew where they were in the therapeutic process. When the patient achieved some goal, no matter how small, they celebrated their victory with some form of acknowledgement such as a star on her chart, a handshake, or simply eye contact and a few words of encouragement. The clinician understood that the patient needed help to get back on track and that she has found the coaching that she needs in the clinician. She also recognized that, if she ignores these psychosocial concerns now, the patient is at risk for becoming increasingly debilitated by chronic pain. Since the clinician was able to see her role as an educator, as well as a clinician who treats patients' physical issues, she was able to assist the patient out of the cycle of chronic pain that she lives with daily.

Once the clinician re-established the therapeutic process, she helped the patient to understand that there is a beginning, middle, and end to all treatment. In doing so, she communicated to the patient that it is up to her to move forward if she wants and that she would accompany the patient on the journey until she meets her goals.

Clinical Case 2-3: *Working with Negative Experiences of Touch or Trauma*

Situation

A 45-year-old man has come to you for treatment. He fatigues easily and moves his body away from even the slightest degree of pressure. In addition, he holds his breath and tenses each time you touch his mid-back, slightly arching his lumbar spine and guarding.

You feel frustrated and cannot find a way to treat this patient's low back. You find yourself tensing and sense a building anger toward this "hard to please" patient.

Issues to Consider

1. What is going on here?
2. What can you do to change the direction of this therapeutic encounter?
3. What self-care strategies can you use in order to manage your own anger?

This patient is demonstrating the hypersensitivity reaction that occurs when someone has an old injury or trauma. The fact that he has come to you for treatment suggests that he believes that massage and manual techniques can help. His history of trauma is, however, hampering his ability to respond positively to interventions. It can be frustrating when a patient responds in this way because his reactivity requires that you treat him differently than other patients. It may require some creativity on your part to establish a treatment plan that helps the patient without activating his hypersensitivity.

Resolution

One way to change your treatment approach would be to acknowledge the patient's discomfort and ask him if there is any way that you could modify your interventions to make him more comfortable. It might be helpful to ask the patient if he has ever injured his back in any way because muscle guarding is a common way that people protect old injuries.

It may also be true that the patient is not that aware of his responses or his own discomfort. The intimacy of the hands-on therapy may feel confusing. Furthermore, his responses may be as much of a surprise to him as they are to you. First principles of "do no harm" suggest that it might be better for you to treat other parts of his body until he is able to receive touch on his back more easily.

The patient would also benefit from some coaching on deep abdominal breathing. You could show him how to breathe through the discomfort before attempting any deeper work on his back. Demonstrating some self-care strategies and acknowledging what is not working will show him that you have his best interests in mind and do not want to harm him. This can only help to ease any discomfort he may feel. Once he begins to trust you, then he can become an ally in the healing experience.

Being angry or frustrated at this does not help you to provide patient-centered care. In the short term, deep breathing and committing yourself to responding professionally and compassionately are better strategies for managing your feelings. Nevertheless, if a patient like this triggers feelings of anger or discomfort, it is best to discuss the case with a peer or supervisor so that you can better understand what is bothering you. Once you understand and can acknowledge the triggers you are reacting to, this behavior will lose the ability to frustrate you.

Clinical Case 2-4: *Maintaining Patient Privacy*

Situation

Patient A became the clinician's patient when she was pregnant with her first child. She found treatment with massage techniques helpful in managing her low back pain and swollen ankles, which were especially troublesome in her third trimester. The clinician even came to the hospital to treat Patient A right after her baby was born. Since Patient A loves everything that the clinician does in the course of treatment, she suggested that her pregnant best friend (Patient B) see the clinician.

Patient A discussed this suggestion with the clinician. In doing so, she explained to the clinician that this was Patient B's first pregnancy and that she was a little worried about how things were going. Patient A confided that Patient B would need extra support during her pregnancy since her husband was overseas.

A few weeks later, Patient B arrived for her appointment. Patient B was quiet and reluctant to share the details of her situation with the clinician. The session progressed as a normal introductory session. The clinician was pleased when Patient B admitted that she felt more relaxed at the end of the session and scheduled another appointment the following week.

A few days later, Patient A arrived for her appointment with the clinician. She asked her how Patient B had liked her session. The clinician, not used to discussing one patient with another, reluctantly shared that the friend seemed shy but that she liked the intervention. Patient A asked the clinician if Patient B had told her that her husband was going to remain overseas for the next 6 months and gave her the details of how her friend was responding. The clinician was unaware of this and told her so. After listening to Patient A, the clinician decided to speak to Patient B about how her husband's absence was affecting her.

Issues to Consider

1. What is going on here?
2. How would you describe the clinician's behavior?
3. What actions does the clinician need to take to ensure that she maintains her patient's friend's (Patient B) right to privacy?

Every therapeutic relationship needs to be founded on patient safety and confidentiality so that the patient may trust the therapeutic process. The patient needs to know that what she says or experiences is not discussed with anyone else, except in very specific confidential situations such as peer supervision.

Health care often mixes physiological responses with personal, social, or emotional information. Although individuals' responses to treatment may vary, they are all most definitely private. The confidentiality that cloaks therapeutic encounters is like a boundary around the patient. Only the patient may discuss her experience or health care with friends or family. A clinician must never share a patient's condition, confidences, responses to treatment, and other personal information, or the patient's trust will be broken.

In this case, Patient A initiated the contact between Patient B and the clinician. She hopes that her friend will receive the help she needs during her pregnancy, and she shares these hopes and expectations with the clinician. As a health-care professional, the clinician wants to help Patient B, but she makes a mistake in considering Patient A's perspective.

First, by listening to Patient A talk about Patient B's problems, the clinician communicates indirectly to her that they are equally responsible for Patient B's health care. The clinician does not stop Patient A from discussing her friend, and she does nothing to create a boundary between her as the clinician, who should maintain complete confidentiality for all patients, and Patient B.

Second, the clinician resolves to discuss the information from Patient A with Patient B. This confirms that there is now a triangle between the three women. This is a breach of trust since it will confirm to Patient B that the clinician has discussed her with Patient A. This action, although well intentioned, ignores the nature of the friendship between Patient A and Patient B. The clinician has no knowledge of how their friendship works and may appear to be siding with Patient A against Patient B. This type of triangulating damages the therapeutic process.

Third, by not allowing the therapeutic process to unfold naturally with Patient B, the clinician has compromised her objectivity and her ability to assess and address Patient B's needs for treatment.

Resolution

The clinician stopped all discussions about Patient B with Patient A. She also chose not to mention the information that Patient A gave her because this would enhance the triangle relationship. This was difficult to establish after the fact, but in this case, it was necessary to be direct and truthful. The clinician used an "I" statement to clarify to Patient A, without pointing fingers, what exactly had to change:

When I listened to you the other day as you described your friend's circumstances, I felt uncomfortable because my job as a clinician is to maintain confidentiality for all my patients. I appreciate your comments, but I will not discuss your friend with you again.

The clinician also discussed the situation with one of her peers to get guidance on how to ensure Patient B's privacy. Above all else, the clinician committed to ensure Patient B's complete confidentiality regarding her health care.

REVIEW SECTION

TAKEAWAYS

1. The therapeutic relationship is a trust relationship because of the client's vulnerability and the clinician's responsibility not to exploit or harm the client through this vulnerability.
2. The clinician sets the tone of the therapeutic relationship based on her willingness to share information, support client goals, and empathize with the client's circumstances or condition. The clinician must, therefore, hold the best interests of the client above all other aspects of the interaction.
3. Clients need safety, predictability, patience, clear and explicit interpersonal processes, healthy boundaries, and responsible closure within the therapeutic relationship.
4. Client-centered care looks beyond the mere delivery of services to the client to include advocacy, empowerment, respect for the client's autonomy, and the client's participation in decision-making. This approach is essential in Outcome-Based Massage™.

5. The therapeutic contract is the end product of the negotiation of the clinical care that the client will receive. Both the client and the clinician have rights and responsibilities within the therapeutic contract.
6. There are three phases in the therapeutic process: building trust, exploring sensation, and healthy closure.
7. Ethical behavior on the part of the clinician is an essential component of the therapeutic relationship. Before the clinician can examine the client or initiate the treatment plan, he requires the client's understanding and consent.
8. Clients and clinicians can have emotional responses to each other and it is the clinician's responsibility to address and manage these responses.
9. It is unethical and abusive for clinicians to engage in personal or sexualized contact with clients because of the power imbalance between clinicians and their clients.
10. Clients may have negative experiences of touch or strong emotional responses to massage. In either case, clinicians need to be prepared for and respond appropriately to client's emotional responses to massage.

Critical Thinking Questions

1. What type of therapeutic contract would you employ in your practice?
2. If you have a client that does not seem to be getting any better, how might you discover what is affecting her progress?
3. If you feel attracted to a client, what should you do?
4. How would you respond if a client told you she wanted to be your friend?
5. What resources are available to you when you are faced with an ethical dilemma?

6. What type of question would help you encourage a client to talk about her condition? Give an example.
7. When should you employ "I," "we," or "you" in a client interview?
8. Why is context important when seeking client's desired goals?
9. How may your assumptions contribute or detract from client outcomes?
10. When is it appropriate to disclose personal information to clients?

References for Chapter 2 begin on p. 449.

CHAPTER 3

Evidence for Massage

OBJECTIVES

After studying this chapter, the reader will have the information required to do the following:

1. List sources of evidence for clinical practice.
2. Describe methods for locating and evaluating evidence for clinical practice.
3. Explain different research methods and designs.
4. Describe the steps required to critically read a research article.
5. Discuss trends and issues in massage therapy research and understand how to apply best available evidence in clinical practice.

Evidence is information on clinical care that researchers and therapists collect in a systematic manner. It is typically about the outcomes and, occasionally, the process of clinical care. As both providers and consumers of health-care information and services, therapists are bombarded daily with evidence in a variety of forms, ranging from professional journals to the Internet and public discussion. Clients also deal with the same bewildering array of opinions and information. Rather than answering questions, this information often raises new questions such as: "What is good evidence?" and "What constitutes best evidence when making clinical decisions?" This chapter addresses these questions. It also describes how evidence helps therapists who are using Outcome-Based Massage™ to serve their clients better. Finally, it introduces concepts related to the steps of finding, understanding, critically evaluating, and applying best evidence to clinical practice.

Evidence

WHY THERAPISTS NEED EVIDENCE

An evidence-based approach is a key component of Outcome-Based Massage™. Menard[1] suggests that an evidence-based approach is essential in health care and provides several reasons for using evidence to inform clinical practice. First and foremost, therapists need evidence in order to provide the best possible care to their clients. Evidence supports the theoretical foundation of a discipline and helps therapists to be critical thinkers. It also helps them to distinguish between useful and safe practices and those that might be harmful to clients. Furthermore, it assists them in educating themselves and their clients about what massage and other health-care interventions can and cannot do. Second, evidence fosters public acceptance of massage and other complementary health-care modalities and provides a common language that facilitates communication about massage techniques. Third, evidence enables therapists to stay current, to be lifelong learners, and to be better consumers of health-care resources themselves.

Increasingly, as massage becomes more widely accepted,[2-6] consumers, health-care practitioners, government agencies, professional associations, and researchers are asking important questions about the safety and effectiveness of massage as a health-care intervention.[7-10] Furthermore, increased use of and reimbursement for massage interventions bring an increased requirement for accountability. Consequently, therapists need to know which massage techniques work best for which clients and under which conditions.[10]

On a more personal level, therapists are also ethically committed to being lifelong learners who participate in self-reflection and the continuous development of skills, knowledge, and attitudes in professional practice. In this arena, evidence can guide clinical decision-making and professional growth.

EVIDENCE-BASED PRACTICE

The systematic use of evidence in clinical decision-making is the basis of evidence-based practice (EBP), or what David Sackett first identified as evidence-based medicine (EBM). Sackett[11,12] defines EBM as "… the integration of best research evidence with clinical expertise and client values." Within this definition, best research evidence means the best available clinical, client-centered research that examines the accuracy, safety, efficacy, and cost effectiveness of diagnostic and assessment tests, prognostic markers, and therapeutic interventions. Clinical expertise is the therapist's ability to use clinical skills and past experience to identify each client's unique health status and the potential risks and benefits of interventions that could be used in each case. Client values refer to the unique preferences, goals, and expectations that each client brings to the therapeutic relationship. Sackett[11,12] proposes that therapists need to integrate all of these components in order to become proficient in EBP. To guide them in doing so, Sackett[11,12] suggests that therapists follow five steps for integrating evidence into clinical practice: (1) ask an answerable question, (2) collect evidence systematically, (3) appraise evidence critically, (4) apply the results of their analysis of the evidence to practice,

and (5) evaluate the results that they obtain when they apply the evidence to practice.

Greenhalgh[13] further defines evidence-based medicine as "… the enhancement of a therapist's traditional skills in diagnosis, treatment, prevention, and related areas through the systematic framing of relevant and answerable questions and the use of mathematical estimates of probability and risk." This extends two important concepts in Sackett's definition. First of all, it emphasizes the importance of therapists learning how to ask clinical questions that are answerable, something that is not as straightforward as it initially sounds. Second, it suggests that therapists have to understand the basic concepts of designing and conducting research.

In addition, several authors on EBP discuss why it is sometimes difficult to base clinical decision-making on "best evidence."[14-16] They maintain that, at times, there is very little evidence and, at other times, there is too much of it. In addition, they suggest that therapists do not have enough time, or do not make enough time, to find research papers, read them, and distinguish the bad papers from the good. Finally, they point out that interpreting how to put the new information into clinical practice can also seem daunting. Notwithstanding these complexities, Outcome-Based Massage™ considers the adoption of EBP to be essential for therapists.

Initiating Evidence-Based Practice

For students and therapists, the first step in engaging in EBP can be to develop their ability to use evidence from different sources. The four essential competencies for research literacy are the ability to find, understand, critically evaluate, and apply research evidence to practice (Key Points 3-1).[1] Although it is beyond the scope of this book to provide comprehensive information on how to develop research literacy skills, we will use this list of essential competencies and the clinical case to guide the introduction to EBP.

FINDING THE EVIDENCE FOR PRACTICE

Evidence can come from primary or secondary sources.[1,17] The primary source documents the primary research, which is the original research conducted by therapists or researchers. Primary sources are typically professional journals, conference presentations, and, occasionally, textbooks. A secondary source is a summary of the information presented in a primary source. Secondary sources can include secondary research studies, which summarize and draw conclusions from primary studies, such as nonsystematic literature reviews, systematic literature reviews, and meta-analyses. There are also a wide variety of other secondary sources, such as textbooks, the popular media, the Internet, professional courses, and professional journals. Evidence from both primary and secondary research can be evaluated through a ranking system. There are many different ranking models which will be covered in more detail in this chapter. Some models utilize a traditional hierarchy that creates levels of evidence based on what are considered to be the most rigorous and least rigorous research designs. Other systems utilize non-hierarchical approaches, such as the evidence house and evidence funnel, that propose incorporating many different kinds of research methods in order to make the best informed decision.

Evidence from Primary Sources

The most accurate and direct representation of the evidence is the researcher's original documentation. Therapists can locate primary sources through databases for scientific and health-related information (Key Points 3-2). Within

ERIC

Content: The Education Resources Information Center (ERIC) is a digital library of education-related resources sponsored by the Institute of Education Sciences of the U.S. Department of Education. The collection consists of electronic bibliographic records describing journal and nonjournal literature selected by ERIC from 1966 to 2003 and full-text articles.

CHID

Content: CHID is a bibliographic database produced by agencies of the National Institutes of Health. This database provides titles, abstracts, and availability information for health information and health education resources.

PEDro

Content: PEDro is the Physiotherapy Evidence Database. It has been developed by the Centre for Evidence-Based Physiotherapy to give rapid access to bibliographic details and abstracts of randomized controlled trials (RCT), systematic reviews, and evidence-based clinical practice guidelines in physical therapy.

primary sources, there are a variety of methods of gathering and analyzing data. These range from individual case studies to systematic reviews of multiple studies based on the relative strength of the data or combined data to answer questions on safety and effectiveness. Research published in a peer-reviewed professional journal is considered to be the gold standard of quality. Peer review is a prior-to-publication process in which a group of experts from a profession independently review research articles for scientific merit, participant safety, ethical considerations, and other rigorous criteria. The peer reviewers make recommendations on whether or not the articles meet the criteria for publication. Peer-reviewed journals state their criteria for inclusion, thereby enabling therapists to make informed choices about some of the underlying assumptions or potential biases a publication may have. Although peer review increases the likelihood that the research information published is of high quality, it is still useful for therapists to read all publications with a thoughtful and critical eye. By contrast, the review process is less rigorous for journals without peer review, conference presentations, and professional courses.

Evidence from Secondary Sources

Secondary sources of evidence are often easier to locate than primary sources. Searching the Internet, in popular and social media sites (Google Scholar, Facebook, blogs, chat rooms, etc.), is often the first step a student or therapist who is new to EBP will take in finding evidence for practice. However, one cannot assume that these secondary sources accurately report the original findings of the studies

they describe. As a result, there are several cautions to using secondary sources. First, therapists must read information in the popular media, such as newspapers and magazines or online, carefully because the findings of the original research study can be manipulated or distorted by publication bias and reporting techniques. Second, although the Internet continues to be the fastest growing public repository of information, it requires knowledge of good search techniques to find relevant resources. Fortunately, therapists are becoming increasingly savvy about how to access and critically assess information on the Internet. However, there is a persistent myth that all information on the Internet is one keyword and one click away. Anyone who has tried to find quality research on massage on the Internet by typing the key word "massage" into a search engine will understand how challenging it can be to find good evidence. Furthermore, the quality of information on the Internet varies from researchers' own accounts of their work to members of the general public posting information that is of personal interest. Therefore, therapists are encouraged to examine Internet content to critically review the source and reputation of the information.

Finally, although selected groups of peers review textbooks with greater rigor than the popular media is reviewed, there is no standard for judging the evidence textbooks present and the accuracy with which they quote primary sources. The same issue applies to secondary sources in professional journals and professional courses.

UNDERSTANDING THE EVIDENCE FOR PRACTICE

Understanding evidence requires that therapists gain a basic understanding of research methods and evaluate the underlying assumptions and biases of research studies. There are two primary approaches to conducting research: quantitative and qualitative.[1,17-19] Quantitative research methods evolved from basic science research and use the collection and analysis of numerical data. Qualitative research methods, from the social sciences research tradition, use the collection and analysis of word-based experiential and observational data, rather than numbers.

Basics of Quantitative and Qualitative Research

Qualitative and quantitative research goals and methods differ in a variety of ways.[20] Quantitative research is based on the belief that researchers can stand back from reality in order to observe and measure it using objective instruments. Qualitative researchers consider themselves to be part of the reality they are observing. Consequently, qualitative researchers propose that it is hard to distinguish between the observer and what he or she observes and that researchers change reality as they study it.

These key differences provide the foundation for what quantitative and qualitative researchers consider to be "truth": the relationship between facts and values, and the goals of investigation.[20] The cornerstone of quantitative research is to find a measurable representation of reality that can be duplicated by other researchers following the same process which is carefully controlled for observer or other forms of bias. Qualitative research allows for and acknowledges various forms of potential bias or subjectivity and proposes multiple theories on the phenomenon being studied, each of which is an equally acceptable "truth" seen from a variety of vantage points. In quantitative research, the goal of the researcher's methodology is to test and to determine which theory comes the closest to approximating the "truth" or reality. Furthermore, quantitative researchers use specified scientific methods to control for and try and rule out various forms of bias and to demonstrate that results of the research did not occur by chance. These techniques include manipulating the clinical setting and participants, measuring phenomena, controlling the environment as much as possible, and using statistical analyses. This strategy supports the principle that quantitative researchers can reproduce results of other studies if they use the same objective procedures. Qualitative researchers are less concerned with being able to replicate results and more concerned with observing phenomena in their natural setting and documenting their insights about their observations, utilizing data from interviews, direct observations, and artifacts such as journals.

Finally, the goal of quantitative researchers is to discover laws about the causes and effects of phenomena that can be generalized to other situations. The goal of qualitative researchers is to gain a deep or "rich" understanding of the subject that they are observing. These differing goals result in different methods for collecting and analyzing data.[18,19,21]

Quantitative, Qualitative, and Mixed Methods Research Designs

There are many types of quantitative research study designs.[1,9,17,19] Researchers can use these designs to form hypotheses or statements that researchers can show to be true or false by collecting and analyzing data. Descriptive studies provide a record or description of events or activities. Descriptive study designs include surveys, case reports, case series, and correlational studies. On the other hand, explanatory studies try to explain the connections between events or variables and examine cause and effect. Researchers use these studies to test hypotheses. Explanatory study designs are either experimental or quasi-experimental. Experimental studies include randomized controlled trials and other variations on designs with randomization and control groups. By contrast, quasi-experimental studies are those that lack randomization and control groups, such as studies in which an individual acts as his own control. Textbooks on research methods[1,17,22] contain a more detailed discussion of terminology, procedures, and statistics associated with quantitative research designs for massage and allied health care.[9,19]

There are also many types of qualitative studies, the most common of which are grounded theory, ethnography, and phenomenology.[1,9,17,20,23-26] Data collection most often takes place in the natural environment where the behaviors or phenomena that are the subject of the research actually take place, rather than in the laboratory or the highly controlled clinical environment, as is the case in quantitative research. Grounded theory, developed by Glaser and Strauss,[27] involves the generation of theory from participants' responses. In other words, researchers transcribe, categorize, and sort participants' responses to identify patterns and develop theory. An ethnography describes and interprets the activities of a group of people who have a common feature. Finally, phenomenologic studies are those that describe a specific aspect of a group's experiences and are concerned with how individuals interpret and make sense of their experiences, as opposed to simply describing those experiences. Textbooks on the methods and terminology of qualitative research outline the specifics of the different approaches.[19,20,27]

Mixed methods research is defined as "research that collects both qualitative and quantitative data in one study and integrates these data at some stage of the research process" (pp. 9-10).[28] Massage therapy is a complex intervention consisting of physiological, psychological, social, and spiritual components, and many other factors can affect massage outcomes such as the intent of the therapist and the clients' experiences, beliefs, and values. Consequently, using both quantitative and qualitative methods in a study can add richness and depth and provide a more complete picture than one research method or the other alone. Mixed methods research is particularly useful when the different kinds of data gathered from quantitative and qualitative methods can be meaningfully analyzed in relationship to each other; in other words, integrated in such a way that the whole is greater than the sum of the parts.[21,28] There are a variety of reasons for a mixed methods approach such as identifying areas in which data from different methods support or contradict a given conclusion or using the results from one method to develop the other method. The most common designs for mixed methods research are concurrent studies, in which they use both qualitative and quantitative methods simultaneously, or sequential studies, in which researchers use one type of method (qualitative or quantitative) followed by the other. Details of mixed methods research principles are found in a variety of research textbooks.[10]

Designs for Massage Research

Massage research may be either primary or secondary research.[1,20] A study in which the researchers collect original data from their subjects on the phenomena that they are investigating would be considered primary research. Types of primary research include clinical trials, surveys, ethnographies, and a variety of other research designs. By contrast, those studies that compile and analyze data from existing primary research studies are called secondary research. This section examines some of the ways in which primary and secondary research can be used in massage.

Primary Research

Massage is a complex intervention with physiological, psychological, and social components. It is challenging to try to separate the specific effects of massage, such as neurological and cardiovascular effects, from the nonspecific effects, including the therapeutic relationship, environment, the process of therapy, and the beliefs and attitudes of both the client and the therapist.[29,30] So which research method is more appropriate for primary research on massage techniques: qualitative or quantitative? That depends on the research question one is asking.[9,31] Some research questions benefit from one method or the other; however, we can best answer some research questions using a combination of qualitative and quantitative research methods.[21] Consider the research question about the effectiveness of a particular massage intervention for a particular population: "Do daily interventions of massage improve the gestational date achieved of women with high-risk pregnancies who are on bed rest?" Researchers could answer this question best using a quantitative design. Whereas researchers can answer a research question about the meaning of the massage experience for the client (such as "What are the perceptions and experiences of daily massage interventions of women with high-risk pregnancies who are on bed rest?") better using qualitative research methods. Furthermore, the use of mixed methods research can extend the information gathered on a variety of questions. More and more, individuals conducting research on massage techniques are recognizing that existing research methodologies fail to address critical aspects of massage and choose to use both quantitative and qualitative—or mixed—methods in their studies to address a variety of questions. In addition, researchers are developing research methods for interventions that are complex systems of treatment with multiple kinds of interventions in one treatment such as traditional Chinese medicine. Whole systems research, for example, is an approach for examining the complex interrelationship between the specific and nonspecific effects (the interplay between client, provider, treatment, and context) of various types of interventions or a massage therapy practice as a whole system.[21,32]

Secondary Research

The sheer volume of research evidence available can be daunting. Some researchers and professional journals attempt to collect, summarize, and comment on recent articles to make it easier for therapists to observe the trends in the research and stay current. Some forms of this secondary research use rigorous criteria to evaluate all related studies on a particular subject and can be a useful way for therapists to review the conclusions of a number of related studies simultaneously. Sackett et al.[11,12] and others such as the Cochrane Collaboration (http://www.cochrane.org/) and the CONSORT Group (http://www.consort-statement.org/) provide guidelines for a systematic analysis and reporting of research articles to determine their rigor.

Systematic reviews and meta-analyses are two common types of secondary research.[18] A systematic review is an approach that is used to identify, appraise, and synthesize all the relevant empirical evidence that meets pre-specified eligibility criteria to answer a given research question.

Researchers who are conducting systematic reviews use specific methods to minimize bias and produce more reliable findings that can be used to guide decision-making. On the other hand, performing meta-analyses involves the use of statistical methods to combine results of similar individual studies in order to increase the power of the analysis and understand whether the treatment effects are similar in similar situations. The validity of the results of meta-analysis is determined in part by whether the studies used are similar enough to be combined.

EVALUATING THE EVIDENCE FOR PRACTICE

When asked, "What is good evidence?" a wise person replied, "It depends on who is asking." By this, they meant that evidence is not neutral or unbiased. People generate evidence under specific historical and social conditions. Consequently, like all other forms of knowledge, this information is not entirely free of biases or errors. Knowing that real people, under real and often less-than-ideal circumstances, generate evidence does not mean that therapists cannot rely on evidence to help them make sound clinical decisions. It does mean, however, that they need to use the best evidence available in an educated and critical manner. To do so, therapists need to go beyond evaluating the methodology used to obtain the evidence. They should also consider how research questions get asked and why, how evidence is obtained and by whom, who funds and conducts research, and who stands to benefit from the research. This weighing of the relative strengths, weaknesses, and biases of evidence is a critical component in the clinical decision-making process.

Levels of Evidence

Guidance on how to evaluate evidence comes from multiple sources. Sackett et al.[11,12] have created a hierarchy of research designs, called levels of evidence, and a systematic approach for evaluating evidence (Key Points 3-3). This hierarchy ranks several different types of studies.[11,12,33] Meta-analyses use statistical techniques for combining results from different studies to obtain a quantitative estimate of the overall effect of a particular intervention or variable on a defined outcome, producing a stronger conclusion than can be provided by any individual study.[34] Systematic reviews also evaluate findings from individual studies and combine these findings using statistical techniques. Randomized controlled trials use control groups and the random assignment of participants into experimental or control groups. In cohort studies, researchers follow the outcomes of a group of participants who they identify as having received the intervention and a group with similar characteristics who did not. Case–control studies are those in which researchers identify individuals who have similar outcomes and examine their history to determine if they received the same intervention. Finally, a case series is a summary of findings on a group of participants with similar characteristics or who received the same intervention without reference to findings on a control group. Studies at the top of Sackett's hierarchy provide

| | | Key Points: 3-3 |

Sample of Sackett's Levels of Evidence

Grade of Recommendation	Level of Evidence	Type of Study
A	1a	Systematic reviews of randomized controlled trials
	1b	Individual randomized controlled trials with a narrow confidence interval
	1c	All or none case series
B	2a	Systematic reviews of cohort studies
	2b	Individual cohort studies and low-quality randomized controlled trials
	2c	Outcomes research
	3a	Systematic reviews of case–control studies
	3b	Individual case-controlled studies
C	4	Case series and poor-quality cohort and case–control studies
D	5	Expert opinion without explicit critical appraisal, or based on physiology, bench research, or "first principles"

Adapted with permission from Sackett D, Straus SE, Richardson WS, Rosenberg W, Haynes B. *Evidence-Based Medicine: How to Practice and Teach EBM.* Edinburgh: Churchill Livingstone; 2000:7-8[12]; Glaros S. All evidence is not created equal: a discussion of levels of evidence. *PT Mag.* 2003;11:42-49, 52.[33]

the strongest evidence of a cause-and-effect relationship between the intervention and the outcome and vice versa.

A variety of points of view exist about the concept of a hierarchy of research designs.[13-16] At the top of Sackett's[11,12] levels of evidence, after the meta-analysis and systematic review, that combine findings from research, is the randomized controlled trial, which is considered the most rigorous of the experimental design methods because of its level of experimental control and randomization of participants. At the bottom of Sackett's hierarchy is descriptive research, which does not use a high degree of control and randomization. This traditional hierarchy of evidence is a concern for research on massage techniques because it suggests that much of the evidence for massage comes from traditions of research that rank lower on the levels of evidence and are, thus, less rigorous. To address this issue, Jonas[16] proposes building an "evidence house" and Finch[14] proposes an "evidence funnel." The evidence house describes a number of rooms, all equal in importance, that include many kinds of rigorous research methods, both qualitative and quantitative, rather than a hierarchical model.[16] The evidence house allows therapists to review evidence from each room and apply it to practice. The evidence funnel takes information gathered from different sources and channels it into a relevant evidence section whereby the therapist, after carefully assessing the information, can make the best informed decision.[14] Both Jonas and Finch suggest that including a variety of research methodologies can provide a more balanced and complete picture of what constitutes massage and how it works. The methods used depend on the question or questions that the researcher is trying to answer.

Reading and Evaluating Research Articles

Therapists must resist the temptation to read the Introduction and then skip to the Discussion and Conclusions of a research article. A systematic assessment of the credibility of the conclusions of a research study enables therapists to determine the degree to which it is appropriate for them to apply that evidence to their own clinical practices. The section in this chapter entitled How to Read a Research Article Critically outlines a basic process that can provide a starting point for using the evidence in the research literature for Outcome-Based Massage™. Although an in-depth treatment of the process for analyzing research articles is beyond the scope of this book, the chapters on treatment techniques will introduce brief analyses of samples of evidence to illustrate this approach.

APPLYING EVIDENCE TO PRACTICE

Applying best evidence to practice is one set of threads in the complex tapestry of professional practice. Sackett et al.[11,12] outline how an evidence-based approach to practice integrates best available research evidence, clinical expertise, and client values. Adopting an evidence-based approach to practice is a process that requires that therapists become aware of and reflect on their own assumptions, biases, and knowledge base.[35] An ethical therapist continuously examines and develops knowledge, skills, and attitudes throughout their professional career. They seek out and critically evaluate the best evidence for practice and then apply relevant information to confirm, modify, or alter their approach to practice. Since they recognize that

future research may show that some of today's accepted practices are ineffective, they feel comfortable challenging conventional wisdom and thinking for themselves. Finally, a reflective therapist understands that acquiring research literacy and developing an evidence-based approach to practice is not about learning a specific set of skills for a single use. Instead, it is about integrating critical thinking into all aspects of professional life and using best available evidence from a variety of sources to enhance professional accomplishment and clients' safety and well-being. Key Points 3-4 outlines some activities that therapists can use to facilitate their development of an evidence-based approach to practice.[35]

Key Points: 3-4

Activities That Facilitate EBP

- Pose specific questions of practical value to clients
- Search for best evidence
- Critically evaluate best evidence
- Take action guided by that evidence
- Reflect
- Formulate thoughtful questions
- Read critically
- Discuss and learn with others
- Confirm, alter, or modify practice
- Continuously learn and self-evaluate
- Set aside time to journal and reflect on practice
- Set aside time to search the Internet; set up "Alerts" for new information
- Subscribe to journals/newsletters
- Join a peer supervision group
- Join your professional association
- Take professional development courses in research literacy and research capacity
- Find professional supervision or a mentor
- Join an evidence-based professional group
- Critically evaluate your own performance
- Commit to lifelong learning
- Create an evidence-based newsletter for clients
- Give talks/information-sharing sessions in your community
- Write and publish case reports and critiques of best evidence
- Get involved with research initiatives by collaborating with established academic researchers

Adapted with permission from Gibbs LE. *Evidence-Based Practice for the Helping Professions: A Practical Guide with Integrated Multimedia.* Pacific Grove, CA: Thompson, Brooks, Cole; 2003:19.

TRENDS IN THE EVIDENCE ON MASSAGE

The volume of research on massage continues to grow. The number of high-quality studies is also increasing. For the greater part, these studies have investigated the safety and benefits of massage. Most of this work focuses on pain relief, psychological effects, and effects on specific populations and conditions, across the lifespan from infants to the elderly. However, there are few rigorous studies on the effects of massage on specific tissues, muscle tension, connective tissue integrity, or fluid. There is still very little known about optimal dosage and frequency of massage treatment or the effects of specific massage techniques for specific conditions and populations. Finally, given the range and diversity in massage research methods and outcomes, there are only a handful of meta-analyses and other systematic reviews of massage research that are useful in helping us to identify the most commonly reported and substantiated effects of massage.[36-39]

Regardless of the source and type of research, we can consider the research in massage within four categories: established, promising, unsubstantiated, and needed. Established research refers to those research findings that have been substantiated by multiple studies and which we feel most comfortable using to guide practice. Promising research includes those findings that have some support from research, but not to the same degree as the substantiated research. These are in sharp contrast to the unsubstantiated research which consists of anecdotal findings or those from a few, poorly designed studies. Finally, needed research represents those areas for which there is a lack of evidence. This section outlines selected research that can be described as established or promising, while the section entitled Issues in Massage Research identifies some areas for which research is needed.

Effects of Massage on Pain Including Low Back Pain

A small, but growing, number of clinical trials suggest that massage can reduce pain in people with headaches and migraines,[40-43] low back and other orthopedic pain,[2,44-48] neck and shoulder pain,[49,50] osteoarthritis (OA),[29,51] pregnancy and labor,[30,52] and adult and pediatric cancer.[36-39,53-56] Furlan et al.[57] offer several conclusions in their Cochrane systematic review on massage and chronic, nonspecific low back pain. They concluded that, for chronic, nonspecific low back pain, massage is effective for pain and function and that massage is

similar to exercise, and it is superior to joint mobilization, relaxation therapy, physical therapy, acupuncture, and self-care education. Studies, they also noted, varied in methodological quality, heterogeneous population, massage techniques, and comparison groups. The majority of studies assessed improvements in pain and function immediately after the sessions or in the short term. Fewer studies measured outcomes at long-term follow-up. Massage was clearly most effective when it was delivered with exercise and education.[26,58-60]

In one study, Cherkin et al.[37] found that massage interventions may save money by reducing the number of health-care provider visits, the use of pain medications, and the costs of back care services.[37] Furthermore, they report that the beneficial effects of massage appear to be long-lasting (at least 1 year post-intervention) for clients with chronic low back pain (CLBP). More recently, a large-scale longitudinal study by Cherkin and colleagues[44] compared two different types of massage therapy with each other and with standard care. After 10 weeks of treatment, subjects in the relaxation massage and structural massage groups had fewer symptoms of back pain and experienced less associated disability than those in the standard care group. Most of these gains were still observed at the 52-week follow-up. However, at follow-up, the researchers stated that they observed no clinically meaningful difference between relaxation and structural massage in terms of relieving disability or symptoms. Findings like these should lead to more outcome studies that compare two or more types of massage techniques for a given population or condition.

Effects of Massage on Mood

There is promising evidence that massage therapy produces significant psychological benefits such as the reduction of anxiety and depression in both adults and children with a variety of conditions.[36,61-64] Moyer et al.[36,65] have provided detailed descriptions of studies on the effects of massage on anxiety and depression. They conclude that multiple applications of massage may reduce perceived pain. In addition, they point out that trait anxiety and depression are among the best documented psychological effects of massage, with a course of interventions using massage techniques providing benefits similar in magnitude to those of psychotherapy.[36,65]

Other Effects of Massage

The following is a selection of other possible physiological effects of massage therapy on which there is a limited amount of research.

A number of studies suggest there may be specific effects of particular benefit to patients with cancer, including reductions of anxiety, nausea, and pain, and improvements in appetite and sleep.[53,66-83] In addition, some research suggests that massage techniques may improve venous and lymphatic return, but much more research is needed to support this.[68,74-78,84-109] This is similar to the situation for the use of massage to increase arterial flow; the body of research is small and contradictory.[90,110-118] Furthermore, a small amount of recent research tends to confirm the traditional use of percussion for airway clearance,[119-123] although mechanical devices are probably equally effective, and massage for symptom relief and pulmonary function.[56,124] Another promising finding is massage therapy's effect on oxytocin. Oxytocin is a neuropeptide that plays a key role in mammalian social attachment and affiliation.[125] Massage therapy may, under certain conditions, lead to an increase of oxytocin that would be consistent with feelings of well-being, pro-social behavior, and the promotion of health and may help to explain some of the complex effects of massage on clients' perceptions of well-being post-massage.[126] Finally, some research studies have found a significantly positive effect of massage on the various indices of immune function, but this finding has not been uniform.[36,48,63,64,127-141] For example, there is an ongoing debate on whether biochemical indicators of stress, such as cortisol, serotonin, and dopamine levels, change following massage therapy. Several studies from the University of Miami's Touch Research Institute have shown that cortisol levels decrease following massage, whereas other studies have not demonstrated these findings, suggesting that further research is needed in this area.

Oddly enough, there are no readily available studies on the effect of massage on reducing the resting tension of healthy muscle, which is a commonly quoted reason for intervention in the general population. This may be due to a poor understanding of what physiological processes contribute to resting tension in healthy muscle and the problems inherent in reliably assessing resting tension.[142] Finally, there is limited evidence to support the use of massage to reduce elevated tone associated with some neurological conditions.[143-145]

A lack of evidence for the effects of massage is more of a reflection of methodological limitations than of a lack of potential treatment effectiveness. Therapists can still benefit from reading the existing research on massage as long as they are aware of its strengths and limitations. Dryden and Moyer.[10] provide a thorough analysis of research in massage therapy by population and condition such as those areas noted in Table 3-1.

Table 3-1	Some Areas of Research on Massage
	Youth
Infants	■ Infant development ■ Infants with low birth weight
Children and adolescents	■ Cancer ■ Sleep ■ Anxiety ■ Depression ■ Autism spectrum disorders ■ Attention deficit hyperactivity disorder ■ Aggression ■ Pulmonary function
	Adults—Physical
Athletes	■ Architectural and neural effects ■ Blood flow and lactate clearance ■ Muscle force and power production ■ Muscle soreness
Cancer	■ Anxiety ■ Depressed mood ■ Fatigue ■ Nausea ■ Pain
Headache	■ Migraine ■ Tension headache
Pain	■ Fibromyalgia ■ Low back pain ■ Neck pain ■ Shoulder pain
Pregnancy	■ Pregnancy ■ Labor
Scar	■ Burns ■ Hypertrophic scars
	Adults—Psychosocial
Mood	■ Depression (autonomic nervous system activation, neurotransmitter influences, muscle tension) ■ State anxiety ■ Trait anxiety
Trauma	■ History of sexual trauma
	Geriatric
Healthy	■ Balance ■ Constipation ■ Flexibility ■ Pain
Chronic conditions	■ Arthritis ■ Dementia ■ Insomnia ■ Palliative care

Dryden T, Moyer CA, eds. *Massage Therapy: Integrating Research and Practice.* Champaign, IL: Human Kinetics; 2012.

ISSUES IN MASSAGE RESEARCH

Many of the same methodology issues faced by research on complementary and alternative health care, and by healthcare research in general, currently plague the research on the effects of massage. The issues include the following:

- A lack of relevant outcome measures
- Weak research methods
- Poorly defined procedures for interventions
- Heterogeneous or small samples

However, these limitations should not deter progress in this area. Instead, an understanding of the current limitations can fuel advances in research on massage therapy. Furthermore, therapists should note that there is an ever-increasing number of well-designed studies, including randomized controlled trials, that systematically document the positive effects of massage.

Issues in Current Research Methodologies

The Cochrane systematic review by Haraldsson et al.[39] of the effects of massage for people with mechanical neck disorders illustrates some of the current limitations of massage research. First, they found that the methodological quality of the studies was low and classified 12 of the 19 studies as low-quality studies. In addition, the heterogeneity of the participants in the studies prevented statistical pooling of results across studies. On the positive side, the characteristics of participants in the studies were well reported. By contrast, the studies had poor descriptions of the massage intervention and the experience of the treating therapists. Descriptions of interventions often combined multiple techniques and omitted descriptions of the specific interventions and their rationale. Some studies included massage interventions that many therapists would not consider appropriate for the conditions under investigation. In addition, only 11 of the 19 studies provided sufficient detail to determine who was actually delivering the intervention. Finally, the variations in the massage techniques and research methods made it impossible for these authors to draw conclusions about the effectiveness of massage for improving neck pain and function.

Directions in Designing and Reporting Research for Massage

In acknowledgment of the existing limitations in the research, there is a movement underway to develop clearer guidelines for designing and reporting research on massage. Several of these efforts are intended to cross disciplines and journals with the aim of enhancing the overall quality of evidence on massage therapy.

In the realm of research design, several key issues are targeted for improvement. These include the following:

- Increasing the number of studies on effectiveness
- Providing clear definitions of massage protocols or interventions that include the dosage and frequency of interventions
- Evaluating specific massage techniques, rather than using global interventions that combine multiple techniques
- Outlining the qualifications of treating therapists and other study personnel
- Examining the complex nonspecific effects of massage such as the therapeutic relationship and clinical setting
- Creating and using outcome measures that can measure the potential effects of massage
- Increasing the number of participants in studies or using methodologies that are appropriate for studies with small sample sizes
- Using more systematic and rigorous research designs for qualitative, quantitative, or mixed methods studies

Peer-reviewed journals provide guidelines for reporting research. In addition, some organizations are developing standards that apply to multiple journals and disciplines. The CONSORT statement, for example, takes an evidence-based approach to improving the quality of reports of randomized trials.[146] This statement is available in several languages and has been endorsed by prominent medical journals such as *The Lancet, Annals of Internal Medicine,* and *Journal of the American Medical Association.* CONSORT is comprised of a checklist and flow diagram to offer researchers a standard way to report trials. The checklist includes items, based on evidence, that researchers need to address in their reports. To supplement this, the flow diagram provides researchers with a clear picture of the progress of research participants in the trial, from the time of randomization to groups until the end of their involvement in the project. The intent is to make reports of the experimental process more clear so that users of the data can evaluate it effectively.

As stated previously in this chapter, ethical therapists continuously examine and develop their knowledge, skills, and attitudes throughout their professional careers. Critically evaluating the methodology we use in massage studies is another key component that is necessary for enhancing the quality of research studies on massage and the evidence to support the use of massage in clinical practice.

IN CONCLUSION

Massage is known for its integration of body, mind, and spirit. Few therapists today continue to wonder if integrating available best evidence into clinical practice undermines the importance of a therapist's ability to feel and use intuition. Understanding the evidence for practice, critical thinking, and being aware of one's own feelings and lessons learned from clinical experience, along with the careful consideration of the unique needs and preferences of clients is the integration of the art and science of massage. One enhances the other. Many brilliant and creative solutions arise from hunches, intuition, and feelings. For effective Outcome-Based Massage™, EBP works best when therapists develop their capacity to think critically, to feel, and to attend to their intuition simultaneously. For these reasons, therapists are wise to develop the ability to find, understand, critically evaluate, and apply research to practice.[10,147-156] They must select research from primary and secondary sources with a critical eye. When consuming that research, they must familiarize themselves with research methodologies from qualitative, quantitative, and mixed methods approaches and consider the appropriateness of the research methods and levels of evidence used to answer the research question(s) asked. Finally, they must be lifelong learners who continue to apply new evidence to their clinical practices throughout their careers.

Practice

Notes: This section contains instructions and clinical cases that demonstrate how to use some of the approaches to using evidence for massage that were introduced in this chapter.

HOW TO READ A RESEARCH ARTICLE CRITICALLY

Clinicians can assess the relative strengths and weaknesses of a research study for themselves by asking good questions while reading research articles.[1,11,12,16,39,68,157,158] Table 3-2 includes some questions that clinicians can use to guide their reading.

The Introduction

Clinicians can glean the purpose of the study from the Introduction. This is also the section in which quantitative studies will outline the hypothesis the study is testing. In reading the Introduction, clinicians can determine if there is a clear clinical problem or gap in the research that provides a sound rationale for the study. In addition, they can examine the clinical population and clinical issues that the study addresses and decide if they are relevant for their own clinical practice.

Research Methods

Whether the study is qualitative or quantitative, the Methodology section often holds the key to the credibility of the study. There are several important issues for novice clinicians to consider. First, clearly defined procedures for interventions, and the training of the clinicians providing interventions, will assist clinicians in determining (a) whether the interventions are relevant for their clinical populations, (b) whether researchers delivered them correctly, and (c) whether they could reproduce them in their own clinical practice. Second, clinicians can consider the characteristics of the study sample and judge whether they are a good representation of the clinical population or if researchers selected them in a manner that may distort the results. Third, clinicians can peruse the research procedures to identify if they are well described, are logical, and enable the researchers to answer the question or purpose they stated in the Introduction. Finally, clinicians need not shy away from the Data Analysis section. Even without advanced statistical knowledge, clinicians can make sense of the basic intent of the analysis and evaluate whether the researchers analyzed the relevant data. For example, did the researchers use some means of determining a correlation between scores if they claim to be identifying relationships? Or, did they use tests that show differences between the scores of groups if they state that they are comparing the performance of those groups?

Research Results

Whether results are in a narrative, tables, charts, or other diagrams, they must be well organized and easily

Table 3-2	**Some Questions to Consider When Reading Research Articles**

Introduction

- ■ Is the clinical issue/problem or gap in the research clearly stated?
- ■ Do the authors provide a complete and up-to-date literature review?
- ■ Did the authors examine other studies that focus on similar designs, populations, and outcomes?
- ■ Does the literature review provide support for clinical problem or research gap?
- ■ Is the problem clinically relevant?
- ■ Do the authors provide a stated model or paradigm that forms the theoretical basis for the study?
- ■ Are the purposes or research questions clearly stated and supported by the literature?
- ■ Does the quantitative study provide an identified hypothesis or expectation?

Methods

Quantitative studies
- ■ Are the participants well described and a good representation of the clinical population?
- ■ Do the authors give sufficient information on the sample and sampling approach for you to determine whether there is any bias in recruiting?
- ■ Do the research methods allow the researcher to address the purpose of the study?
- ■ Does the research design address threats to internal validity such as history, maturation, and testing?
- ■ Are the interventions (independent variables) and anticipated response or outcomes (dependent variables) clearly described so you know what the authors are trying to measure?
- ■ Do the authors describe the measures clearly and provide information on their reliability, validity, and other psychometric properties?
- ■ Is it clear what questions the authors are answering with each measure?
- ■ Do the authors control or deliver the intervention (independent variable) systematically?
- ■ Are the treatment procedures and training of the people delivering the intervention described clearly enough so that you could reproduce them?
- ■ Do the authors describe the research procedures clearly so that you can evaluate whether they are logical and reproducible?
- ■ Do the authors analyze all of the important data?
- ■ Does the data analysis match the design and purposes of the study?

Qualitative studies
- ■ Are the participants and the context in which they live well described?
- ■ Are the researchers qualified to use the methods described in their study? For example, are they experienced interviewers?
- ■ Do the authors clearly describe their sample and sampling approach for you to determine whether there is any bias in recruiting?
- ■ Are the treatment procedures and training of the people delivering the intervention described clearly enough so that you could reproduce them?
- ■ Do the research methods allow the researcher to address the purpose of the study?
- ■ Do the researchers use rigorous and appropriate methods for collecting high-quality data?
- ■ Do the researchers describe techniques they use to increase the quality of their results and interpretations?
- ■ Have the researchers accounted for all of the participants, or did some of them leave the study?
- ■ Does the data analysis match the design and purposes of the study?

Results

- ■ Do the authors clearly report key findings from data analysis or are there missing data?
- ■ Are the findings consistent with the stated purpose and procedures?
- ■ For quantitative studies, do the authors state whether their results are statistically significant or clinically significant?
- ■ Could the researcher have reasonably obtained the reported results using the procedures they outline?
- ■ For quantitative studies, do you believe that changes in outcomes or response (dependent variables) are due to the intervention (independent variable)?
- ■ For qualitative studies, are the results credible, given the question and the methods?

Table 3-2	Some Questions to Consider When Reading Research Articles *(Continued)*
Discussion/conclusions	■ Are the conclusions what you would expect from the authors' stated results and purposes?
	■ In quantitative studies, do the authors state whether the hypothesis was rejected or accepted?
	■ Do the authors relate their findings to existing literature and clinical practice when explaining their conclusions?
	■ Do the authors provide a logical explanation for their results or lack of results?
	■ Do the authors outline limitations of their design and suggested improvements?
	■ Do the authors provide directions for future research suggested by their study?
	■ Would you change the way you practice based on this study?
General questions	■ Is it a peer-reviewed journal with blinded reviewers?
	■ Are the background and experience of the researchers appropriate for the study?
	■ Is there any bias resulting from the agencies that funded the study?

Adapted from Menard MB. *Making Sense of Research: A Guide to Research Literacy for Complementary Practitioners*. Toronto: Curties-Overzet; 2003; Dumholdt E, Malone T. Evaluating research literature: the educated clinician. *Phys Ther*. 1984;65:487-491, with permission.

understood. The main issue for clinicians is whether the researchers could have reasonably obtained their results using the procedures they described. From there, clinicians can locate the positive and negative findings the researchers report. Clinicians are wise to return to the Results section as they read the Discussion and Conclusions to see if the researchers' findings do, in fact, support their conclusions.

Discussion and Conclusions

Armed with a basic analysis of the study, clinicians can review the researchers' conclusions with a critical eye. Do the authors give logical explanations for their findings or lack of findings? Do they use the existing literature to support their arguments? Are there gaps in the logic of their conclusions or limitations to the study design? These are some of the questions clinicians can consider at this point. Finally, they can focus on identifying the relevance of the study's findings for their own clinical practice.

CLINICAL CASES ON EVIDENCE FOR MASSAGE

Clinical Case 3-1 illustrates how clinicians can use evidence when there is a reasonable amount of evidence on the effects of massage techniques for a specific clinical condition. Clinical Case 3-2, on the other hand, demonstrates that sound evidence is not always available and suggests strategies for addressing this situation.

Clinical Case 3-1: *Applying Evidence to Practice for Chronic Low Back Pain (CLBP)*

Patient Profile

A 42-year-old female engineering technologist has been referred by her family physician for massage therapy treatment for nonspecific chronic low back pain. For the previous 2 months, the patient has been experiencing localized, dull constant ache in the low back and general stiffness, which is worse at the end of the day. She spends long hours at her computer at work and at home, sits in her car for a 2-hour daily commute to and from her office, and has little time for exercise. She has been prescribed over-the-counter ibuprofen for pain and is taking no other medications or natural health products.

(Continued)

Initiating EBP

In order to begin to formulate an initial assessment and treatment plan, and prior to the patient's first appointment, the clinician first reviews various articles and texts he has on CLBP and also reflects on the many patients with CLBP that he has already successfully treated over the years, thinking about commonalities and differences. In addition, the clinician develops a clear idea of a good research question he might enter into an online database in order to find the most recent, best available evidence on CLBP and also what kind of key words he might use in a database.

Using the PICO model from Sackett's EBM[11,12] the clinician thinks about the following:

- P, Patient information—For which group do I need information? Adults with nonspecific CLBP.
- I, Intervention—What intervention do I want to use? Massage therapy, exercise.
- C, Comparison—What is the evidence that the proposed intervention produces better or worse results than no intervention? Massage therapy versus no intervention.
- O, Outcomes—What is the effect or outcomes? Pain, sleep, anxiety, depression, mobility.

Sample EBP question: For adults with nonspecific chronic back pain, does massage therapy versus no treatment reduce pain, increase sleep, improve mood, increase mobility?

Finding the Evidence for Practice

Using PubMed (www.Pubmed.com) and other open-access databases, the clinician searches various databases using key words such as "massage" and "low back pain," and the EBP question he has created, to find relevant research online. He finds several peer-reviewed articles[44,45,84] and a recent Cochrane systematic review of the literature.[57]

Understanding the Evidence for Practice

The clinician gained a solid, basic understanding of the various kinds of research methods through course and reading. He understood basic quantitative, qualitative, and mixed methods research methodology, and the relative utility and applicability of the various methods for answering different kinds of questions such as "Is the intervention effective?" (i.e., randomized controlled trials and systematic reviews) and "What is the experience of the patient?" (i.e., qualitative research and case studies). The clinician carefully and critically reads the articles—reading the Abstract, Introduction, Methods, Discussion, and Conclusion sections—looking for whether the information provided is logical, the methods match the question the researchers asked, the procedures and massage protocols are transparent and clear, and the researchers have been very specific and thorough about the probability that the outcomes reported happened by chance or can be attributed to the massage therapy intervention.

Evaluating the Evidence for Practice

Critically reading the articles, the clinician learns that the current best available evidence clearly indicates that massage therapy for CLBP is a safe and moderately effective treatment when compared with no treatment[37,44,45,84] and that is most effective when combined with patient education and exercise.[26] He also understands that there is little consistent evidence in the research on the kinds of massage therapy techniques that are most effective or the frequency and duration of massage therapy treatments. Fortunately, his own clinical experience, and discussions he has with other experienced clinicians in his peer supervision group, helps him to begin to formulate a plan.

Applying Evidence to Practice

Using standardized assessment measures for pain, range of motion, function, and a thorough general health history, including questions on mood, sleep, exercise, and allergies, and a respectful, collaborative discussion with the patient about past experience with massage therapy, patient preferences, and functional goals, the clinician suggests a treatment plan using a variety of massage techniques (relaxation and specific muscle techniques), self-care, and exercise for 1-hour weekly treatment for 6 weeks. He assures the patient that he will be using pre- and post-massage evaluation measures for effectiveness of outcomes throughout the implementation of the treatment plan and will adjust the plan accordingly. He also asks the patient to track her outcomes herself.

After 6 weeks, the patient describes that her CLBP has been reduced (as measured on a Visual Analogue Scale [VAS] for pain), she can bend over and touch her toes without pain and has other improved outcomes as measured on the Roland-Morris disability questionnaire. In addition, she is sleeping better, feeling less stressed in general, and enjoying the exercise program. The clinician discharges the patient and lets her know that she is welcome to come back for additional treatments if her CLBP returns and that she might consider using massage therapy on an as-needed basis, as part of her overall health and wellness maintenance and care.

Clinical Case 3-2: *Applying Evidence to Practice for Osteoarthritis*

Patient Profile

A 65-year-old man who presented to an outpatient clinic with pain in his knees. Other than a history of osteoarthritis (OA) of the hips and knees, he is healthy and active. He does not want to take medication and is hoping that therapy can assist him in managing his pain and returning to his daily walking program.

Initiating EBP

A clinician in an outpatient setting noticed that she had been seeing a growing number of patients with pain secondary to OA of the knees and hips. This patient attracted her attention because she had been treating these patients on a case-by-case basis. She wondered if she could make her intervention for this man with bilateral knee pain more effective by incorporating some new information on OA and the management of that condition.

Finding the Evidence for Practice

The clinician began by consulting her clinical textbooks (secondary sources) to increase her understanding of the pathophysiology and clinical issues related to OA. Then she read about different therapeutic approaches for pain due to OA. She was surprised to see that there were contradicting approaches to using massage techniques for these patients. As a result, she decided to explore the research literature.

Since she was not familiar with database searches, she first found some of the articles cited in the reference sections of the textbooks. These were somewhat dated, and none were specifically on the use of massage techniques for pain due to OA. As a result, she decided to venture into database searches. In preparation for this, the clinician developed a clear idea of a good research question she might enter into an online database in order to find the most recent, best available evidence on OA and also what kind of key words she might use in a database.

Using the PICO model from Sackett's EBM[11,12] the clinician thinks about the following:

P, Patient information—For which group do I need information? Adults with OA

I, Intervention—What intervention do I want to use? Massage therapy, exercise

C, Comparison—What is the evidence that the proposed intervention produces better or worse results than no intervention? Massage therapy versus no intervention

O, Outcomes—What is the effect or outcomes? Pain, mobility

Sample EBP question: For adults with OA, does massage therapy versus no treatment reduce pain and increase mobility?

To perform the search of the literature, she selected PubMed as a starting point since she could access it from her computer at work. Using combinations of the key words "massage," "soft tissue techniques," "osteoarthritis," "pain," "alternative medicine," and "complementary medicine," she found a few articles. She sifted through these until she found a couple current studies on massage interventions for people with OA. She was concerned about the limited amount of research on the effects of massage for people with OA and wondered how much she could base her treatment decisions on such limited evidence.

Understanding the Evidence for Practice

The clinician decided to begin with the randomized controlled trial "Perlman A, Sabina A, Williams A, Njike V, Katz D. Massage therapy for osteoarthritis of the knee. *Arch Intern Med.* 2006;166:2533-2538" because she had heard that randomized controlled trials were more rigorous. She chose not to discard the survey and the case report on a single patient because she felt that they might also have important information to offer.

Before reading the article, she took a look at pointers for reading research in one of her textbooks. She noted that randomized controlled trials were, among other things, intended to test a hypothesis and use randomization and control to decrease the likelihood that the findings were due to chance.

Evaluating the Evidence for Practice

The clinician was relieved to see that the article was only six pages long. On reading the Introduction, she saw that the researchers' purpose was to evaluate the effectiveness of massage therapy for OA. She reviewed the Methods and learned that the study had 66 subjects, men and women aged 35 years and up, who received care for OA on an outpatient basis. She was pleased to see that the researchers had eliminated people who had recent steroid use or confounding health conditions such as fibromyalgia or cancer. This made it easier for her to judge the effects of the massage techniques on the OA pain.

The clinician reviewed the procedures and saw that the researchers had randomly assigned participants into one of two groups. The treatment group received 8 weeks of weekly hour-long

(Continued)

full-body Swedish massage interventions by certified massage clinicians. The control group went on a waiting list to receive the same intervention after the first 8-week period. The study included several measures. The first was the WOMAC (Western Ontario and McMaster Universities Arthritis Index), a questionnaire that assessed pain, stiffness, and functional limitations. The other measures were the VAS for pain, joint range of motion, and time to walk 50 feet.

When she moved on to the Results, the clinician found that all of the participants completed the study and that, at the beginning of the study, both groups were the same on all baseline measures except pain (the treatment group reported higher levels of pain). She had some difficulty following the statistics, but she did figure out that the treatment group showed a statistically significant difference on range of motion, WOMAC score (pain, stiffness, and function), VAS pain reports, and the time to walk 50 feet. After they received the 8-week intervention, the control group showed similar changes.

The researchers, physicians, and physician's assistants attributed the decrease in perceived pain and stiffness and increases in range of motion, perceived functional level, and ability to walk 50 feet to the Swedish massage interventions. The clinician noted that they had selected Swedish massage techniques of petrissage, tapotement, and effleurage because they were commonly used techniques. She was disappointed to see that the authors did not offer any physiological explanation for their findings. Furthermore, they did not give a rationale for delivering a 1-hour full-body massage to individuals who presented with knee pain nor for allowing the clinicians to choose the massage techniques at their discretion. Based on the design of the study, the clinician was not able to identify which of the techniques were contributing to the patients' improvements. She recognized that the fact that it was a randomized controlled trial did not guarantee that it would provide sound evidence for her clinical practice.

Applying Evidence to Practice

The clinician pondered what she had just learned and tried to identify how this information would assist her in treating her patient with OA. She did not want to rely solely on the evidence that she had found because there was scant literature on massage and OA and uncertainty about which techniques were contributing to the positive results. The clinician recalled that EBP consists of evidence, clinical expertise, and patient values. In the light of the limited evidence, she decided to focus on her clinical expertise and her patient's needs. She listed the following guidelines for management from her clinical textbooks and her own clinical experience:

Impairment in Body Structures and Functions for Massage

1. Pain: acute nociceptive and chronic pain
2. Decreased muscle extensibility
3. Muscle spasm
4. Decreased joint mobility and complaints of morning stiffness

5. Increased resting muscle tension
6. Trigger points
7. Postural malalignment
8. Altered sleep patterns secondary to chronic pain
9. Altered body image

Functional Limitations

1. Gait problems
2. Pain with functional activities, such as walking, standing, and transfers
3. Decreased activity tolerance secondary to pain, muscle weakness, and compensatory movements

Possible Clinical Outcomes for Massage Techniques

1. Effleurage
   - Sedation
   - Reduced perception of pain
2. Petrissage
   - Reduced resting muscle tension
   - Sedation
   - Increased muscle extensibility
   - Marginal effect on trigger point reduction resulting in pain reduction
3. Tapotement
   - Not indicated for the key impairments for OA pain
   - Increased alertness
4. Stripping
   - Reduction of trigger point activity resulting in pain reduction
5. Specific compression
   - Reduction of trigger point activity
6. Joint play/mobilization techniques
   - Low-grade techniques for pain reduction resulting in pain reduction
7. Complementary techniques to include
   - Stretching
   - Ice or heat
   - Therapeutic exercise
   - Functional activity

The clinician's first decision based on her clinical experience and her patient's needs was to ensure that her clinical examination addressed the key impairments in body structures and functions for OA to provide her with a better framework for selecting massage and other complementary techniques. The clinician's quandary was that the research on massage and OA did not provide adequate evidence to guide treatment. Nevertheless, she did not want to ignore it all together. She concluded that there was not sufficient justification for her to deliver a 1-hour full-body Swedish massage interventions to a patient with only one or two affected joints and that she could use her treatment time more effectively with a more localized treatment that incorporated other massage and complementary techniques. Based on her clinical knowledge and her patient's needs, the clinician chose petrissage as the most useful of the three techniques for treatment used in the research, since tapotement was primarily for stimulation and effleurage was more useful as an introductory technique. In addition, she chose to add stripping, specific compression, joint play/mobilization techniques, and complementary techniques to the interventions depending on her patients' presenting impairments in body structures and functions. The clinician's final decision was to plan for regular reassessments of her patient's progress so that she could determine the effects of her treatment and modify it appropriately. She also decided to go back to the research literature to get more information on the effects of petrissage, stripping, specific compression, and joint play techniques in general and for patients with OA.

REVIEW SECTION

TAKEAWAYS

1. Evidence supports clinical decision-making, fosters public acceptance of massage therapy, and encourages massage clinicians to be lifelong learners.
2. EBM includes three pillars: best research evidence, clinical expertise, and patient values.
3. Evidence-Based Practice is a key component of Outcome-Based Massage™.
4. Research literacy is the ability to find, understand, evaluate, and apply research evidence to practice.
5. Whether sources are primary or secondary, read all research with a critical eye.
6. Clinicians need to understand the basic concepts of designing and conducting research.
7. Understanding research requires a basic knowledge of quantitative and qualitative research methods.
8. Applying evidence to practice requires the clinicians to reflect on their own assumptions, biases, and knowledge.
9. While the evidence base for massage therapy is growing, certain methodological limitations need to be addressed to produce more rigorous massage studies.
10. Future massage therapy research should include clearly defined massage protocols, larger sample sizes, and more systematic rigor and should focus on effectiveness, dosage, and the nonspecific effects of massage therapy.

Critical Thinking Questions

1. What are (a) the similarities and differences and (b) the advantages and disadvantages of primary and secondary sources?
2. What are examples of research questions that can best be answered using (a) quantitative designs, (b) qualitative designs, and (c) mixed methods designs?
3. How can massage therapy research benefit from (a) quantitative designs, (b) qualitative designs, and (c) mixed methods designs?
4. What are some situations or ways in which randomized controlled trials fail to provide sound evidence for the use of massage techniques?
5. Which of the activities in Key Points 3-4 can you reasonably initiate within the next month? Write out the steps you need to take to implement one of these activities and put that plan into action.
6. In what ways could you incorporate patient values into EBM? Provide examples.
7. What are the advantages and disadvantages of hierarchical and non-hierarchical evidence ranking systems?
8. Why is research literacy important for making evidence-informed decisions?
9. How could clearly defined massage protocols improve massage therapy research?
10. How could biased evidence negatively impact clinical decision-making? Provide examples.

References for Chapter 3 begin on p. 450.

OBM
Clinical
Decision-
Making

Therapeutic
Relationship

Evidence-
Based
Practice

Outcome-
Based
Massage

CHAPTER 4

Client Examination for Outcome-Based Massage™

OBJECTIVES

1. Distinguish between the aims of client examination for medical massage versus wellness massage.
2. Identify the elements of the client interview that are relevant to the assessment of soft tissue dysfunction.
3. Identify the components of the objective examination for massage, including musculoskeletal, psychoneuroimmunologic, multisystem, neurologic, cardiopulmonary, and functional components.
4. Discuss how to perform palpation and identify the impairments that can be assessed using palpation.
5. Describe a variety of nonpalpatory approaches to assessing the impairments that are relevant to massage.

This chapter reviews selected issues for therapists to consider when conducting a client examination prior to using massage techniques. These topics include the focus of an examination for the use of massage techniques, body structures and functions that are relevant to massage, client reports that arise during the course of history-taking that can suggest soft tissue dysfunction, and the use of palpation and nonpalpatory examination techniques. Therapists can integrate this information into a client examination that is appropriate for their scope of practice and their clients' conditions. Numerous clinical texts document client examination techniques for musculoskeletal, neurologic, cardiopulmonary, and psychological conditions for the various health-care professions. Consequently, this chapter assumes that readers will consult those texts for details on the client examination approach and techniques that are within their scope of practice.

Chapter 5 outlines the purpose and steps in the Evaluation Phase of Outcome-Based Massage™ clinical decision-making. To be effective, therapists need to recognize that the focus of the client examination will differ for medical massage and wellness massage as they progress through the Evaluation Phase.

Evidence

FOCUS OF THE CLIENT EXAMINATION FOR OUTCOME-BASED MASSAGE™

Client Examination for Medical Massage

In the International Classification of Functioning, Disability and Health model (see Chapter 1), clinical conditions result in impairments in body structures and functions.[1,2] These impairments are, in turn, associated with limitations in the client's ability to perform activities. There are three primary objectives associated with the treatment of the impairments resulting from clinical conditions:

1. Identification of soft tissue dysfunction related to the client's clinical condition
2. Identification of other primary and secondary impairments that therapists can treat with massage techniques if appropriate
3. Identification of the client's activity and participation limitations that are associated with soft tissue dysfunction

During the client examination, which includes the client interview and objective tests and measures, therapists identify and measure the client's impairments. In particular, they include the assessment of soft tissue function and dysfunction through the use of tests and measures, such as palpation, that directly assess soft tissue.[1-20] In addition, therapists can extend their interpretation of the findings from standard musculoskeletal, neurologic, cardiopulmonary, integumentary, or psychological measures to include an analysis of how soft tissue dysfunction may be contributing to the client's symptoms.

Not all of the impairments identified during the client examination will be suitable for treatment with massage techniques. In addition, therapists' failure to identify impairments may compromise the effectiveness of the treatment that they provide. The task of sorting impairments into those that are or are not amenable to treatment with massage techniques comes later in the treatment-planning process. Nevertheless, it is useful to consider whether a reported or observed impairment may involve soft tissue dysfunction. There are a variety of impairments, outcomes, and examination techniques that are relevant to massage, some of which are summarized in Table 4-1. This chapter discusses the assessment of impairments and activity and participation restrictions in preparation for using massage techniques.

The extent to which therapists will have to modify their customary approach to client examination will depend on how relevant soft tissue dysfunction is to the client's clinical condition. For example, a strong focus on soft tissue dysfunction is less appropriate for the client with a long-standing below-knee amputation and a referral for gait training. By contrast, this focus would be more relevant if the client presents with chronic neck and shoulder pain. Nevertheless, therapists are wise to consider, even briefly, the role of soft tissue dysfunction and potential uses of massage techniques during their client examinations for clients with clinical conditions.

Client Examination for Wellness Massage

The Wellness Interactions Model guides therapists' examinations of clients who request wellness interventions (see Chapter 1). First, therapists determine clients' perceived level of wellness and how this relates to their health status. Table 1-6 outlines some of the domains and relevant outcomes for wellness to assist with this process. There is one primary objective associated with wellness interventions:

1. Identification of the body structures and functions in the client's wellness goals that therapists can treat with massage techniques

Often, clients who have no clinical condition state that they seek only wellness or relaxation present with significant impairments such as anxiety, increased resting muscle tension, postural shortening, muscle weakness, limited range of motion, and pain. If this is the case, therapists may have to explain how these impairments can affect a client's well-being. In this situation, the assessment of impairments and limitations in activity performance may still be relevant. Technically, in a true wellness client, impairments are at grade zero. When this occurs,

Table 4-1	Examples of Outcomes and Examination Techniques for Massage[1-423]

Impairment	Outcome	Tests and Measures
Musculoskeletal		
■ Adhesions/scarring	■ Increased tissue mobility ■ Decreased scarring	■ Visual inspection ■ Measurement of dimensions ■ Palpation ■ Ultrasonography ■ Magnetic resonance imaging ■ Arthroscopy
Impaired connective tissue integrity ■ Fascial restrictions ■ Abnormal connective tissue density ■ Decreased mobility of skin, superficial and deep fascia	■ Separation and lengthening of fascia ■ Promotion of dense connective tissue remodeling ■ Increased connective tissue mobility	■ Visual inspection of static and dynamic postural alignment ■ Palpation ■ Skin mobility
Impaired joint integrity ■ Inflammation of joint capsule or ligaments ■ Restrictions of joint capsule and ligaments	■ Decreased signs of inflammation of joint capsule, tendons, or ligaments ■ Decreased capsular and ligament restrictions ■ Increased joint mobility ■ Increased joint integrity	■ Palpation ■ Selective tissue tension testing ■ Ligament stability tests ■ Magnetic resonance imaging ■ Arthroscopic examination ■ Arthrography ■ Stress radiography ■ Ultrasonography ■ (See measures of impaired joint mobility)
Impaired joint mobility ■ Decreased voluntary range of motion	■ Increased joint mobility ■ Increased voluntary range of motion	■ Universal goniometer ■ Parallelogram goniometer ■ Visual estimation of range of motion ■ Fingers-to-floor distance ■ Schober (tape measure) method ■ Passive accessory motion testing ■ Palpation of end feel on overpressure ■ Two- and three-dimensional computer-aided motion analysis ■ Computerized six–degree of freedom electromagnetic tracker ■ Self-report range of motion measures ■ Cervical range of motion (CROM) instrument ■ Single and double inclinometer ■ Electrogoniometers ■ Palpation meter ■ Arthrometer
Impaired muscle integrity ■ Decreased muscle extensibility ■ Muscle strains and tears	■ Increased muscle extensibility ■ Decreased signs of inflammation and promotion of healing of tendons	■ Muscle extensibility tests ■ Selective tissue tension testing

Table 4-1	Examples of Outcomes and Examination Techniques for Massage[1-423] (*Continued*)	
Impairment	**Outcome**	**Tests and Measures**
Impaired muscle integrity (Continued) ■ Tendinopathies ■ Trigger points	■ Decreased signs of inflammation and promotion of healing of muscle ■ Decreased trigger point activity ■ Increased joint mobility	■ Palpation ■ Trigger point tests: twitch response, presence of taut bands, patterns of pain referral, electromyography ■ Pressure sensitivity testing (pressure algometer) ■ Universal goniometer ■ Isokinetic dynamometer ■ Dynamic ultrasonography
■ Impaired muscle performance (strength, power, endurance)	■ Enhanced muscle performance secondary to the enhancement of muscle extensibility, reduction of pain, reduction of muscle spasm, enhancement of joint mobility, normalization of joint integrity, reduction of trigger point activity, etc. ■ Balance of agonist/antagonist muscle function	■ Manual muscle testing ■ Handheld dynamometer ■ Repeated isotonic motion ■ 1-Repetition maximum test ■ Single-leg hop test ■ Myotome testing ■ Modified sphygmomanometer ■ Pinch meter ■ Self-report measures of perceived exertion ■ Isokinetic dynamometer ■ Isoinertial devices ■ Pedaling devices ■ Electromyogram ■ Kinematic and kinetic gait analysis with two- or three-dimensional computer-assisted motion analysis and force analysis
■ Abnormal resting muscle tension ■ Muscle spasm	■ Decreased muscle spasm ■ Normalized resting muscle tension ■ Increased joint mobility	■ Palpation ■ Tissue compliance meter ■ Continuous electromyography ■ Myotonometer ■ Thermography
■ Postural malalignment	■ Normalized postural alignment ■ Increased postural awareness	■ Visual inspection of static and dynamic posture ■ Functional postural analysis measures ■ Postural grid ■ Posture analysis forms ■ Universal goniometer ■ Plumb line ■ Inclinometer ■ Tape measure ■ Photography ■ Kyphometer ■ Flexible ruler Video image and frame analysis ■ Two- or three-dimensional computer-assisted motion analysis Three-dimensional electrogoniometers ■ X-ray line drawing analysis ■ Force platforms

(*Continued*)

Table 4-1	Examples of Outcomes and Examination Techniques for Massage[1-423] (*Continued*)

Impairment	Outcome	Tests and Measures
■ Postural malalignment (Continued)		■ Functional postural analysis measures ■ Block method
Psychoneuroimmunologic		
■ Stress	■ Systemic sedation ■ Increased perceived relaxation ■ Decreased levels of cortisol, epinephrine, and norepinephrine	■ Interview regarding perceived stress levels and symptoms of stress ■ Self-report stress measures ■ Galvanic skin response ■ Heart rate ■ Blood pressure ■ Finger pressure ■ Blood work: lipid peroxide, prolactin, cortisol, testosterone, glycated hemoglobin ■ Salivary cortisol levels
Multisystem		
■ Pain	■ Pain reduction through primary treatment of dysfunction, e.g., active trigger points ■ Counterirritant analgesia ■ Systemic sedation resulting in decreased perception of pain	*Pain Behavior* ■ Interview regarding location, quality, and behavior of pain ■ Pain diagram (used in conjunction with interview) ■ Self-report measures of pain intensity and affective component ■ Self-report measures of the impact of pain on function ■ Palpation ■ Pressure sensitivity testing (pressure algometer) ■ Selective tissue tension testing ■ Test for allodynia (light touch) ■ Body diagram *Tests and Measures of Pain Syndromes* ■ Neural tissue tension tests ■ Neural provocation tests ■ Trigger point tests: twitch response, presence of taut bands, patterns of pain referral, electromyography ■ Dynamic surface electromyography ■ Electrophysiologic studies ■ Thermography ■ Brain functional magnetic resonance imaging
■ Impaired sensation (secondary to entrapment neuropathy or nerve root compression)	■ Normalized sensation (secondary to the reduction of nerve and nerve root compression due to fascial restrictions and trigger points)	■ Sensory discrimination (kinesthesia, graphesthesia, stereognosis) ■ Vibrometer ■ Dermatome testing: light touch, pin prick, temperature ■ Filament testing (pressure)

Table 4-1	Examples of Outcomes and Examination Techniques for Massage[1-423] (*Continued*)

Impairment	Outcome	Tests and Measures
■ Impaired sensation (secondary to entrapment neuropathy or nerve root compression) (Continued)		■ Palpation of nerve ■ Neurodynamic testing ■ Myotome testing ■ Electrophysiologic (nerve conduction) testing ■ Electroneurotomy ■ Single-frequency vibrometry tests ■ Magnetic resonance imaging
■ Swelling: edema, joint effusion, lymphedema	■ Increased lymphatic return ■ Increased venous return ■ Decreased joint effusion ■ Decreased edema ■ Increased joint integrity ■ Increased joint mobility	■ Visual inspection ■ Volumetric analysis ■ Girth measurements: tape measure, wire, jeweler's ring ■ Palpation ■ Multiple-frequency bioelectrical impedance analysis ■ Magnetic resonance imaging ■ Laser-Doppler flowmetry
Neurologic		
■ Abnormal neuromuscular tone: spasticity, rigidity, clonus	■ Normalized neuromuscular tone ■ Alteration of movement responses through proprioceptive and exteroceptive stimulation techniques ■ Balance of agonist/antagonist muscle function	■ Palpation ■ Graded passive range of motion tests, e.g., Modified Ashworth scale ■ Quick stretch tests ■ Reflexes ■ Pendulum test ■ Isokinetic dynamometer ■ Handheld dynamometer ■ Electromyogram with isokinetic dynamometer ■ Electrophysiologic testing ■ Standardized measures of motor control ■ Standardized measures of self-care ■ Standardized functional measurements
Cardiopulmonary		
■ Impaired airway	■ Increased respiration/gaseous exchange ■ Increased airway clearance/mobilization of secretions ■ Decreased dyspnea	■ Interview regarding frequency and effectiveness of cough ■ Visual inspection of effectiveness of cough ■ Visual inspection of quality and quantity of sputum ■ Visual inspection and palpation of respiration rate and pattern ■ Auscultation of breath sounds ■ Pulse oximetry ■ Self-report dyspnea rating scales ■ Arterial blood gases ■ Pulmonary function tests ■ Self-report measures of quality of life ■ Standardized measures of self-care

(*Continued*)

Table 4-1	Examples of Outcomes and Examination Techniques for Massage[1-423] (*Continued*)

Impairment	Outcome	Tests and Measures
■ Dyspnea	■ Decreased dyspnea due to increased airway clearance ■ Decreased dyspnea due to increased perceived relaxation	■ Visual inspection of respiratory pattern and effort of breathing ■ Self-report perceived exertion and dyspnea rating scales ■ Self-report measures of outcome of dyspnea ■ Six-minute walk test of functional exercise capacity ■ Respiration rate ■ Oxygen saturation ■ Arterial blood gases ■ Capnography
■ Impaired rib cage mobility (other than bony abnormality)	■ Increased rib cage mobility ■ Increased muscle extensibility ■ Increased ventilation	■ Visual inspection and palpation of lateral costal, sternal, and diaphragmatic motion during respiration ■ Palpation of rib cage motion during respiration ■ Changes in girth of rib cage during respiration
Functional		
■ Self-care ■ Health-related quality of life	■ Increased independence in self-care activities ■ Enhanced health-related quality of life	■ Standardized measures of self-care, e.g., Barthel Index ■ Standardized measures of health-related quality of life, e.g., Medical Outcomes Survey—Short Form-36 (MOS SF-36)

therapists still assesses body structures and functions to determine which are amenable to optimized function or to determine when prevention of a potential impairment may be a desired outcome. Furthermore, this examination must also identify the client's current wellness behaviors and any barriers and facilitators to wellness such as social attitudes, available wellness services, education, and the individual's financial status.

PERFORMING THE CLIENT EXAMINATION

The client examination consists of the subjective examination and the objective examination. The subjective examination, also known as the client history or the client interview, refers to the client's report of various aspects of his condition such as his medical history, chief complaint, chronology of symptoms, level of function, preferences, and treatment goals. By contrast, the objective examination, also called the physical examination, consists of objective tests and measures performed by the therapist.

Performing the Subjective Examination

Numerous clinical texts detail the nuances of interviewing or history-taking for various health-care professions. During the course of taking the standard client history, therapists can integrate questions to identify **soft tissue dysfunction**. Examples of client-reported history that suggest soft tissue dysfunction may include[4,6,7,9,21,21-33]

■ Reports of any long-standing musculoskeletal condition that may result in chronic soft tissue tightening
■ A history of prolonged infection near the affected region
■ Reports of a change in pain over time from an initially specific, localized pain to a more diffuse, generalized pain
■ A history of chronic pain
■ A history of pain combined with anxiety or stress or emotional trauma
■ Idiopathic pain with a complex history of multiple injuries
■ Multiple surgeries that might predispose the client to scarring
■ A history of multiple conflicting assessments and ineffective treatments from multiple providers

- Postural changes over time
- A history of symptom relief from massage or stretching
- The client uses words such as "tight," "hard," or "wired" to describe his/her symptoms
- A history of bony changes such as a leg length discrepancy, scoliosis, or dental malocclusion

Performing the Objective Examination

The order and content of the objective examination will vary with the client's presenting issue and the purpose of treatment (medical massage or wellness massage). In addition, therapists develop their own approach to performing the physical examination. This chapter outlines the tests and measures in an order that is appropriate for the associated impairment. For example, the musculoskeletal examination begins with an assessment of posture before the client is on the treatment table. Therapists may use their experience and discretion in determining the order in which they perform the objective examination.

Using Palpation in Client Examination

This chapter contains a separate section on palpation since skilled **palpation** is an art, a required component of many client examination techniques, and a prerequisite skill for the effective execution of all massage techniques.[3-36] Therapists can use palpation to assess and reassess the client's impairments throughout the client examination and treatment process. Furthermore, continuous palpation throughout the application of massage techniques allows therapists to use the client's response to the techniques to guide them in modifying the intervention as it proceeds.

There are many ways to perform palpation that are determined by the purpose of palpation, the object of palpation, the client's condition, and the therapist's skill level.[3-36] Regardless of how therapists are performing the palpation, all forms of palpation share common characteristics. During palpation, therapists attempt to identify subtle characteristics of the selected structure and distinguish between normal and abnormal findings. Since palpation is comparative in nature, it involves movement of the contact surface or of therapists' attention. Although the emphasis of this chapter is on client examination, the comments on palpation are also relevant to re-examination and treatment.

Basic Principles of Palpation

Palpation is moving inquiry that requires attention and concentration, discrimination, identification, inquiry, and intention.[3-36] As therapists perform palpation, they seek answers to a variety of questions that inform effective palpation such as the following: What is this structure or quality? How does this finding differ from other structures or qualities that I have palpated? How does this finding relate to the client's history? How does this structure reflect the client's demonstrated and reported function? After extensive practice, therapists can easily move from conscious questioning to more effective palpation.

Objects of Palpation

Therapists identify the client's impairments in body structures and functions, such as those listed below, through the palpation of specific **objects of palpation**[3-36]:

- Abnormal connective tissue density
- Abnormal levels of resting muscle tension
- Abnormal neuromuscular tone
- Adhesions
- Impaired extensibility of contractile and noncontractile tissues
- Impaired integrity of contractile and noncontractile tissues
- Decreased rib cage mobility
- Fascial restrictions
- Muscle spasm
- Pain
- Scarring
- Swelling: edema, effusion, lymphedema
- Trigger points

These objects of palpation are the focus of therapists' attention during palpation. They are not necessarily physical structures; instead, they may be a characteristic, such as temperature, or a phenomenon, such as resistance to movement. The objects of palpation described in this chapter are anatomical structures, temperature, contour and bulk, texture and consistency, fluid status, body rhythms, tremors and fasciculations, and vibration.

The nature of the object of palpation influences therapists' choice of method of palpation. For example, it is difficult to palpate skin temperature using deep thumb pressure. Similarly, it is less effective to palpate tissue resistance to barriers in the superficial fascia using a fast scanning palmar contact. Consequently, therapists should specify the object(s) of their inquiry prior to beginning palpation and select a suitable palpation technique.

Contact Surfaces Used for Palpation

Therapists' hands must be supple and relaxed at all times during palpation.[3-36] Since therapists' dominant hands are generally more sensitive, they should use that hand for palpating very subtle structures. As they perform palpation, they may use their hands to do similar things such as comparing left and right sides. Conversely, their hands may perform different tasks, as is the case when one hand moves a body segment and the other evaluates the resulting motion.

Therapists can use virtually any surface to palpate: fingers and thumbs, the whole palmar surface, the thenar and hypothenar eminences, or the back of their hands.[3-36] They should select a surface that relates to the particular aim of palpation. For example, the finger and thumb tips and pads have the greatest discriminatory ability and are best for palpating subtle objects. On the other hand, grasping forms of palpation may use the index and thumb together like a pincer or the whole hand.

Force of Palpation

As with massage techniques, therapists should match the force they apply to the tissues during palpation to the task at hand.[3-36] This force can vary in rate, pressure, direction, and duration.

Rate of Palpation

Therapists can use different rates of palpation to obtain different types of information.[3-36] A scanning or stroking type of palpation moves relatively quickly over a large area. Consequently, therapists use this when they want to collect information from a wide area. An example of this would be comparing bilateral tissue contours or assessing resting muscle tension of the client's entire back. A **scanning, or stroking, palpation** works best when static palpation would distort findings. By contrast, **static palpation** involves no movement of the palpating hand and is best suited for palpating moving phenomena such as pulse or respiratory rhythm.

Pressure of Palpation

Lack of concentration, too much pressure, and too much movement are among the other common errors of palpation. Therapists should use the minimum pressure required to contact the chosen tissue or structure.[3-36] In doing so, they should proceed from exerting a lighter force to a greater force, which results in the palpation of superficial tissue layers prior to deeper layers. Therapists do not need to apply pressure slowly. Nevertheless, their touch should be firm, not tentative or abrupt, regardless of the rate at which they are applying pressure. There will be occasions when therapists need to apply a considerable amount of compression to the client's tissues. In such situations, therapists need to gauge how the client's compressed tissues are deforming under the controlled application of their body weight. This type of palpation might be better termed "proprioceptive" palpation, as opposed to "manual" palpation, because therapists use their entire body to sense the movement of tissues.

Direction of Palpation

Therapists can apply the **force of palpation** as a **shearing** force perpendicular to or parallel to the client's tissues.[3-36] Different directions of force result in different responses of the client's tissues.

When the force of palpation is perpendicular to the client's tissues, it produces a vertical compression. This form of palpation has several uses. For example, therapists can use perpendicular forces to palpate a pulse or pitting edema. They can also use them when measuring the sensitivity of a trigger point.

Tension along a tissue layer and **drag** occur when therapists apply the force of palpation in a direction that is parallel to the client's tissues (horizontal force).[3-36] Drag is a term used to describe both the therapist's palpation and the tissue layer's resistance to lengthening in response to that force. External and internal factors can result in an increase or decrease of the amount of drag that occurs during palpation. External factors include the presence of moisture on the skin, which can increase or decrease drag, and the presence of skin oil or lubricant, which can generally decrease it. Internal factors include underlying tissue changes. The assessment of drag is an integral part of therapists' examination of connective tissues such as skin and fascia.

Therapists can also use palpation to exert a shearing force on the client's tissues.[3-36] Shear involves adjacent, parallel tissue layers sliding over one another and displacing adjacent laminar elements. When drag is applied to a specific tissue layer, shear occurs between that layer and the layer that is adjacent and parallel to it. Therapists can use shearing forces, in combination with compression, when assessing muscle tone and bulk.

In practice, any palpation technique or massage technique combines elements of compression, drag, and shear.[3-36] In general, the direction of the force that therapists apply during the palpation of a particular tissue is often the same as the direction that they would use to treat that tissue.

Duration of Palpation

Although therapists should not hurry palpation, their palpation of most structures and characteristics need not take longer than a few seconds.[3-36] Indeed, the effects of prolonged palpation on tissues can confound the client examination. This occurs because maintaining a position or pressure can result in the adaptation of tissue receptors in the therapists' hands. In addition, it can also produce changes in the client's tissues. For example, when palpating a myofascial trigger point located in a deep layer, sustained pressure would have the same effect as the specific compression technique used for treatment of this condition. The palpation of barriers in connective tissue is an exception to this rule because it requires longer than a minute as a result of the biochemical nature of the tissue. In this situation, palpation merges into treatment.

Integration of Information from Other Senses

Effective palpation is the result of appropriate interplay of therapists' senses.[3-36] For example, therapists' vision may be useful in corroborating some of the findings of palpation such as posttraumatic swelling. At the same time, visual inspection may interfere with therapists' ability to palpate subtler objects such as the small intrinsic movements of connective tissue under traction.

Client's Response to Palpation

Therapists must observe and interpret the different verbal and physiologic responses that palpation can evoke in a client.[3-36] **Local reflex signs** include discoloration of the skin (blanching or flushing) or more general autonomic responses such as sweating and nausea. Neuromuscular responses include twitching, spasm, or clonus. Clients may indicate that they are experiencing pain by grimacing, vocalizing, or making sudden involuntary movements.

Therapists must remember that pain is a common response to palpation, which they need to respect and observe carefully. Therapists can also quantify pain with, for example, an 11-point rating scale for grading tenderness or a visual analog scale (VAS). The various types of pain responses differ in their significance and reliability. Tenderness to deep palpation, for example, is an unreliable finding since tenderness can be referred from other sites. Pain on percussion may have specific meaning for certain musculoskeletal conditions. Finally, during palpation, therapists need to be aware that palpation itself can sometimes produce negative or positive changes in the tissues that they are palpating.

Documentation of the Client Examination

Repeated client re-examination, close monitoring of the client's response to treatment, and ongoing assessment of the client's progress toward the stated outcomes are cornerstones of Outcome-Based Massage™. Documentation of the client examination and treatment are, therefore, critical components of Outcome-Based Massage™. There are a variety of approaches to the documentation of the findings of the client examination including SOAP, ASTER, and Focus Charting. In addition, whether the documentation is written or electronic, there are a variety of issues to consider, such as client confidentiality and right to access their medical records, legal and regulatory requirements for documentation, and facility-specific guidelines for timing, frequency, and comprehensiveness.[37] For these reasons, therapists should consult books and other information on the requirements and procedures for documentation that are pertinent to their treatment settings.

MUSCULOSKELETAL EXAMINATION

Posture

Definitions and Etiology

Posture

Posture is the positioning and alignment of the skeleton and associated soft tissues in relation to gravity, the body's center of mass and base of support.[6,21,25-27,38-53]

Postural Malalignment

Postural malalignment is abnormal joint alignment or deformity within a bone.[6,21,25-27,38-53] Since all tissue growth and repair can be influenced by mechanical loading and body posture, postural malalignment can contribute to the development of neurovascular and musculoskeletal dysfunction. This contribution can be direct or as a result of the compensatory motions or postures that can accompany postural malalignment. For example, chronic placement of the head anterior to the body's center of gravity is a common postural malalignment that is associated with neurologic and musculoskeletal dysfunction.

Overview of Examination Techniques

There are a variety of approaches to assessing posture.[6,21,25-27,38-53,54-60] Soft tissues exert a stress on bony structures; consequently, pathologic changes in the tension of muscles and connective tissue can affect postural alignment. The purpose of the postural analysis is, therefore, to document alignment of both soft tissue and bony structure. This information provides objective data that therapists can use to corroborate or refute findings from the client's functional limitations and other examination techniques. This assists in the identification of appropriate outcomes.

Visual inspection of the symmetry of bony landmarks, muscle contours, and other tissues with the client in static postures, such as sitting, standing, or lying, is the common clinical approach to assessing postural alignment.[6,21,25-27,38-53] Visual inspection of dynamic posture is of greater importance in the assessment of fascial restrictions. The technique of visual inspection can be refined through the use of postural grids, photography, and various posture analysis forms such as the Portland State University Posture Analysis Form. In addition, therapists can obtain information on the client's postural awareness during the client interview.

Goniometry, plumb lines, inclinometers, tape measures, and video image and frame analysis are among the tools that are available for quantifying postural malalignment.[6,21,25-27,38-53] For example, sagittal plane postural alignment of the head and shoulder in relation to the lateral malleolus can be measured using a carpenter's tri-square with a line level attached to the horizontal arm or a goniometer with a line level attached to the horizontal arm.

More sophisticated measures of postural alignment include three-dimensional electrogoniometers, such as the Metrecom Skeletal Analysis System, a force platform; X-ray line drawing analysis for sagittal plane spinal displacement; and visual estimation of lumbar lordosis from radiographs (which can be inaccurate and unreliable).[6,21,25-27,38-53] Dynamic postural analysis can be performed using three-dimensional computer-assisted motion analysis, with or without electromyography (EMG). Finally, postural alignment during functional activity can be assessed using measures such as the Ovako Working Analysis System.

Joint Integrity

Definitions and Etiology

Joint Integrity

Joint integrity is the extent to which a joint conforms to the expected anatomical and biomechanical norms.[38,39,61-83]

Capsular Restrictions

Capsular restriction is anatomical or pathological shortening of the joint capsule.[38,39,61-83] Capsular restrictions occur as a result of a variety of clinical conditions such as disuse, immobility, venous congestion, and diabetes. "Frozen shoulder" or adhesive capsulitis, for example, is a common capsular lesion seen in rehabilitation. This adherence of the shoulder capsule to the humeral head may be the consequence of altered supporting structures of and around the shoulder or autoimmune, endocrine, or other systemic diseases.

Capsular Laxity

Capsular laxity is anatomical or pathological lengthening of the joint capsule.[38,39,61-83] For example, global (anterior, inferior, and posterior) excessive laxity of the glenohumeral joint capsule leads to multidirectional instability of the shoulder.

Capsulitis and Synovitis

Capsulitis and synovitis describe inflammation of the synovium and the joint capsule and associated internal ligaments.[38,39,61-83] This can be associated with capsular distention secondary to increased levels of fluid in the joint, for example, as in rheumatoid arthritis.

Ligament Insufficiency

Ligament insufficiency is anatomical or pathological shortening of the capsular ligament.[38,39,61-83] For example, anterior capsular ligament length insufficiency in the glenohumeral joint can contribute to altered glenohumeral joint mechanics and shoulder pain.

Ligament Laxity

Ligament laxity is anatomical or pathological lengthening of the capsular ligament.[38,39,61-83] Anterior cruciate ligament laxity, for example, is a common cause of knee instability, pain, and functional limitations in athletes.

Nonmyofascial Trigger Points

A nonmyofascial trigger point is a hyperirritable spot in scars, fascia, periosteum, ligaments, and joint capsules that is associated with a hypersensitive palpable nodule in a taut band.[21,34,38-40,61-84]

Overview of Examination Techniques

There are a variety of approaches to assessing joint integrity.[21,34,38-40,61-84,85-88] Cyriax[78] defined "capsular patterns," which are clinical signs of capsular lesions that are demonstrated during selective tissue tension testing that are supported by recent research. Selective tissue tension testing involves the performance of a specific sequence of active range of motion, passive range of motion, and resisted isometric testing of the joint in question, during which therapists observe sequences of pain and limitations of motion. Therapists can identify clinical conditions with high levels of reliability (kappa = 0.875) using selective tissue tension testing.

The integrity of ligaments is best assessed clinically using a variety of static stability tests that demonstrate the stability of the ligaments of selected joints.[21,34,38-40,61-84] An example of these tests is the Lachman test of knee collateral ligament stability. Laboratory or instrumented tests of impaired joint integrity include magnetic resonance imaging (MRI), arthroscopic examination, arthrography, stress radiography, and ultrasonography.

Joint Mobility

Definitions and Etiology

Joint Range of Motion

Joint range of motion is the capacity of the joint to move within the anatomic or physiologic range of motion that is available at that joint based on its arthrokinematics and the ability of the periarticular connective tissue to deform.[38,89-130] Range of motion reflects the function of the contractile, nervous, inert, and bony tissues and the client's willingness to perform a movement.

Impaired joint mobility can be the result of numerous primary impairments, such as impaired muscle extensibility, altered muscle tone, capsular restriction or inflammation, tendinopathy, neurologic deficit, pain, or bony deformity.[38,89-130]

Passive Range of Motion

Passive range of motion is the amount of joint motion available when an examiner moves a joint through its anatomic or physiologic range, without assistance from the client, while the client is relaxed.[38,89-130]

Active Range of Motion

Active range of motion is the amount of joint motion that can be achieved by the client during the performance of unassisted voluntary joint motion.[38,89-130]

Accessory Joint Motion

Accessory joint motion is the range of motion within synovial and secondary cartilaginous joints that is not under voluntary control. Consequently, therapists can only obtain this measure passively.[38,89-130] These motions, also known as joint play movements, are essential for full and pain-free active range of motion.

End Feel

End feel is the quality of motion or sensation that therapists "feel" in the joint during overpressure at the end of passive range of motion.[38,89-130]

Overview of Examination Techniques

There are a variety of approaches to assessing joint mobility.[38,89-139] Goniometry is the established approach to measuring joint range of motion for peripheral joints, and the universal goniometer is accurate and efficient. Numerous studies have documented high degrees of intrarater reliability using intra-class correlations (ICCs of 0.88 to 0.93) and relatively lower levels of interrater reliability (ICCs of 0.80 to 0.85) for the universal goniometric measurements of a variety of upper and lower extremity joints by novice and experienced therapists. Less sophisticated techniques for range of motion testing include visual estimation of range of motion. The findings from this technique may be more variable for many peripheral joints, regardless of therapists' level of experience, but more reliable in joints, such as the forefoot, that are more difficult to measure with goniometry. Two- and three-dimensional computer-aided motion analyses can provide information on the range of motion of multiple joints in static and dynamic postures, which can be more reliable than goniometry, particularly in complex joints. Therapists have used a variety of tools for the measurement of the range of motion of the cervical and lumbar spine and pelvis.[38,89-130] There are simplistic measures of spinal range of motion that involve the measurement of various distances using a tape measure. The use of measured distances of the client's fingers to the floor in the testing of spinal range of motion may be the least reproducible approach and also reflects the range of motion of joints other than the spine. Another approach, the Schober method of using a tape measure placed on spinal landmarks to evaluate the motion of the spine, may be associated with considerable error. Pelvic range of motion can be difficult to measure. Consequently, therapists can use devices such as the palpation meter, a caliper–inclinometer combination, or basic inclinometry to facilitate accurate measurement.

Therapists measure accessory, or joint play, movements with the joint in the loose-packed position.[155,246-289] One technique described by Kaltenborn involves the palpation of glide and traction/compression ranges of motion during passive movements and the use of a 6-point grading system as follows: hypomobile (0-2), normal (3), or hypermobile (4-6). Accessory movement testing has shown poor to fair intrarater ($r = 0.75$) and interrater ($r = 0.45$) reliability. Laboratory or instrumented measures of accessory joint motion are now available. For example, therapists use arthrometers to measure anterior-posterior translation (glide) in the knee joint.

The quality of movement is as important as the quantity of range that is available.[38,89-130] Therefore, therapists should assess the quality of the movement throughout the range and at the end of the range as they perform passive range of motion. In doing so, they should apply overpressure at the end of the range and note whether the "end feel" is normal (bone-to-bone, soft tissue approximation, or tissue stretch) or abnormal (muscle spasm, hard capsular, soft capsular, bone-to-bone, empty, or springy block) for that joint.

Muscle Integrity

Definitions and Etiology

Muscle Integrity
Muscle integrity is the extent to which a muscle conforms to the expected anatomical and biomechanical norms.[21,25-27,38,140-156]

Muscle Extensibility
Muscle extensibility is the ability of the muscle and fascia to deform during the movement of a joint through its anatomical range.[21,25-27,38,140-156]

Contracture
Contracture is a permanent muscular shortening due to a variety of physiologic changes in muscle such as fibrosis or loss of muscular balance.[21,25-27,38,140-156] Physiologic contractures are permanent muscular contractions or shortening that does not involve motor activity. The shortening of involved muscles in Volkman ischemic contracture, for example, involves prolonged ischemia, myonecrosis, proliferation of fibroblasts, scar contraction, and formation of myotendinous adhesions. Muscle contractures may be associated with muscle imbalances that result from neurologic disorders such as the presence of hypertonia in cerebellar lesions. They can also be associated with atrophy and fibrosis, as is the case in Duchenne muscular dystrophy in which biopsies of contractures in selected muscles show a combination of muscle fiber atrophy with perimysial and endomysial fibrosis.

Muscle Strain or Tear
Muscle strain or tear is a lesion or inflammation of muscle fibers that can occur in response to trauma.[21,25-27,38,140-156]

Tendinitis
Tendinitis is inflammation of the peritendinous tissues that can occur in response to repetitive mechanical trauma.[21,25-27,38,140-156]

Tendinosis
Unlike tendinitis, which is an inflammatory condition, tendinosis refers to common overuse tendon conditions with a histopathology consistent with noninflammatory, degenerative conditions of unknown etiology.[21,25-27,38,140-156]

Myofascial Trigger Point
A myofascial trigger point is a hyperirritable spot in skeletal muscle that is associated with a hypersensitive palpable nodule in a taut band.[21-25,34]

- Active trigger points are painful even when no one palpates them.[21-25,34]
- Latent trigger points are not painful in and of themselves unless therapists palpate them.[21-25,34]

Overview of Examination Techniques
There are a variety of approaches to assessing muscle integrity.[21-25,34,157-166] Impaired muscle extensibility is measured clinically using stretch tests, defined as passive range of motion tests in which the muscle in question is placed in a stretched position, that have been defined for the given muscle group. Extensibility of the hamstring muscles, for example, can be measured using goniometric measures of passive knee extension with the pelvis stabilized; this test can be reliable ($r = 0.99$) and performed with little associated pelvic motion. The Sit-and-Reach Test is another commonly used measure of hamstring extensibility. It is less accurate than the measurement of hip joint angle in this test position because the Sit-and-Reach Test also appears to reflect spinal mobility and anthropometric factors. Laboratory or instrumented measures of muscle extensibility include the use of force/angle data from isokinetic dynamometers, such as the KinCom to measure muscle extensibility with high levels of reliability (ICC = 0.81 to 0.95) for selected muscle groups, and dynamic ultrasonography.

Tendinopathies, muscle strains, and muscle tears are assessed using the methods of selective tissue tension testing outlined earlier in this chapter.[21-25,34,157-164]

In this case, therapists are looking for a relatively strong contraction of the muscle, with pain on contraction of the muscle (active movement in one direction), pain on stretch of the muscle (passive movement in the opposite direction), pain on isometric movement, and a possible decrease in range of motion if there is a gross hematoma. The distinction between tendinous and muscular lesions depends on the location of pain during testing and the results of palpation of tenderness. Therapists can use MRI when they require additional diagnostic information.

Impaired muscle integrity is also associated with impaired muscle performance and pain that other sections describe in detail.[21-25,34,157-164]

Muscle Performance

Definitions and Etiology

Muscle Performance

Muscle performance is the muscle's capacity to do work based on its length, tension, and velocity.[21,25-27,38,65-77,79-84,90,91,109,156,167-192] Neurologic stimulus; fuel storage; fuel delivery; and balance, timing, and sequencing of muscle contraction all influence integrated muscle performance.

Muscle Strength

Muscle strength is the force or torque produced by a muscle or group of muscles to overcome a resistance during a maximum voluntary contraction.[21,25-27,38,65-77,79-84,90,91,109,156,167-192]

Muscle Power

Muscle power is the work produced by a muscle per unit of time (strength × speed).[21,25-27,38,65-77,79-84,90,91,109,156,167-192]

Muscle Endurance

Muscle endurance is the muscle's ability to contract, or maintain torque, over a number of contractions or a period of time.[21,25-27,38,65-77,79-84,90,91,109,156,167-192] Conversely, fatigue is a muscle's inability to maintain torque or the loss of power over time.

Because of the multiple inputs required for integrated muscle performance, impaired muscle performance can be the result of adhesions, impaired muscle integrity, abnormal neuromuscular tone, impaired joint mobility, impaired joint integrity, swelling, impaired connective tissue integrity, pain, and postural malalignment, which are described in detail in other sections of this chapter.[21,25-27,38,65-77,79-84,90,91,109,156,167-192] This chapter does not describe muscle weakness, a primary cause of impaired

muscular performance, because massage techniques do not have a direct effect on increasing muscle strength.

Overview of Examination Techniques

There are a variety of approaches to assessing muscle performance.[21,25-27,38,65-77,79-84,90,91,109,156,167-195] Muscle strength can be measured isometrically, isotonically, and isokinetically. The graded manual muscle test is a long-standing clinical approach to isotonic strength testing that has questionable interrater reliability but good intrarater reliability ($r = 0.88$). Other options for isotonic testing include the one-repetition maximum test. Handheld dynamometers are an accurate and reliable means of measuring isometric muscle strength and have become the mainstay of clinical practice. Therapists typically perform hand strength testing with the grip strength dynamometer, the modified sphygmomanometer, and the pinch meter. They can measure isokinetic strength in a variety of ways using isokinetic dynamometers such as peak torque, mean peak torque, and force–frequency relationship. Muscle power is described in terms of peak power, mean power, instantaneous power, and torque–velocity relationships achieved through isokinetic testing. Isoinertial devices produce constant resistance to a movement that enables therapists to measure isoinertial performance, particularly in trunk muscle testing.

Muscle endurance can be assessed using simple clinical measures, such as the number of repetitions performed, the single-leg hopping test, or more complex tests that include endurance time to limit of endurance and mean power frequency derived from an electromyogram.[21,25-27,38,65-77,79-84,90,91,109,156,167-192] The client's perceived rate of exertion can be measured using rate of perceived effort tests, such as the Borg Perceived Effort Test, and correlated with objective measures of fatigue.

Clients with certain clinical conditions may require modifications to the usual muscle performance testing measures.[21,25-27,38,65-77,79-84,90,91,109,156,167-192] The modified sphygmomanometer is a reliable means (ICCs for interrater reliability of up to 0.85) of assessing isometric strength, particularly in geriatric clients and those with rheumatoid arthritis. Therapists can also use pedaling activities to measure mechanical work and joint power generation patterns in clients who have had cerebrovascular accidents (CVAs).

Therapists can also assess the impact of an individual's muscle performance on his ability to perform functional tasks.[21,25-27,38,65-77,79-84,90,91,109,156,167-192] The Sit-to-Stand Test, for example, shows the impact of lower extremity strength on the client's ability to perform a functional transfer. The functional capacity evaluations used in occupational medicine measure a client's ability to perform work-related tasks such as pulling, lifting, carrying, and handling weights that reflect muscle performance. Kinematic and kinetic gait analysis using two- or three-dimensional computer-assisted motion analysis and force analysis show the impact of muscle performance on gait.

Resting Muscle Tension

Definitions and Etiology

Resting Muscle Tension

Resting muscle tension is the firmness to palpation at rest observed in muscles with normal innervation or the perceived texture of muscle during palpation.[21-25,30,34,38,101,183-192,196-209] The section "Scientific Basis of Soft Tissue Examination" offers a more detailed definition of resting muscle tension.

Muscle Spasm

Muscle spasm is an involuntary contraction of a muscle that results in increased muscular tension and shortness that cannot be released voluntarily.[21-25,30,34,38,183-192,196-205] Research suggests that increased excitability of alpha-motor neuron pools contributes to the occurrence of muscle spasm.

Overview of Examination Techniques

There are a variety of approaches to assessing resting muscle tension and muscle spasm.[21-25,30,34,38,183-192,196-205,210-214] Nevertheless, research suggests that palpation is still an important method for measuring these. The other tests for resting muscle tension are the tissue compliance meter (static measure of consistency of soft tissue), badismography, continuous EMG, the myotonometer (dynamic measure), and thermography.

Adhesions and Scarring

Definitions and Etiology

Scar

A scar is the fibrous tissue that replaces normal tissues that a burn, wound, surgery, radiation, or disease has destroyed.[38]

Adhesions

As with scars, adhesions result from the replacement of normal tissue with connective tissue after a burn, wound, surgery, radiation, or disease destroys the original tissues.[3-36,38] Adhesions may be fibrous or fibrinous. Fibrinous adhesions have fine bands of fibrin that form as a result of an exudate of plasma or lymph or an extravasation of blood. Fibrous adhesions come from the organization of fibrinous adhesions into fibrous strands. Unlike scarring, adhesions are characterized by a loss of mobility of tissues that normally glide or move in relation to each other. Adhesions can contribute to impaired muscle, joint, and connective tissue integrity, which are described in detail in other sections of this chapter.

Overview of Examination Techniques

There are a variety of approaches to assessing adhesions and scarring.[3-36] Adhesions are of greater clinical significance than scars since they are associated with impaired tissue mobility. The measurement of adhesions through observation and palpation is, unfortunately, less accurate than that of scars. Therapists can confirm the presence of scar through visual inspection and by objective measurements of dimensions. Ultrasonography, MRI, and arthroscopy are more accurate, although clinically less practical, approaches.

Connective Tissue Integrity

Definitions and Etiology

Fascial Restrictions

Fascial restrictions are the adhesion of one fascial layer to another with the associated development of elasto-collagenous cross-links and loss of fluid consistency of fascial ground substance.[23,38,61,215-232] Fascial restrictions may be caused by trauma, adhesion, inflammatory or infectious processes, osseous restrictions, chronic fascial compartment syndromes, neurologic or circulatory compression syndromes, or postural malalignment such as leg length discrepancy, pelvic malalignment, and dental malocclusion. Finally, fascial restrictions may cause pain, impaired motion, and general dysfunction throughout the body. These symptoms may occur at a distance from the restriction and may result in impaired cellular metabolism, nutrition, elimination, respiration, or lymphatic flow.

Abnormal Connective Tissue Density

Abnormal connective tissue density is irregular connective tissue remodeling that occurs during the consolidation and maturation stages of connective tissue healing.[23,38,61,215-232] This can be associated with chronic orthopedic injuries, including strains, fractures, and repetitive strain injuries, such as tendinosis, tenosynovitis, bursitis, and plantar fasciitis, in which there is ongoing microtrauma, low-grade inflammation, and tissue remodeling.

Overview of Examination Techniques

There are a variety of approaches to assessing connective tissue integrity.[3-36,61,217-232] Techniques for evaluating connective tissue impairments include visual inspection of the client's static and dynamic postural alignment; palpation of tissue, skin mobility, and vasomotor response. Therapists need to evaluate the client's entire body, regardless of the client's complaint, because imbalances in the fascial system can have significant effects at locations other than the site of the restriction.

PSYCHONEUROIMMUNOLOGIC EXAMINATION

Stress

Definitions and Etiology

Chronic Stress

Chronic stress is a prolonged and heightened state of arousal that has negative physiologic and psychological consequences.[157-164,196,233-264] Chronic stress responses occur over the cognitive, physiologic, affective, or behavioral domains and may have consequences, such as impaired cognitive function, depression, anxiety, muscle tension, and impaired social functioning.

Stress Response

Stress response is the individual's cognitive, physiologic, affective, or behavioral response to the stressor or stress-provoking situation.[157-164,196,233-264]

Cognitive Transactional Model of Stress

The **Cognitive Transactional Model of Stress** views stress as the condition that results when a person's interactions with his environment leads him to perceive a discrepancy, whether real or not, between the demands of the situation and the resources of his biological, psychological, or social systems.[157-164,196,233-264]

Physiologic Model of Stress

Hans Selye discovered that the adrenal cortex and neuroendocrine and immune systems interact during stress, a finding that current research supports.[157-164,196,233-264] He defined stress as the body's automatic response ("fight or flight") to a demand that is placed on it. Selye also made the distinction between negative and positive stress (distress and eustress, respectively).

Life Events Model of Stress

Holmes and Rahe defined a model of stress that examined the nature and consequences of negative life events and proposed that interpersonal stressors are predictive of increases in disease activity.[157-164,196,233-264]

Overview of Examination Techniques

Chronic psychosocial stress has numerous pathophysiologic effects that may stem from excessive sympathetic nervous system activation.[157-164,196,233-264] In particular, adrenal glucocorticoid hormones may play a major role in the stress response because of their profound effects on mood, behavior, neurochemical transmission, and neuroendocrine control. The pathophysiologic effects of chronic stress include insulin resistance, hyperinsulinemia, coronary heart disease risk, infertility in females, therapy-resistant periodontitis, and impaired hippocampus-mediated memory processes. In children, chronic stress may be associated with impaired mental and affective stability, integrity, and development.

There are a variety of approaches to assessing chronic psychosocial stress.[157-164,196,233-264] Because of the subjective nature of stress, clients' perceptions of their symptoms and stress levels are a critical component of the client examination. Client interviews can elicit clients' reports of physical, mental, emotional, and behavioral symptoms of stress and descriptions of the situations that they perceive to be stress provoking. Therapists can use a verbal or visual analog scale to obtain a basic rating of the client's perceived stress level. There are also numerous standardized self-report stress-rating questionnaires that therapists can use to assess their clients' perceived level of stress and the factors contributing to the stress that their clients experience. These tests provide a well-defined set of information and are usually designed and validated for a specific population. Therapists who wish to use a standardized measure of stress should consult the manual for details of the professional training required prior to administering the measure. This will enable them to determine whether their training and scope of practice allow them to administer the measure. Some of these measures use dominant models of stress as their basis. For example, the Schedule of Recent Experience, Impact of Events Scale, and Social

Readjustment Ratings Scale are classic measures based on Holmes and Rahe's Life Events Model of Stress. The Cognitive Transactional Model of Stress provides the basis for the Hassles and Uplifts and the Ways of Coping Questionnaire from Folkman and Lazarus.[95] In addition, there are health-related stress questionnaires such as the Cardiac Event Threat Questionnaire. Buros Mental Measurement Yearbook[265] is a useful source of information on standardized stress questionnaires that includes the test population, test purpose, test details, and reviews.[164] Key Points 4-1 lists some of the many tests described in Buros.[164]

Therapists can also use any of the range of physiologic measures of chronic stress that are available.[157-164,196,233-264] Clinical measures include heart rate, systolic and diastolic blood pressure, finger pulse rate, skin conductance levels, and finger temperature. EMG, especially lateral frontalis electromyogram responses, is an indicator of stress. Laboratory measures of blood samples include levels of lipid peroxides in venous blood samples; levels of the stress-related hormones prolactin, cortisol, and testosterone; and glycated hemoglobin levels. Finally, analysis of saliva identifies salivary cortisol levels, a common physiologic indicator of stress.

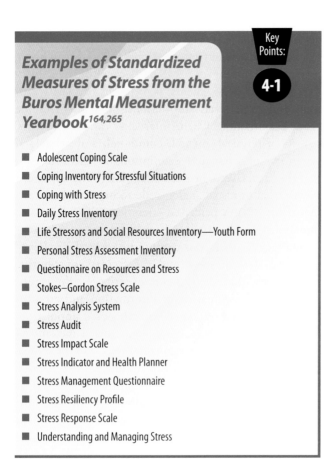

Key Points: 4-1

Examples of Standardized Measures of Stress from the Buros Mental Measurement Yearbook[164,265]

- Adolescent Coping Scale
- Coping Inventory for Stressful Situations
- Coping with Stress
- Daily Stress Inventory
- Life Stressors and Social Resources Inventory—Youth Form
- Personal Stress Assessment Inventory
- Questionnaire on Resources and Stress
- Stokes–Gordon Stress Scale
- Stress Analysis System
- Stress Audit
- Stress Impact Scale
- Stress Indicator and Health Planner
- Stress Management Questionnaire
- Stress Resiliency Profile
- Stress Response Scale
- Understanding and Managing Stress

MULTISYSTEM EXAMINATION

Pain

Definitions and Etiology

Pain

Pain is an unpleasant sensory and emotional experience associated with actual or potential tissue damage and described in terms of damage.[266]

Acute Pain

Acute pain is provoked by noxious stimulation from injury, surgery, and/or disease and is often a warning sign to stop movement and seek medical help.[267]

Chronic Pain

Chronic pain persists beyond the normal healing time and includes aspects of peripheral and central sensitization and psychological components.[268,269]

Note: Different pains have different generators and need different treatment strategies. This section describes the characteristics of somatic, neuropathic, and psychological pain.

Somatic Pain

Somatic pain is caused by a stimulus to tissue in a person with an intact nervous system. There are several types of somatic pain[21,25-27,62,89,215,217,270-312]:

- **Inflammatory Pain** is caused by tissue response to an injury or irritant and should resolve when the irritant ceases with healing.
- **Nociceptive Pain** is caused by noxious stimuli of nociceptive receptors in the skin or muscles: touch, pressure, temperature. It is the sensitization of peripheral nociceptors as a result of injury that causes an increased release of neurotransmitters in the dorsal horn of the spinal cord. The sensitized dorsal horn neurons demonstrate an increased background activity, an increased receptive field size, and increased responses to peripherally applied stimuli.

Neuropathic Pain

Neuropathic pain is caused by an injury, dysfunction, or change within the sensory nervous system, with the presence of neurologic signs that can include motor and autonomic changes. Central nervous system (CNS) sensitization causes neuroplastic changes in the spinal cord and brain.[270] There are several types of neuropathic pain[21,25-27,62,89,215,217,270,272-313]:

- **Central Pain Syndrome** is caused by a lesion in the CNS that affects the pain regulation systems in the spinal cord and brain such as injury, CVA, tumor, or disease. Thalamic lesions are the most common and present on the contralateral side in a nondermatomal distribution.

- **Complex Regional Pain Syndrome (CRPS)**, previously known as Reflex Sympathetic Dystrophy, is a syndrome that affects both the sensory and motor parts of the CNS through sensitization and neuroplastic changes. It will have a sympathetic component at some stage of its presentation, but is distinct from Sympathetically Maintained Pain.

- **Fibromyalgia** is sensitization of the sensory nerves within the muscles causing central sensitization. It is often associated with depression and poor sleep secondary to neurotransmitter dysfunction, which mediates pain, mood, and sleep.

- **Phantom Pain** involves central changes prior to loss of body part that cause subsequent incongruity of sensory and motor input. Typically, clients will perceive pain in body parts that are no longer present.

- **Radiculopathy** is a pathologic condition caused by blockage or pressure on nerve root(s) that results in sensory abnormalities, pain, and motor loss within the nerve root distribution. Symptoms are usually within nerve root distributions: dermatomes for sensory function and myotomes for muscle function.

- **Radicular Pain** is pain caused by stimulation of nociceptive afferent fibers in spinal nerves, nerve roots, or ganglia. It is caused by spontaneous ectopic nerve discharge and is different from radiculopathy, although both are often present at the same time.

- **Referred Pain** is pain that the client perceives as coming from an area away from the source because of the proximity of different afferent sensory nerves. Visceral and trigger point pain are examples of referred pain.

- **Visceral Pain** is pain from organs innervated by the autonomic nervous system, which is both a sensory and motor system. The pain is usually a combination of nociceptive and neuropathic pain. Organ pain refers to somatic pain fields because of lack of separate visceral sensory pathways and the low number of visceral afferent fibers. For example, cardiac ischemia is associated with pain in left arm, neck, and face. Visceral pain usually follows a sclerotomal distribution.

- **Dermatomal Pain**: A **dermatome** is an area of skin supplied by one dorsal nerve root. Injury of a dorsal root can result in sensory loss in the skin or can be experienced by the client as a burning or electric pain. For example, irritation of the C7 nerve root can lead to sensory changes in the C7 dermatome: lateral arm and forearm to the index, long, and ring fingers on the palmar and dorsal aspect.

- **Myotomal Pain**: This is pain in a myotome, a group of muscles supplied by one nerve root. For example, injury to the teres minor can result in referred pain near the insertion of the deltoid.

- **Sclerotomal Pain**: This is pain in a sclerotome, an area of bone or fascia innervated by one segmental nerve root. For example, hip pain can be referred to the groin, sacroiliac joints, lumbar spine, knee, or ankle.

- **Referred trigger point pain** arises in a trigger point, but the client feels it at a distance that is often entirely remote from its source. The pattern of referred pain relates to its site of origin. The distribution of referred trigger point pain rarely coincides entirely with the distribution of a peripheral nerve or dermatomal segment. Untreated trigger points can be associated with pain syndromes that include, but are not limited to, radiculopathy, tennis elbow, tension headache, occipital headache, and frozen shoulder.

Psychological Pain

Psychological pain is physical pain that is caused, increased, or prolonged by mental, emotional, or behavioral factors.314 It can include the following:

- **Chronic Pain Syndrome/Somatization Disorder** is a pattern of recurring, multiple, clinically significant pain complaints that results in medical treatment and causes significant social and occupational dysfunction.

- **Pain Disorders** is pain, causing distress and/or functional impairment, where psychological factors play an important part in its onset, severity, and continuation. This is not conscious or intentional. Hypochondriasis, which is the excessive or unreasonable fear of having a serious disease that is often caused by misinterpretation of body symptoms, falls within this category.

Overview of Examination Techniques

There are a variety of approaches to assessing pain.[21,25-27,39-53,157-164,233-250] Pain is a subjective experience. Consequently, the pain interview is an important means of eliciting information on the different components of the client's experience of pain, such as pain intensity, pain location, pain behavior, and the client's response to pain. Through the pain interview, therapists can determine the nature and the behavior of the client's symptoms over a 24-hour period. General guidelines for a pain interview appear in this chapter. Therapists should modify the number of issues they cover in the pain interview based on the clinical setting and the client's clinical condition. For example, a more detailed pain interview may be appropriate for a client with chronic back pain in an occupational medicine clinic than it would be for a client with an acute episode of shoulder pain. Readers can refer to the texts on client examination for their health-care profession to locate guidelines on issues related to pain assessment for specific clinical conditions. Therapists can use the information from the pain interview during the evaluation phase of clinical decision making to confirm or refute their hypothesis about the client's clinical condition. They can also use the pain interview findings to clarify the impact of the client's pain on his/her functional level and to guide their identification of functional outcomes.

Therapists can use a pain threshold meter or pressure algometer to measure tissue sensitivity to pressure.[21-25,34,157-164,196,246-249] There are a variety of types of pressure algometers available. Typically, these devices consist of a component for applying pressure, such as a hard rubber tip, attached to a pressure (force) gauge. The dial of the gauge shows pressure readings in kg/cm^2 or lbs/cm^2. Therapists obtain pressure sensitivity readings by using the algometer to apply a gradually increasing force on the client's tissues and noting the pressure reading at the time at which the client reports experiencing pain or discomfort. Interrater reliability for pressure algometer scores varies (ICCs of greater than $r = 0.78$ and Pearson correlation coefficients of $r > 0.82$). The pressure algometer is valuable for documenting and reassessing the effects of trigger point therapy and other interventions that change tissue sensitivity because it provides a means of quantifying the client's subjective complaints.

There are a number of assessment tools to test the interplay of pain and a client's psychological reaction to pain. Many are time consuming to administer and to interpret with limited value to our treatment strategies. The one area that affects our treatments is catastrophizing by clients and it can be measured by The Pain Catastrophizing Scale.

Pain behavior is a normal way of people to communicate to others they are in pain. It only becomes a problem when it is excessive and disruptive to the clinic or the treatment. Tools to measure pain behavior take hours of special observational training and are not practical for most therapists.

There are several appropriate neurologic tests. For example, neural tension, reflexes, and sensation need to be tested. In addition, therapists can test for allodynia (pain with normal nonpainful light touch) and summation (repeated nonpainful touch that causes pain that increases exponentially), which are signs of neuropathy, loss of inhibition, centralization of pain, and neuroplastic changes.

There are many pain assessment tools for adults; a selection of these are outlined in this section.[315] There are also a number of tools for assessing infants, children, adolescents, geriatric clients, and people with limited ability to communicate, but they are not discussed here. Self-reporting scales include the following:

- **Numeric Rating Scale:** A 0 to 10 response scale, with 0 being no pain and 10 being pain bad as can get. This can be verbal 0 to 10 or visual with marking one of the 11 choices.
- **Verbal Categorical Rating Scale:** 4-point scale of 1—no pain, 2—mild pain, 3—moderate pain, 4—severe pain.
- **Visual Analog Scale/Graphic Rating Scale:** A written rating scale of pain intensity that is widely used both clinically and in research because of the ease with which therapists can administer it.[113-155] The VAS consists of a straight line measuring 10 cm in length. "No pain" is at the left end of the line, and "the worst pain I have ever experienced" is at the right end. Test–retest reliability for the VAS has been reported as $r = 0.99$. Concurrent validity between the VAS and the Numeric Pain Rating Scale ranged between $r = 0.77$ and $r = 0.91$.
- **Face Picture Scale:** Pictures or drawings of facial expressions of people with different levels of pain. This can be used for different age ranges from children to geriatric clients, clients with cognitive impairments, and clients who speak a different language.
- **Neuropathic Pain Scale:** Pain quality, verbal or written, scale with 10 items that are rated on a 0 to 10 scale. The 11th item allows a client to report the pattern of his/her pain as constant, intermittent, or constant with intermittent increases.
- **Body Diagram:** A pain drawing that a client produces on a body diagram can serve several purposes. First, therapists can use it as an adjunct to the pain interview as a means of facilitating the client's discussion of her symptoms. It is a simple and reliable method of identifying the location of a client's pain and associated symptoms such as paresthesia and tightness. In addition, they can also use it to guide treatment planning and to document the client's response to treatment.
- **The McGill Pain Questionnaire (short form or short form-2):** Therapists can administer this as a written test or verbally by reading the items to clients. It is discriminating enough to help in differential diagnosis of pain syndromes and client's psychological stressors. It is often used in research, because it is reliable, valid, and sensitive.

Special tests that can be conducted on clients with pain vary with the suspected cause of the pain. Therapists can perform thermography with an infrared device that is used to detect house-heating leaks and is sensitive, valid, and reliable. This is very useful for CRPS and Thoracic Outlet Syndrome. Although nerve conduction tests can identify which nerves are damaged from the limb to the nerve root and whether healing is occurring, they are not particularly useful for diagnosing specific pain syndromes. In addition, clients with pain have difficulty tolerating nerve conduction studies. Brain functional MRIs are sometimes used since clients with pain who have similar diagnosis have similar brain activity, but functional MRIs are not yet sufficiently developed to be used to diagnose an individual client's pain syndrome.

Impaired Sensation Secondary to Entrapment Neuropathy

Definitions and Etiology

Entrapment Neuropathy

Entrapment neuropathy is nerve compression that can result from muscle and connective tissue shortening and inflammation associated with trigger point activity, fascial restrictions, overuse syndromes, and other clinical conditions.[21,25-27,52,215,316-325] The client with an entrapment neuropathy will present with pain, paresthesia, numbness, or loss of range of motion. Common peripheral entrapment neuropathies include carpal tunnel syndrome, cubital tunnel syndrome, and tarsal tunnel syndrome. Less common entrapment neuropathies include posterior interosseous nerve syndrome and anterior interosseous nerve syndrome.

Overview of Examination Techniques

There are a variety of neurologic and musculoskeletal approaches to assessing entrapment neuropathies.[21,25-27,52,215,316-325] Dermatome testing includes light touch, hot/cold, pinprick, and filament testing. Myotome testing uses isometric movements and reflexes. In addition, therapists can use sensory discrimination testing (kinesthesia, graphesthesia, and stereognosis), palpation of the nerve in the area of possible compression, vibrometer testing, and neural tension testing.

Electrophysiologic testing (nerve conduction studies) evaluates late responses (F waves and H reflexes) and long-latency reflexes.[21,25-27,52,215,316-325] These studies enable therapists to identify the location and severity of the neuropathy. Electroneurometry (skin surface electrical stimulation of the motor nerve), single-frequency (120 Hz) vibrometry tests, and MRI are also of value in the diagnosis of entrapment neuropathies.

Swelling

Definitions and Etiology

Swelling

Swelling is an abnormal enlargement of a segment of the body.[25,38,326-336]

Edema

Edema is an accumulation of fluid in cells, tissues, or serous cavities.[25,38,326-336] Edema has four main causes: increased permeability of capillaries, decreased plasma protein osmotic pressure, increased pressure in capillaries and venules, and lymphatic flow obstruction.

Effusion

Effusion is excessive fluid in the joint capsule, indicating irritation or inflammation of the synovium.[25,38,326-336]

Lymphedema

Lymphedema is accumulation of abnormal amounts of lymph fluid and associated swelling of subcutaneous tissues that results from the obstruction, destruction, or hypoplasia of lymph vessels.[25,38,326-336]

Dependent Edema

Dependent edema is an increase in extracellular fluid volume that is localized in a dependent area such as a limb.[25,38,326-336] Dependent edema can be associated with swelling or pitting.

Pitting Edema

Pitting edema is edema that retains the indentation produced by the pressure of palpation.[25,38,326-336]

Solid Edema

Solid edema is the infiltration of subcutaneous tissues by mucoid material.[25,38,326-336]

Overview of Examination Techniques

There are a variety of approaches to assessing swelling.[25,38,326-336] Therapists can obtain the client's description of her swelling and related symptoms through the client interview, in conjunction with the use of a body diagram. Visual inspection of swelling can assist therapists in determining how best to measure it. Palpation of swelling provides data on the quality of the swelling and the degree of edema that is present. Grading scales for edema include a 4-point scale for the degree of pitting and a 3-point scale for stage of lymphedema. Therapists can measure the girth of swollen body segments using a flexible tape measure, jeweler's ring, or wire. Volumetric analysis, in which the amount of fluid displaced by the limb is measured, provides a simple means of quantifying the extent of swelling that is more appropriate for swelling of the extremities. Comparison of volumetric analysis and estimation of limb volume using measurements of the limb perimeter showed that there was no significant difference between the two measures of limb volume for the arm but that volumetric analysis was more reliable and accurate for the hand. Laboratory or instrumented measures of swelling include multiple-frequency bioelectrical impedance analysis, MRI, and laser-Doppler flowmetry.

NEUROLOGIC EXAMINATION

Neuromuscular Tone

Definitions and Etiology

Muscle Tone

Muscle tone is resting tension and responsiveness of muscles to passive elongation or stretch.[38,183-192,197-205,325,337-361]

Postural Tone

Postural tone is the development of muscular tension in skeletal muscles that participate in maintaining the positions of different parts of the skeleton.[38,183-192,197-205,325,337-361]

The cerebellum regulates postural tone. Unlike resting muscle tension, constant muscle activation is required for the maintenance of postural tone. Furthermore, the self-sustained firing of motor neurons may reduce the need for prolonged synaptic input.

Hypertonia

Hypertonia is a general term used to refer to muscle tone that is above normal resting levels, regardless of the mechanism for the increase in tone.[38,183-192,197-205,325,337-361]

Hypotonia or Flaccidity

Hypotonia, or flaccidity, is a general term used to refer to muscle tone that is below normal resting levels, regardless of the mechanism for the decrease in tone.[38,183-192,197-205,325,337-361]

Spasticity

Spasticity is increased muscular tone that is a result of an upper motor neuron lesion that may or may not be associated with reflex hyperexcitability.[38,183-192,197-205,325,337-361] Spastic muscle exhibits a velocity-dependent increase in

tonic stretch reflexes. The quicker the stretch the therapist uses, the more pronounced the resistance of the spastic muscle being tested.

Rigidity

Rigidity is increased muscular tone that occurs as a result of brainstem or basal ganglia lesions.[38,183-192,197-205,325,337-361] Rigidity involves a uniformly increased resistance in both agonist and antagonist muscles, resulting in stiff, immovable body parts, independent of the velocity of the stretch stimulus. Clients exhibit two types of rigidity: (1) cogwheel rigidity, which is a ratchet-like response to passive movement, alternating between giving way and increased resistance, and (2) lead pipe rigidity, which is constant response to passive movement.

- **Decorticate rigidity** occurs as a result of brainstem lesions.[38,183-192,197-205,325,337-361] It presents clinically as sustained contraction and posturing of the trunk and lower limbs in extension and the upper limbs in flexion.
- **Decerebrate rigidity** occurs as a result of brainstem lesions.[38,183-192,197-205,325,337-361] It presents clinically as sustained contraction and posturing of the trunk and lower limbs in extension.
- **Parkinsonian rigidity** occurs as a result of basal ganglia lesions.[38,183-192,197-205,325,337-361] It presents clinically as a tight contraction of both agonist and antagonist muscles throughout the movement (lead pipe rigidity). Clients with Parkinson disease will eventually present with rigidity.

Clonus

Clonus is a cyclical, spasmodic hyperactivity of antagonistic muscles that occurs at a regular frequency in response to a quick stretch stimulus.[38,183-192,197-205,325,337-361]

Overview of Examination Techniques

There are a variety of approaches to assessing abnormal muscle tone.[38,183-192,197-205,325,337-361] The measurement of abnormal muscular tone requires an understanding of neurologic lesions. Manual passive motion testing and the use of tone grading scales, such as the Ashworth scale, are central to the examination of abnormal tone. The client examination for spasticity can also use the pendulum test (using isokinetic dynamometers or a goniometer), torque/electromyogram curves for ramp and hold or sinusoidal oscillation, or the use of handheld or isokinetic dynamometers to measure resistance to passive movement.

Some standardized assessments of motor control, such as the Fugl-Meyer assessment and the Montreal Evaluation, include sections on manual testing of muscle tone.[38,183-192,197-205,325,337-361]

In addition to manual passive motion testing, spasticity can be evaluated using electrophysiologic measures that measure the electrical and mechanical features of hypertonic muscle. These measures include electromyographic testing of reflexes such as the T reflexes, H reflexes, F responses, long-latency stretch reflexes, the tonic vibration reflex, and flexor reflexes. Research suggests, however, that there is a stronger correlation between Ashworth scale scores and spasticity than with laboratory or instrumented tests of reflex activity. Therapists can also test for exaggerated or clonic deep tendon reflexes in hypertonic individuals or absent or decreased reflexes for hypotonic states.

In light of the impact that neurologic conditions can have on an individual's functional level, there are numerous functional measures that are used in client examination.[38,183-192,197-205,325,337-361] These measures are similar in their emphasis on motor recovery and the functional tasks that are most often affected in individuals who have had strokes. They differ, however, in the philosophical principles on which they are based. For example, the measures that reflect neurodevelopmental therapy principles include the Rivermead Motor Assessment Protocol and the Montreal Assessment. The Fugl-Meyer assessment uses Brunnstrom's sequence of motor recovery. The Functional Test for the Hemiparetic Upper Extremity is based on both Brunnstrom and neurodevelopmental therapy principles. The structure of other measures, such as the Motor Assessment Scale, the Physical Assessment for Stroke Patients, and the Arm Function Test, is not based on either philosophy.

CARDIOPULMONARY EXAMINATION

Dyspnea

Definitions and Etiology

Dyspnea

Dyspnea is shortness of breath, labored or difficult breathing, or an uncomfortable awareness of one's breathing.[38,362-382] Dyspnea is usually an indication of inadequate ventilation or insufficient amounts of oxygen in the circulating blood. Dyspnea is a complex sensation that involves (a) the physiologic and psychological events or stimuli

preceding the development of dyspnea, (b) the characteristics of an individual or his/her environment that mediates his/her response to the dyspnea, and (c) the outcomes that result once the individual has reacted to the dyspnea.

Overview of Examination Techniques

There are a variety of approaches to assessing dyspnea.[38,362-384] Clinical examination of a client with dyspnea can include visual inspection for posture used during respiration; quality, rate, and pattern of breathing; accessory muscle use; color; and affect. Laboratory tests of decreased ventilation include arterial blood gases, which show oxygenation, acidosis, alkalosis, compensatory mechanisms, and buffer systems, and capnography, which determines levels of carbon dioxide.

There is only a fair association between perceived dyspnea and actual physiologic lung function, possibly because of the different components that are the antecedents, mediators, and outcomes of dyspnea outlined earlier.[38,362-382] For this reason, self-report measures of dyspnea are important. Measures such as the British Medical Research Council Questionnaire, the American Thoracic Questionnaire, and the Dyspnea Interview Schedule can assess the events or stimuli that precede the dyspnea. The American Thoracic Questionnaire, the Chronic Respiratory Questionnaire, the Dyspnea Interview Schedule, the Pulmonary Functional Status Scale, and the Therapy Impact Questionnaire may measure characteristics that mediate the dyspnea. The Dyspnea Visual Analog Scale, the Therapy Impact Questionnaire, and the Borg Perceived Exertion Scale measure an individual's reactions to dyspnea. In addition, the Therapy Impact Questionnaire, the Baseline Dyspnea Index, the Transition Dyspnea Index, the Chronic Respiratory Questionnaire, the Oxygen Cost Diagram, the Dyspnea Interview Schedule, and the Modified Medical Research Council Dyspnea Scale measure the consequences of an episode of dyspnea. Finally, since decreased exercise capacity is one of the consequences of dyspnea, measures of functional exercise capacity, such as the 6-minute walk test, can be a valuable inclusion.

Rib Cage Mobility

Definitions and Etiology

Rib Cage Mobility

Rib cage mobility is the capacity of the rib cage to move within the available anatomical range of motion during respiration, based on the arthrokinematics of the joints of the rib cage and the thoracic spine, and the ability of the associated soft tissues to respond to the movement.[38,362-382]

Overview of Examination Techniques

There are a variety of approaches to assessing rib cage mobility.[38,362-382,54-60] Examination of rib cage mobility involves both visual inspection and palpation. The visual inspection performed by therapists should include general posture, breathing pattern, chest wall shape, symmetry of chest wall movement, accessory muscle use, and muscle contours. Palpation of chest wall excursion during respiration should address lateral costal and diaphragmatic excursion, thorough palpation of the intercostal spaces, sternal motion, and apical motion. Therapists can also use palpation to assess the mobility of the thoracic spine, the costovertebral joints, and the sternocostal joints. Palpation of muscle tension in the accessory muscles of breathing, such as the sternocleidomastoid and the intercostal muscles, will complete the palpation process. Finally, therapists can quantify rib cage mobility by measuring rib cage excursion during respiration with a tape measure using a consistent measurement site and position.

Airway Clearance

Definitions and Etiology

Airway Clearance

Airway clearance is the ability to move pulmonary secretions effectively through the use of normal mechanisms of cough and the mucociliary escalator.[38,362-382]

Chronic Obstructive Pulmonary Disease

Chronic obstructive pulmonary disease is a pulmonary disorder characterized by the presence of increased airway resistance.[38,362-382] These disorders are associated with increased sputum production and cough that can predispose the individual to recurrent bronchial infection. Examples of chronic obstructive pulmonary disease include emphysema, chronic bronchitis, and asthma.

Chronic Restrictive Pulmonary Disease

Chronic restrictive pulmonary disease is a pulmonary disorder characterized by the restriction of lung expansion, such as interstitial fibrosis.[38,362-382]

Overview of Examination Techniques

There are a variety of approaches to assessing impaired airway clearance.[38,362-382] Therapists base the clinical examination of impaired airway clearance on a number of clinical signs and symptoms. The Respiratory Nursing Diagnosis Scale, which defines major and minor characteristics of impaired airway clearance, summarizes many of these clinical signs and symptoms. According to this scale, the most important characteristic of impaired airway clearance is an ineffective cough. The minor characteristics include tenacious sputum; subjective complaints of inability to cough up secretions; increased or copious sputum; absent, decreased, or abnormal breath sounds; air hunger; abnormal respiratory pattern; nasal flaring; anxiety; dyspnea at rest; cyanosis or other change in color; and restlessness. Characteristics deemed less relevant to impaired airway clearance include asymmetric chest excursion, abnormal inspiratory-to-expiratory ratio, dyspnea on exertion, diaphoresis, and pain.

A number of clinical tests collect the data on which to base the identification of impaired airway clearance.[38,362-382] Visual inspection of cough, visual inspection of the volume and quality of sputum, respiration rate and pattern, color, and accessory muscle use are essential starting points. Pulse oximeters measure oxygen saturation, which is the degree to which arterial blood is oxygenated. Unfortunately, the reliability of this measure decreases when clients' skin has darker pigmentation. Breath sounds and heart rate are assessed using auscultation. Finally, therapists can use self-report measures to elicit a client's perception of breathlessness (measured on a VAS), rating of dyspnea on a Dyspnea Rating Scale, or perceived exertion on a Perceived Exertion Rating Scale.

There are several laboratory tests of symptoms associated with impaired airway clearance.[38,362-382] Arterial blood gases show oxygenation, acidosis, alkalosis, compensatory mechanisms, and buffer systems. Pulmonary function tests show inspired volume, respiratory exchange ratio, forced expiratory volumes, inspiratory capacity, and vital capacity. In addition, there are a variety of measures of oxygen consumption. Finally, laboratory measures of actual particle clearance rates are not yet appropriate for use with humans, although they are common in animal research.

A variety of self-report functional measures, such as the Nottingham Health Profile for quality of life and the Self-Efficacy for Functional Activities questionnaire, measure the client's perception of the impact of impaired airway clearance and chronic respiratory disease on his/her functional level and quality of life.[38,362-382]

FUNCTIONAL EXAMINATION

Self-Care Activities

Definitions and Etiology

Self-Care Activities

Self-care activities refer to those daily tasks that an individual needs to perform in order to be independent.[385-400] These tasks include dressing, feeding, grooming, hygiene, functional mobility, and functional communication. Therapists consider an inability to perform any of these tasks a limitation in level of activity or participation, otherwise known as a functional limitation.

Overview of Examination Techniques

There are a variety of approaches to assessing independence in self-care.[385-400] Self-care activities are more frequently measured using standardized measures of self-care to assess the clients' functional limitations and their progress on the identified functional outcomes. For example, the Barthel Index is a self-care measure that consists of the following 10 items that represent basic self-care activities: feeding, wheelchair transfer, grooming, bathing, walking on level surface, climbing stairs, dressing, bowel control, bladder control, and toilet use. Although it is one of the oldest self-care measures, ongoing studies are evaluating its validity and reliability. The Barthel Index is still widely used for the examination of clients with strokes, hip fractures, liver transplants, Parkinson disease, amputations, and other clinical conditions.

Health-Related Quality of Life

Definitions and Etiology

Health-Related Quality of Life

Health-related quality of life is the client's perception of the impact that his clinical condition is having on his quality of life.[401-420] It can be an issue to address in the client examination for massage since the impairments described earlier can have an impact on the client's level of activity and participation in society.

Overview of Examination Techniques

There are a variety of approaches to assessing health-related quality of life.[401-420] Measures of health-related quality of life have a broader focus than self-care measures and they typically cover the domains of physical, psychological, emotional, and social function. For example, the Medical Outcomes Survey—Short Form-36 (MOS SF-36) is a frequently used health-related quality of life measure that researchers have validated for several diseases and translated into other languages. The following are selected health-related quality of life measures, which assess different components of quality of life.[401-420]

In addition, therapists are using disease-specific quality of life measures, such as the Rheumatoid Arthritis Quality of Life Scale, more frequently in clinical examination and studies. Other measures include

- Medical Outcomes Study Health Status Questionnaire
- Duke-UNC Health Profile
- The Sickness Impact Profile
- McMaster Health Index Questionnaire
- Functional Status Questionnaire
- Nottingham Health Profile

SCIENTIFIC BASIS OF SOFT TISSUE EXAMINATION

Therapists can use a deeper understanding of the anatomy and physiology related to soft tissue examination to increase the effectiveness of their soft tissue examination. This section outlines the basic anatomy of the soft tissue layers and possible mechanisms for the behavior of soft tissue in preparation for a more detailed discussion of how to perform palpation within the client examination for Outcome-Based Massage™. There are ongoing debates around many of the issues in this area and therapists can consult textbooks and research articles devoted to these topics for more comprehensive information.

Soft Tissue Layers

Traditionally, the term **soft tissue** describes any tissue that is not bone or articular surface.[9,23,24,421] More specifically, soft tissue includes the **epithelium**, fascial and other **connective tissues**, and the skeletal muscle **contractile tissues**. Therapists frequently sense a succession of layers of tissue that are oriented from surface to deep as they palpate clients' bodies. In doing so, they can use differences between the characteristics of these layers, such as hardness, density, texture, and mobility, to distinguish between tissue layers.

Anatomically, there are several distinct tissue layers.[9,23,24,421] The most superficial is the thin, denser epithelium, which consists of closely packed columnar or squamous cells that have little intercellular material between them. The lower part of the skin or dermis is also dense and consists of collagen bundles supporting blood vessels, nerves, sweat glands, and hair follicles. Subcutaneous fascia and connective tissue underlie the skin layers and have greater mobility. They consist of several different types of cells such as fibroblasts and fat cells, and elastin and collagen fibers embedded in a matrix of gelatinous material, the consistency of which varies by the depth and in response to many factors. Nerves, blood vessels, and lymph vessels lie in the connective tissue. The deepest level is the myofascial contractile tissue, comprised of muscle, its enveloping fascial layers, its associated tendon(s), and its periosteal attachments.

As Figure 4-1 shows, the skin consists of a layer of epithelium, the epidermis, and the dermis, which is the first layer of connective tissue.[9,23,24,421] Deep in the skin lies the **superficial fascia**, which houses fat and water, provides a path for nerves and vessels, and sometimes contains thin strains of striated muscle that can control the movement of the skin. The investing layer of the **deep fascia** is dense connective tissue that lies between the superficial fascia and muscle. The investing layer of the deep fascia is continuous with the superficial fascia and the thin fibrous layer covering muscles (epimysium) and extending between their bundles (perimysium). The primary functions of the deep fascia are to allow muscles to move freely, to carry nerve and blood vessels, to fill the space between muscles, and to provide an origin for muscles. For example, aponeuroses, retinacula, and interosseous membranes are all deep fascia. The deep fascia around muscle is continuous with the periosteum. In areas in which there is no muscle, the investing layer of the deep fascia is continuous with the periosteum. Finally, connective tissue exists in synovial joints; for example, the synovial membrane and the extrinsic ligaments are modified connective tissue.

Soft Tissue Mobility and Restrictive Barriers

Normal Soft Tissue Range of Motion

Soft tissues have an available range of motion that may be comparable to the range of motion available in joints.[4,8,9,22-24,421] Within this range of motion, normal soft tissue has three barriers, or resistances, that can limit movement (Figure 4-2). Therapists are "engaging" these tissue barriers at the point when they palpate a resistance to tissue motion. The physiologic barrier (Ph) is the resistance that determines the range of motion that is available under normal conditions. In other words, the tissue's range of motion lies between the two physiologic barriers, with the least amount of resistance being apparent at the midrange (M). The elastic barrier (E) is the resistance that therapists feel at the end of the passive range of motion, when they have taken the "slack" out of or are "engaging" the tissue. The anatomical barrier (A)

FIGURE 4-1 Skin layers. (From Thomson JS. *Core Textbook of Anatomy*. Philadelphia, PA: J. B. Lippincott Company; 1977:15. Used with permission of Lippincott Williams & Wilkins.)

FIGURE 4-2 Normal tissue barriers. A, anatomical barrier; E, elastic barrier; Ph, physiologic barrier; M, midrange. (Reprinted with adaptations from Greenman PE. *Principles of Manual Medicine*. 2nd ed. Philadelphia, PA: Lippincott Williams & Wilkins; 1996:43. Used with permission of Lippincott Williams & Wilkins.)

is the final resistance to normal range of motion that the bone, ligament, or soft tissue can provide. Motion beyond the anatomical barrier results in tissue damage.

Restrictive Barriers

Restrictive, or pathologic, barriers in soft tissue occur when soft tissue dysfunction is present.[4,8,9,22-24,421] Restrictive barriers may occur in skin, fascia, muscle, ligament, joint capsule, or a combination of these tissues. They can be located anywhere between the normal physiologic barriers, can limit the available range of motion within the tissues, and can alter the position of the midrange. Furthermore, the presence of a restrictive barrier will change the quality of the movement and the "feel" at the end of the tissue range of motion. This is similar to the abnormal "end feels" therapists palpate in joints. An example of a restrictive barrier (R) and its impact on the position of the midrange (M2) appears in Figure 4-3.

Barrier-Release Phenomenon

Therapists engage the tissue barrier at the point at which they palpate a resistance to tissue motion.[4,8,9,22-24,421] If therapists sustain the pressure on the tissue barrier, a "release" may occur after a latency period that will vary with the nature of the tissue and its state of health. This release results in a reduction of the resistance that will enable therapists to move the tissue beyond the location of the original barrier without increasing the pressure of palpation. This phenomenon is called the **barrier-release phenomenon**.

Different types of tissue respond differently to sustained pressure.[4,8,9,22-24,421] For example, connective tissue is most responsive to sustained pressure and will demonstrate a slow, palpable stretch of tissues called creep or viscoelastic creep. This stretch occurs beyond the elastic barrier (E) shown in Figure 4-3. In the case of pathologic or restrictive barriers, this release can last up to 30 seconds or longer and can result in normalized tissue mobility and pain reduction. Since connective tissue forms a portion of all soft tissues, some creep is evident in all soft tissues in proportion to the amount of connective tissue that is present in that structure.

Resting Muscle Tension

Definition

Human resting muscle tension, or resting myofascial tone (HRMT) is the passive tonus or tension of skeletal muscle that derives from its intrinsic (EMG-silent) molecular viscoelastic properties. The word tone has been used to convey varying clinical and physiologic features that have led to confusion and controversy. HRMT is the vital low-level, passive tension, and resistance to stretch that makes an important contribution to the maintenance of postural stability in balanced equilibrium positions or when the body is supported against gravity. In contrast, co-contraction of muscle is an active neuromotor control that provides greater levels of tonus for increased stabilization. Functionally, HRMT is integrated with other passive fascial and ligamentous tensional networks of the body to form a **biotensegrity system**, in which the biomechanical forces allow both movement and the maintenance of static postures.

Poorly defined terminology and a lack of differential clarity on the source of passive versus low-level activated muscle tension hamper the understanding of musculoskeletal pain, particularly of postural muscle pain.[21-25,31,34,38,89,183-192,196-205] Therapists often develop an

FIGURE 4-3 Restrictive tissue barriers. A, anatomical barrier; E, elastic barrier; Ph, physiologic barrier; R, restrictive barrier; M, midrange; M2, pathologic midrange. (Reprinted with adaptations from Greenman PE. *Principles of Manual Medicine*. 2nd ed. Philadelphia, PA: Lippincott Williams & Wilkins; 1996:43. Used with permission of Lippincott Williams & Wilkins.)

informal language for describing states of resting tension in otherwise healthy individuals. Some words such as "hard," "tight," "soft," "wiry," and "ropy" directly describe the texture of the muscle at rest. Expressions like "normally toned," "well-toned," or "hypertonic" make a judgment about both the physical properties and the implied function. Descriptors like "boggy," "dry," or "leathery" have unspoken implications about tissue health. Terms like "taut band" or "facilitated segment" link palpatory findings to complex theories about pathology of muscle or other tissue. Therapists need to use these terms with caution, since the literature has not defined them systematically.

Conceptual Framework

The literature describes two physiologic components of passive resting muscle tension: the intrinsic biomechanical properties of muscle and the CNS-activated contractile component of muscle tension. While both components have mechanical properties of stiffness, viscoelasticity, and tension, they differ in their characteristics and underlying basis. Most authors include low-level, nonvoluntary contractile activity in the definition of resting tension, particularly of axial or postural muscles. Mechanically, the low-level, CNS-activated component is an addition to the intrinsic material properties. The preceding differences in descriptions of resting (passive) and low-level, CNS-activated muscle tension are not well discriminated in the literature.[89]

Therapists know that the firmness and texture of skeletal muscle varies greatly from person to person.[21-25,31,34,38,183-192,196-205] Moreover, different muscles in the same client or in the same muscle at different times can also vary in resting tension. The contribution of low-level CNS contractile activity to the variability in resting tension is not well known. Therapists often observe how massage techniques can change palpable resting tension. These changes in resting tension may relate to decrease in a client's pain, involuntary muscle guarding, psychological stress, or other factors contributing to the level of muscle activation. Any contribution of massage techniques to intrinsic passive muscle tone is not currently known.

One prevalent theory, as inferred above, was that resting tension arises from a constant low-level contraction of skeletal muscle fibers, although recent research questions that theory.[21-25,31,34,38,183-192,196-205] The emerging conceptual framework is that [truly] passive resting muscle tension results from a complex contribution of several intrinsic material components: (1) actin and myosin (actomyosin) myofibril low-level cross-bridge cycling; (2) the giant structural proteins of striated muscle, titin, on stretching, and (3) other proteins, like connectin. Each

of these intrinsic muscle elements contributes to the passive resting tension, independent of CNS contraction or evidence of activation on EMG monitoring. The contribution of low-level CNS activation to static (not passive) muscle tone is difficult to determine clinically. However, it can be monitored and differentiated from truly passive tone by sensitive surface EMG technique, similar to methods used in feedback relaxation. The framework described in this section takes into account the following observations about skeletal muscle[21-25,31,34,38,183-192,196,205] that therapists can notice during palpation:

- Therapists can change the shape of muscle during applied force.
- A deformed muscle reverts quickly to its former size and shape, although the muscle's shape and resting tension may change slightly if it were in a state of guarding or spasm.
- The texture of the same muscle can differ temporally. Sometimes, it feels softer, more flexible, and more fluid; at other times, it may feel harder, stiffer, and more solid. This texture is partly dependent on the muscle's position and state of activation.
- The texture of a muscle can differ spatially. Relatively soft areas in a muscle may surround harder "knots."
- Therapists can observe a wider range of textures across a sample of healthy clients than may occur in the same person over time. This range is along the same soft-to-hard continuum.
- Muscle fascicles may be palpable at rest, particularly when tensed. These fascicles are similar to, but less well-defined than, those therapists may feel when a muscle contracts.
- Sometimes, a muscle that is "at rest" feels as though it is contracting, due to its increased tension or spasm.
- Palpation or massage can provoke a low-grade transient muscle activation and contraction. Therapists can sometimes observe a similar involuntary contraction or "twitching" (fasciculation) of muscle at rest.
- After an injury, therapists may find that the characteristic texture of muscle tissue is obscured. In the early period after an injury, it may feel as though it contains fluid, whereas in the later period after injury, it may feel considerably firmer, like modeling clay.

Biomechanical Contributions to Passive Resting Tension

This category of resting tension has been termed viscoelastic tone or passive tone. It refers to the contribution made by the physical and material substances contained in muscle tissue, independent of CNS activation.[200,206-209,422] This is an important distinction that is not made in common definitions of resting tone, which suggest that the latter is a combination of true passive muscle tension and low-level active muscle tension.[21-25,31,34,38,89,183-192,196-205]

Muscle is a tissue composed of "subtissues": water, smaller organic molecules, larger complex organic molecules, and even more complex biopolymers. Each of these elements has different physical or material properties, such as density, stiffness, and deformability. The behavior of muscle during palpation reflects the properties of these components (Figure 4-4).

Water

Water associated with muscle tissue exists in several locations[21-25,31,34,38,89,183-192,196-205]:

1. Contained in associated vessels, such as arteries, veins, or lymphatics;
2. In the interstitium, restrained in compartments formed by connective tissue;
3. Freely in the interstitium; and
4. Loosely bonded to the hydrophilic molecules of the connective tissue matrix.

Water normally flows relatively freely between these areas.[21-25,31,34,38,89,183-192,196-205] Changing a muscle's position passively from a shortened position to a lengthened one results in increased fluid tension within the muscle, which causes the muscle to feel firmer during such palpation. Pathology or injury may also shift water balance toward or away from one location, resulting in palpable changes in resting tension. For example, excess interstitial water may feel soft during initial stages of edema and lymphedema, or it may feel hard in compartment syndromes. The latter occurs when pressure increases as a result of the water being restrained within the thick fasciae. Some therapists believe that it is also possible through palpation to identify when the matrix is dehydrated.

Connective Tissue

Fascia contributes to a varying proportion of the firmness of muscles at rest, as assessed by palpation.[21-25,31,34,38,89,183-192,196-205] This firmness results from two components: collagen fiber bundles and the connective tissue soft matrix in which the collagen fibers are embedded. Denser modeling of the connective tissue within the muscle, like fibrosis and scarring, is one of several processes that may contribute to the increased firmness and stiffness that therapists may palpate in the chronic stages of orthopedic injuries.

Muscle Tissue

When the muscle is not activated, its contractile elements—myofibrils, composed of actin and myosin (actomyosin), within sarcomeres in series—afford low-level resistance to compression or stretching.[200,206-209,422] These low-level biomechanical interactions are independent of the far greater muscle tension and tone which results from CNS-activated contraction.[21-25,31,34,38,89,183-192,196-205] A discussion of the contributions of active contraction to truly resting (passive) tension follows. Muscle also contains variable amounts of embedded fat (the marbling seen in meat), which gives little resistance to pressure during palpation under normal circumstances.

Biomechanical Behavior of Muscle as a Whole

The mechanical behavior of noncontracting, passive muscle is complex.[200,206-209,422] A force that therapists apply quickly to muscle, such as a stretch or digital compression, will produce an initial deformation known as elastic

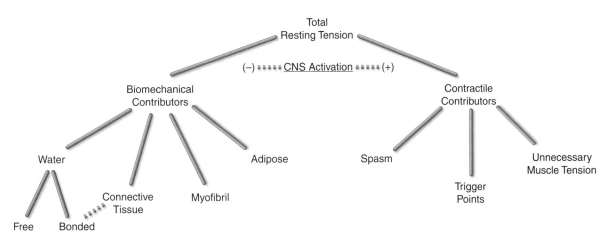

FIGURE 4-4 Components of resting muscle tension. (Adapted from Mense S, Simon DG. *Muscle Pain: Understanding Its Nature, Diagnosis, and Treatment.* Philadelphia, PA: Lippincott Williams & Wilkins; 2001.)

deformation. When they apply the same force slowly, it produces another deformation called viscous (or plastic). Furthermore, the amount of deformation of the tissues depends on the rate of application of the force. In addition, muscle tissue shows the property of thixotropy. After initiating movement, muscle becomes less resistant to stretching and less stiff. Such change can be noted in the stirring of certain gels, like honey, which stiffens on standing, but becomes less viscous as the flow (shear) increases. These behaviors depend on complex molecular interactions between the several components listed earlier that are discussed in detail in specialized texts.

Contribution of Low-Level Actomyosin Myofibril Cycling to Passive Resting Tension

Physiologically, non–CNS-activated resting tension is contributed by low-level cycling of myosin head cross-bridging to actin filament sites in the sarcomeres, which make up the myofibril.[200,206-209,422] Passive, CNS-independent muscle tension can be demonstrated in isolated tissue from experimental animals.[200] It also occurs in humans during anesthesia[89] or when fully relaxed and supported from gravity. In attempting to become fully relaxed, complete independence of CNS activation is difficult to achieve and varies among individuals.[21,34,89] Therapists often note differences in myofascial tension or stiffness among individuals. The challenge is to interpret if variations may be due to the passive biomechanical properties, which differ by age and sex, or if the clients are not fully relaxed. Unrecognized and involuntary guarding or tensing reactions contribute to the activated tension (Figure 4-4).

Active Tone

Most authors define the CNS-stimulated muscle contraction as **active tone** or hypertonicity. This contractile activity is minimal in relaxed, normally innervated healthy muscle tissue. However, as previously noted, it is difficult to relax muscle completely without any CNS contribution. Figure 4-4 shows examples of ways in which contractile activity causes increased resting tension.

Unnecessary or Extraneous Muscle Tension

Unnecessary or extraneous muscle tension refers to "unwitting muscular contraction" or muscle tension that is potentially under voluntary control.[21-25,31,34,38,89,183-192,196-205] Therapists commonly see clients with increased muscle tension due to situational stress. Such clients with unnecessary muscle tension often request massage for wellness or to address their effects of stress.

Trigger Points

Trigger points involve myofibril shortening and activity, possibly as a result of calcium leakage at dysfunctional motor end plates.[21-25,31,34,38,89,183-192,196-205] Therapists in this situation may observe that motor neuron and EMG activity are absent.[423] The contraction knots and taut bands of trigger points frequently cause elevated resting tension in the surrounding muscle fibers.

Spasm

Spasm involves involuntary contractile activity that is associated with motor neuron and EMG-monitored activity.[21-25,31,34,38,89,183-192,196-205] Spasm produces pain in one of three ways: (1) by overloading parts of the muscle; (2) by subjecting nociceptors between active and nonactive parts of the muscle to shearing forces; or (3) through ischemia. Spasm is a common result of orthopedic injuries.

IN CONCLUSION

Client examination plays a critical role in Outcome-Based Massage™ by providing the clinical findings on which therapists can base the confirmation of their clinical hypothesis and their treatment planning. Consequently, therapists who are conducting client examinations with a view to using massage as a primary or complementary treatment modality need to expand the focus of their standard approach to examination to include the assessment of soft tissue dysfunction and the impairments that are relevant to the use of massage techniques.

Palpation provides an important means of assessing a variety of aspects of soft tissue function that can suggest the presence of impairments, such as temperature, tissue mobility, fluid status, tissue texture, and tissue consistency. In addition, the client's response to palpation can give therapists other information about the client's presenting impairments. However, palpation is not the only means of assessing a client's impairments. Therapists can also extend their interpretation of the findings from standard musculoskeletal, neurologic, cardiopulmonary, and psychological tests and measures to include an analysis of the contribution of soft tissue dysfunction. Finally, the client examination conducted by therapists should also address the client's level of ability to perform functional activities and quality of life, so that therapists have data on which to base the identification of appropriate functional outcomes.

Practice

Note: This section contains instructions and clinical cases that demonstrate how to use some of the examination techniques and approaches that were introduced in this chapter.

PRACTICAL ASPECTS OF PALPATION

Clinicians need to match palpation techniques to the object of palpation, whether it is a physical structure or a characteristic. The following are examples of objects of palpation and appropriate palpation techniques:

Anatomical Structures

The ability to palpate anatomical structures systematically is an absolute prerequisite for clinicians who use massage,[3-36] because this ability has a direct impact on the accuracy of the clinicians' examination using palpation, the effectiveness of the massage techniques they perform, and whether the patient achieves treatment outcomes. The palpation of anatomical structures, detailed in comprehensive texts on this topic, involves the ability to discriminate between tissue types and to distinguish a structure from its surrounding structures with accuracy. Through palpation, clinicians can identify bone, joint space (joint line), ligament, tendon (including junctions to both periosteum and to muscle), aponeurosis, fascia (septae, sheathes, retinacula), nerves, vessels, and viscera. Each anatomical structure has a characteristic "feel," which stems from its structure and histology. Clinicians need to use compressive contact when they palpate anatomical structures. They also need to select contact surfaces and levels of pressure for palpation based on the structure that they are palpating

Layer palpation, the palpation of soft tissue layers, is central to massage. It involves the palpation of the skin, superficial fascia, deep fascia, muscle, and periosteum.

Skin

Clinicians should use minimal force and note the following characteristics as they palpate patients' skin.[4,8,9,22-24,421] First, there are normal variations in skin thickness, for example, the thickness of the sole versus the dorsum of the foot. Second, skin has elastic rebound that varies with age. Third, there are variations in the tightness of the attachment of the skin, for example, the tightness of the attachment of the skin of the elbow versus the skin of the scalp. Clinicians can also assess the level of moisture on the skin surface and the hydration of the skin itself because these may reflect a patient's circulatory, trophic, or nutritional status. Finally, clinicians may also be able to distinguish between the epidermis and the dermis by using gentle horizontal drag at the very surface of the skin.

Superficial Fascia

Clinicians can engage the superficial fascia and the fat deposits it contains by increasing the compressive force they apply.[4,8,9,22-24,421] They can try to gauge the "turgor," or fluid pressure, of the tissues since edema often deposits into this tissue layer. They can also estimate the thickness of the superficial fascial layer by comparing different regions. The tissue mobility tests outlined in this chapter are also appropriate for assessing the superficial fascia. In addition, clinicians can test the mobility of the superficial fascia by folding it or by lifting and rolling it over the surface of the underlying tissues (see Skin Rolling in Chapter 10). Clinicians should compare the results they obtain for superficial fascia with those that they obtain for the skin.

The Investing Layer of the Deep Fascia

The investing layer of the deep fascia is smooth, firm, and continuous and lies between the superficial fascia and muscle.[4,8,9,22-24,421] Consequently, clinicians may need practice to locate it precisely. The client examination procedure for connective tissue massage includes the assessment of the investing layer of the deep fascia. Clinicians use techniques similar to those for the more superficial layers, described earlier, to assess the mobility of this connective tissue layer. The difference between these two approaches is that assessing the investing layer of the deep fascia requires more refined palpation skills because there is more intervening tissue. Tissue restrictions identified by clinicians often correlate with the restrictions that they find in the more superficial layers. These restrictions may indicate underlying muscle tension, segmental dysfunction, or visceral imbalance.

Muscle

Clinicians assess resting muscle tension during palpation by noting a muscle's response to the compressive and shearing forces that they deliver with their finger(s) or hands.[4,8,9,22-24,421] During palpation, their hand(s) may compress the whole muscle or bend it. They can also slowly enter the muscle tissue and tease its fibers apart using their fingers or thumbs. The higher the resting level of tone, the denser and harder the tissue will be on palpation. Increases and decreases in resting muscle tension are relative states because degrees of tone vary greatly from one person to another and between one segment of an individual's body and another. Spasm is more dramatic and, thus, more readily distinguished by clinicians. Elevated resting tone can result from a wide variety of clinical conditions, including injury, degenerative diseases, and stress.

In addition to assessing resting muscle tension during the palpation of muscle, clinicians can note whether high turgor (fluid distention) is present since this can indicate a postexercise condition or an inflammatory condition.[4,8,9,22-24,421]

Periosteum

This tissue layer is only accessible to palpation in areas where there is no overlying muscle.[4,8,9,22-24,421] Clinicians can use compressive fingertip force to palpate the thin, dense, spongy layer superimposed on the hardness of the underlying bone.

Tissue Mobility and Restrictive Barriers

Barrier-Release Phenomenon

Clinicians can observe the barrier-release phenomenon in tissues during their application of horizontal drag, vertical compression, or shear forces to the tissues using either small or large contact surfaces.[4,8,9,22-24,421] Consequently, they can use palpation to identify the feel at the end of the available range of motion of tissue using a variety of palpation techniques including digital compression or a palmar drag on the superficial fascia. The barrier-release phenomenon is most useful when palpating connective tissue, but clinicians can also apply it to any tissue or structure.

Palpation of Tissue Mobility

Clinicians can apply a compression or drag force, or a combination of the two, to a given tissue or structure

within a patient's body and observe the resulting movement.[4,8,9,22-24,421] In doing so, they can observe whether the normal range of motion is present in the tissues or whether restrictive barriers exist. If clinicians palpate a restrictive barrier, they must note the available range of motion in the tissues, the quality of movement through the range of motion, and the feel of the point at which they engage the restrictive barrier.

Temperature

The palpation of temperature can provide information about the status of inflammation, circulation, and organ function.[3-36] There are several approaches to palpating temperature. In one method, clinicians place the back of their hands in direct contact with the patient's skin. The pressure used for this method must be very light; otherwise, vasodilatation will occur and confound the findings.

Contour and Bulk

Contour and bulk refer to the gross shape and size of the body region. Clinicians can best examine these characteristics with a relatively fast-moving scanning palpation using a large contact surface such as the entire palmar surface of their hand.[3-36] Clinicians should correlate the information they obtain from their palpation of contour and bulk with the findings from their visual inspection of the patient's body.

Texture and Consistency

Texture and consistency refer to variations in the density of tissues, regardless of the depth of the layer in which the tissues occur.[3-36] In other words, they describe the density of superficial tissues, such as the skin, or deeper tissues, such as the hamstring attachment to the ischial tuberosity.

There are two categories of tissue texture that are important because they reflect the presence of inflammation.[3-36] The first is acute inflammation, which generally produces different degrees of tissue softness that reflect the presence of extravasated fluid in the tissues. The terms "distended," "spongy," or "boggy" describe this texture. The second is chronic inflammation, which typically produces varying degrees of tissue "hardness" as a result of the deposit of collagen into the tissues. Some descriptors for the tissue "hardness" associated with chronic inflammation are "indurated," "ropy," and "stringy."

Fluid Status

Clinicians can use palpation to measure turgidity, which is fluid pressure or fluid tension.[3-36] Palpation of fluid involves the use of large contact surfaces to palpate excess fluid and push it from one place to another. These tests enable clinicians to gauge the amount of excess fluid in an area and the pressure of the fluid. They can also assess whether the fluid is located in the intra- or extra-articular space, that is, whether it is an edema or an effusion. Finally, clinicians can use sustained digital compression to determine whether "pitting" is present.

Viscosity refers to the "thickness" or "stickiness" of semi-liquid materials.[3-36] Clinicians can assess viscosity using palpation. This is valuable because muscle and connective tissue commonly become less viscous in response to interventions such as the local application of neuromuscular or connective tissue massage techniques or heat.

Body Rhythms

Clinicians assess **pulses** and **respiratory rhythms** using static palpation with minimal to moderate compression and a contact surface of appropriate size.[3-36] The amount of force they apply during the palpation of pulses is important because the use of excessive compression can result in inaccurate findings. Clinicians assess pulses using a single hand. By contrast, they can use two hands, placed on opposite sides of the rib cage, to produce a three-dimensional test when they are palpating respiratory rhythms. Clinicians can palpate both pulse and respiration at a distance to the site, although this technique sometimes confuses novices. Clinicians with advanced skills or specialized training can palpate subtler pulsations of inherent tissue motions using a broad-contact static palpation.

Tremors and Fasciculations

Fasciculations are localized, subconscious muscle contractions.[3-36] They do not involve the entire muscle because they result from the contraction of the muscle cells innervated by a single motor axon. **Tremors**, by contrast, are rhythmic movements of a joint that result from involuntary contractions of antagonist and agonist muscle groups. Clinicians can palpate both tremors and fasciculations statically with minimal to moderate compression and contact surfaces of varying sizes.

Vibration

Clinicians can palpate two types of vibration: crepitus and fremitus.[3-36] Crepitus is a vibration of variable fineness that is associated with a roughened gliding surface of a tendon, a tendon sheath, or the articulating surfaces of a joint. Clinicians can sometimes hear crepitus, in addition to palpating it. Fremitus is another palpable vibration. Clinicians can palpate this pulmonary vibration over the rib cage as the patient speaks or vocalizes.

PRACTICAL ASPECTS OF THE MUSCULOSKELETAL EXAMINATION

This section contains examples of how to perform different aspects of the musculoskeletal examination of body structures and functions including posture, scar, fascial mobility, joint integrity, joint mobility, muscle integrity, muscle performance, and trigger points.

Posture: Visual Postural Analysis

Clinicians can use the following steps to perform visual postural analysis.

Clinician's Position for the Postural Analysis

- Anterior view: The clinician stands directly in front of the patient at a distance of approximately 5 to 8 feet, with the patient standing or sitting.[6,21,25-27,38-53] If the patient is in supine position, the clinician stands at the foot of the treatment table. Standing on a stool may offer a clearer view.
- Posterior view: The clinician stands directly behind the patient at a distance of approximately 5 to 8 feet, with the patient standing or sitting. If the patient is prone, the clinician stands at the foot of the treatment table. Standing on a stool may offer a clearer view.
- Lateral view: The clinician positions himself to the side of the patient in alignment with the patient's external auditory meatus for the examination of the lateral view with the patient standing or sitting. If the patient is in side lying position, the clinician is positioned at the side of the treatment table. Standing on a stool may offer a clearer view. In addition, standing at the side of the treatment table may provide a less obstructed view of the patient's upper body, compared with the anterior view, if the patient has a large abdomen or considerable amounts of pectoral or breast tissue.

Patient's Position for the Postural Analysis

Observation of the patient from different views and in different positions can provide the clinician with a greater understanding of the patient's postural alignment. For example, a patient whose postural alignment differs in standing versus supine may have a pelvic malalignment, a leg length discrepancy, muscular weakness, or an impaired postural awareness. In addition, the clinician can also identify whether the patient has a pelvic malalignment or a leg length discrepancy by comparing the patient's postural alignment in sitting and standing. If the patient is nonambulatory, the clinician may use sitting and supine positions for this purpose.

Steps in Performing a Postural Analysis

1. Ask the patient to remove her shoes and don clothing or a gown that allows the clinician to view landmarks, while ensuring appropriate draping.
2. Select a view to assess, for example the anterior view, and identify the appropriate position for doing so.
3. Position the posture grid or plumb line.
4. Position the patient in relation to the posture grid or plumb line so that the selected view of the patient is unobstructed and the posture grid or plumb line provides an appropriate frame of reference.
5. Ask the patient to assume a relaxed posture, rather than what she thinks is "good" posture. Allow the patient to settle into that position for a minute to get a more accurate representation of her usual posture. If this is painful, then decrease the amount of time the patient spends in this position.
6. Assume the appropriate position from which to observe the landmarks for the selected view.
7. Perform the visual inspection of the selected view, identifying the positions of the landmarks listed in Landmarks for Visual Postural Analysis and noting the symmetry of body contours and muscle bulk throughout the patient's body. Ensure that you perform a bilateral comparison wherever this is appropriate.
8. Confirm or refute the findings of visual analysis with palpation.
9. Document the findings of visual analysis.
10. Note findings that will be an indication for further patient examination using other tests and measures.
11. Reposition the patient for the next view in the assessment.

Anterior Landmarks for Visual Postural Analysis

Head and Neck
1. Orientation of the end of the nose with the manubrium, xiphoid process, and umbilicus (the umbilicus is often not in vertical alignment with these other landmarks)
2. Vertical alignment of the head, for example, excessive lateral flexion or rotation
3. Level of the eyes
4. Vertical alignment of the jaw
5. Contours of trapezius muscle

Upper Extremities
1. Carrying angle of elbows (5° to 15° is the normal range of the carrying angle for an elbow)
2. Levels of hands (used in identifying asymmetrical shoulder levels)
3. Direction of palms (used in identifying asymmetrical shoulder rotation)

Trunk
1. Trunk in vertical alignment (note asymmetry of skin folds or the distances of the patient's arms to her trunk)
2. Level of acromioclavicular joints
3. Level and length of clavicles
4. Sternum and costocartilage aligned (note superior, inferior, or lateral deviations of these landmarks)
5. Ribs aligned and symmetrical bilaterally
6. Differences in weight bearing on the lower extremities as reflected by the position of the trunk over the extremities

Lower Extremities and Pelvis
1. Levels of the anterior superior iliac spines
2. Torsion of the tibia or femurs
3. Orientation of the knees, for example, varus or valgus
4. Orientation of the patellae
5. Levels of the fibular heads
6. Levels of lateral malleoli
7. Levels of the medial malleoli
8. Foot angle (10° of external rotation or toeing out is normal)
9. Orientation of the arches of the feet, for example, neutral, pronated, supinated, pes cavus, or pes planus with the feet in their usual posture and then with the great toes aligned; if the patient wears orthotics, it may be appropriate to also observe foot position with the patient's shoes on

Lateral Landmarks for Visual Postural Analysis

1. Deviation from an imaginary vertical line running through the following landmarks: ear lobe through the bodies of the cervical vertebrae, through the acromion process, through the lumbar vertebrae, through the highest point of the iliac crest, through the hip joint, anterior to the knee joint, and anterior to the ankle joint
2. Position of the glenohumeral joint
3. Position of the sternum: note if it is overly prominent or depressed
4. Tilt of the pelvis
5. Alignment of the knees: note recurvatum or excessive flexion

Posterior Landmarks for Visual Postural Analysis

Head and Neck
1. Vertical alignment of the head

Upper Extremities
1. Level of the shoulders

Trunk
1. Levels and alignment of the spines and inferior angles of the scapulae (the scapulae should rest on the thorax between the levels of T2 and T8; note whether the scapulae are abducted, adducted, elevated, or depressed)
2. Position of the scapulae against the thorax: note if they are winging
3. Distance of the vertebral borders of scapulae from the thoracic vertebrae
4. Vertical alignment of the spine (note any lateral curvature)
5. Distance between the twelfth rib and the iliac crest

Lower Extremities and Pelvis
1. Level of the iliac crests
2. Level of the posterior superior iliac spines
3. Levels of the gluteal folds
4. Levels of the knee joints
5. Angle of Achilles tendons (should be vertical)
6. Position of the hindfoot with the feet in their usual posture and then with the great toes aligned (note whether the hindfoot is in varus or valgus). If the patient wears orthotics, it may be appropriate to also observe foot position with the patient's shoes on

Note: Pelvic malalignment or a small hemipelvis can present as changes in thoracic alignment in sitting. In addition, consider a more detailed examination of pelvic misalignment if the patient's anterior superior iliac spines or posterior superior iliac spines are asymmetrical. Clinicians can refer to other sources for detailed guidelines on the examination of pelvic alignment.

Joint Integrity: Capsular Pattern Testing

Clinicians can use the following steps to assess a capsular pattern in a restricted shoulder:

1. Determine if your universal goniometric measurements of AROM match the capsular pattern for the glenohumeral joint.
2. Capsular pattern for the glenohumeral is as follows:

   - external rotation—greatest limitation
   - abduction—moderate limitation
   - internal rotation and flexion—least limitation

Joint Mobility: Thoracolumbar Flexion Range of Motion

Clinicians can use the following steps to perform thoracolumbar flexion range of motion using a tape measure:

1. Have the patient in standing position.
2. Patient keeps the knees and elbows straight.
3. Have the patient bend forward toward the ground with arms in front reaching toward the floor.
4. Measure from the tip of the patient's third finger to the floor using a tape measure.

Muscle Integrity: Thomas Test

Clinicians can use the following steps to perform the Thomas Test for hip flexor shortness:

1. Have the patient lie supine.
2. Check for lordosis, which is a predictor of a tight hip flexor.
3. Passively flex one of the patient's hips, bringing the knee to the chest.
4. Ask the patient to hold the knee to help stabilize the pelvis and flatten out the lumbar region.
5. If the leg that you are testing (the leg on the table) does not have a hip flexion contraction, it will

remain on the testing table. If a contracture is present, the leg will raise off of the table.

6. Lack of full hip extension with knee flexion less than 45° indicates iliopsoas tightness. If full extension is reached in this position it would indicate rectus femoris tightness. If any hip external rotation is observed it may indicate iliotibial band tightness.

Muscle Integrity: Palpation of Trigger Points

Clinicians can use the following steps to perform palpation for trigger points[21-25,34,157-164]:

1. Explain the purpose of palpation and the procedures to be followed to the patient.
2. Ask the patient to inform you when she experiences tenderness, a referral of pain, or tingling or any other symptoms as a result of your palpation.
3. Determine the muscle you will palpate for the presence of trigger points. This may include a review of the patient's reported pain behavior in the subjective examination for references to possible trigger point referral zones. Other potential locations of trigger points include muscles that showed limited range of motion on examination.
4. Ensure that your hands are warm and dry.
5. Position the patient with the muscle that you will be examining in approximately two-thirds of its normal stretch position. Refer to Travell[21] and Simons' Myofascial Pain and Dysfunction: The Trigger Point Manual for the test positions for specific trigger points.
6. Drape the patient appropriately (see Chapter 6).
7. Ensure that the patient is warm and that the muscle you plan to palpate is relaxed.
8. Identify the possible location of the trigger point.
9. Palpate the location of the trigger point using one of the following approaches:
   a. Flat palpation: Slide your finger or thumb along the taut band in the patient's muscle until the patient reports that you have reached the location of maximum tenderness, which represents the trigger point.
   b. Pincer palpation: You can use this for muscles that you can lift easily. Grasp the belly of the muscle between your fingers and thumb. Squeeze and roll the muscle tissue between your fingers to locate the taut band in the muscle. You can repeat this maneuver along the muscle belly until you locate the trigger point.
   c. Snapping palpation: Once you locate the taut band using pincer palpation, roll the taut band

quickly under your fingers to produce a local twitch response.

10. During palpation, determine whether the following are present:
    a. Taut bands. The fiber direction and the pain referral pattern will enable you to identify the involved muscle.
    b. Local hardness. The trigger point itself may present as a very small area of focal hardness (palpable nodule) in the taut band. Compress this area against the underlying tissues, and determine whether you reproduce the characteristic pain referral pattern for the trigger point in question.
    c. Twitch responses. You can palpate twitch responses in superficial muscles.
    d. Jump sign. A patient may produce a large involuntary contraction and other gross affective signs of pain if you palpate the trigger point too forcefully.
    e. Generalized hardness. If there are adjacent trigger points in overlapping layers, the practitioner may find it difficult to palpate anything other than a generalized hardness. For example, this commonly occurs between the scapulae.
11. During palpation, have the patient compare the pain you produce by palpating the trigger point to her presenting symptoms. The patient should be able to recognize the pattern of pain referral if the trigger point is the contributing cause of her pain.

Muscle Performance: Isometric Strength Testing

Clinicians can use the following steps to perform isometric strength testing of the quadriceps:

1. Have the patient long sit with a small folded towel under the knee.
2. Have patient perform "quad setting" by pressing the back of his knee into towel.
3. Observe and palpate the contraction of the quadriceps.

Scar: Scar Assessment

Clinicians can use the following steps to perform the examination of scar:

1. Position the patient so that the scar is not in a stretched position and is readily accessible to you.
2. Prior to initiating palpation, explain the purpose and procedures of palpation to the patient. In particular,

instruct the patient to tell you when she feels any discomfort. In doing so, inform her that you will cease applying pressure as soon as she indicates discomfort, so that she does not experience undue discomfort. This is especially important if the patient has reported that the scar is painful.

3. Begin palpation using light pressure. Then, gradually increase the depth of palpation.
4. Assess whether the scar tissue moves as freely as the surrounding tissues. As you palpate the scar, identify differences in the mobility of different areas of the scar tissue. In addition, note areas in which the scar appears to be adherent to adjacent or deeper tissues. Document this information using the positions of a clock, for example, 3:00 (with 12:00 being in the cephalad direction).
5. During palpation, ask the patient to report when she experiences pain at the site of the scar or elsewhere during palpation. Movement of the scar should be pain free.
6. Identify areas of the scar that are puckered, and document this information.
7. Adjuncts to palpation used to assess changes in the dimensions of scars include the measurement of the depth of the scar using a ruler and photography. Follow your facility's guidelines for obtaining the patient's written permission for photographs.

Fascial Mobility: Connective Tissue Mobility

Clinicians can use the following steps to assess connective tissue mobility:

1. Stretch the skin horizontally in one direction at a time without gliding or engaging underlying issues.
2. Let the skin recoil.
3. Stretch the skin, and sustain this position at the barrier.
4. Note how soon the skin begins to elongate.

PRACTICAL ASPECTS OF THE PSYCHONEUROIMMUNOLOGIC EXAMINATION

This section contains examples of how to perform different aspects of the psychoneuroimmunologic examination of body structures and functions including self-reported symptoms of chronic psychosocial stress and self-reported levels of stress.

Stress: Self-Reported Symptoms of Chronic Psychosocial Stress

Clinicians can use the following steps to perform the measurement of self-reported symptoms of chronic psychosocial stress:

1. During the subjective examination ask the patient whether he has experienced any changes in the following areas and to describe the symptoms:

   ■ Mental and Emotional Signs of Stress: These are changes in emotions and mental function that result from chronic stress. Some examples of emotional and mental changes that are associated with chronic stress include forgetfulness, poor concentration, anxiety, anger, and depression.
   ■ Physical Signs of Stress: These are changes in bodily functions that may occur when people are under stress. Some examples of physical signs of stress include muscle tension, stomach problems, changes in sleep patterns, and fatigue.
   ■ Behavioral Signs of Stress: These are changes in behavior that may occur when stress levels are too high. They are often the easiest signs of chronic stress to spot. Some common examples of behavioral changes include disorganization, withdrawing from relationships or usual activities, or neglect of personal appearance.

Stress: Self-Reported Levels of Chronic Psychosocial Stress

Clinicians can use the following steps to perform the measurement of self-reported levels of chronic psychosocial stress:

1. During the subjective examination, ask the patient to rate her perceived level of stress using a 5-point numeric rating scale. You may use descriptors to assist patients in selecting a number to represent their levels of stress such as those in this example:
   ■ 1: No stress
   ■ 2: I rarely have stress
   ■ 3: I sometimes have stress, I can handle it
   ■ 4: I have a lot of stress, sometimes I have difficulty coping
   ■ 5: I have too much stress, I can't cope

PRACTICAL ASPECTS OF THE MULTISYSTEM EXAMINATION

This section contains examples of how to perform different aspects of the multisystem examination of body structures and functions including pain and swelling.

Pain: Pain Interview

During the pain interview, clinicians elicit information about the patient's pain including: location of pain and 24-hour pain behavior, positions that aggravate pain, activities that aggravate pain, self-management of pain, and ergonomic issues. Clinicians can use the following steps to perform the pain interview:

Location of Pain and 24-Hour Pain Behavior

Discuss the following issues with the patient as a means of outlining the behavior of the patient's pain over a 24-hour period.[6,21,25-27,26,34,38-53,163,196,233] Bear in mind that the relevance of these issues will vary with the patient's clinical condition.

1. Location of symptoms: The patient clarifies any locations marked on the pain drawing that are unclear.
2. Priority of symptoms: The patient distinguishes between primary and secondary symptoms noted on the pain drawing.
3. Nature of pain: The patient selects a pain identifier, such stabbing or burning, that best describes the pain in a particular location.
4. Intensity of pain: The patient defines the intensity of pain that has occurred during a specified time period. The practitioner may use a numeric rating scale of 0 to 10, in which 0 represents the absence of pain and 10 represents the most pain the patient has ever experienced.
5. Additional symptoms: The patient describes associated symptoms, such as paresthesia, that has been noted on the diagram.
6. Frequency and duration of symptoms: The patient indicates whether pain is constant or intermittent. The patient also indicates how frequently and for how long the symptoms occur. A distinction between the duration of symptoms that occur during the day versus the night may be relevant to the patient's clinical condition. The frequency of the symptoms may be stated as a percentage, such as "50% of waking hours," or in relation to a time of day or an activity, such as "pain starts after 11:00 AM and persists until bedtime" or "burning sensation occurs after 30 minutes of keyboarding."

Positions That Aggravate Pain

1. Ask the patient to list the positions, such as sitting or standing, in which she notices an increase in her pain and associated symptoms.
2. For each position, elicit the following information:
   a. How long can the patient maintain the position before noticing that the symptoms start or before they increase when there is a constant baseline level of pain?
   b. How long can the patient maintain the position before the symptoms reach a level of intensity that necessitates moving out of the position?
   c. When the symptoms change, as a result of being in the position, what is the change in level of intensity of the symptoms? Use the scale of 0 to 10 discussed earlier to show the difference.
   d. What does the patient do to ease pain and other symptoms once the position aggravates them? For example, note the positions, modalities, exercises, and medications the patient uses to ease pain.
   e. Once the patient has moved out of the position and used some means of pain relief, how much time elapses before the patient notices that the symptoms have returned to the original level?

Activities That Aggravate Pain

1. Ask the patient to list the activities during which she notices an increase in her pain and associated symptoms. These activities can include the following:
   a. Self-care activities such as grooming, feeding, and functional mobility
   b. Community management activities (instrumental activities of daily living) such as driving, taking the bus, and grocery shopping
   c. Work-related activities such as lifting, keyboarding, and telephone use
   d. Leisure activities such as sexual activity, walking, watching television, and playing sports
   e. Sleeping. Since patients' symptoms are frequently aggravated during sleep, this activity usually warrants additional discussion of issues such as sleep position, bed type, and sleeping behavior
2. For each activity, elicit the following information:
   1. What is the time period for which the patient can perform the activity before noticing that the

symptoms start (or increase if there is a constant baseline level of pain)?

2. What is the time period for which the patient can perform the activity before the symptoms reach a level of intensity that causes cessation of the activity?

3. When the symptoms change as a result of performing the activity, what is the change in level of intensity of the symptoms (use a scale of 0 to 10 to show the difference)?

4. What does the patient do to ease pain and other symptoms once performing the activity aggravates them? For example, note the activities, modalities, exercises, and medications the patient uses to ease the pain.

5. Once the patient has ceased the activity and used some means of pain relief, how much time elapses before the patient notices that the symptoms have returned to the original level?

Self-Management

1. Ask the patient to describe the strategies she uses to manage symptoms. Include details of the frequency, duration, and effects of these activities.

2. Ask the patient if she has received a self-care program in the past. Determine whether she is still performing it. If so, discuss the frequency, duration, and effects of this self-care program.

Ergonomics

1. Ask the patient to describe and demonstrate the following:
   a. Usual positions in which she performs her work
   b. Any repetitive activities that are associated with performance of the job
   c. Positions that she uses at work that she feels are safe and comfortable
   d. Positions that she uses at work that she feels cause her pain
   e. Positions that she uses at work that she feels are adaptations to pain or that she uses to minimize pain

2. Ask the patient whether the placement of the furniture and equipment in her work area appears to be contributing to her pain.

3. Ask whether the patient has had an ergonomic evaluation of her work place by a qualified professional. If so, what were the results?

Pain: Visual Analog Scale and Body Diagram

Self-reporting on the location and characteristics of pain is an important component of the pain assessment. Clinicians can use the body diagram (Figure 4-5) and VAS (Figure 4-6), a pain intensity scale, to assess the patient's present and ongoing pain levels. Be consistent and use the same scale for each subsequent examination. As the patient completes the diagram and the scale, the clinician can elaborate on different aspects of the pain outlined in the Pain Interview, for example, asking the patient, "What makes it worse and better?" or cueing the patient with some of the terms listed in the McGill Pain Questionnaire (SF-MPG-2) such as

- Continuous Pain: Throbbing, aching, heavy, cramping
- Intermittent Pain: Shooting, stabbing, electric-shock, piercing
- Neuropathic Pain: Burning, caused by light touch, itching, tingle, numbness
- Affective: Tiring, exhausting, sickening, fearful, punishing, cruel

The Body Diagram

Clinicians can use the following steps when using the body diagram (Figure 4-5) in the pain interview:

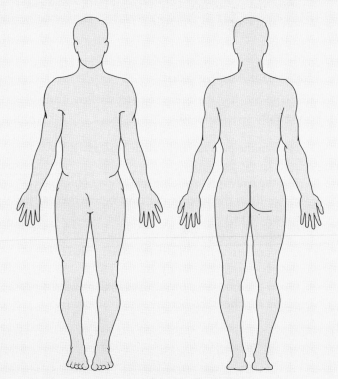

FIGURE 4-5 Body diagram for the pain drawing.

1. Provide the patient with a diagram of the human body (Figure 4-5) and colored pens.
2. Explain the purpose of the pain drawing and any predefined symbols, such as dotted lines, that represent pain and associated symptoms.
3. Inform the patient what time period the pain drawing is intended to represent. For example, this may be pain and symptoms experienced over the previous 24 hours. This time period will vary with the nature of the patient's clinical condition.
4. Ask the patient to indicate the location of any pain and associated symptoms that she has experienced during the specified time period on the diagram, using colors and predefined symbols. If the patient is unable to complete this task independently, the practitioner may provide the appropriate level of assistance.
5. When the patient has completed the pain drawing, discuss the drawing to clarify and expand on the information that the patient has provided. Clinicians can do this as part of the pain interview.
6. Document this supplemental information on the pain drawing or elsewhere in the patient's chart. The section on general pain behavior in the pain interview notes some issues that may be worthy of additional attention depending on the patient's clinical condition.
7. The clinician may wish to identify asymptomatic areas that are immediately adjacent to the symptomatic area on the pain drawing.

The Visual Analog Scale

Clinicians can use the following steps when using the VAS (Figure 4-6) in the pain interview:

1. Explain the pain rating levels at both extremes of the scale to the patient.
2. Ask the patient to mark the line at the point that corresponds to the intensity of pain experienced at the time at which she is completing the VAS.
3. Measure the distance from the beginning of the line to the patient's mark; this is the value that represents the patient's intensity of pain.
4. On re-examination, present the patient with a new diagram rather than her previous pain rating.

Pain: Palpation for Pain

Clinicians can use the following steps to perform palpation for pain:

1. Ensure that your hands are warm and dry.
2. Position the patient in a comfortable position in which the area to be palpated is readily accessible to you.
3. Drape the patient appropriately (see Chapter 6).
4. Explain the purpose of palpation and the procedures to be followed to the patient.
5. Ask the patient to inform you when she experiences tenderness, a referral of pain, or tingling or any other symptoms as a result of your palpation.
6. Select the location where you will begin palpation based on the patient's reports of the locations of pain, patterns of referred pain, or areas of tissue tightness that may be contributing to a postural dysfunction.
7. Begin palpation using light pressure. Gradually increase the depth of palpation because a rapid change of depth may elicit a guarding response.
8. As you palpate each location, ask the patient if pressure on a given area causes any tenderness, localized pain, or referred pain. Move between locations slowly to avoid eliciting a painful spasm.
9. Observe the patient for twitching, vasomotor responses, and changes in breathing.
10. As you progress with palpation, identify and palpate areas in which there are abnormalities of tissue texture such as bogginess or taut tissue bands.
11. Increase the depth of palpation and repeat the process if palpation with light pressure does not reproduce the patient's symptoms or the results of this palpation are inconclusive.
12. In addition to palpating the locations of pain the patient has reported, you may also wish to palpate the following:
    a. Trigger points that may refer to the painful areas
    b. Related dermatomes
    c. Related sclerotomes
13. Document all locations in which the palpation reproduces the patient's symptoms, and note the patterns of referred pain that result from palpation.

Note: Tenderness on palpation of a given area may be referred tenderness from another area and may not be a reliable finding. The practitioner needs to corroborate the findings of palpation for pain with other clinical tests and measures.

No pain ⌐   ⌐ The worst pain I have
                                                          ever experienced

FIGURE 4-6 Visual analog scale for pain measurement.

Pain: Tissue Sensitivity with Pressure Algometer

Clinicians can use the following steps when using a pressure algometer to test tissue sensitivity in patients with suspected trigger points:[21-25,34,157-164,246-249]

1. Stand in a position that will enable you to apply an even pressure to the patient's tissues when the pressure algometer is positioned perpendicular to the patient's skin.
2. Position the patient in a relaxed and well-supported position.
3. Explain the overall procedure to the patient, and demonstrate the application of the pressure algometer on an unaffected area of the patient's body. In particular, instruct the patient to say "Yes" when she first feels discomfort and explain that you will cease the application of pressure as soon as she does so to ensure that she does not experience undue discomfort. Explain that rubor and capillary breakage can occur following tissue sensitivity testing with a pressure algometer, and provide basic instructions for the application of ice to the affected areas.
4. Identify the location where you want to test tissue sensitivity. For example, in the case of a trigger point, palpate for a taut band and an area of tenderness in the location specified for that trigger point. Once you have located the area to be tested, you may wish to mark it.
5. Ensure that the pressure gauge is at zero. Place the contact surface of the pressure algometer on the location you wish to test.
6. Hold the pressure algometer so that the shaft of the instrument is at a 90° angle to the surface of the patient's skin.
7. Using your free hand, gradually apply pressure on the patient's tissues with the pressure algometer. Continue to increase the pressure gradually until the patient reports feeling discomfort.
8. Cease applying pressure as soon as the patient reports discomfort, and note the pressure algometer reading at that point.
9. Reset the gauge to zero prior to the next episode of testing.

Swelling: Girth Measurement

Clinicians can use the following steps to perform girth measurements of the ankle using the "figure 8" technique:

1. Have the patient long sitting with lower leg beyond end of table.
2. Using a 1/4-inch tape measure, place the end of the tape measure midway between the tibialis anterior tendon and the lateral malleolus, drawing the tape medially across the instep.
3. Pull the tape across the arch of the foot proximal to the base of the fifth metatarsal, around the ankle joint just distal to the medial malleolus, across the Achilles tendon, then distal to the lateral malleolus returning to the starting position. This will form a figure 8.
4. Repeat this measurement three times and then take the average of the measurements.

PRACTICAL ASPECTS OF THE NEUROLOGIC EXAMINATION

This section contains examples of how to perform different aspects of the neurologic examination of body structures and functions including muscle tone and clonus.

Muscle Tone: Spasticity Testing

Clinicians can use the following steps to perform spasticity testing with the Modified Ashworth Scale:

1. Place the patient in a supine position.
2. If testing a muscle that primarily flexes a joint, place the joint in a maximally flexed position and move to a position of maximal extension over 1 second (count "one thousand one").
3. If testing a muscle that primarily extends a joint, place the joint in a maximally extended position and move to a position of maximal flexion over 1 second (count "one thousand one").
4. Score based on the following scale:
   - 0: No increase in muscle tone
   - 1: Slight increase in muscle tone, manifested by a catch and release or by minimal resistance at the end of the range of motion when the affected part(s) is moved in flexion or extension
   - 1+: Slight increase in muscle tone, manifested by a catch, followed by minimal resistance throughout the remainder (less than half) of the range of motion
   - 2: More marked increase in muscle tone through most of the range of motion, but affected part(s) easily moved
   - 3: Considerable increase in muscle tone, passive movement difficult
   - 4: Affected part(s) rigid in flexion or extension

Clonus: Babinski Reflex

Clinicians can use the following steps to test the Babinski Reflex:

1. Coarsely run the end of a reflex hammer up the lateral aspect of the foot from heel to big toe.
2. The normal reflex is toe flexion. If the toes extend and separate, this is an abnormal finding called a positive Babinski sign.

PRACTICAL ASPECTS OF THE CARDIOPULMONARY EXAMINATION

This section contains examples of how to perform different aspects of the cardiopulmonary examination of body structures and functions including rib cage mobility.

Rib Cage Mobility: Chest Expansion Testing

Clinicians can use the following steps to measure chest expansion:

1. Have the patient short sit.
2. Place a tape measure around the patient's chest at the level of the fourth intercostal space.
3. Ask the patient to exhale maximally and take a measurement of the chest expansion.
4. Ask the patient to inhale maximally and hold his/her breath.

5. Take a second measurement of the chest expansion.
6. The normal difference between chest expansion during inhalation and exhalation is 3 to 7.5 cm or 1 to 3 in.

PRACTICAL ASPECTS OF THE FUNCTIONAL EXAMINATION

This section contains examples of how to perform different aspects of the functional examination such as self-care.

Self-Care: Barthel Index

Clinicians can use the following steps to adminster the Barthel Index:

1. The scale consists of 10 common ADLs, 8 of which represent activities related to personal care and 2 of which are related to mobility.
2. The Barthel Index can be completed through either direct observation or self-report.
   a. Direct observation: Ask the patient to perform the tasks on the measure. Observe and rate his performance on the tasks.
   b. Self-Report: Read the patient each of the tasks on the measure and ask him to rate his ability to perform each task.
3. The index yields a total score out of 100, with higher scores indicating greater degrees of functional independence.

Clinical Case: *Client Examination for Neck and Upper Back Pain*

Patient Profile

Your patient is a 45-year-old female violinist with a symphony orchestra. Her primary complaint is a painful tightness bilaterally in her neck and upper back. The symptoms come on when she plays for more than 15 minutes during both practice and performance, when she reads, and when she runs for exercise. She has had this problem intermittently for about 1 year. X-rays ordered by her doctor show mild degeneration of the intervertebral joints at levels C5-C7. Otherwise she is in good health.

Relevant Examination Techniques and Clinical Findings

Subjective

Examination Technique
- Patient reported history

- Patient interview

Finding
- The patient uses words such as "tight," "hard," or "wired" to describe her symptoms
- Rates pain at 2/10 at rest
- Rates pain at 7/10 during practice and performance

Objective

Examination Technique
- Palpation of soft tissue (skin gliding and skin rolling)

Finding
- Hypertonic upper trapezii bilaterally

- Measurement of cervical active range of motion with universal goniometer

- Active range of motion:
  - Flexion: limited into flexion—20°
  - Rotation: limited bilateral rotation—30° bilaterally

Analysis

Impairment in Body Structure and Function
- Impaired connective tissue integrity/ decreased fascial mobility

Activity Limitation
- Decreased ability to practice or perform with instrument greater than 15 minutes

Outcomes
- Increased connective tissue mobility

Functional Outcomes
- Able to practice and perform for 45 minutes pain free

REVIEW   SECTION

TAKEAWAYS

1. Client examination plays a critical role in Outcome-Based Massage™.
2. Use of the ICF model provides the clinician with a structured framework for examining a patient.
3. A detailed subjective examination provides clinicians with crucial patient information about possible soft tissue dysfunctions.
4. The pain interview is an important means of eliciting information on the different components of the patient's experience of pain, such as pain intensity, pain location, pain behavior, and the patient's response to pain.
5. There are a multitude of reliable and valid tests and measures available to clinicians for examination and assessment of patients with clinical conditions and wellness goals.
6. Clinicians can perform and analyze tests and measures when examining the musculoskeletal, psychoneuroimmunologic, multisystem, neurologic, and cardiopulmonary systems, including an analysis of the contribution of soft tissue dysfunction.
7. Skilled palpation is a required component of many client examination techniques, and a prerequisite skill for the effective execution of all massage techniques. Clinicians can use palpation to assess and reassess the patient's impairments throughout the client examination and treatment process.
8. The ability to identify subtle characteristics of the selected structure will help clinicians distinguish between normal and abnormal findings.
9. Postural analysis is used to document alignment of both soft tissue and bony structure. This information provides important objective data that can be used to identify the patient's potential functional limitations.
10. Clinicians should also address the patient's level of ability to perform functional activities and quality of life, so that they will have data on which to base the identification of appropriate functional outcomes.

Critical Thinking Questions

1. What specific modifications do you need to make in your approach to a patient with clinical conditions versus wellness goals, so that your examination findings will guide your choice of massage techniques?

2. How do you guide your specific interview questions to begin to develop a hypothesis of soft tissue dysfunction for a patient with pain symptoms?

3. Do you need to examine the different systems even if the patient is only describing musculoskeletal symptoms? If so, why?

4. How does examination of the patient's posture contribute to the identification of potential areas of soft tissue dysfunction?

5. What are the similarities and differences between the range of motion available in joints and the range of motion of soft tissue?

6. How do clinicians use their senses to determine a patient's soft tissue dysfunctions?

7. What palpation techniques do clinicians use to assess each of the soft tissue layers?

8. What are the common "objects of palpation"? Which palpation techniques and types of force of palpation do clinicians use to assess these structures?

9. Why do you need to know what type of pain your patient may be presenting with at the outset of the client examination?

10. What outcome measures are available to you to identify improvements in the patient's symptoms, function, and perceived quality of life?

References for Chapter 4 begin on p. 453; see Further Reading list on p. 461.

Outcome-Based Massage™ Clinical Decision-Making

OBJECTIVES

After studying this chapter, you will have the information that you need to do the following:

1. Describe the four phases of the Outcome-Based Massage™ clinical decision-making process: evaluation phase, treatment planning phase, treatment phase, and discharge phase.
2. List impairments that clinicians can treat with massage techniques and the outcomes that they can achieve by doing so, then outline how to select massage techniques required to remediate impairments, enhance wellness, and achieve identified functional outcomes.
3. Identify the process by which clinicians use the findings from the client examination and re-examinations to develop the plan of care and then modify, refine, and progress interventions.
4. Describe how to identify the client's discharge needs, plan for discharge, and discharge a client.
5. Describe the relationships between Outcome-Based Massage™ clinical decision-making, evidence-based practice, and the therapeutic relationship.

The clinical decision-making process guides the therapist through the examination, treatment, and discharge of the client. Outcome-Based Massage™ (OBM) clinical decision-making, the decision-making process proposed for Outcome-Based Massage™, addresses issues that are specific to the integration of massage techniques into clinical practice. This chapter discusses Outcome-Based Massage™ clinical decision-making over four phases: the evaluation phase, the treatment planning phase, the treatment phase, and the discharge phase. It provides guidelines for therapist to use to enhance the appropriateness and adequacy of the client examinations, plans of care, and interventions they plan and provide. In addition, it shows the relationship between Outcome-Based Massage™ clinical decision-making and evidence-based practice and the therapeutic relationship.

Note: The numbers 1 through 9 in the titles of the Evidence section correspond to the numbers of the steps in Figure 5-1.

Evidence

THE OUTCOME-BASED MASSAGE™ CLINICAL DECISION-MAKING PROCESS

The terms clinical decision-making, clinical reasoning, and clinical problem solving are used to describe the process by which therapists analyze client information and formulate and progress therapeutic regimens for their clients.[1-8] Outcome-Based Massage™ clinical decision-making (Figure 5-1), the **clinical decision-making process** for Outcome-Based Massage™, integrates clinical reasoning models with the frameworks for massage discussed in the earlier chapters.

Although we present this process graphically as a series of steps, we do not intend therapists to use it in a linear, sequential manner. In reality, as research indicates, therapists who are engaged in the clinical decision-making process often perform several steps of the process concurrently.[4] In addition, therapists use an iterative decision-making process, rather than a linear process. In other words, they cycle through the same steps of the decision-making process several times and each time that they repeat the steps they expand on their information and refine their conclusions.

Phases in Outcome-Based Massage™ Clinical Decision-Making

The Outcome-Based Massage™ clinical decision-making process has four phases: the **evaluation phase**, the **treatment planning phase**, the **treatment phase**, and the **discharge phase**, each with its distinct purpose and procedures. Together, these phases lead the therapist through a systematic process that enhances the fit between the client's presenting issues and the treatment techniques that the therapist selects. This will ultimately improve the quality of care that therapists deliver, their clients' outcomes, and client satisfaction.

The evaluation phase provides the foundation of the clinical treatment process. The steps in the evaluation phase revolve around formulating and confirming a **clinical hypothesis** about the client's clinical problem or wellness goals. This phase begins with data gathering through the **client examination** and also involves confirming the **clinical problem** or articulating the **wellness goals**, creating a summary of clinical findings, and deciding whether to pursue treatment.

The steps in the treatment planning phase involve identifying body structures and functions that are appropriate for treatment, and selecting treatment techniques

Evaluation
1. Review the client's reason for seeking treatment
2. Conduct the subjective and objective client examination
3. Analyze findings and confirm the client's presenting issue

Treatment planning
4. Identify client impairments/wellness goals and specify outcomes
5. Select appropriate treatment techniques and create plan of care

Treatment
6. Deliver the treatment outlined in the plan of care
7. Conduct client re-examination and modify treatment (ongoing)

Discharge
8. Identify client's discharge needs and formulate discharge plan
9. Discharge the client when appropriate outcomes are met

FIGURE 5-1 Outcome-Based Massage™ clinical decision-making process.

that will produce improvements in the client's impairments in body structures and functions, functional limitations, or overall wellness.[8] The treatment planning phase for Outcome-Based Massage™ begins with the summary of clinical findings from the evaluation phase and ends with a written **plan of care**.

The treatment phase is an ongoing cycle of treatment, **re-examination**, and treatment progression that begins after the therapist completes the plan of care. The end of this phase is not clearly delineated; instead, there is a gradual transition from treatment phase to discharge phase.

The final phase is the discharge phase. **Discharge** involves the transition of the client from the therapist's care to self-care or to treatment by another therapist. The discharge phase begins before the client's discharge date; it spans the period from the initiation of discharge planning to the actual discharge date.

Outcome-Based Massage™ Clinical Decision-Making for Wellness versus Medical Massage

Therapists can use the four-phase Outcome-Based Massage™ clinical decision-making process for both medical massage and wellness massage, although interventions for wellness and the treatment of **impairments** differ in several ways (Table 5-1). Massage for both the treatment of impairments in body structure and function following a clinical condition and wellness require a clinical reasoning process

in which therapists perform a systematic client examination and establish outcomes to guide the intervention.

For Outcome-Based Massage™ clinical decision-making, the primary distinction between medical massage and wellness massage is whether or not the focus of **treatment** is on an impairment in the client's body structure or function. Medical massage, the treatment of impairments, takes place after an individual has experienced a clinical condition. Clients' impairments can be any loss or abnormality of the client's body structures or functions that occur as a result of the **pathophysiology** of a clinical condition.[5,9] The aim of medical massage is to reduce the impairments associated with clinical conditions. During the Outcome-Based Massage™ clinical decision-making process, the therapist creates a list of impairments and a list of outcomes that are focused on the treatment of primary impairments, **recovery**, and the prevention of **secondary impairments**.

This is in contrast to wellness massage, in which the client does not present with impairments in body structures and function that are secondary to a clinical condition. Instead, the client has several body structures and functions that are free of impairments and goals for wellness. The aim of wellness massage is to achieve the client's wellness goals in the absence of impairments in body structure or function. During the Outcome-Based Massage™ clinical decision-making process, the therapist will examine these structures and functions to ensure that they are free of impairments prior to embarking on a wellness intervention that targets these areas. Then the

Table 5-1	**Comparison of Interventions for Medical Massage and Wellness Massage**	
	Treatment of Impairments	**Wellness Interventions**
Timing of intervention	■ After the clinical condition occurs	■ At any time in the individual's life
Focus of intervention	■ Signs and symptoms of the clinical condition ■ Impairments in body structures and functions with grades 1–4	■ Body structures and functions with impairments of grade 0 (no impairment)
Client examination	■ Examine body structures and functions ■ Identify impairments resulting from the clinical condition	■ Examine body structures and functions ■ Identify body structures and functions that are relevant to the individual's goals for wellness
Overall goal of intervention	■ Identify and manage impairments resulting from the clinical condition	■ Optimize well-being across physical, mental, spiritual, and social domains
Clinical reasoning process	■ Complete clinical reasoning process	■ Complete clinical reasoning process
Outcomes	■ Specified outcomes related to identified impairments in body structures and functions ■ Based on specific therapeutic effects of massage	■ Specified outcomes related to identified body structures and functions ■ Based on specific therapeutic effects of massage

therapist will create a list of those body structures and functions that are related to the client's wellness goals and determine outcomes for optimizing these structures and function.

Of note is that despite this distinction between the treatment of impairments and wellness interventions, in day-to-day practice, many therapists call the treatment of stress-related disorders wellness. By definition, this treatment of stress-related disorders, such as anxiety or increased muscle tension, is the treatment of impairments, whereas stress-management interventions that prevent impairments and optimize function are "wellness" interventions.

The clinical case of the client with neck pain, later in this chapter, will illustrate the detailed steps in Outcome-Based Massage™ clinical decision-making for the treatment of a clinical condition. Readers can apply this information on the distinction between clinical decision-making for treatment of impairments versus wellness interventions to arrive at the guidelines for the latter.

EVALUATION PHASE

We cannot emphasize the importance of the evaluation phase enough. When a client presents for clinical care it is often because she has a problem. Through the client examination and the **evaluation** of the clinical findings, the therapist clarifies the client's clinical problem and identifies the client's relevant impairments and functional limitations. She will then use this information for outcome identification and treatment planning. Consequently, an appropriate, accurate, and comprehensive evaluation phase can enhance the potential effectiveness of an intervention.

Review Treatment Reason and Conduct Subjective and Objective Client Examination (Steps 1 and 2)

The evaluation phase begins with a review of the client's reason for seeking treatment since the latter will provide a focus for the client examination. The client examination follows and involves collecting information on the client's health status and clinical condition through history-taking, a general systems review, and tests and measures.[9] Therapist and client characteristics can influence the scope of the examination a therapist performs. Relevant therapist characteristics include her scope of practice, her area of specialization, and the type of examination she selects. Client characteristics include the client's diagnosis, general health status, the nature of the clinical setting, and the acuity, severity, complexity, and stability of the client's condition (see Table 5-2). The initial multidisciplinary neurologic examination for a geriatric client with Parkinson's disease in an inpatient setting, for example, would be broader in scope and cover the issues in more detail than an interim examination of an adolescent with chondromalacia patellae in an outpatient orthopedic clinic.

Conduct Subjective Examination

Prior to taking the client history, the therapist identifies whether or not there is a specific diagnosis on the client's referral. If there is a specific diagnosis, then the therapist's **history-taking** and **subjective examination** will include questions relating to that diagnosis and will focus on eliciting information to confirm or refute the client's presenting diagnosis. If, on the other hand, the client has a referral without a **medical diagnosis**, the therapist begins by eliciting general information that will serve to clarify the client's presenting problem and suggest a clinical diagnosis. Chapter 4 provides suggestions for issues to consider in history-taking for massage. Therapists can document the client's history within the written plan of care or separately.

Generate Preliminary Clinical Hypothesis

Existing clinical decision-making processes all include some form of data gathering and the formulation and testing of a clinical hypothesis.[1-4,8] In the current process, the therapist forms a preliminary clinical hypothesis about the client's presenting issues, based on the diagnosis on the client's referral and the information she has gathered from the history and subjective examination. This clinical hypothesis helps the therapist select appropriate tests and measures and provides a focus for the client examination. The following are some pointers for avoiding common errors in generating and using clinical hypotheses in the client examination.

- Generate a few possible hypotheses about the client's clinical problem early in the examination as a guide.[3,4]
- Have less than three hypotheses so that you can use a focused set of tests and measures.
- Avoid making hypotheses very general so that they will fit inconsistent findings.
- Include both objective data and information on the clients' perception of their clinical condition and functional limitations.[2]

Table 5-2   Scope and Content of Client Examinations

	Initial Examination	Interim Examination or Re-examination	Discharge Examination	Follow-Up Examination
Scope	■ Detailed exploratory examination	■ Focused examination related to the identified outcomes related to impairments and functional limitations	■ Detailed examination related to the intervention provided and the outcomes related to impairments and functional limitations the client has achieved	■ Focused examination related to (a) the maintenance of previously achieved outcomes related to impairments and functional limitations or (b) the identification of ongoing treatment needs
Timing	■ Performed prior to the initiation of treatment	■ Performed at intervals following the initiation of treatment	■ Performed at the end of the intervention period and prior to discharge of the client	■ Performed following discharge from an episode of care
Objectives	■ Confirm or refute the client's presenting diagnosis ■ Identify and measure the client's impairments, functional limitations, and functional areas to provide a basis for treatment planning and a baseline for interim examinations ■ Identify and measure the client's prior and presenting level of function to provide a basis for identifying reasonable functional outcomes	■ Identify and measure changes in the client's impairments and functional level from the baseline established at the initial examination ■ Determine the client's achievement of outcomes ■ Determine the client's readiness for treatment progression ■ Determine the need to modify the plan of care or outcomes	■ Determine the client's readiness for discharge through measurement of progress on outcomes ■ Identify and measure client's discharge needs ■ Identify and measure changes in the client's impairments and functional level from the baseline established at the initial examination	■ Identify and measure changes in the client's health status, impairments, and functional level from the baseline established at the most recent discharge examination ■ Determine client's level of safety and adaptation to their environment ■ Determine client's ongoing treatment needs
Components	■ History to elicit information to confirm or refute the presenting diagnosis or to establish a diagnosis if none is given ■ Tests and measures to (a) confirm or refute the presenting diagnosis or to establish a diagnosis if none is given (b) Identify and measure impairments and functional limitations	■ Tests and measures to determine changes in impairments and functional limitations	■ History to summarize treatment ■ Discussion of the client's perceived discharge needs ■ Tests and measures to determine client's impairments and functional level at discharge	■ History to elicit information on changes in health status, safety, and adaptation to the environment ■ Tests and measures to determine changes in impairments and functional limitations

- Be selective in the data that gathered and use the referring diagnosis as a guide when possible.
- Be flexible and depart from a standard examination framework to seek clarification on issues that arise during the examination.
- Stay focused on the main clinical hypothesis to prevent becoming overwhelmed by a large amount of irrelevant data.
- Avoid exaggerating findings to justify an existing hypothesis.
- Be willing to acknowledge that an existing hypothesis is incorrect and seek a new hypothesis.

Conduct Objective Examination

Observe Client

Once the therapist has formed her preliminary clinical hypothesis, she observes the client to identify observational cues that may support her hypothesis. At this early stage of the examination, the therapist needs to avoid having too narrow a focus. The observation of the client should be general enough to provide data that may suggest an alternative hypothesis, yet still enable the therapist to identify specific clinical signs that are consistent with the hypothesis. This observation can include postural alignment, muscle bulk and contours, and other areas outlined in chapter 4 and the individual techniques chapters. Based on her observations, the therapist may be able to refine her hypothesis about the client's clinical problem.

Select Tests and Measures

The therapist then proceeds to the next step in gathering data to confirm or refute her clinical hypothesis: the selection and application of **tests and measures**. The types of tests and measures, and the order in which the therapist conducts them, will differ with the client's characteristics and condition. In other words, therapists use different examination approaches for clients with neurologic, musculoskeletal, cardiopulmonary, or psychoneuroimmunologic conditions. For example, a musculoskeletal examination may consist of postural analysis, visual inspection, range of motion testing, muscle performance testing, and palpation. By contrast, a cardiopulmonary examination may consist of visual inspection, palpation, and percussion. Additional modifications exist for examinations of adult, pediatric, and geriatric clients.

The selection of appropriate tests and measures is one of the most difficult components of the examination. The problem lies not in a lack of information, but in the possibility of being overwhelmed by the considerable number of possible special tests and clinical signs. The therapist faces the challenge of recalling appropriate examination techniques, noting the client's response, and making a correct interpretation of the findings. Having one or two hypotheses about the client's problem can assist the therapist in refining her choice of examination techniques.

Examine the Client

To keep data at a manageable level, the therapist may find it effective to first select and carry out a few tests that therapists commonly used to confirm or refute a given condition. If the findings are positive, the therapist can then collect more general information about the client's impairments, functional limitations, and areas of function. If the findings from these confirmatory tests are negative, the therapist can decide whether she needs additional tests or to change her hypotheses. In situations in which the therapist does not have a clear clinical hypothesis, scanning examinations provide a means of quickly determining the integrity of several systems and assessing the nature of the client's symptoms.[10] Chapter 4 provides information on some examination techniques for massage that the reader can use to guide her selection of examination techniques.

Analyze Findings and Confirm the Client's Presenting Issue (Step 3)

Confirm the Clinical Hypothesis

At the conclusion of her client examination, the therapist analyzes the impairments stemming from the client's clinical condition and either confirms or refutes her clinical hypothesis. Some health-care professions call the process and result of analyzing and organizing the findings from the client examination into clusters or syndromes the **therapy diagnosis**.[9] If the findings from the client examination do not support the therapist's clinical hypothesis, she will have to re-formulate her hypothesis and repeat the process of selecting and carrying out appropriate tests and measures. There are situations in which the client may not present with a clearly defined clinical condition. In that case, it may be appropriate for the therapist to focus the treatment planning process on the general goal of improving the client's presenting impairments and functional limitations, rather than on identifying and treating a specific clinical condition.[9]

Summarize Pertinent Clinical Findings

Once the therapist confirms her clinical hypothesis, she produces a summary of the impairments and functional limitations with which the client presents. This summary can be documented within the written plan of care or separately. In Outcome-Based Massage™, as with other clinical approaches, failure to identify the impairments that are contributing to the client's functional limitations can lead to the development of an intervention that is not effective in achieving the established **functional outcomes**. In the clinical example, had the therapist assumed that the client was presenting with functional limitations secondary to a radiculopathy, he would have provided a regimen that would not have relieved the client's symptoms nor improved the client's functional level.

Determine Appropriateness for Treatment

Not all clients who receive a referral for treatment will actually require treatment. Therapists must, therefore, review the findings from the client examination and determine whether the client would benefit from treatment such as the direct application of treatment techniques, and education, and coordination of services. Once the therapist has confirmed that treatment is appropriate, and before beginning treatment planning, she needs to determine whether she has a **legal right to treat** and the **clinical competence to treat** the client's clinical condition.

Legal Right to Treat

Legal right to treat refers to whether the clinician's professional scope of practice includes the treatment of the client's clinical problem, the examination techniques, and the treatment techniques which the clinician wishes to use. Professional scope of practice is dictated by the laws of the jurisdiction in which the clinician practices. Health-care professions have practice acts that protect public health and safety by regulating the qualifications, registration, and discipline of members of the profession. For each profession, these practice acts outline the qualifications; licensing or registration requirements; treatments that can be applied by, grounds for discipline; and sanctions that will be applied to violators of the practice act. Legal right to treat can be a gray area where the practice of massage is concerned. Clinicians from a range of health-care professions can use some massage techniques within their scope of practice without advanced training or certification, while others cannot. For example athletic trainers, massage therapists, nurses, occupational therapists, physical therapists, chiropractors, and other bodyworkers can

incorporate superficial reflex techniques, such as stroking applied to facilitate relaxation, into the interventions for clients with a variety of clinical conditions. By contrast, the application of manual lymph drainage techniques for the management of lymphedema may be outside the scope of practice of several of these health-care professionals. In addition, the clinician needs to determine whether the client has other therapeutic needs that a clinician from a different health-care profession could address more appropriately. This situation would warrant a referral to that health-care professional for treatment of those clinical problems that are outside of the clinician's scope of practice. In light of the complexity of issues related to the scope of practice, clinicians need to consult the practice acts for their professions to determine their legal right to use massage techniques for the different clinical conditions they encounter in clinical practice.

Ethical Right to Treat

In addition to legal issues related to right to treat, the therapist also has to make an ethical decision regarding her competence to treat the client's presenting clinical problems. This is a subjective decision that requires a balance of confidence in one's clinical skills and an objective assessment of the limitations of one's clinical expertise. In other words, it is not sufficient that the therapist's practice act permits the provision of interventions for a condition or the application of selected techniques; the therapist must also have sufficient training to administer this care appropriately, safely, and effectively.

TREATMENT PLANNING PHASE

The treatment planning phase is the critical point in Outcome-Based Massage™ clinical decision-making at which the therapist consolidates examination findings into the clinical problem list and uses the latter as the basis for establishing the treatment outcomes that will form the foundation of the intervention.

Identify Client Problems/Wellness Goals and Specify Relevant Outcomes (Step 4)

Analyze Findings and Generate the Clinical Problem List

Before the therapist can begin selecting treatment techniques, she needs to organize the clinical findings on the client's impairments and functional limitations into a **clinical problem list** to guide treatment planning. First of all, it is important for the therapist to distinguish between the client's areas of function and dysfunction or those areas that will respond to the direct application of treatment techniques and those that will not. Rather than dismissing areas of function because they do not require treatment, the therapist is wise to identify which of these areas she can use to compensate for impairments that are not amenable to active treatment. An example of this strategy occurs later in this chapter.

Once the therapist has identified the areas of dysfunction, it is important for her to differentiate between the client's impairments and functional limitations. Impairment can be any loss or abnormality of the client's body structures or functions, while functional limitations refer to the individual's ability to execute tasks within his environment.[11] The strategy used in treatment planning for Outcome-Based Massage™ will be to select treatment techniques to treat the identified impairments and to use the identified functional limitations as a baseline for setting functional outcomes. Once the therapist completes these tasks, she can compile the clinical problem list.

Identify Functional Outcomes

The therapist can now focus on identifying relevant functional outcomes in collaboration with the client and predicting the amount of time needed to achieve these outcomes. These outcomes should be consistent with the functional limitations that she documented during the client examination. Table 1-5 gives examples of functional outcomes. The therapist will base the outcomes and the time needed to achieve them on several factors:

- The client's current and prior level of function
- The severity, complexity, stability, and acuity of the client's condition
- The client's discharge destination
- The literature on the prognosis for an individual with that condition
- The therapist's judgment, from clinical experience, of what the client has the potential to achieve[9]

In addition, therapists can seek guidance from articles on clinical practice and research in professional journals, clinical texts, general practice guidelines for professions, or the numerous practice guidelines that are available for specific clinical conditions. In some health-care professions, this process of predicting the client's level and timing of improvement is known as the **therapy prognosis**.[9]

It is not sufficient to identify the long-term functional outcomes for the client; the therapist must also identify short-term outcomes and predict what level of improvement the client can achieve in a given time frame. This is necessary because while long-term functional outcomes are useful for gauging the client's readiness for discharge, they are of little value in evaluating the client's immediate and ongoing response to treatment. A short-term outcome that the client can achieve within a few sessions provides a useful early benchmark of the effectiveness of the intervention and can be an invaluable aid to the ongoing modification and progression of treatment. The time period for achieving these short-term outcomes will vary with the acuity, severity, complexity, and stability of the client's condition; the expected rate of change in the client's functional level; the frequency of interventions; the anticipated duration of the treatment; and the clinical setting. The therapist's goal is to set outcomes in measurable and meaningful increments that the client can reasonably achieve in the allocated time period. It may be appropriate, for example, to set weekly, or even daily, outcomes for a client in an acute care or outpatient setting whom she expects to have significant functional gains over a short course of treatment. By contrast, monthly outcomes may be more meaningful for a geriatric client in a skilled nursing setting who receives treatment for a chronic condition.

A common question is: "How can the therapist determine whether the functional outcomes are appropriate for massage?" In reality, the issue is whether the impairments that the therapist must address to achieve the functional outcome are appropriate for treatment with the use of massage as the primary treatment technique. This decision about the relevance of the impairments for massage comes later in this phase of the decision-making process.

Identify Treatable Impairments and Relevant Outcomes

Once the therapist has established functional outcomes, she works backward to identify the following:

- Which impairments need to be treated to facilitate the achievement of the functional outcomes
- Which of these impairments are amenable to active treatment
- Which impairments require compensations because they are not amenable to active treatment
- The **impairment-related outcome** for each impairment that she will treat

Traditionally, therapists established treatment goals and selected treatment techniques based solely on the impairments that they observed during the client examination. The adoption of models of functioning, disability, and health in health care has expanded this focus to include the impact of treatment on clients' body structures, body functions, their level of activity, and functional limitations.[11] Therapists now identify and treat clients' underlying impairments and address their level of activity and functional limitations. What remains unclear is whether there is a direct relationship between improved impairments and improvements in functional level. A balanced approach to treatment planning is to identify and treat the client's impairments as a means of facilitating the achievement of the functional outcomes, rather than focusing solely on impairments or functional limitations.

Although the therapist will use the identified functional outcomes as the primary means of judging the client's progress, it is still beneficial for her to identify outcomes related to impairments. The therapist can then use the client's progress, or lack thereof, on the outcomes related to the client's impairments as a basis for determining whether the client is responding to the treatment techniques that she is applying. Table 1-4 contains some examples of outcomes related to impairments.

Plan Compensatory Strategies

The therapist also distinguishes between the impairments that are amenable to active treatment and those for which she must plan a means of compensation. The clinical scenario of the client with myofascial cervical pain is admittedly a straightforward one in which all of the client's impairments are amenable to active treatment. A more complex case would be, for example, a 65-year-old who is 3 months post a right-sided cerebrovascular accident. The therapists treating this client have identified a left drop foot, left-sided weakness, primitive movement patterns, increased tone in the trunk and involved extremities, painful left shoulder subluxation, and edema in the left hand as the primary impairments. Of these, the drop foot has shown no further signs of recovery and no longer appears amenable to active treatment. Consequently, the therapists do further examination to rule out a peripheral nerve injury or other localized damage to the tibialis anterior muscle. They then consider the drop foot to be an impairment for which they can use a **compensatory strategy** of an ankle–foot orthosis and ambulatory aids. The therapists can also use one of the client's available functional areas to compensate for this impairment in addition to using external orthoses and devices. An example is gait training in the use of the more functional pelvic and lower extremity muscle groups to compensate for the drop foot during ambulation.

Select Appropriate Treatment Techniques and Create Plan of Care (Step 5)

Identify Impairments Appropriate for Massage Techniques

In Outcome-Based Massage™ clinical decision-making, the treatment planning phase also includes the identification of those impairments that are most appropriate for the application of massage techniques. The therapist bases this decision on her knowledge of the expected outcomes of massage techniques and whether massage techniques can have a direct or secondary effect on the impairment. There are three possible options: massage has a **direct effect** on the impairment; massage has a **secondary effect** on the impairment; and massage has no effect on the impairment. Identifying between massage techniques that have a direct effect on the impairment and those that do not assists the therapist in creating an intervention that will result in improved functional outcomes and prioritizing treatment techniques within an intervention. If the massage technique has no documented or demonstrated effect on the impairment, the therapist has little justification for including it in the intervention. Table 1-4 presents a general summary of expected outcomes of massage techniques to assist the therapist in determining when it is appropriate to treat an impairment using massage techniques.

Since the decision regarding the relevance of impairments for massage is a critical one, here are further examples of how clinicians can make this decision. Consider the case of a client who presents with the impairments of pain, adhesions, and decreased muscle extensibility in the later stages of therapy following surgical repair of the Achilles tendon. The clinician can use connective tissue techniques to increase muscle extensibility and promote remodeling of dense connective tissue. Consequently, massage techniques are appropriate as primary treatment techniques for adhesions and decreased muscle extensibility. In this situation, the massage technique will have a direct effect on the impairment and the clinician can use other techniques in a complementary manner.

There are also circumstances in which massage techniques can have a secondary or indirect effect on an impairment, for example a client who presents with decreased muscle performance secondary to pain, guarding, and muscle spasm following the reduction of a glenohumeral dislocation. In this situation, the clinician can use superficial reflex techniques to reduce pain, guarding, and muscle spasm and thus facilitate improvements in muscle performance. If a massage technique has a secondary effect on the impairment, the clinician may choose to use that technique in a complementary manner within the intervention. In this case, the primary treatment techniques would be therapeutic exercise. Finally, if the client presented with the impairment of muscle weakness secondary to a peripheral neuropathy, then the impairment would not be appropriate for massage because massage techniques do not have a documented effect on neurologically based muscle weakness. Once the therapist has identified which impairments are appropriate for treatment with massage, he is able to proceed to treatment selection.

Select Treatment Techniques

Once the therapist has identified the impairments for which massage techniques have a direct effect or secondary effect, she can proceed with selecting the techniques she will use in the intervention. The therapist matches appropriate massage techniques to impairments by considering three factors:

1. Match of expected outcome, related to impairments, of the massage technique to the client's impairment
2. Identification of **contraindications** or **cautions** in the application of that technique given the client's clinical condition
3. The therapist's legal right and competence to use the technique

The chapters on massage techniques describe the expected outcomes of each massage technique to assist therapists in selecting massage techniques.

Simply matching impairments to the outcomes of massage techniques is not, however, sufficient to guarantee that a technique is appropriate for that client's condition. Before performing any massage technique, the therapist needs to consider the general cautions and contraindications to the application of that technique for the client's clinical condition (Table 5-3).[12-25] The techniques chapters cover the relevant clinical considerations, cautions, and contraindications for specific massage techniques.

While this list is a necessary starting point for the consideration of cautions and contraindications to treatment, the therapist should also use her judgment about the application of massage techniques to the client at

hand. A useful rule of thumb is that if a client's condition requires ongoing management by another health-care professional, then it is appropriate for the therapist to consult that health-care professional for guidelines regarding cautions and contraindications to treatment.

The therapist also needs to consider whether there are any anatomical structures that can be damaged during the application of massage techniques.[12-26] For example, the application of friction or specific compression over a peripheral nerve in a location where it is close to the skin may produce a neuropraxia.[27] While some sources describe '**Endangerment Sites**' (see Table 5-4) as areas of the human body over which the use of direct or sustained pressure is contraindicated,[12,28] the therapist may also use her judgment in determining whether these areas are contraindicated for other massage techniques. Students and novice therapists who are not experienced in applying treatment techniques should take a conservative approach to applying massage techniques in "Endangerment Sites" and situations in which there are specific cautions or contraindications to the use of a technique.

Generate the Plan of Care

It is unlikely that a plan of care will consist only of massage techniques. The therapist must also select other treatment techniques such as therapeutic exercise, electrotherapeutic modalities, education, and training on functional activity, which she will need to use in order to achieve the identified outcomes. These treatment techniques will vary depending on the scope of practice of the health-care professionals.

A list of treatment techniques does not constitute a plan of care; the therapist also needs to specify and document the treatment parameters within the client's written plan of care. The duration of the episode of care (the current treatment period) and the frequency of interventions should be consistent with the severity, stability, complexity, and acuity of the client's clinical condition; the client's treatment tolerance; the client's prognosis; and the identified outcomes. Other factors that can influence the duration of care and frequency of treatment sessions include the client's cognitive status, pre-existing conditions, potential discharge destination, overall health status, and probability of prolonged impairment.[9] The therapist must also determine the scope, frequency, and duration of the massage techniques in the intervention. Chapter 14 provides further information about these issues. Finally, the therapist also needs to consider the client's home or work environment, social context, and personal goals for treatment to ensure that the intervention

Table 5-3	Suggested Cautions and Contraindications for Reflex and Mechanical Massage Techniques[12-28]

Local Conditions

Contraindications

- Acute flare-up of inflammatory arthritis: rheumatoid arthritis, systemic lupus, Reiter's syndrome, etc.
- Acute neuritis
- Aneurysms
- Areas of altered or impaired sensation
- Baker's cyst
- Ectopic pregnancy
- Esophageal varicosities
- Frostbite
- Local contagious skin condition
- Local infection
- Local irritable skin condition
- Malignancy
- Open wound or sore
- Peripheral neuropathy
- Phlebitis, thrombophlebitis, and arteritis
- Post anti-inflammatory injection (24–48 h)
- Recent burns
- Undiagnosed lump

Cautions

- Acute disk herniation
- Acute inflammatory condition
- Allergies to lubricants and cleansers
- Anti-inflammatory injection site
- Buerger's disease
- Chronic abdominal or digestive disease
- Chronic arthritic conditions
- Chronic diarrhea
- Chronic or longstanding superficial thrombosis
- Contusion
- Endometriosis
- Flaccid paralysis
- Fracture—while casted and immediately post cast removal
- Hernia
- Joint instability or hypermobility
- Kidney infection or stones
- Mastitis
- Minor surgery
- Pelvic inflammatory disease
- Pitting edema
- Portal hypertension
- Presence of pins and staples
- Prolonged constipation
- Recent abortion or vaginal birth
- Trigeminal neuralgia

General Conditions

Contraindications

- Acute conditions requiring first aid: anaphylaxis, epileptic seizure, pneumothorax, myocardial infarction, syncope, status asthmaticus, cerebrovascular accident, diabetic coma, insulin shock, appendicitis
- Advanced kidney failure[a]
- Advanced respiratory failure[a]
- Anemia (depending on the cause)[a]
- Diabetes with complications[a]
- Eclampsia
- Hemophilia[a]
- Hemorrhage
- Highly metastatic cancers
- Intoxication
- Liver failure[a]
- Sepsis
- Severe atherosclerosis[a]
- Shock
- Significant fever (>101.5°F or 38.3°C)
- Systemic contagious/infectious condition
- Unstabilized cerebrovascular accident
- Unstable hypertension
- Unstabilized myocardial infarction

Cautions

- Asthma
- Atherosclerosis
- Cancer
- Chronic congestive heart failure
- Chronic kidney disease
- Client taking medications that alter neurological, cardiovascular, psychological, or kidney function
- Coma
- Drug withdrawal
- Emphysema
- Epilepsy
- Hypertension
- Hypotension
- Immunosuppression
- Inflammatory arthritis
- Major or abdominal surgery
- Multiple sclerosis
- Osteoporosis
- Post-cerebrovascular accident
- Post-myocardial infarction
- Pregnancy and labor
- Psychiatric conditions
- Recent head injury
- Spasticity or rigidity

[a]Skilled clinicians with advanced training may consider these to be cautions, rather than contraindications.

Table 5-4	Selected Endangerment Sites[12,13,15]	
Head and Neck	**Trunk**	**Extremities**
■ Neck, including anterior and posterior triangle	■ Axilla	■ Ulnar nerve at medial epicondyle
■ Eye	■ Xiphoid process	■ Femoral artery, nerve, and vein in the area of the inguinal triangle
■ Trachea	■ 12th (floating) rib	
■ Styloid process of the temporal bone	■ Kidneys in the area of the 12th rib	
	■ Umbilicus	
	■ Linea alba	
	■ Sciatic notch	

adequately addresses these factors. Failure to do so may have a negative impact on the level of the client's adherence with self-care and participation in the plan of care.

TREATMENT PHASE

With the plan of care in hand, the therapist embarks on the treatment phase. This is an ongoing cycle of treatment and client re-examination, in which the findings of the client examinations are used to modify and progress the treatment regimen.

Deliver the Treatment Outlined in the Plan of Care (Step 6)

Select Treatment and Re-examination Techniques

The therapist is ready to initiate treatment once she has completed the plan of care. First of all, she selects a subset of the prioritized massage and **complementary treatment techniques** from the plan of care as a starting point. The aims of the first stage of treatment are to gauge the client's treatment tolerance and to ascertain whether the treatment techniques can affect the client's impairments. It is, therefore, advisable for the therapist to select those techniques that are most likely to have a direct effect. At the outset of the episode of care, the therapist also identifies which subjective and objective examination techniques she can use to determine whether the client is having a positive response to treatment. In doing so, she includes questions that seek the client's perspective on her progress and the intervention. This information is invaluable since these factors can signal problems that the client is having with the intervention and can provide the therapist with

guidance on how to improve client adherence to or participation in the plan of care.

Carry Out Initial Intervention

As mentioned above, during the first stage of treatment the therapist is evaluating the appropriateness of the plan of care and gauging the client's treatment tolerance. She bases the intensity of the interventions on the level of acuity of the client's condition, using less intense treatments for a more acutely ill client and vice versa. In addition, she is cautious not to introduce too many treatment techniques at once since that will make it difficult for her to identify the techniques to which the client had a positive or adverse response. The therapist also conducts formal and informal client examinations to determine the client's response to treatment.

Conduct Client Re-examination and Modify Treatment (Step 7)

Conduct Client Re-examination

The therapist can perform informal client examinations at any time during the interventions. Palpation and the massage techniques themselves can provide information on the client's response to the technique the therapist is applying and to the intervention as a whole (see Chapter 4). These informal examinations can be interspersed throughout the interventions. Once the client has reached a point at which the therapist can reasonably expect a measurable clinical change, the therapist carries out a more formal re-examination using the tests and measures she selected for this purpose. This re-examination focuses on the identification and measurement of changes in the client's impairments and functional level from the baseline established at the initial examination.

Assess Client Progress

The therapist uses the re-examination as a means of determining the client's progress toward the achievement of the identified outcomes and the client's readiness for treatment progression. She can also use this information as the basis for her decision on whether to modify the plan of care or the identified outcomes.

Address Lack of Change

If the result of the client re-examination is that the client does not demonstrate any clinical change, the therapist must first determine whether it may be too early to observe a change. If this is the case, she re-attempts treatment with the original set of techniques and may consider the addition of another treatment technique before the next formal re-examination. If, however, the therapist believes that the client has had ample time to demonstrate a clinical change, then the therapist must re-evaluate the appropriateness of the plan of care. Possible causes for the client's failure to respond to interventions for the therapist to consider are an incorrect clinical hypothesis, an inappropriate treatment technique, or an incorrect application of a technique. If the therapist's clinical hypothesis was incorrect, she will need to revisit the evaluation phase and repeat the client examination to identify the client's clinical condition. The therapist can remedy the choice of inappropriate treatment techniques by selecting more appropriate techniques and modifying the plan of care. Finally, if the therapist's choice of clinical hypothesis and treatment techniques appears to be accurate, then she needs to refine her application of the treatment techniques.

Progress Plan of Care and Assess Progress through Re-examination

Once the therapist is confident that the direction of the plan of care is appropriate, then the cycle of treatment progression and informal or formal re-examination begins. Throughout this cycle, the therapist ensures that she assesses both the client's impairments and functional level at appropriate intervals. Ideally, each intervention should incorporate an element of informal examination and progression or modification of either the treatment techniques or client education. Chapter 14 "Designing Interventions and Discharge Planning" discusses these issues in greater detail. During the application of each treatment technique,

the therapist informally evaluates the client's response and uses this information to fine tune the intervention and her application of treatment techniques. The therapist can also use these informal examinations to identify when the client has a flare-up of her clinical condition that results in an increase in her impairments and functional limitations. The timing of formal examinations of the client's progress on functional outcomes will depend on the time frames that the therapist has defined for those outcomes.

DISCHARGE PHASE

The therapist and client gradually transition into the discharge phase as the end of the treatment regimen draws close. During this phase, the activities that occur during treatment sessions shift in emphasis from the therapist delivering care to the client performing self-care.

Identify Client's Discharge Needs and Formulate Discharge Plan (Step 8)

Identify Postdischarge Needs

There is, unfortunately, no exact formula to use for determining when to initiate the discharge process. Consequently, the therapist can initiate discharge planning as early as the first session or much later in the treatment process. There are many factors that can influence the therapist's decision on when to begin the discharge phase. First of all, the therapist must also consider the client's characteristics such as the client's progress with her functional outcomes, her psychological and educational readiness for discharge, and the resources needed and available to the client following discharge. In addition, the therapist cannot ignore the constraints to discharge planning imposed by the nature of the clinical setting and the predicted length of the episode of care. For example, in cases 5-1 to 5-4 clinical scenario, the therapist can begin discharge planning in earlier sessions because of the relative brevity of the client's course of treatment. While one can argue that every intervention is preparing the client for discharge, there are specific activities that are associated with facilitating an effective discharge.

Initiate Postdischarge Education and Referrals

As the client approaches achievement of 75% of her functional outcomes, the therapist needs to initiate a discussion of the client's discharge concerns and needs. This may occur earlier if the client appears to have complex needs that will require more discharge planning or the clinical setting dictates shorter **episodes of care**. Although the therapist may not be able to address all of the client's discharge needs, a complete list of discharge needs is valuable for planning self-care education, referrals to other health-care professionals, and other client resources.

By the time the client is close to achieving her functional outcomes, the therapist should have initiated referrals, identified equipment needs and initiated purchases, finalized the content of home programs, and begun discharge self-care education. The emphasis of the final sessions prior to discharge will shift to include a larger educational component. Chapter 2 also discusses the psychological preparation of the client for discharge. If the therapist refers the client to another health-care professional, for example, a sub-acute unit or home health care, the discharge process will also include written and verbal communication with the other therapists.

Discharge Client When Appropriate Outcomes Are Met (Step 9)

Progress Plan of Care and Determine Readiness for Discharge

As the client approaches the final stages of treatment, the therapist ensures that she has appropriately completed the progression of the various components of the plan of care. She uses the results of her ongoing client re-examinations to guide the rate at which she progresses interventions. These clinical findings also indicate when the client has achieved 90% of her functional outcomes.

Finalize Discharge Plans and Review Home Program

As the client nears completion of the course of treatment, the therapist ensures that the client is competent in her postdischarge self-care program. She also confirms that she has finalized all postdischarge arrangements.

Conduct Discharge Examination and Discharge Client

The final, or discharge, client examination provides the therapist with a confirmation of the client's readiness for discharge. It is also a record of the status of the client's impairments and functional level at the time of discharge.

Special Discharge Issues

Can you discharge a client if he has not met the outcomes defined for his intervention? There is much discussion and controversy about whether clinicians can terminate treatment for reasons other than the clients' achievement of their clinical outcomes such as the end of reimbursement or the client's request. Ideally, the clinician will use the extent to which the client achieves his clinical outcomes as the guide for discharge. There are circumstances, however, in which the client need not meet the established functional outcomes before discharge. These situations include the following:

- When the clinician recognizes that the outcomes were not achievable given the client's condition and health status
- When the client's functional level reaches a plateau before achieving the outcomes but he carries out his daily activities sufficiently to justify discharge
- When the client is unable to progress toward the outcomes because of medical or psychological complications
- When the client refuses ongoing treatment
- When the clinician or client believes that the client cannot benefit from further treatment[9]

Ultimately, the clinician must use her clinical judgment, input from the client, and examination findings to guide decisions about the timing of discharge. In all situations, appropriate documentation of the rationale for discharge is necessary.

Another concern is whether you can justifiably continue to treat a client after he has met the identified outcomes. If the client's clinical outcomes were consistent with the severity, complexity, stability, and acuity of his clinical condition, then the clinician cannot ethically justify ongoing treatment. If a clinician is uncertain whether treatment should end, she should re-evaluate the client's clinical outcomes within the context of her scope of practice. This will assist her in determining whether the client has ongoing therapeutic needs that she can address or whether she needs to refer the client to another health-care professional for care.

ONGOING CARE

Therapists must modify the four-phase clinical decision-making process for clients who require ongoing episodes of care because of their clinical condition or the nature of their clinical care. Clients who require ongoing episodes of care include the following:

- Pediatric clients with developmental disabilities
- Clients with chronic or terminal conditions who are at risk for deterioration of health status
- Geriatric clients who are at risk for falls or deterioration of health status
- Clients who have ongoing disability and health-care needs as a result of spinal cord injury, head injury, amputation, or other traumatic injury
- Clients who are receiving wellness interventions

The clinical decision-making process does not end at the discharge phase when a client requires ongoing episodes of care. First of all, the therapist's discharge planning must include organization, or at the very least a discussion, of the follow-up care. Second, the therapist must plan and implement a follow-up client examination and thus initiate the evaluation phase once more.

The follow-up examination (see Table 5-2) is a focused client examination in which the therapist determines whether the client has demonstrated a deterioration of impairments or functional level since the prior examination. Based on the clinical findings she obtains from this examination, the therapist identifies whether the client has new treatment needs. If the client does not require ongoing care, the therapist documents this finding and organizes further follow-up if warranted. On the other hand, if the client does demonstrate a deterioration in status, the therapist initiates the treatment planning phase of the clinical decision-making process and then moves onto the treatment and discharge phases. In the case of wellness interventions, the therapist does not base the need for ongoing care on a deterioration of health status but on the identification of the client's need for interventions to maintain or improve his current level of wellness.

INTEGRATING THE THERAPEUTIC PROCESS AND EVIDENCE

Outcome-Based Massage™ Clinical Decision-Making and Evidence-Based Practice

As previously noted, evidence-based practice provides therapists with a framework for using the evidence to guide the client evaluation, treatment planning, and treatment

in Outcome-Based Massage™. Let us examine how that works in practical terms.

In evidence-based practice, Sackett et al.[29] propose five steps to guide the therapist through the process of using evidence in practice (Figure 5-2). The therapist can use these steps as he proceeds through the four phases of Outcome-Based Massage™ clinical decision-making.

Ask an Answerable Question

When the therapist reviews the reason for the client seeking treatment during the evaluation phase, this often results in questions about the client's presenting condition and the appropriate treatment approach. At this point, the therapist can "ask an answerable question" about the client's condition and associated treatment issues.

Collect Evidence Systematically

Prior to and during the subjective and objective examination of the evaluation phase, the therapist can use the answerable question as a basis for systematically collecting evidence about the client's condition, relevant examination techniques, appropriate treatment approaches, and other aspects of the client's care.

Appraise Evidence Critically

Typically, the therapist will have evidence of different types such as literature reviews, clinical trials, and case reports. He will need to appraise this evidence critically in order to identify which evidence will be used to guide this treatment approach.

Apply Results to Practice

Once the therapist is comfortable with his choice of evidence, he will summarize the key findings and apply these results to practice by using them to guide him during the evaluation, treatment planning, treatment, and discharge phases of Outcome-Based Massage™ clinical decision-making.

Evaluate Performance

During the ongoing cycle of client treatment and re-examination, the therapist evaluates how the client responds to the treatment regimen based on the evidence. He notes which evidence is consistent with his clinical findings and which evidence his treatment outcomes contradicts. As part of this process, the therapist forms his own conclusions about his client's condition, examination, and treatment and, in doing so, generates new evidence that integrates his findings with the earlier evidence. Whenever possible, the therapist closes the loop between evidence and clinical practice by sharing this new

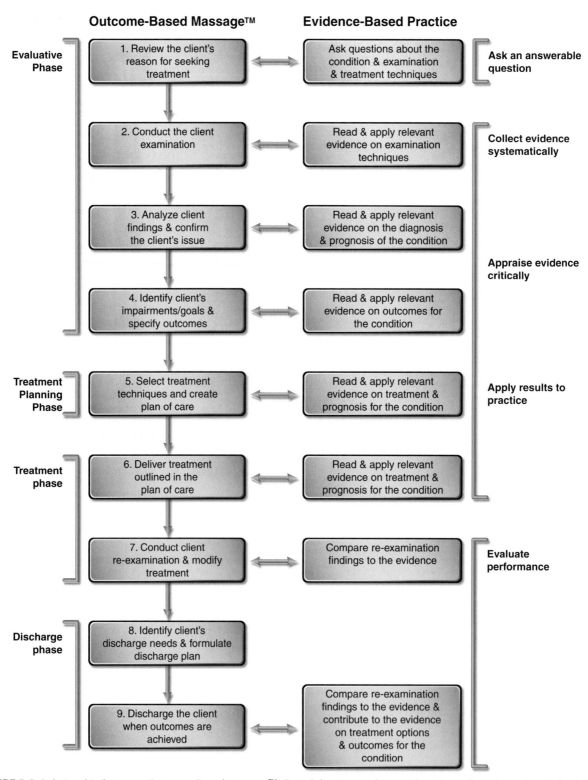

FIGURE 5-2 Relationship between Outcome-Based Massage™ clinical decision-making and evidence-based practice. (Adapted from Dryden T, Moyer CA, eds. *Massage Therapy: Integrating Research and Practice.* Champaign, IL: Human Kinetics; 2012 with permission of Human Kinetics.)

OBM Clinical Decision-Making

Environmental phase

↓

Treatment planning phase

↓

Treatment phase

↓

Discharge phase

Therapeutic Process

Building trust

↓

Exploring sensation

↓

Creating healthy closure

FIGURE 5-3 Relationship between Outcome-Based Massage™ clinical decision-making and the therapeutic process.

evidence with the clinical community through informal discussions with peers, clinical inservices, conference presentations, or written articles.

Outcome-Based Massage™ Clinical Decision-Making and the Therapeutic Process

The therapeutic process is a trust relationship that occurs between the therapist and the client in the context within which therapists provide Outcome-Based Massage™. The therapeutic process has a beginning, middle, and end, as does Outcome-Based Massage™ clinical decision-making. The three phases of the therapeutic process—building trust, exploring sensation, and creating healthy closure—occur as the clinician progresses through the evaluation, treatment planning, treatment, and discharge phases of Outcome-Based Massage™ clinical decision-making (Figure 5-3).[30]

Building Trust

During the evaluation and treatment planning phases of Outcome-Based Massage™ clinical decision-making, the therapist has the dual goals of building trust with the client and determining an appropriate plan of care. Managing these concurrent goals requires a delicate balance. Therapists who focus solely on accurate clinical decision-making and devalue the importance of close collaboration with the client and development of the therapeutic relationship run the risk of making the client uncomfortable with the treatment process. Conversely, therapists who emphasis relationship building at the expense of a thorough client examination and treatment planning process

will have difficulty generating a viable plan of care. Ideally, the therapist will establish a safe collaborative relationship with the client and a plan of care that is based on a sound examination and treatment planning process.

Exploring Sensation

Throughout the treatment phase, the client may experience a variety of physical and emotional sensations that result from the application of massage techniques. Once the client has developed trust in the therapist, she will be better prepared to explore these sensations in a manner that contributes to a better understanding of her body and achievement of her therapeutic outcomes. In both exploring sensation and the treatment phase, the client may cycle back and forth between periods of improvement and plateau or decline. Typically, the client will make more consistent progress during later stages of the therapeutic and treatment processes.

Healthy Closure

Client discharge from treatment represents the end of OMB clinical decision-making and the therapeutic process. During the discharge phase and healthy closure, the therapist's aim is to transition the client from care by the therapist to self-care. As the therapist manages the technical aspects of patient education and discharge planning, he also needs to ensure that he addresses the client's emotional needs and brings the therapeutic relationship to a positive closure. Healthy closure contributes to client satisfaction and ongoing adherence to self-care, which are critical outcomes for Outcome-Based Massage™.

IN CONCLUSION

Therapists can use the clinical decision-making process proposed for Outcome-Based Massage™ as a guide through the evaluation, treatment planning, treatment, and discharge phases of clinical care. The aim of this process is to enable the therapist to integrate massage techniques effectively into clinical care, as the primary or complementary treatment technique. Although the steps in Outcome-Based Massage™ clinical decision-making are presented in a linear sequence, the process is an iterative one in which the therapist may perform several steps concurrently. The decision-making process proposed in this chapter provides guidelines for enhancing the appropriateness and adequacy of the examinations, plans of care, and interventions provided by therapists. It is also related to the processes of evidence-based practice and the therapeutic relationship.

Practice

Note: This section contains instructions and clinical cases that demonstrates how to use some of the approaches to Outcome-Based Massage™ Clinical Decision Making that were introduced in this chapter.

Clinical cases 5-1 to 5-4 of a client with neck pain will illustrate in more detail the steps in Outcome-Based Massage™ clinical decision-making for the treatment of clinical conditions. Readers can apply the information on the distinction between clinical decision-making for treatment of clinical conditions versus wellness interventions to arrive at the guidelines for the latter.

1. The numbers of the steps in Figures 5-4, 5-5, 5-6, and 5-7 correspond to the step numbers 5-1 through 5-27 that appear in the Clinical Cases 5-1 to 5-4.
2. We have written a clinical scenario that is broad enough to apply to multiple professions. Readers need to use the scope of practice for their professions to guide their use of the examination and treatment techniques noted in this scenario.

Clinical Case 5-1: *Evaluation Phase*

Patient Profile

The patient is a 28-year-old woman who works as a cashier in a supermarket, with a 2-month history of neck pain of gradual onset. Her referral states "neck pain." Her treatment process follows the steps in Figure 5-4.

Step 1: Conduct Subjective Examination

Since the referral does not provide a specific diagnosis, the Clinician includes questions aimed at clarifying whether the patient has radiculopathy or soft-tissue injury. These questions include the following:

- Radiation of pain
- 24-Hour pain behavior
- Effect of position on pain
- Presence of paresthesia

The patient's responses about her neck pain do not include radiating pain below the elbow, paresthesia, or pain increasing with cervical extension or lateral flexion.

The patient reports the following:

- An insidious onset of localized neck and shoulder pain
- Stiffness and decreased active cervical range of motion
- Neck muscle tightness
- Neck muscle spasm
- Transient headaches

Step 2: Generate Preliminary Clinical Hypothesis

Based on the findings of the history and subjective examination, the Clinician hypothesizes that the patient's symptoms are due to the presence of active myofascial trigger points. A myofascial trigger point is a hyperirritable spot within a skeletal muscle that is associated with a hypersensitive palpable nodule in a taut band.[10] Trigger points may refer pain, create nerve entrapment, contribute to muscle weakness, and significantly limit the range of motion. Active trigger points, which are painful even when they are not being palpated, contribute to the following:

- Decreased muscle flexibility and muscle strength
- Increased referred pain during compression. In this case, they will produce referred pain in a pain pattern specific to that trigger point and can produce referred motor and autonomic responses.
- Local twitch response in the muscle fibers in the area of the active trigger point when stimulated.

Step 3a: Observe Client

The Clinician gathers observational data to initiate the identification of whether the patient has myofascial neck pain, rather than a radiculopathy.

The Clinician's observations include the following:

- No neck or shoulder girdle muscle wasting
- Forward head posture
- Visible muscle spasm in the region of the right upper trapezius

Using this information, the Clinician refines the clinical hypothesis to state that the patient has active myofascial trigger points in the right upper trapezius and possibly levator scapula muscles.

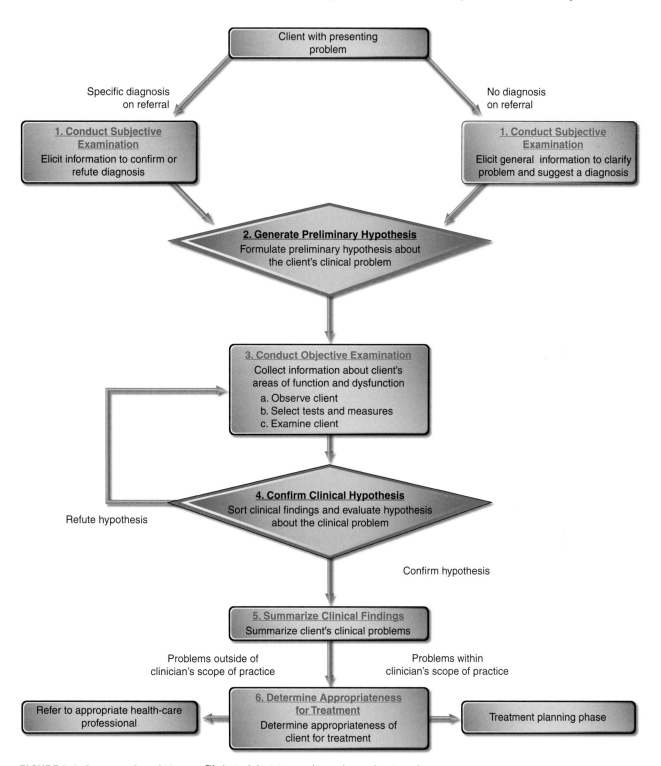

FIGURE 5-4 Outcome-Based Massage™ clinical decision-making: the evaluation phase.

(Continued)

Step 3b: Select Tests and Measures

The Clinician selects tests and measures that will provide information that will confirm or refute the presence of myofascial trigger points. These include the following:

- Palpation of trapezius and levator scapulae muscles
- Cervical range of motion
- Upper extremity dermatomes
- Upper extremity myotomes
- Cervical compression and distraction
- Performance of functional activities

Step 3c: Examine the Client

1. The Clinician examines the patient for signs of trigger points through palpation of the patient's trapezius and levator scapulae muscles for the following:
   - The presence of taut bands or nodules
   - The occurrence of a twitch response
   - Specific patterns of pain referral
2. The Clinician examines the patient's cervical spine with the following tests:
   - Range of motion: The Clinician notes that the patient presents with decreased active cervical range of motion.
   - Strength: The Clinician documents decreased strength of the right scapular elevation and retraction (trapezius and levator scapulae).
3. The Clinician rules out the presence of a radiculopathy by testing
   - Upper extremity dermatomes and myotomes
   - Cervical compression
   - Cervical distraction
     The Clinician records the negative findings on these tests.
4. The Clinician assesses the patient's functional level since he can use the patient's functional areas to compensate for areas of dysfunction. In doing so, he notes the patient's difficulty performing the functional tasks associated with her job as a cashier, including
   - Driving to work
   - Lifting and transferring objects with her right arm
   - Reaching objects above her head

Step 4: Confirm the Clinical Hypothesis

The Clinician identifies the critical impairments stemming from the patient's clinical condition. The Clinician also confirms the clinical hypothesis that the following clinical signs are secondary to active myofascial trigger points in the right upper trapezius and right levator scapulae muscles:

- Neck pain and headaches
- Spasm
- Muscle tightness
- Decreased range of motion
- Decreased strength
- Inability to lift and reach

Step 5: Summarize Pertinent Clinical Findings

Subjective
Pain:

- Neck pain at rest, at the end of range of motion, and during functional activity; reported pain intensity of 8/10 on a visual analog scale
- Reported inability to drive or check out groceries at the cash register for >10 minutes secondary to increased neck pain
- Tightness of neck muscles on waking and with fatigue
- Transient headaches (temporal region)

Functional Limitations:

- Inability to drive for >10 minutes secondary to increased neck pain
- Inability to perform repetitive upper extremity movements in standing using the right arm for >10 minutes (as required for checking out groceries at the cash register) secondary to neck pain
- Inability to perform lifting and transferring tasks required for her job

Objective Findings
Observation:

- Forward head posture

Palpation:

- Palpable muscle spasm in the right trapezius
- Palpable taut bands in trapezius and levator scapulae
- Reported positive pattern of pain referral on palpation of the right trapezius trigger point
- Reported positive pattern of pain referral on palpation of the right levator scapulae trigger point
- Twitch response on palpation of trigger point locations in upper trapezius and levator scapulae muscles

Range of Motion:

- Decreased active cervical range of motion: Flexion 50%, extension 75%, right rotation 75%, and left lateral flexion 50%
- Tightness of the right trapezius and the right levator scapulae muscles
- Range of motion of shoulder, elbow, wrist, and hand within normal limits

Strength:

- Decreased strength: Right levator scapulae—scapular elevation = grade 4, right trapezius—scapular elevation, scapular retraction = grade 4
- Strength of other shoulder, forearm, and hand muscles = 5/5

Functional Activities

- Inability to reach objects placed 1 foot above head with the right arm (as required for retrieving items from overhead shelves) secondary to neck pain
- Inability to lift a 5-lb object above shoulder level using the right arm (as required for placing boxes of dried goods on overhead shelves) secondary to neck pain
- Inability to lift and transfer a 15-lb object using the right arm (as required for placing customers' purchases into shopping carts) secondary to neck pain
- Inability to perform more than three repetitions of lifting and transferring a 3-lb object at waist level using the right arm (as required for checking out customers' groceries and placing them in shopping bags) secondary to neck pain.

Step 6: Determine Appropriateness for Treatment

The Clinician in this clinical scenario has training in trigger point therapy and considers the treatment of this patient with myofascial neck pain to be within the professional scope of practice and clinical competence. If this patient with neck pain had signs of an underlying metabolic disorder, significant radiculopathy, or any unusual clinical findings, it would be appropriate for the Clinician to refer the patient to a physician for further examination and treatment.

Clinical Case 5-2: *Treatment Planning Phase*

Patient Profile

The Patient is described in Clinical Case 5-1. Her treatment process follows the steps in Figure 5-5.

Step 7: Analyze Findings and Generate the Clinical Problem List

Impairments

- Pain: Neck pain and temporal headaches
- Decreased muscle extensibility: Tightness of trapezius and levator scapulae muscles
- Postural malalignment: Forward head posture
- Resting muscle tension: Muscle spasm in the right trapezius
- Decreased active cervical range of motion
- Decreased muscular performance: Decreased right trapezius and right levator scapulae strength and endurance
- Decreased muscle integrity: Active trigger points in the right upper trapezius and levator scapulae

Functional Limitations

- Inability to drive for >10 minutes secondary to increased neck pain
- Inability to perform repetitive upper extremity movements in standing using the right arm for >10 minutes secondary to neck pain
- Inability to reach objects placed 1 foot above head with the right arm secondary to neck pain
- Inability to lift a 5-lb object above shoulder level using the right arm secondary to neck pain
- Inability to lift and transfer a 15 lb object using the right arm secondary to neck pain

- Inability to perform more than three repetitions of lifting and transferring a 3-lb object at waist level using the right arm secondary to neck pain

Step 8: Identify Functional Outcomes

The Clinician identifies the functional outcomes outlined below based on (a) the patient's presenting functional limitations and (b) the observation that the patient is a young woman who is in good health, besides the myofascial neck pain, and who had normal functional ability before the onset of pain 2 months prior to the examination.

Functional Outcomes
Short-Term Outcomes (2 weeks)

1. Able to drive for 1/2 hour without complaints of pain
2. Able to work checking out groceries at the cash register for 1/2 hour, with appropriate breaks, without complaints of pain
3. Able to lift a 5-lb object and place it on shelf at shoulder level—one repetition without complaints of neck pain
4. Able to reach objects placed 1 foot above head with the right arm without complaints of neck pain
5. Able to lift and transfer an 8-lb object at waist level with the right arm without complaints of pain
6. Able to perform five repetitions of transferring a 5-lb object at waist level using the right arm without complaints of pain.

(Continued)

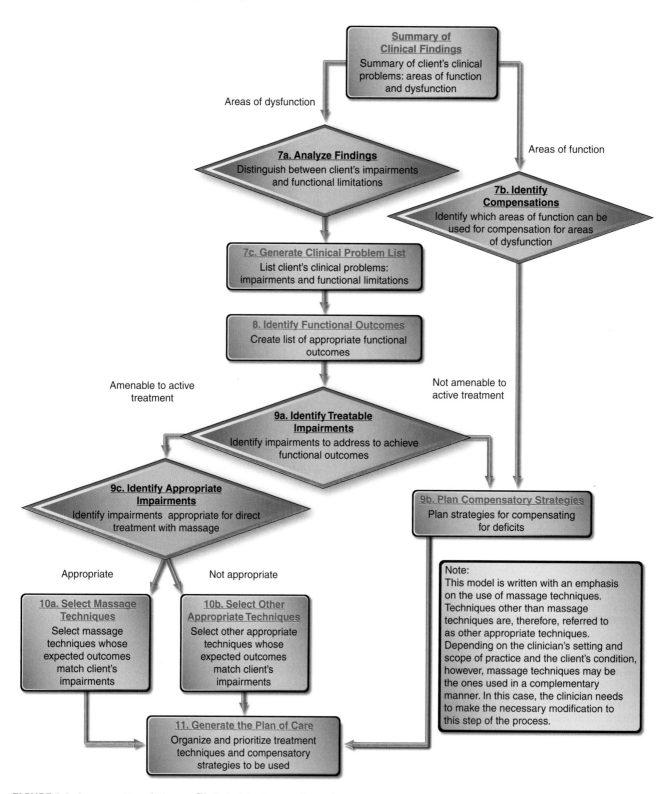

FIGURE 5-5 Outcome-Based Massage™ clinical decision-making: the treatment planning phase.

Long-Term Outcomes (Discharge: 4 weeks)

1. Able to drive for 1.5–2 hours without complaints of neck pain
2. Able to work checking out groceries at the cash register for 2 hours, with appropriate breaks, without complaints of pain
3. Able to lift an 8-lb object and place it on shelf at shoulder level—five repetitions without complaints of neck pain
4. Able to reach objects placed 2 feet above head with the right arm without complaints of neck pain.
5. Able to lift and transfer a 15-lb object at waist level with the right arm without complaints of neck pain
6. Able to perform 15 repetitions of transferring a 5-lb object at waist level using the right arm without complaints of neck pain

Functional Limitation	Associated Impairments
Inability to Perform Lifting Tasks (continued)	■ Decreased muscle extensibility: Tightness of trapezius and levator scapulae ■ Muscle spasm in the right trapezius ■ Decreased muscular performance: Decreased right trapezius and right levator scapulae strength and endurance ■ Decreased muscle integrity: Active trigger points in the right upper trapezius and levator scapulae

Step 9a: Identify Treatable Impairments and Relevant Outcomes

Functional Limitation	Associated Impairments
Inability to Perform Driving Tasks	■ Pain: Neck pain and temporal headaches ■ Postural malalignment: Forward head posture ■ Decreased active cervical range of motion ■ Muscle spasm in the right trapezius ■ Decreased muscle integrity: Active trigger points in the right upper trapezius and levator scapulae
Inability to Perform Repetitive Upper Extremity Movements in Standing	■ Pain: Neck pain and temporal headaches ■ Postural malalignment: Forward head posture ■ Decreased active cervical range of motion ■ Muscle spasm in the right trapezius ■ Decreased muscular performance: Decreased right trapezius and right levator scapulae strength and endurance ■ Decreased muscle integrity: Active trigger points in the right upper trapezius and levator scapulae ■ Decreased muscle extensibility: Tightness of trapezius and levator scapulae
Inability to Perform Lifting Tasks	■ Pain: Neck pain and temporal headaches

Step 9b: Identify Treatable Impairments and Relevant Outcomes

Impairment	Outcome
■ Pain: Neck pain and temporal headaches	■ Pain reported is 0/10 on a visual analog scale
■ Postural malalignment: Forward head posture	■ Normalized cervical and head posture
■ Decreased muscle integrity: Active trigger points in the right upper trapezius and levator scapulae	■ No signs of active trigger points on palpation of trapezius and levator scapulae muscles; no palpable taut bands, positive pattern of pain referral, or twitch signs
■ Decreased active cervical range of motion	■ Active cervical range of motion: Flexion 100%, extension 100%, right rotation 100%, and left lateral flexion 100%
■ Muscle spasm in the right trapezius	■ No palpable muscle spasm in the right trapezius muscle
■ Decreased muscular performance: Decreased right trapezius and right levator scapulae strength and endurance	■ Muscle strength: Right levator scapulae—scapular elevation = grade 5; right trapezius—scapular elevation, scapular retraction = grade 5
■ Decreased muscle extensibility: Tightness of trapezius and levator scapulae muscles	■ Normal extensibility of the right trapezius and the right levator scapulae muscles

(Continued)

Step 9c: Identify Impairments Appropriate for Massage Techniques

Impairments

- Pain: Neck pain and headaches

- Decreased muscle extensibility of trapezius and levator scapulae

- Postural malalignment: Forward head posture

- Spasm in the right trapezius

- Decreased active cervical range of motion

Role of Massage

- Direct effect on pain due to presence of active trigger points

- Direct effect on muscle extensibility

- Direct effect on the lengthening of shortened anterior neck and trunk muscles

- There will also be a secondary effect resulting from the inactivation of the trigger points since the decrease in pain will minimize the compensatory postural changes that are due to trigger point pain

- Direct effect on muscle spasm

- Direct effect on the lengthening of shortened anterior neck and trunk muscles that contribute to decreased range of motion

- There will also be a secondary effect from the inactivation of the trigger points since the decreased range may be due, in part, to a combination of trigger point pain and compensatory muscle guarding

Impairments

- Decreased muscular performance: Decreased right trapezius and right levator scapulae strength

- Decreased muscle integrity: Active trigger points in the right upper trapezius and levator scapulae

Role of Massage

- Secondary effect since weakness is likely secondary to trigger point pain and disuse

- Direct effect on the active myofascial trigger points

Step 10a and 10b: Select Treatment Techniques

Massage Techniques

- Specific compression
- Superficial effleurage
- Superficial stroking
- Petrissage
- Broad-contact compression
- Stripping
- Self-care—specific compression with a hand-held massage device

Other Appropriate Treatment Techniques

- Moist heat for trigger point pain
- Ice for acute spasm
- Specific stretches for trapezius and levator scapulae muscles
- Postural re-education
- Active range of motion exercises
- Strengthening exercises
- Self-care education
- Functional activity

Step 11: Generate the Plan of Care

Note: Item to document

Plan of Care

Subjective History of Present Illness:

- Two months ago, the patient had insidious onset of localized neck and shoulder pain, right side greater than the left, with stiffness, decreased active cervical range of motion, neck muscle tightness, neck muscle spasm, and transient headaches
- Seen by MD and given muscle relaxants with little effect
- Is right handed

Current Medication: Acetaminophen for pain
Current Functional Status: On reduced hours secondary to neck pain and difficulty performing job-related tasks

Subjective
(*Continued*)

Past Medical History: Unremarkable; no prior history of neck or upper extremity injuries; no prior therapy

Pain: Neck pain at rest, at the end of range of motion, and during functional activity; reported pain intensity of 8 on a visual analog scale; transient headaches (temporal region)

Muscle Tightness: Tightness of neck muscles on waking and with fatigue

Functional Limitations: Reported inability to drive or check out groceries at the cash register for >10 minutes secondary to increased neck pain

Prior Functional Level: Full-time cashier at supermarket; able to perform all job-related tasks without difficulty

Objective

Posture: Forward head posture

Palpation:

- Palpable muscle spasm in the right trapezius
- Palpable taut bands in the right trapezius and levator scapulae
- Reported positive pattern of pain referral on palpation of the right trapezius trigger point
- Reported positive pattern of pain referral on palpation of the right levator scapulae trigger point
- Twitch response on palpation of trigger point locations in the right upper trapezius and the right levator scapulae muscles

Range of Motion:

- Decreased active cervical range of motion: Flexion 50%, extension 75%, right rotation 75%, and left lateral flexion 50% with pain at the end of range of motion; other ranges full and pain free
- Full and pain-free active range of motion of shoulder, elbow, wrist, and hand bilaterally

Muscle Extensibility: Tightness of trapezius and levator scapulae muscles

Strength:

- Decreased strength of the right levator scapulae—scapular elevation = grade 4
- Decreased strength of the right trapezius—scapular elevation, scapular retraction = grade 4
- Strength of other shoulder, wrist, and finger motions = grade 5

Functional Limitations:

- Inability to drive for >10 minutes secondary to increased neck pain
- Inability to perform repetitive upper extremity movements in standing using the right arm for >10 minutes (as required for checking out groceries at the cash register) secondary to neck pain
- Inability to reach objects placed 1 foot above head with the right arm (as required for retrieving items from overhead shelves) secondary to neck pain
- Inability to lift a 5-lb object above shoulder level using the right arm (as required for placing boxes of dried goods on overhead shelves) secondary to neck pain
- Inability to lift and transfer a 15-lb object using the right arm (as required for placing customers' purchases into shopping carts) secondary to neck pain
- Inability to perform more than three repetitions of lifting and transferring a 3-lb object at waist level using the right arm (as required for checking out customers' groceries and placing them in shopping bags) secondary to neck pain

Analysis

Trigger points in right upper trapezius and levator scapulae muscles with associated muscle tenderness, muscle tightness, and decreased cervical spine range of motion

Impairments:

- Pain: Neck pain and temporal headaches
- Decreased muscle extensibility: Tightness of trapezius and levator scapulae muscles
- Postural malalignment: Forward head posture
- Resting Muscle tension: Muscle spasm in the right trapezius
- Decreased active cervical range of motion
- Decreased muscular performance: Decreased right trapezius and right levator scapulae strength and endurance
- Decreased muscle integrity: Active trigger points in the right upper trapezius and levator scapulae

(*Continued*)

Analysis Functional Limitations:
(continued)
- Inability to drive for >10 minutes secondary to increased neck pain
- Inability to perform repetitive upper extremity movements in standing using the right arm for >10 minutes secondary to neck pain
- Inability to reach objects placed 1 foot above head with the right arm secondary to neck pain
- Inability to lift a 5-lb object above shoulder level using the right arm secondary to neck pain
- Inability to lift and transfer a 15 lb object using the right arm secondary to neck pain
- Inability to perform more than three repetitions of lifting and transferring a 3-lb object at waist level using the right arm secondary to neck pain

Outcomes (related to impairments):

- Pain reported is 0/10 on a visual analog scale
- Normalized cervical and head posture
- No palpable muscle spasm in the right trapezius muscle
- No signs of active trigger points on palpation of trapezius and levator scapulae muscles: Palpable taut bands, positive pattern of pain referral, or twitch signs
- Active cervical range of motion: Flexion 100%, extension 100%, right rotation 100%, and left lateral flexion 100%
- Normal extensibility of the right trapezius and the right levator scapulae muscles
- Muscle strength: Right levator scapulae—scapular elevation = grade 5; right trapezius—scapular elevation, scapular retraction = grade 5

Functional Outcomes

Short-Term Outcomes (2 weeks):

- Able to drive for 1/2 hour without complaints of pain
- Able to work checking out groceries at the cash register for 1/2 hour, with appropriate breaks, without complaints of pain
- Able to lift a 5-lb object and place it on shelf at shoulder level—one repetition without complaints of neck pain
- Able to reach objects placed 1 foot above head with the right arm without complaints of neck pain
- Able to lift and transfer an 8-lb object at waist level with the right arm without complaints of pain
- Able to perform five repetitions of transferring a 5-lb object at waist level using the right arm without complaints of pain

Long-Term Outcomes (Discharge: 4 weeks):

- Able to drive for 1.5–2 hours without complaints of neck pain
- Able to work checking out groceries at the cash register for 2 hours, with appropriate breaks, without complaints of pain
- Able to lift an 8-lb object and place it on shelf at shoulder level—five repetitions without complaints of neck pain
- Able to reach objects placed 2 feet above the head with the right arm without complaints of neck pain
- Able to lift and transfer a 15-lb object at waist level with the right arm without complaints of neck pain
- Able to perform 15 repetitions of transferring a 5-lb object at waist level using the right arm without complaints of neck pain
- Independent in self-care and therapeutic exercise program

Plan Treatment: Two times a week for 4 weeks
Massage Techniques:

- Specific compression (trigger point release)
- Superficial effleurage
- Superficial stroking
- Petrissage
- Broad-contact compression
- Stripping
- Self-care–specific compression with a hand-held massage device

Plan
(*Continued*)

Therapeutic Exercise:
- Specific stretches for trapezius and levator scapulae muscles
- Postural re-education
- Active range of motion exercises for cervical spine
- Strengthening exercises for cervical and scapular muscles

Modalities:
- Moist heat in the location of the trigger points to reduce trigger point activity and pain
- Ice for acute muscle spasm

Functional Training:
- Functional training in lifting and transferring required for effective job performance as a cashier

Education:
- Self-care education in pain and trigger point management

Clinical Case 5-3: *Treatment Phase*

Patient Profile

The patient is described in Clinical Case 5-1. Her treatment process follows the steps in Figure 5-6.

Steps 12a and 12b: Select Treatment and Re-examination Techniques

Massage Treatment Technique
- Superficial stroking on the site of the acute spasm
- Broad-contact compression

Complementary Technique
- Specific stretches for trapezius and levator scapulae muscles
- Ice for spasm
- Self-care education for pain control

Examination Techniques
Subjective
- Pain reports
- Perceptions of treatment and progress made

Objective
- Muscle spasm
- Trigger point pain referral pattern
- Range of motion

Steps 13, 14, and 15: Carry Out Initial Treatment, Conduct Client Re-examination, and Assess Client Progress

Patient's Response to Initial Interventions (1 week)
Treatment Technique
- Superficial stroking on the site of the spasm
- Broad-contact compression on the location of the trigger points and off the site of the spasm
- Petrissage off the site of spasm
- Specific stretches for trapezius and levator scapulae muscles
- Ice on the location of the muscle spasm
- Self-care education for pain control

Results of Informal Examination
- The patient had negative response to use of ice for spasm; this exacerbated trigger point pain. Superficial stroking was used for spasm.
- Moist heat applied to the trigger point location may be more effective for pain relief.
- Patient's trigger points were initially too sensitive to tolerate specific compression; broad-contact compression was used.

(*Continued*)

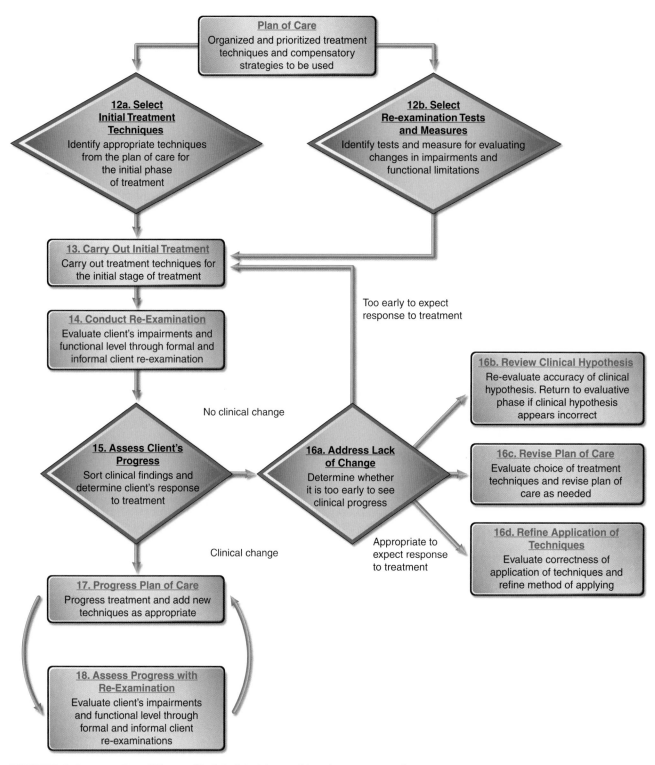

FIGURE 5-6 Outcome-Based Massage™ clinical decision-making: the treatment phase.

■ The patient was able to perform specific stretches for trapezius and levator scapulae muscles appropriately.

Results of Formal Examination

■ Decreased reports of pain during functional activity—reported pain intensity of 6.5 on a visual analog scale

■ Decreased muscle spasm
■ Pattern of pain referral—unchanged

Clinician's Conclusions

Patient is responding to treatment. Trigger point therapy is appropriate.

Steps 17 and 18: Progress Plan of Care and Assess Progress through Re-examination

	Week 2	Week 3
Treatment Techniques	Massage Techniques ■ Broad-contact compression ■ Petrissage ■ Specific compression (trigger point release) Other Appropriate Treatment Techniques ■ Specific stretches for trapezius and levator scapulae muscles ■ Heat to location of trigger points for pain ■ Postural re-education ■ Active range of motion exercises ■ Functional activity ■ Self-care education—add home range of motion and stretching program	Massage Techniques ■ Broad-contact compression (decreased duration) ■ Petrissage (decreased duration) ■ Stripping (increased duration and depth) ■ Specific compression (increased duration and depth of trigger point release) Other Appropriate Treatment Techniques ■ Specific stretches for trapezius and levator scapulae muscles ■ Heat for preparation for stretching ■ Postural re-education ■ Functional activity ■ Strengthening exercises ■ Self-care education—add self-care–specific compression with a hand-held massage device
Results of Patient Re-Examination	Functional Outcomes ■ Reports being able to drive for 0.5 hours without complaints of neck pain ■ Able to perform repetitive upper extremity movements while standing 0.75 hours without complaints of neck pain ■ Able to lift a 5-lb object and place it on shelf at shoulder level—five repetitions without complaints of neck pain ■ Able to reach objects placed 1 foot above head with the right arm without complaints of neck pain ■ Able to lift and transfer a 5-lb object at waist level with the right arm without complaints of neck pain ■ Able to perform 10 repetitions of transferring a 5-lb object at waist level using the right arm without complaints of neck pain Other Examination Findings ■ Reported recent flare-up of pain following attempts to increase work time ■ Reported pain intensity of 5 on a visual analog scale by end of week ■ Pattern of pain referral—decreased intensity of pain on palpation of trigger points ■ Active cervical range of motion: Flexion 75%, extension 90%, right rotation 90%, and left lateral flexion 75% ■ Strength: Right levator scapulae—scapular elevation = grade 4; right trapezius—scapular elevation, scapular retraction = grade 4	Functional Outcomes ■ Reports being able to drive for 1 hour without complaints of neck pain ■ Able to perform repetitive upper extremity movements while standing 1.25 hours without complaints of neck pain ■ Able to lift a 10-lb object and place it on shelf at shoulder level—one repetition without complaints of neck pain ■ Able to reach objects placed 1.5 feet above head with right arm without complaints of neck pain ■ Able to lift and transfer a 10-lb object at waist level with the right arm without complaints of neck pain ■ Able to perform 15 repetitions of transferring a 5-lb object at waist level using the right arm without complaints of neck pain Other Examination Findings ■ Reported pain intensity of 3.5 on a visual analog scale ■ No pain referral on palpation of upper trapezius trigger point; minimal reports of pain for levator scapulae trigger point ■ Active cervical range of motion: Flexion 90%, extension 100%, right rotation 100%, and left lateral flexion 75% ■ Strength: Right levator scapulae—scapular elevation = grade 4+; right trapezius—scapular elevation, scapular retraction = grade 4+

Clinical Case 5-4: *Discharge Phase*

Patient Profile

The patient is described in Clinical Case 5-1. Her treatment process follows the steps in Figure 5-7.

Steps 19, 20, and 21: Identify Postdischarge Needs and Initiate Postdischarge Education and Referrals

Impairment/Functional Limitation	Discharge Need
■ Pain	■ Pain management self-care education
	■ Self-care–specific compression with a hand-held massage device
■ Difficulty performing job-related activities	■ Ergonomic education and work site assessment
■ Decreased muscle extensibility	■ Home stretching program
■ Decreased range of motion	■ Home range of motion program

Steps 22 and 23: Progress Plan of Care and Assess Progress through Re-examination

Week 4

Treatment Techniques

Massage Techniques
- ■ Petrissage (decreased duration)
- ■ Broad-contact compression (decreased duration of trigger point release)
- ■ Specific compression (increased duration)
- ■ Stripping (increased duration and depth)

Other Appropriate Treatment Techniques
- ■ Postural re-education
- ■ Functional activity
- ■ Strengthening exercises
- ■ Self-care education—add ergonomics education, review education on identifying and managing flare-ups

Results of Patient Re-examination

Discharge concerns:
- ■ Cashier station is not ergonomically correct, and this aggravates pain. Patient is concerned about how to manage flare-ups
- ■ Patient is able to demonstrate all self-care activities correctly
- ■ Reported pain intensity is 1 on a visual analog scale
- ■ There is no pain referral on palpation of upper trapezius or levator scapulae trigger points

Steps 24 and 25: Finalize Discharge Plans and Review Home Program

The Clinician outlines a self-care program that addresses the patient's discharge needs. It contains components that reflect the patient's presenting impairments and functional limitations.

Week 4: Self-Care Program

- ■ Pain management
- ■ Ergonomics
- ■ Home stretching
- ■ Home range of motion
- ■ Self-care–specific compression with a hand-held massage device

Steps 26 and 27: Conduct Discharge Examination and Discharge Client

The Clinician documents the clinical findings on the discharge examination. These findings indicate that the patient has achieved her outcomes and is ready for discharge.

Discharge Examination Findings: Functional Outcomes

- ■ Able to drive for 2.5 hours without complaints of neck pain using stretches and postural checks
- ■ Able to work checking out groceries at the cash register for 2 hours without complaints of neck pain; takes appropriate breaks and uses stretches and postural checks; has had ergonomic adjustments to cashier station; occasional complaints of neck tightness with fatigue
- ■ Able to perform lifting tasks required for work as a cashier:
1. Able to lift an 8-lb object and place it on shelf at shoulder level—five repetitions without complaints of neck pain
2. Able to reach objects placed 2 feet above head with the right arm without complaints of neck pain
3. Able to lift and transfer a 15-lb object at waist level with the right arm without complaints of neck pain
4. Able to perform 20 repetitions of lifting and transferring a 5-lb object at waist level using the right arm without complaints of neck pain

Other Examination Findings

- ■ Reported pain intensity of 0.5 on a visual analog scale
- ■ Normalized cervical and head posture
- ■ No palpable muscle spasm in the right trapezius muscle

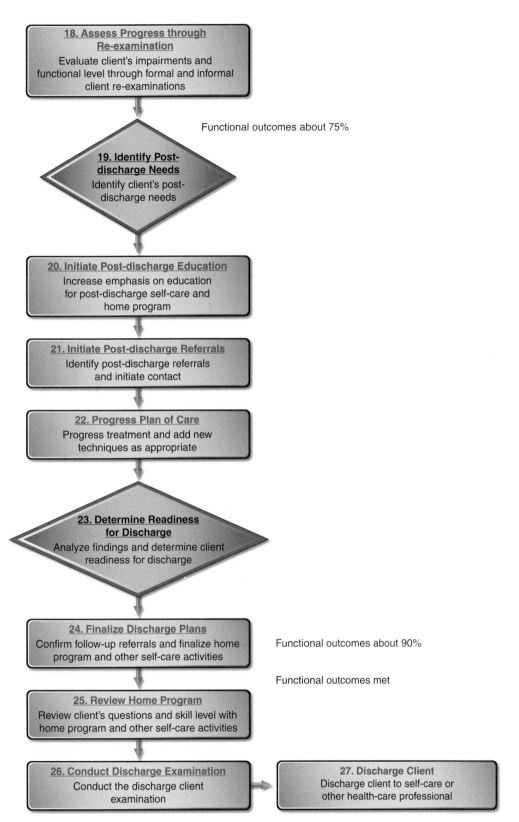

FIGURE 5-7 Outcome-Based Massage™ clinical decision-making: the discharge phase.

(*Continued*)

- No signs of active trigger points on palpation of trapezius and levator scapulae muscles: Palpable taut bands, positive pattern of pain referral, or twitch signs
- Active cervical range of motion: Flexion 100%, extension 100%, right rotation 100%, and left lateral flexion 100%

- Normal extensibility of the right trapezius and the right levator scapulae muscles
- Muscle strength: Right levator scapulae—scapular elevation = grade 5; right trapezius—scapular elevation, scapular retraction = grade 5

REVIEW SECTION

TAKEAWAYS

1. Therapists who are engaged in the Outcome-Based Massage™ clinical decision-making process often perform several steps of the process concurrently and cycle through the same steps of the decision-making process several times and each time that they repeat the steps they expand on their information and refine their conclusions.

2. The Outcome-Based Massage™ clinical decision-making process has four phases: the evaluation phase, the treatment planning phase, the treatment phase, and the discharge phase.

3. The steps in the evaluation phase revolve around formulating and confirming a clinical hypothesis about the client's clinical problem or wellness goals.

4. The steps in the treatment planning phase involve identifying body structures and functions that are appropriate for treatment, and selecting treatment techniques that will produce improvements in the client's impairments in body structures and functions, functional limitations, or overall wellness.

5. The treatment phase is an ongoing cycle of treatment, re-examination, and treatment progression that begins after the therapist completes the plan of care.

6. Discharge involves the transition of the client from the therapists to self-care or to treatment by another therapist.

7. Therapists can use the four-phase Outcome-Based Massage™ clinical decision-making process for both medical massage and wellness massage, although interventions for wellness and the treatment of impairments differ in several ways.

8. For Outcome-Based Massage™ clinical decision-making, the primary distinction between medical massage and wellness massage is whether or not the focus of treatment is on an impairment in the client's body structure or function.

9. In evidence-based practice, Sackett et al.[29] proposed five steps to guide the clinician through the process of using evidence in practice (Figure 5-2). The clinician can use these steps as he proceeds through the four phases of Outcome-Based Massage™ clinical decision-making.

10. The three phases of the therapeutic process—building trust, exploring sensation, and creating healthy closure (Figure 5-3)—occur as the clinician progresses through the evaluation, treatment planning, treatment, and discharge phases of Outcome-Based Massage™ clinical decision-making.

Critical Thinking Questions

1. What are the similarities and differences between the clinical decision-making and treatment process for clients receiving medical massage versus wellness massage?

2. What role does the client's reason for seeking treatment play in Outcome-Based Massage™ clinical decision-making?

3. List three common errors in formulating a clinical hypothesis and describe how you would prevent those errors in your own clinical decision-making?

4. Your client presents with a referral stating "back pain" after a recent fall. During your history-taking you suspect that he may have both a back injury and a

hamstring strain. What are the steps that you would follow in the evaluation phase to address these two issues?

5. Your client has met all of the functional outcomes and outcomes for impairments that you established for her intervention. She has, however, made little progress with her self-care education and home program. What process can you use to facilitate a timely discharge for this client?

6. How would you modify the steps in the four-phase clinical decision-making process if your client presented with wellness goals, rather than a clinical condition?

7. Your client is a 16-year-old boy who is non-verbal and fully dependent for all care following a severe head injury. In your examination you identify multiple impairments, including decreased muscle extensibility, decreased joint range of motion, and decreased skin integrity. On the other hand, you are finding it difficult to identify functional outcomes

and compensatory strategies for this client. What process would you use to develop a balanced plan of care for this client and what might this plan include?

8. Your objective examination shows that your client is making significant improvements on the outcomes for the key impairments that you selected. Nevertheless, she reports little progress with her functional outcomes. What steps could you use to identify what to correct in your intervention?

9. Describe how you would use the steps in evidence-based practice during the examination and treatment planning phases of Outcome-Based Massage™ clinical decision-making.

10. What are some of the possible negative consequences of failing to follow the steps in the therapeutic process as you progress your client through the four phases of Outcome-Based Massage™ clinical decision-making?

References for Chapter 5 are on p. 461.

PART II

Application of Outcome-Based Massage™ to Clinical Conditions and Wellness

OVERVIEW OF CHAPTERS IN PART II

The chapters in Part II, Applications of Outcome-Based Massage™ to Clinical Conditions and Wellness, show therapists (a) how to perform massage techniques and (b) how to use the principles of Outcome-Based Massage™ to develop interventions using massage techniques for clients with clinical conditions or wellness goals.

Chapter 6: Preparation and Positioning for Outcome-Based Massage™

This chapter outlines the two frameworks that guide the practical application of the massage techniques in Outcome-Based Massage™. It also provides guidelines for therapists on how to prepare themselves physically and mentally before they begin to interact with the client; how to select and prepare a variety of treatment materials such as tables, lubricants, and linen; and how to position themselves and their clients during treatment.

Chapter 7: Superficial Reflex Techniques

Superficial reflex techniques are those massage techniques that engage only the skin and primarily affect the level of arousal, autonomic balance, and the perception of pain. These techniques include static contact, superficial stroking, and fine vibration. This chapter describes these techniques, how to perform them, and how to apply them in a practice sequence. It also discusses relevant outcomes and evidence, cautions and contraindications, and how to use the technique in treatment.

Chapter 8: Superficial Fluid Techniques

Superficial fluid techniques are massage techniques that therapists apply to tissues superficial to muscle to increase the return flow of blood or lymph. These techniques include superficial effleurage and superficial lymph drainage. This chapter describes these techniques, how to perform them, and how to apply them in a practice sequence. It also discusses relevant outcomes and evidence, cautions and contraindications, and how to use the technique in treatment.

Chapter 9: Neuromuscular Techniques

Neuromuscular techniques are those massage techniques that palpate muscle, affect the level of resting tension of muscles, and have additional psychoneuroimmunological effects. These techniques include broad-contact compression, petrissage, muscle stripping, and specific compression. This chapter describes these techniques, how to perform them, and how to apply them in a practice sequence. It also includes a discussion of relevant outcomes and evidence, cautions and contraindications, and how to use the technique in treatment.

Chapter 10: Connective Tissue Techniques

Connective tissue techniques are those massage techniques that palpate, lengthen, and promote remodeling of connective tissue. These techniques include skin rolling, myofascial release, direct fascial technique, and friction. This chapter describes these techniques, how to perform them, and how to apply them in a practice sequence. It also discusses relevant outcomes and evidence, cautions and contraindications, and how to use the technique in treatment.

Chapter 11: Passive Movement Techniques

Passive movement techniques are those massage techniques that primarily palpate the movement of tissues and structures, as opposed to palpating their substance or texture. These passive motion techniques, such as shaking, rhythmic mobilization, and rocking, are also used to treat restrictions in tissues and structures. This chapter describes these techniques, how to perform them, and how to apply them in a practice sequence. It also discusses relevant outcomes and evidence, cautions and contraindications, and how to use the technique in treatment.

Chapter 12: Percussive Techniques

Percussive techniques are those massage techniques that use controlled striking of the body to quickly deform and release tissues. These techniques enhance airway clearance, reduce or increase neuromuscular tone, and increase alertness. This chapter describes the various percussive techniques, how to perform them, and how to apply them in practice sequences. It also includes a discussion of relevant outcomes and evidence, cautions and contraindications, and how to use the techniques in treatment.

Chapter 13: Sequencing Massage Techniques for Outcome-Based Massage™

This chapter builds on the Outcome-Based Massage™ clinical decision-making model and earlier chapters on techniques by explaining how to create basic sequences of massage techniques. In doing so, it outlines the principles for selecting and ordering massage techniques to achieve specific clinical outcomes.

Chapter 14: Application of Outcome-Based Massage™ to Clinical Conditions and Wellness

The first section of this chapter provides practical guidelines for developing and progressing interventions for wellness and the treatment of the clinical conditions that use massage techniques to achieve specific clinical outcomes. The other sections outline examples of interventions and progressions that achieve outcomes related to a variety of impairments. The clinical cases in this chapter give additional examples of how to apply the principles of Outcome-Based Massage™ for medical massage (treatment of clinical conditions) and wellness massage. Finally, Quick Treatment Guides for 16 clinical conditions and wellness issues that therapists reported that they commonly treated with massage techniques are included in the insert.

Definitions of Components of Massage Techniques

The following components of massage techniques are outlined within Chapters 7 through 12 on massage techniques.

Contact Surface: The portion of the therapist's hand or arm that is used to execute the stroke.

Pressure: The amount of force per unit area of contact surface that the therapist applies. We define categories of pressure as "minimal" when it engages the skin, "light" when it engages subcutaneous fascia and fat, "moderate" when it engages superficial muscle layers, and "heavy" when it engages deeper muscle layers.

Tissues Engaged: The target tissues or layers of tissue to which the therapist directs the pressure of the stroke and which are mechanically deformed by the application of the technique.

Direction: The direction of the applied force. The direction given in the description of techniques is the direction in which the greatest force is applied during the pressure phase of the stroke. Directions that are commonly specified include centripetal (toward the heart), centrifugal (away from the heart), and transverse or parallel to the fibers of a reference structure.

Amplitude: An indication of the size of the area that is covered by a technique.

Rate: An indication of how fast the force is applied. This is a critical component, since many desired effects occur only at certain rates of application. The rate may describe the speed of the movement of the therapist's hand over the client's skin (distance per second), the frequency of repetitions of a described technique (repetitions per second), or both rates.

Duration: An estimate of a reasonable length of time for which a single technique may have to be applied by a competent therapist in order to achieve the specified impairment-level outcomes of care. This text provides a minimum duration that can be exceeded at the discretion of the therapist, for example, "10 minutes or greater." If a longer duration of application of a technique can result in side effects or risks, this text provides a suggested upper limit, for example, "1 to 10 minutes," and discusses how to determine an appropriate duration of treatment in the accompanying text.

Intergrades with: When one technique is said to "intergrade" with another, the two techniques can be performed consecutively and will merge gradually one into another since there are intermediate hybrid forms of the technique that lie between and resemble both techniques.

Combines with: When one technique is said to "combine" with another, it means that the two techniques may be executed simultaneously.

Context: A brief description of how the technique is conventionally sequenced in relation to other techniques.

Preparation and Positioning for Outcome-Based Massage™

OBJECTIVES

After studying this chapter, you will have the information that you need to do the following:

1. Identify six basic categories of massage techniques and describe how each category affects different types of tissues.
2. Describe techniques for physical and psychological preparation for the therapist.
3. Outline the materials used to perform massage and how to prepare them.
4. Outline and demonstrate how to position a client for massage of different regions of the body.
5. Describe and demonstrate how to perform appropriate draping techniques for different regions of the body.

Using massage techniques in treatment requires more than a laying-on of hands during a treatment session. Several other important activities are involved. First, therapists need to understand the two frameworks that guide the practical application of the massage techniques in Outcome-Based Massage™ (OBM). Second, they need to prepare themselves physically and mentally before they begin to interact with the client. In addition, they must also select and prepare a variety of treatment materials such as tables, lubricants, and linen. During the intervention, they need to ensure that they have positioned the client appropriately and draped the client both prior to and during the massage. Finally, they need to ensure that they have positioned themselves well and use correct body mechanics during the intervention.

Evidence

THERAPIST'S PREPARATION FOR DELIVERING OUTCOME-BASED MASSAGE™ INTERVENTIONS

Prior to beginning their physical and psychological preparation for client care, therapists need to review the two frameworks that provide the foundation for the clinical use of the massage techniques in Outcome-Based Massage™. First of all, the taxonomy of massage techniques, presented in this chapter, is a novel approach to categorizing massage techniques that is consistent with the aims of Outcome-Based Massage™. Second the concepts of intelligent touch define the skills that therapists need for successful application of massage techniques.

Taxonomy of Massage Techniques

Several systems name classical (Swedish) massage techniques in reference to the motions of the therapist: gliding, kneading, rubbing, shaking, and hitting. Therapists have added many "modern" terms to these basic terms, which often reference an originator's name or a foreign language descriptor. We believe that the final effect is without a sound clinical rationale. The classification system retained from the first edition of *Outcome-Based Massage™* seeks to avoid some of the limitations of these two approaches to classification.

This text intentionally avoids the division into "classical" and "modern" service-marked methods. In doing so, we recognize that several innovative massage or "body work" methods have influenced the contemporary practice of massage substantially and we duly acknowledge these methods. Nevertheless, we can organize almost all modern and classical techniques into six clusters of related techniques (Superficial reflex techniques, Superficial fluid techniques, Neuromuscular techniques, Connective tissue techniques, Passive movement techniques, and Percussive techniques), to which we have applied names that we trust make sense to readers.

Therapists apply the structured touch of massage in a specific manner in order to achieve selected therapeutic outcomes. Consequently, the therapeutic effects or possible outcomes of techniques are important when classifying massage techniques. Techniques cannot, however, be classified based solely on their therapeutic effects because a given technique can produce multiple outcomes. For this reason, we base our taxonomy for massage techniques on anatomy, operational requirements, and outcomes. First, we present those techniques that are directed toward superficial tissues. Second, we present those techniques that affect deeper tissues. Third, we present those techniques that affect multiple tissue layers. In addition, we group methods that require the therapist to palpate and observe similar phenomena together. Finally, we place those techniques that require therapists to acquire simpler skills before those techniques that require complex skills.

We use these criteria to define four broad categories of massage techniques that engage particular types of tissue: superficial reflex techniques, superficial fluid techniques, neuromuscular techniques, and connective tissue techniques. These criteria also produce two categories of techniques that engage multiple tissue layers: passive movement techniques and percussive techniques. Techniques in each of these six categories have specific therapeutic effects. In addition, the techniques in the first five categories may produce psychoneuroimmunologic effects, such as the reduction of stress.

Superficial Reflex Techniques

These techniques engage only the skin and may produce reflex effects, such as hyperstimulation analgesia, but no mechanical effects.

Superficial Fluid Techniques

These techniques engage skin, superficial fascia, and subcutaneous fat down to the investing layer of the deep fascia. They produce mechanical effects on superficial lymphatics and possibly the venous circulation.

Neuromuscular Techniques

These techniques engage muscle and the tissues it contains. They affect the function of the contractile element, connective tissue hydration, and lymphatic return. They may also produce complex reflex effects.

Connective Tissue Techniques

These techniques engage superficial and deep layers of connective tissue. They mechanically affect the hydration, extensibility, and modeling of connective tissue. They may also produce complex reflex effects.

Passive Movement Techniques

These techniques produce substantial tissue or joint motion without effort on the part of the client. They engage multiple tissues and structures and have wide-ranging effects on fluid flow, connective tissue, and the neural control of muscle tone.

Percussive Techniques

These techniques deform and release tissues quickly. They engage different tissues depending on the force with which therapists apply them. Therapists use them primarily in cardiopulmonary rehabilitation to assist bronchial drainage and airway clearance mechanically. They may also produce useful reflex neuromuscular effects.

Intelligent Touch

The framework of "intelligent touch" defines six skills that we believe therapists must master before they can use massage techniques successfully. These skills are attention and concentration, discrimination, identification, inquiry, and intention. The premise of this model is that therapists who lack, or are deficient in their ability to perform, any of these skills may be unable to achieve the identified outcomes of the techniques consistently. Consequently, we suggest that an effective therapist should not only learn these skills but also practice them continuously.

Attention and Concentration

Attention and concentration refer to therapists' capacity to focus on the sensory information that they receive primarily, but not exclusively, through their hands. Therapists must learn to focus their awareness on selected aspects of the sensory field at hand and to constantly analyze and organize the many types of information that they obtain. Tissue temperature, texture, and tension are the most basic characteristics that therapists can sense and compare through multiple tissue layers and in different anatomical structures. Massage that therapists perform mechanically or mindlessly, without continuous attention to a broad spectrum of sensory information that is available, produces less than optimal results.

Discrimination

Discrimination, within the context of Outcome-Based Massage™, refers to therapists' ability to distinguish fine gradations of sensory information. With practice, therapists can begin to identify more refined types of sensory information such as tissue characteristics and responses to movement or applied force. Discriminative ability varies widely among novice therapists and can improve with education. Furthermore, although discriminative ability is a fairly common gift, novice therapists may require numerous hours of practice performing massage techniques before their discriminative ability is adequate for independent clinical practice.

Identification

Therapists must be able to distinguish between healthy and dysfunctional tissue states. In addition, they must be able to identify structures and their response to applied forces. Identification is the component of intelligent touch that benefits the most from formal training in anatomy, including the examination of skeletons, palpation of live bodies, and, ideally, the exploration of cadavers while referencing a well-illustrated anatomical atlas.

Inquiry

Intelligent touch is inquiring touch. Good therapists are constantly asking questions. The use of massage is no exception to this requirement. Using inquiring touch does not imply that the therapist's touch feels tentative to the client or that it lacks firmness. Instead, it reflects the never-ending set of questions that inform intelligent touch such as the following: What is this tissue? How does the feel of this tissue relate to the client's history? How does this relate to the client's symptoms? How does this compare to the feel of this type of tissue in other places in the client's body? How does this compare to other healthy and dysfunctional tissues that I have palpated in the past? The process of inquiry requires that therapists make a constant comparison among the tissues they are palpating, other tissues in the client's body, and their memory of other tissues they have palpated.

Intention

The final element of intelligent touch is intention. Intention refers to the therapist's aim of using massage techniques to produce a more normalized response of the client's tissues or other structures. Consequently, intention depends on the therapist having a clear notion of the feel of improvements in the function of tissue and other structures that can arise during the application of any given massage technique. Therapists also need to understand how this improved feel relates to outcomes for body structures and functions, as well as functional outcomes. Therapists who have clear intentions know how both healthy and dysfunctional tissues respond to massage. In addition, they work to produce as close to the ideal tissue response as possible, given the constraints of the client's characteristics and the clinical setting.

Intelligent Practice of Massage Techniques

We advise novice therapists to consider the following guidelines when practicing the application of the massage techniques outlined in this book.

- Locate the tissues selected for treatment through palpation and be specific in your contact of these tissues.
- Palpate continuously for the response of the client's tissues to your application of the technique.
- Frequently observe and elicit feedback on the client's response to your application of techniques.
- First attempt to achieve penetration to deeper tissue layers through repetition of the technique rather than by increasing the pressure of application.
- Decrease the rate of application when you are treating deeper tissue layers in order to provide a sufficient amount of time for the displacement of fluid and the intervening tissues.
- Obtain feedback on the client's level of comfort after changes of position to eliminate positioning as a source of discomfort during the application of techniques.
- Minimize client discomfort during treatment by modifying your application of techniques to ensure the client's comfort.
- Adapt your application of each technique to the region of the body to which you are applying it.
- Practice each technique individually to achieve competence in the execution of that technique before attempting to combine techniques into massage sequences. Unthinking repetition of any sort of routine may result in an inflexibility of treatment approach that may later impede your appropriate use of techniques in clinical situations.

Receipt of Skilled Massage

In recent years, as various forms of massage have received growing attention in scientific and public forums, there has been a trend toward allowing students to perform massage with little or no personal experience with skilled massage or related forms of structured touch. This lack of on-the-table experience can make it difficult for students to acquire more than the most basic proficiency in massage. Students cannot rely on each other to demonstrate refined touch in classroom exchanges. In addition, the brief exposure to the touch of qualified teachers in the classroom does not demonstrate overall flow, pacing, and rhythm to the students. Furthermore, although watching experienced therapists work is extremely useful, it fails to convey the subtleties of touch. In addition, the authors have observed that students who have received touch from competent professionals prior to studying massage techniques often demonstrate much more rapid improvement in their manual skills. On this basis, the authors propose that few preparations will facilitate students' achievement of mastery of the craft of massage as much as the repeated receipt of massage or other manual techniques from competent, experienced professionals. This repeated exposure to "intelligent touch" can impart certain kinesthetic essentials that cannot be conveyed in words, ideas, or images.

THERAPISTS' PHYSICAL PREPARATION FOR TREATMENT (SELF-CARE)

The practice of massage places considerable strain on your body. In particular, the soft tissues of the back and the upper limb are prone to muscular fatigue, tightness, **trigger point syndromes**, and **repetitive strain injury**. Anyone who uses massage techniques extensively in treatment must develop a comprehensive exercise program that includes aerobic, flexibility, resistance, and balance training in order to maintain a trouble-free level of function and to prevent ongoing damage. Failure to pursue an exercise program can place you at greater risk of injury and increases the likelihood that you will experience burnout. Comprehensive programs are beyond the scope of this book and are detailed elsewhere.[1-3] The following is a selection of exercises that are of particular relevance for therapists who use massage techniques in treatment.

Movement

Therapists can use different types of **active exercises** for different purposes. Brisk active exercise increases heart rate, local blood flow, tissue temperature, and tissue **extensibility**. You can use active exercise prior to stretching exercises to warm up at the beginning of the workday and after breaks. Figures 6-1 to 6-4 show several shaking and "swinging" exercises for the whole body, which you can use to loosen the muscles of the shoulder girdle, back, and hips in preparation for performing massage.

Very slow, active movements are excellent for tension release and relaxation (Figures 6-5 and 6-6). When performing these exercises, sit or recline comfortably to promote relaxation throughout your body. Then choose a single isolated motion, such as shoulder abduction, and perform it very slowly and at a consistent rate. The rate of movement should be sufficiently slow that it takes 30 to 60 seconds to complete movement through the available range. At the end of the movement, relax completely and rest for several seconds. You may then either repeat that movement or perform a movement for another joint. This procedure is most effective when you use it on several joints.

Stretching

Stretching techniques are an excellent way to maintain and improve soft tissue **flexibility**, relieve neuromuscular tension, improve capacity for activity, and relieve pain and soreness related to activity.[4-7] There are many different stretching techniques. The following are the basic guidelines for effective static stretching:[5,6]

1. Warm up first with slow active movement.
2. Move to the end of range to the point at which a comfortable stretch is experienced.
3. Breathe deeply throughout the stretch.

A

B

FIGURE 6-2 **A.** Circumduct each arm vigorously 10 to 20 times. This movement opens the shoulder girdle and pushes blood in a centrifugal direction to the hand. **B.** Perform the movement in both directions. Coordinate bending your knees as your arm descends and straightening your knees as your arm ascends.

FIGURE 6-1 Shaking the hands, wrists, and forearms is a good way to relieve local neuromuscular tension immediately before or after massage. You can do this slowly and in a relaxed fashion or more briskly.

FIGURE 6-3 Swing the arms from side to side in the frontal plane; lift both arms up to one side, then relax and allow them to drop passively back down and in front of the body. Then swing them up to the other side, and then relax down again to the center. Produce a continuous movement back and forth like a pendulum.

4. Hold the stretch position for 15 to 30 seconds.
5. Gently move farther into the range without bouncing.
6. Hold the stretch position for an additional 30 seconds.
7. Stretch both sides equally.
8. Never stretch to the point of experiencing pain.

These stretches target areas that are frequently of concern to therapists who use massage in treatment. You can assemble these into short routines to use at the beginning or end of the workday or even in the brief intervals that arise between clients (Figures 6-7 to 6-25).

Self-Massage

Once you acquire some expertise with performing the different massage techniques described later in this text, you can perform them on yourself. Self-massage is particularly useful for relieving the tension that accumulates in your forearms and hands during treatment. You can also incorporate these techniques into your warm-up and cool-down routines (Figures 6-26 to 6-33).

FIGURE 6-4 A. Swing the arms in the horizontal plane around the body in one direction and then back again. Allow the movement of the arms to be as loose as possible, so that the hands swing round to tap the opposite shoulder and hip at the end of each movement. **B.** You can power the movement of the arms by generating a forceful rotation of the trunk and pelvis in one direction and then back again (like a washing machine); the arms follow this movement.

FIGURE 6-5 Lie supine on the floor in this position. Keep hands, arms, and shoulders as relaxed as possible and maintain maximum contact with the floor without forcing. Slide the arm(s) up very slowly as if reaching "over the head" and then back down. Pause occasionally to relax totally and take a full breath. Allow at least 2 minutes to go through the entire cycle up and down. Repeat the entire movement or concentrate on less fluid portions of the joint range of motion.

FIGURE 6-6 Lie supine on the floor in this position. Keep hands, arms, and shoulders as relaxed as possible, and maintain maximum contact with the floor without forcing. Slide the hands very slowly beside the body up toward the armpits (the elbows move out to the side) and then back down. Pause occasionally to relax totally and take a full breath. Allow at least 2 minutes to go through the entire cycle up and down. Repeat the entire movement, or concentrate on less fluid portions of the joint range of motion.

FIGURE 6-7 Active flexion of the neck—"chin to chest."

FIGURE 6-8 Active extension of the neck. Attempt to elongate the entire neck as cervical extension occurs, rather than just moving the occiput toward the first thoracic vertebra.

FIGURE 6-9 Active cervical rotation.

FIGURE 6-10 Cervical side-bending with gentle overpressure. You can stabilize the shoulder girdle by holding under the edge of the chair.

A

B

FIGURE 6-11 A. The "in doorway" stretch for pectoral muscles (the sides of the door frame are represented by the bars). The therapist pushes gently through the door frame toward the viewer, without arching the lower back. This position stretches the clavicular fibers of the pectoralis major. **B.** The "in doorway" stretch with the arms in the upper position stretches the sternal fibers of the pectoralis major.

FIGURE 6-12 To stretch the posterior deltoid, draw the arm across the front of the body toward the opposite shoulder.

FIGURE 6-13 You can stretch the biceps brachii in several positions as long as you extend your shoulder and elbow and pronate your forearm. In this position, extending the thoracic spine will intensify the stretch.

FIGURE 6-14 To stretch all of the triceps brachii you need to flex your shoulder and your elbow.

FIGURE 6-15 A. This behind-the-back clasped-hand position lengthens internal and external rotators of the shoulder on opposite sides. **B.** A towel can help a less flexible person attain the position. The hands can pull up or down to stretch the opposite shoulder.

FIGURE 6-16 Hang from a bar of suitable height (or a door or door frame) to lengthen the entire torso. Maintain contact with ground. Perform a posterior pelvic tilt (tuck the pelvis) to stretch the latissimus dorsi.

FIGURE 6-18 If done carefully, this yoga pose is an excellent stretch for the mid-trapezius. Wrap your arms around each other and simultaneously depress the shoulder girdle, raise your elbows, and push your hands away from your face.

FIGURE 6-19 Arch upward to stretch the extensors of your spine. You can shift your weight forward over your arms or back over your knees to focus the stretch more toward the thoracic or the lumbar extensors, respectively.

FIGURE 6-17 To stretch the interscapular area, assume this position, round the thoracic spine, and push through the sixth thoracic vertebra toward the ceiling.

FIGURE 6-20 "Child's pose"—a most relaxing position for the back. The buttocks rest on the heels. A less flexible person can place one or two pillows over the posterior calves or the thighs for support.

FIGURE 6-21 A. "Knee to chest" provides a unilateral stretch of the gluteus maximus in supine. **B.** "Knee to opposite chest" also stretches the gluteus maximus. To stretch the piriformis, bring the hip down from this position to exactly 90° of flexion.

FIGURE 6-22 To stretch the wrist extensors, extend the elbows and use a gentle pressure of the dorsum of the hands against a vertical or horizontal surface to move the wrist into flexion. Do not lean on the wrists in this position.

FIGURE 6-23 To stretch the wrist flexors, extend the elbows and use a gentle pressure of the palms against a vertical or horizontal surface to take the wrists into extension.

FIGURE 6-24 Another flexor stretch. Interlock the fingers and push the hands as far away as possible.

FIGURE 6-25 "Finger-splits" stretch the intrinsic muscles of the hand. You can perform a maneuver between each pair of adjacent digits.

FIGURE 6-26 Compression administered to the extensors of the forearm with a tennis ball and body weight. See Chapter 9.

FIGURE 6-28 Near the common extensor origin is a frequent trouble spot for repetitive strain injuries. From this position, the therapist can apply stripping, direct fascial technique, or friction. See Chapters 9 and 10.

FIGURE 6-27 **A.** Self-administered direct fascial technique applied to the extensor surface of the forearm. See Chapter 10. **B.** Self-administered direct fascial technique applied to the flexor surface of the forearm. See Chapter 10.

FIGURE 6-29 Thumb kneading applied to the muscles of the thenar eminence. You can continue this with good effect for 5 to 10 minutes or more per hand. See Chapter 9.

FIGURE 6-30 Specific digital compression applied with a reinforced thumb to the muscles of the thenar eminence. See Chapter 9.

FIGURE 6-31 The index finger and the thumb (hidden) work on opposite sides of the intermetacarpal space to free the intrinsic muscles of the hand. Techniques that you can apply in this position include specific compression, stripping, and direct fascial technique. See Chapters 9 and 10.

FIGURE 6-33 You can perform distraction at the metacarpophalangeal joints and all other joints of the hand.

FIGURE 6-32 Performing massage exerts considerable compressive force on joints of the wrist and hand that you can counter with the use of self-mobilization. Here, distraction of the wrist includes both proximal and distal carpal joints.

THERAPISTS' PSYCHOLOGICAL PREPARATION FOR TREATMENT

Burnout Prevention

Chronic stress is excessive or prolonged levels of stress that can cause physical, psychological, and behavioral problems. "**Burnout**" is the exhaustion and loss of interest in work and personal life that can result from chronic stress. While there are often warning signs of burnout, therapists often miss these as a result of lack of awareness of the signs of chronic stress. Each person has her own response to stress. Table 6-1 includes some common signs of chronic stress, which are often preventable and reversible. Therapists are advised to consult a health care

Table 6-1	Common Signs of Chronic Stress

Mental/Emotional Signs	Behavioral Signs	Physical Signs
These are changes in your emotions and mental function. What emotions do you feel and how do your thoughts change when you are under stress?	These are changes in your behavior. They are often the easiest signs of chronic stress to spot. What do you do when you are under stress?	These are changes in your body that you experience. What do you notice happening in your body when you are under stress?
■ Forgetfulness ■ Poor concentration ■ Racing thoughts ■ Anxiety ■ Hopelessness ■ Anger ■ Depression	■ Experience poor decision-making ■ Become short-tempered or irritable ■ Become disorganized ■ Sleep more or less ■ Withdraw or have trouble with relationships	■ Muscle tension ■ Stomach problems ■ Headaches ■ Altered sleep patterns ■ Change in energy level ■ Frequent illness

professional if they are concerned about their signs of chronic stress or other symptoms.

Using Stress Busters

The goal during busy, stressful times is to decrease levels of destructive chronic stress and maintain healthy levels of "good stress" or challenges that make life interesting. This strategy can help therapists to avoid burnout. Stress busters can help therapists achieve this goal.

A stress buster is any activity that therapists can use to control their stress levels. It doesn't have to be complicated. A successful stress buster can be as simple as eating a leisurely breakfast, mentally complimenting yourself on your performance, or taking a few deep breaths before you make a phone call. There are seven types of stress busters:

1. Personal Support: Personal contact with living things—people, pets, even plants—helps you feel supported, enhances your self-esteem, and helps you lower your stress levels.

2. Organizational: These are activities that ease tension by building structure into your personal life.
3. Physical: Activities that enhance your physical well-being will give you more stamina, make you more resilient, and lift your spirits.
4. Emotional: Acknowledging and expressing your emotions will improve both your mental and physical well-being.
5. Mental: Because these are activities you do in your mind, they have the advantage of being portable and private.
6. Diversionary: Taking a break can restore your energy and help you to see your situation from a fresh perspective.
7. Spiritual: Tending to your spiritual life can help you maintain a sense of direction. Remember that spirituality goes beyond religion to embrace Nature and the things that inspire us in our lives.

Table 6-2 shows some examples of stress busters that therapists may use to prevent burnout.

Table 6-2	**Examples of Stress Busters**
Type of Stress Buster	**Sample Stress Buster**
Mental strategies	■ Remember the rewards you get from your work and personal life. ■ Collect information or get training. ■ Pause to pull your thoughts together. ■ Problem solve: Be Prepared. Take the situation apart, examine your options, and develop a plan. ■ Look for a silver lining: Try to find something positive in the situation. ■ Rehearse mentally: Imagine yourself successfully responding to the situation. ■ Build your confidence: Remind yourself of your strong points. ■ Learn by teaching: Teach a new skill to a colleague or someone you know.
Physical strategies	■ Take a deep breath: A slow breath in through your nose and out through your mouth. ■ Relax: Perform a relaxation technique. ■ Eat a healthy meal. ■ Sleep: Have a nap or a good night's sleep. ■ Move: Walk, stretch, dance, jog, cycle, anything goes. ■ Laugh! ■ Massage your tense areas.
Personal support strategies	■ Get guidance from a friend, family member, or any confidant. ■ Talk to or spend time with someone whom you care about. ■ Make a gift for or write a letter to someone. ■ Share a meal with someone. ■ Allow someone to help you. ■ Nurture something: A pet, a plant... ■ Spend some time alone.

(Continued)

Table 6-2	Examples of Stress Busters (*Continued*)

Type of Stress Buster	Sample Stress Buster
Emotional strategies	■ Let yourself feel your emotions—don't block out those feelings. ■ Release your emotions. ■ Hold your tongue if you think you are about to say something you'll regret. ■ Write a letter expressing your feelings to someone who has upset you but don't mail it. ■ Talk to someone about the challenges that you are facing. ■ Work off your strong emotions with vigorous physical activity. ■ Apologize for something that you've done.
Organizational strategies	■ Clean your work area: Sort your paperwork, throw out junk, unclutter your desk. ■ Choose one important goal to work on. ■ Make a "To Do" list and prioritize it before you go to bed. ■ Create a backup plan. ■ Set yourself a schedule. ■ Take it one small step at a time. ■ Identify how you can delegate tasks to other people.
Diversionary strategies	■ Play a game or sport for fun. ■ Listen to something relaxing: Music, audiobooks, nature sounds, chimes... ■ Take a mini vacation using mental imagery. ■ Make or fix something: Furniture, crafts, jigsaws, food, cars... ■ Pamper yourself: A haircut, warm bath, massage, afternoon nap... ■ Do something familiar and comforting: Read a book, daydream, work on a hobby... ■ Do something you've never tried before: Walk in the rain, try a new hobby, go somewhere new...
Spiritual Strategies	■ Engage in a spiritual activity or ceremony. ■ Go to your place of worship or any place where you feel peaceful. ■ Pause to reflect. ■ Enjoy Nature. ■ Speak to someone who can offer spiritual guidance. ■ Give thanks. ■ Remind yourself that you are a part of Nature and that tomorrow brings a chance to start afresh.

Adapted from Andrade C. *60 Stress Busters for Helping Professionals and 60 Stress Busters for Volunteers*, with permission.

Choosing Positive Stress Busters

Some stress busters offer short-term relief and long-term problems. Relying on drugs or alcohol are two obvious examples. Yet even seemingly harmless activities, such as exercise or daydreaming, can have negative effects on therapist personal lives if they use them in excess. A good stress buster must be appropriate for the time and place you need to use it. For example, while chanting aloud may be relaxing at home, this may not be appropriate in public. In addition, therapists need to identify whether they need a short-term or long-term stress buster. There is nothing wrong with using short-term stress busters. Therapists who find themselves facing the same problem repeatedly, may find a longer-term solution—one that seeks and addresses the source of the problem—to be more beneficial.

Time Management

You must ensure that you allot adequate time to perform the types of treatment you have scheduled, to review clients' files, to check reference material, and to think about each client. Ideally, you should be able to manage your own treatment schedule. This will enable you to consider and address clients' needs, the facility's policies, charting requirements, reimbursement issues, and your own capacity for performing treatments as you schedule clients. If another individual is responsible for booking, you will need to state your guidelines for booking clearly to that person so that they do not impose an unreasonable and rushed schedule on you.

Using Physical Modalities for Psychological Preparation

Once you ensure that you have adequate time for treatment and other supporting activities, you can use some of the physical modalities previously described, such as gentle stretching, to assist your psychological preparation. In the same manner, conscious diaphragmatic breathing, correct body mechanics, and the use of controlled repetitive movement during the performance of massage techniques can deepen your level of relaxation.

Spiritual Preparation

Professions that use massage are usually service-oriented professions. You may draw upon a number of different resources for informing and deepening your ethical commitment to others and cultivating an attitude of peaceful, fulfilling service to others. These include a variety of forms of nonsectarian and sectarian spiritual practice such as the use of autogenic or visualization exercises for relaxation or drawing upon an established faith. It is invaluable for you to practice some routine of calming the mind throughout the workday, especially in the few minutes preceding sessions. Since isolation contributes to the experience of "**burnout**" that is so common in service-oriented professions, it is also wise to include in your clinical practice

opportunities for interactions with colleagues, such as continuing education courses, review of clients, and professional meetings. Finally, service to others should not be at the expense of taking care of yourself.

THERAPISTS' PREPARATION OF MATERIALS FOR TREATMENT

Tables

The treatment table or massage table is an essential tool in the practice of massage. Since treatment tables come in a variety of makes and styles, you should consider your anticipated needs carefully prior to purchasing a table. Any table that you use for massage techniques must be solid, stable, easy to clean, at least 28 × 72 in., and adjustable for height to accommodate different clients and types of work. Ideally, the table will have high-density foam padding on both the top and sides of the tabletop because you may frequently lean or brace yourself against the sides of the table. A well-designed, adjustable face cradle or head support is a desirable addition to the basic treatment table. This is an appropriate alternative to the use of face holes, since the latter rarely fit all clients equally well.

Stationary tables are preferable for the clinic or office setting, since they are extremely strong and stable, although heavy and not easily moved (Figure 6-34). A hydraulic or electric height-adjustable table provides quick adjustment to the different heights that are required for the most efficient application of different techniques.

If you travel frequently to provide care, there are many styles of well-built portable tables from which to choose (Figure 6-35). These tables weigh between 10 and 20 kg, are strong and attractive, are equipped with face cradles and arm shelves, and only lack quick height

FIGURE 6-34 A metal-frame stationary table with face hole and adjustable legs that you can tilt partially.

FIGURE 6-35 A portable table.

adjustments. As a result, you may choose to use a portable table for your primary place of practice.

If you select a table that lacks a mechanism for quickly adjusting height, set the table up at a lower height. The use of a lower table height requires you to have training and practice in the correct use of your legs. Novice therapists frequently set their tables too high, which predisposes them to make many errors in body mechanics. When you are performing work that requires use of a substantial amount of body weight, such as **neuromuscular** and **connective tissue techniques**, you may set the height of the table to the level of your extended fingertips or even lower (Figure 6-36). For lighter work, such as superficial reflex and passive movement techniques, you may set the table height to the level of your wrist or even higher.

Portable massage chairs are specifically designed for "on-site" or "mobile" practices of massage (Figure 6-37A). These chairs offer comfort and ease of access to common problem areas for the office worker. They are not, however, very versatile, and some clients may find the half-kneeling position difficult to assume (Figure 6-37B).

Before and between clients, therapists should clean the table, bed, or chair surfaces that come in contact with clients with commercially available disinfectants, and draping should be washed with soap and hot water and rinsed with a 10% bleach solution.[8]

A

FIGURE 6-36 Correct table height varies with the technique that is being performed and the size of the client. Usually, the working height of the table lies between the height of the therapist's wrist and the tips of the extended fingers. Occasionally, the optimal height may be as low as the therapist's knees or as high as the waist.

B

FIGURE 6-37 A. Portable massage chair with a strong, light, upholstered frame that folds into an easily carried unit. **B.** It offers good access to the back and neck.

FIGURE 6-38 The therapist will require supports in a variety of shapes and sizes.

Supports

You can use either a commercially designed set of bolsters or a set of pillows when positioning clients on a bed or the floor. In addition, you need a large selection of pillows and bolsters of various sizes and shapes, including at least six standard-sized pillows (Figure 6-38). If necessary, you can place foam- or kapok-filled mats on the floor. The physical demands of working on the floor are extreme, however, and the repertoire of techniques that can be adapted for floor work is limited. Before and between clients, therapists should clean mat surfaces that come into contact with clients with commercially available disinfectants, and draping should be washed with soap and hot water and rinsed with a 10% bleach solution.[8]

Linen

Sturdy, bleachable, opaque, cotton sheeting in white or pastels are common for clinical use. Although single (twin) flat sheets ensure ample coverage, a slightly narrower width of 50 to 54 in. is easier to handle and can reduce bunching of excess draping. Pillow cases, small and large towels, and blankets are among the basic linen supplies. You must launder any linen that comes into contact with clients after each use with detergent and hot water. Some facilities also use bleach and commercial degreaser. Whenever possible, use professional laundering.

Lubricants

Therapists use lubricants to control the amount of **glide**, **friction**, and **drag** that occurs between their moving hands and their clients' skin. Although you may apply lubricants to the client's skin, they affect your ability to palpate and produce changes in the client's subcutaneous tissues. Consequently, you require lubricant for some techniques, avoid it for others, and obtain potential benefit for other

techniques only when you carefully choose and apply the lubricant. Because of the different requirements for lubricants, you should have on hand a selection of lubricants to facilitate application of a range of techniques. Any lubricant that you use must be hypoallergenic and dispensed in a hygienic manner that does not contaminate the supply, such as through a squeeze bottle, pump, or shaker. Clients must **consent** to the choice of lubricant and must consent before you add scent to the lubricant as, for example, in **aromatherapy**.

Oils

Oils continue to be the lubricant of choice for classic **neuromuscular techniques**. You can use virtually any high-quality vegetable oil, including olive, sunflower, safflower, almond, jojoba, and coconut oils. Mineral oil, on the other hand, is considered to be less nutritious for the skin.[9] Each oil has a slightly different density, stickiness, and rate of absorption. Oil has two drawbacks: it goes rancid, and it stains. In addition, you must remove unabsorbed oil from the client's skin with disposable towels, which you can moisten with alcohol.

Lotions

Lotions are opaque, liquid suspensions of particles in either oil or water. Since lotions are readily absorbed into the client's skin, their lubricating qualities decline quickly with time. This rapid absorption can be an advantage when you are preparing the client's tissues for deeper neuromuscular or **connective tissue techniques**.

Creams

Creams are thicker suspensions, often oil based, that fall midway between oils and lotions in terms of their rate of absorption. Creams can be quite oily and promote glide. Alternatively, they may contain sticky ingredients, such as lanolin and beeswax, which reduce glide and increase your tendency to drag the client's skin. The ability of some creams to reduce glide may be useful for connective tissue techniques.

Powders

Use fine powder in the form of French chalk, cornstarch, or unscented baby powder for techniques that require glide and when clients refuse oil. Furthermore, powder is the preferred lubricant for most **lymph-drainage techniques**.

CONCLUSION

The correct preparation for treatment is a critical component of Outcome-Based Massage™. A sound understanding of the taxonomy and principles of intelligent touch that guide the clinical use of the massage techniques in Outcome-Based Massage™ is the first step. In Outcome-Based Massage™, the taxonomy of massage techniques organizes techniques based on anatomy, operational requirements, and outcomes. In addition, the six components of intelligent touch—attention and concentration, discrimination, identification, inquiry,

and intention—define the skills that therapists need for successful application of massage techniques. Therapists can increase their skill in performing Outcome-Based Massage™ by performing intelligent practice of massage techniques and receiving skilled massage in order to learn the correct application and flow of techniques. Personal preparation of the therapist needs to address both psychological and physical needs in order to prevent burnout and injury and increase one's personal satisfaction as a therapist. Finally, therapists need to prepare and maintain proper hygiene of their tools, such as treatment tables or chairs, supports, linen, and lubricants.

Practice

Note: This section contains instructions that demonstrate how to perform some of the strategies for preparation and positioning that were introduced in this chapter.

POSITIONING AND DRAPING THE PATIENT DURING TREATMENT

Positioning

In selecting the position for massage, consider the aims of treatment, the areas you wish to access, and your patient's preferences and comfort. Prone, supine, side-lying, seated, seated inclined, and long-sitting are common options, each of which has its own specific requirements for pillow placement and support. Key Points 6-1 summarizes which muscles, tissues, and regions are readily accessible in the common positions used for treatment.

Once you have positioned the patient correctly on the treatment table, adjust, add, or remove the pillows, bolsters, or rolled towels used for support to ensure that the patient is comfortable. Figures 6-39 to 6-45 illustrate some common positions and how you can support them with pillows. In practice, place pillows beneath the bottom sheet so that you can reuse them without having to recover them. Many other configurations are possible and will be required if you work in a hospital, rehabilitation, sports, or office setting.

Key Points: 6-1

Treatment Positions for Various Muscles

Prone Is an Excellent Treatment Position for

- Posterior cervical muscles
- Latissimus dorsi
- Rhomboids
- Mid and lower trapezius
- Spinal extensors
- Gluteus maximus
- Hamstrings
- Triceps surae
- Intrinsic foot muscles

Supine Is an Excellent Treatment Position for

- All muscles of the head and neck
- Pectorals
- All muscles of the arm
- Abdominals
- Quadriceps
- Muscles of the anterior compartment

Side-Lying Is an Excellent Treatment Position for

On Uppermost Side of the Patient's Body

- Scalenes
- Rotator cuff
- Pectoralis minor

- Serratus anterior
- Abdominals
- Quadratus lumborum
- Iliocostalis
- Gluteus medius and minimus
- Iliotibial tract
- Peronei

On Lower Side of the Patient's Body
- Adductors of the hip
- Triceps surae

Seated Upright Position Is an Excellent Treatment Position for
- Upper trapezius

Seated Inclined Position Is an Excellent Treatment Position for
- All muscles of the posterior aspect of the head and neck
- All muscles of the upper back
- All muscles of the posterior aspect of the upper arms

FIGURE 6-40 Legs can be elevated for drainage with **(A)** a tilted treatment table or **(B)** a mound of pillows.

Draping

Draping does more than place the patient in a safe, warm, modest, and comfortable position in which to receive the intended massage. Appropriate draping can also serve to achieve and maintain appropriate patient–clinician boundaries that clinicians need in all practice settings, including the classroom. Because draping sets a symbolic and an actual boundary between you and the patient during treatment, you must make draping comfortable yet precise and secure when exposing the patient's body for treatment purposes.

FIGURE 6-39 A. Typically therapists use one or two pillows under the knees when a client is supine to reduce the strain on the lower back. **B.** You may need an additional pillow or towel roll under the cervical spine for the comfort of clients who have an anterior-head posture.

FIGURE 6-41 In prone position, a single pillow under the ankles takes pressure off the knees.

FIGURE 6-42 A, B. Prone, an additional small pillow placed under the abdomen can raise the lumbar spine into a less lordotic position. This may reduce the back pain of some clients with low back pain such as those with acute facet derangement.

FIGURE 6-43 A, B. Add another towel roll under the upper chest to improve comfort for large-breasted women or to take the pressure off the thyroid cartilage.

FIGURE 6-44 A. In side-lying position, use pillows for the head and legs. **B.** Place one or two pillows between the client's knees to enhance comfort. **C.** To access the medial tissues of the thigh and leg nearest the table, flex the hip and knee of the upper leg to 90°, and use pillows to support the upper leg so that the pelvis does not rotate.

Your scope of practice, the professional code of conduct, and local laws will dictate what is permissible in terms of exposing the patient's body during treatment. When undraping the patient, adhere to these rules:

1. Only undrape one body segment at a time.
2. Only undrape areas that are to be treated.
3. Do not undrape the gluteal cleft, perineum, genitals, and female breast.

FIGURE 6-45 Several pillows support a relaxed seated position that offers good access to the upper back, shoulders, and posterior neck.

There are three possible legitimate exceptions to these rules.[10,11] In each case, you must know whether your local laws supersede the exception.

1. You may expose the female breasts if breast massage is clinically indicated and the patient has provided voluntary **informed consent** to this exposure prior to treatment.
2. You may undrape the pelvis if the patient has provided voluntary informed consent to massage for the purposes of labor support and/or delivery. Clinicians who have the treatment of pelvic floor dysfunction in their professional scope of practice should consult their professional organization for guidelines on draping.
3. You may treat infants undraped with parental consent.

Use the following steps for carrying out draping when massage is a primary modality and you are in a clinical setting with individual treatment rooms and tables. You may modify these procedures if you use massage techniques as an adjunct to other manual or exercise techniques or if you practice in a hospital, rehabilitation, sports, or other setting. Once you have negotiated the plan of care with the patient, identify the articles of clothing and jewelry that she will need to remove and explain the rationale for doing so. If the patient chooses to remain clothed or partially clothed, you must explain the technical consequences of this choice to the patient. Then give the patient clear instructions on how to position herself on the table and how to arrange the draping and supports that you have provided. Once you are sure that you have answered the patient's questions, leave the room so that the patient can undress in privacy.[10] If the patient requires assistance undressing or getting onto the table, you must clearly explain which items of the patient's clothing—if any— you will be removing and where you will be touching or moving her; you also need to obtain and record consent for this assistance before assisting the patient. Clean your hands and other contact surfaces thoroughly with soap and hot water or alcohol-based hand sanitizer for at least 10 seconds prior to beginning draping procedures and subsequent massage.[8,10]

Students must practice the process of appropriate draping repeatedly and extend appropriate respect to each other during classroom practice. In addition, it is useful for students to perform initial classroom practice with the practice partners clothed until they develop a reasonable level of skill in draping.

The draping sequences in Figures 6-46 to 6-59 all use two single (twin) flat sheets and a few towels. Clinicians can also perform the sequences with sheets as narrow as 4 feet wide. When clinicians perform these draping sequences as described, the draping will be comfortable and secure and will ensure privacy for unclothed patients. You can easily modify the sequences for the legs should the patient choose to wear her underwear. In addition, you will need to modify the draping if you are using massage as an adjunct to other modalities and if the clinical setting or patient preference requires the use of a gown.

Following a clinical session, if there is sufficient time, invite the patient to rest before rising. Then instruct the patient on how to get off the table safely, using statements such as "roll onto your side, let your legs drop off the table, and slowly come to a sitting position, using your arms to push up." If the patient has physical limitations, you may also be required to give the patient discreet assistance to sit up, stand, or dress after the session.

FIGURE 6-46 A. Starting position for undraping the female torso in supine. **B.** Place a folded towel on top of the sheet over the breasts. The client holds the top edge of the towel while the therapist withdraws the sheet from under the towel. **C.** Tuck the towel under the torso or arms, and then expose the abdomen. **D.** In the final position, the drape is securely tucked, and the client's abdomen is exposed from the xiphoid process to the anterior superior iliac spine.

FIGURE 6-47 For women, the chest towel can be folded back to undrape one or both breasts if informed consent has been obtained and massage of breast tissue or the pectoral muscles is clinically indicated.

FIGURE 6-48 A. For men, the issue of consent to treat the anterior torso is less delicate. If you are to perform extensive work on a male client's torso, he can be undraped to the waist. If you only plan for abdominal massage, you should offer him a chest towel for warmth. **B.** The final drape tucked at the level of the anterior superior iliac spine.

FIGURE 6-49 A. Undraping the anterior leg. You expose the client's leg and gather the extra sheet between the legs. **B.** You then pull the extra sheet underneath the exposed leg back toward the side of the table. Here, the weight of the leg securely anchors the sheet. **C.** You can tuck the top edge of the drape under the gluteal at the level of the greater trochanter. **D.** Or you can roll the edge of the sheet higher to expose the anterior superior iliac spine and tuck it under the client's lower back.

FIGURE 6-50 **A.** Turning to prone. The basic procedure is similar for turning from supine to prone, from prone to supine, or from either position to or from side-lying. Use the front of your thigh to pin the sheets against the near edge of the table while your hands secure both sheets across the table. Instruct the client to turn. **B.** Throughout the turn, maintain control of both sheets at both sides of the table. Failure to do this will result in exposure of the client or a migrating bottom sheet that bunches uncomfortably under the client. Take care to minimize inadvertent touching of the client during the turn.

FIGURE 6-51 **A.** Starting position for undraping the torso in prone position. **B.** For general back massage, the back is exposed to just below the level of the posterior superior iliac spine. **C.** The drape is securely tucked. **D.** The client may choose to position her arms at her sides. **E.** Or the client may position her arms overhead.

FIGURE 6-51 (*Continued*)

FIGURE 6-52 This angled draping unilaterally exposes the superior gluteal insertions. Clinicians must work on these extensively when treating many lumbar conditions.

FIGURE 6-53 **A.** The procedure for undraping the posterior leg is similar to that for the anterior leg. Expose the client's limb and gather the extra sheet between the legs. **B.** Pull the extra sheet underneath the exposed thigh back toward the side of the table. Here, the weight of the leg securely anchors the sheet. **C.** For a low drape, tuck the upper edge of the sheet under the anterior thigh at the level of the greater trochanter. **D.** A more common and much more useful technique is to roll the edge of the sheet toward the gluteal cleft and securely tuck it above the anterior superior iliac spine, thus exposing the bulk of the gluteals.

FIGURE 6-54 A. To expose the back and the flank of a side-lying female client, first instruct the client to clasp a standard-sized pillow in front. **B.** Undrape the back to the desired level. **C.** Then securely tuck the drape. The upper arm can be raised overhead, while the lower arm maintains the pillow in position.

FIGURE 6-55 The side-lying position potentially offers unparalleled access to the uppermost rotator cuff, serratus anterior, quadratus lumborum, and portions of the pectorals and spinal extensors.

A   B   C

FIGURE 6-56 A. To undrape the bottom leg in side-lying position (for work on the adductors, triceps surae, and tibialis posterior), first flex the knee and hip of the top leg to 90° and use pillows to keep it forward and out of the way (see Figure 6-44C). Then expose the bottom leg from behind and gather the extra sheet between the legs. **B.** Then pull the extra sheet underneath the exposed leg back toward the posterior side of the table at the level of mid-thigh or slightly higher. Here, the weight of the leg securely anchors the sheet. At this point, instruct a male client to move his genitals in a superior direction (e.g., "Adjust yourself."). **C.** The top edge of the drape is then rolled and pushed as close to the ischiopubic ramus as possible, and the posterior edge is tucked under the greater trochanter. You may best perform techniques on the adductor attachments onto the ramus through the sheet, for reasons of discretion.

A   B   C

FIGURE 6-57 A. To expose the top leg in side-lying position, fold the posterior portion of the sheet forward. Move as much of the extra sheet as possible out of the way in a superior direction. **B.** Pull the edge of the drape back under the leg. The drape now surrounds the leg to be exposed, as in a pant leg. The other leg is not exposed at any time during the procedure. Again, move as much of the extra sheet as possible out of the way in a superior direction. **C.** Keeping it tight to the leg, gradually work the "pant leg" drape up the thigh. **D.** Finally, pull the superior edge of the drape toward the groin and toward the gluteal cleft and roll it over the iliac crest. It takes practice to get this draping tight and secure. **E.** Gently lift the leg, and place a pillow under the knee for support.

FIGURE 6-57 (Continued)

FIGURE 6-58 The preferred position in which to work on the piriformis is with the knee and hip both flexed to 90°. If you have applied the drape correctly, it will be possible for you to move the leg without the drape loosening.

FIGURE 6-59 Wrap-around draping is useful for seated massage of the head, neck, and shoulders in a seated inclined position.

CLINICIANS' POSTURE, ALIGNMENT, AND BODY MECHANICS DURING TREATMENT

Efficient posture and movement constitute the physical foundation of effective execution of massage techniques. The outcomes and characteristic "feel" of well-performed massage techniques depend as much on correct use of your feet, legs, pelvis, and respiratory apparatus as they do on the motion of your upper limbs. Students and clinicians who aspire to achieve expertise in performing massage strokes may have postural habits that they must systematically retrain. Furthermore, this retraining must start before instruction in manual technique begins, since attention to your posture will decrease once you begin to learn manual technique. If you have habitually poor body mechanics that are not corrected, then you will experience fatigue and pain when performing massage strokes. For many, this unpleasant result can occur in as little as a few hours or weeks.

The following general principles of body mechanics apply during massage:

1. Keep your posture aligned and as upright as possible, except during controlled transfer of body weight.
2. Keep both feet in contact with the floor.
3. Reduce the vertical distance between yourself and the patient by bending your knees, rather than by bending at the waist.
4. Reduce the horizontal distance between yourself and the patient by repositioning your legs or shifting your weight onto your forward leg, rather than by bending at the waist or reaching excessively.
5. Point your navel area toward the body segment of the patient that you are treating.
6. Increase pressure through the controlled use of body weight, rather than through muscle strength.
7. You may lean in a controlled way toward the point of contact with the patient. When doing so, control the amount of your body weight that you are transferring to the patient precisely and continuously.
8. Position your joints as close to neutral as possible and do not load them when they are in a close-packed position.
9. Change position (e.g., from sitting to kneeling) frequently to vary the mechanical stress that is being placed on your body.

The chapters on techniques use the postures and movements described in this chapter[8,9,12,13] during the application of massage techniques. Ideally, practice them until they have become habitual before attempting to learn the manual parts of massage techniques. These exercises will assist you in developing the relaxation, awareness, balance, coordination, flexibility, and strength that are required to perform massage. A lack of familiarity with these or comparable exercises can compromise the quality of your manual technique and increase risk of injury. Furthermore, these exercises are worthwhile in their own right, and you can incorporate them into your daily warm-up or cool-down.

Standing Aligned Posture

This deceptively simple posture can actually be quite difficult to maintain because it often reveals and accentuates chronic patterns of tension in the body when you first begin to use it. The steps for performing this posture follow (see Figures 6-60A and 6-60B).

Stand with your feet positioned shoulder-width apart. Use the glenoid fossa as a landmark, rather than the lateral surface of the deltoid.

1. Breathe deeply and relax.
2. Let the weight settle down through your legs and into your feet.
3. Explore the manner in which your feet contact the ground by rocking from front to back, shifting from left to right, and shifting the inside to the outside.
4. Attempt to find the foot position in which you distribute the weight of your body evenly through your feet.
5. Let the top of your head rise up gently. You may want to have someone check whether you are incorrectly positioning your head by flexing or extending your neck.
6. Try to hold a standing aligned posture for 10 minutes, progressively refining both your foot contact with the ground and your sense of vertical alignment.

Standing Aligned Posture with Diaphragmatic Breathing

The following are the steps for performing this posture (Figure 6-60C):

1. Assume a standing aligned posture until you feel very stable and relaxed.
2. Focus your attention on your breathing.

A   B   C

FIGURE 6-60 A. Lateral view of standing posture shows a forward lean; a shortening in this therapist's lumbar muscles, with an accompanying anterior pelvic tilt; and an anterior-head posture. These may be due to postural habit or chronic fascial shortening. **B.** The therapist's lumbar spine is in a more neutral position, and the whole posture is better aligned after he balanced the weight on his feet, softened his knees, let his sacrum drop, and let his head rise. Here, the therapist has overcompensated by bending his knees more than necessary. **C.** Using the diaphragm to breathe produces a passive rise of the abdomen on inhalation. Use standing aligned posture when you perform superficial reflex techniques that do not require application of pressure and that you need to sustain for some time.

3. Let your upper chest remain still, and breathe using your diaphragm so that your abdomen passively moves out during the inhalation and passively moves back during the exhalation.
4. Remain in this position and continue to focus on the passive movements of your abdomen. Gradually increase both the duration and depth of the inhalation.
5. Sustain focused breathing for 10 minutes, and periodically check the alignment of your body.

Standing Pelvic Tilt

The following are the steps for performing this posture (Figure 6-61):

1. Assume a **standing aligned posture** until you feel very stable and relaxed.
2. Ensure that your knees are not hyperextended.
3. Focus your attention on your pelvis.
4. Keeping the legs and upper body motionless, perform a posterior pelvic tilt by letting your sacrum drop and rolling your anterior superior iliac spine in a posterior direction.

FIGURE 6-61 During a standing slow pelvic tilt, the pelvis is tucked under, while the thorax remains in the same position. This results in a lengthening of the lumbar region and a reduction of the normal lordosis. This movement is a prerequisite for later movements that involve bending the knees.

5. Place a hand on your lumbar spine and note whether you feel it flatten slightly; this indicates that the posterior pelvic tilt has occurred.
6. Hold the pelvic tilt and breathe deeply using your diaphragm in the manner outlined in the previous section.
7. Relax.
8. Perform this tilt and relax movement 10 to 20 times.
9. Vary your practice of this posture by making the movement larger or subtler or by varying the amount you bend your knees.

Proper performance of a posterior pelvic tilt in standing requires some flexibility. If it is difficult to perform, practice this posture lying supine on a flat surface with your knees and hips flexed, progress to lying supine with your knees and hips extended, and then attempt to perform it standing with your back against a wall before reattempting the posture in unsupported standing.

Seated Aligned Posture

The following are the steps for performing this posture (Figure 6-62):

1. Sit upright on a level, firm, well-padded chair that allows your knees and hips to rest at 90° of flexion. Place your feet on the floor, shoulder-width apart or slightly wider.

FIGURE 6-62 Use seated aligned posture when applying many different techniques. Note the feet flat on the floor and the erect upper body supported by the ischiopubic rami.

2. First touch and then focus your attention on your ischial tuberosities.
3. Allow your spine to flex until you feel the weight of your upper body resting on your ischial tuberosities.
4. While maintaining your upper body in an upright position, slowly roll the contact point of your pelvis with the chair forward so that it shifts from being on the ischial tuberosities to being along the ischial rami in the direction of the symphysis pubis.
5. Since that movement should extend your lumbar spine, place your hand in the small of your back and note whether you feel the erector spinae muscles tighten in your lumbar region.
6. Very slowly rock back and forward several times and locate the point on your pelvis, between your ischial tuberosities and symphysis pubis, at which your upper body feels upright and most comfortably balanced over the pelvis (somewhere around the perineum). The erector spinae muscles in your lumbar region should not be engaged in that position.
7. Breathe deeply using your diaphragm.
8. Let the top of your head rise up gently. You may want to have someone check whether you are incorrectly positioning your head by flexing or extending your neck.
9. Sit for 10 minutes, progressively refining both the contact of your pelvis with the chair and your sense of vertical alignment.

Lunge

This position is also known as walk-standing, bow stance, or archer stance. The following are the steps for performing this posture (Figures 6-63A and 6-63B):

1. Stand with your feet together.
2. Externally rotate your left hip to 20° to 45° so that your left foot is turned out.
3. With your right foot, step forward and to the right of the left foot a comfortable distance.
4. Maintaining an upright torso, slowly straighten your left (back) leg without hyperextending your knee, and bend your right (forward) leg as you move your body over your forward foot.
5. Straighten your right (forward) leg and bend your left (back) knee as you shift your weight onto your back leg. Slowly shift your weight back and forth from your left to right foot, while keeping your torso perfectly poised and upright. Your head should remain equidistant from the floor throughout the movement.

A   B

FIGURE 6-63 A. Lunge position with the weight over the back leg. **B.** Lunge position, shifting the weight toward the front leg (the rear leg can still be straightened some more). As you shift your weight back and forth, your torso remains balanced and motionless in relation to the moving legs. This basic leg movement, used for many techniques, requires some quadriceps strength.

6. You may also synchronize your breathing with the movement by inhaling as you shift your weight in the posterior direction and exhaling as you shift your weight in the anterior direction.

7. Continue for 5 minutes, and then repeat the exercise with the other foot forward.

8. Vary your practice of this posture and make it more challenging by gradually increasing the distance between your feet and the degree to which you flex your knees.

Lunge and Reach

The following are the steps for performing this posture (Figures 6-64A and 6-64B):

1. Begin by performing the steps in the **lunge** movement previously described.

2. As you shift your weight onto your forward leg, extend both arms straight ahead at navel level without fully extending your elbows. As you shift your weight onto your back leg, flex your elbows and shoulders and bring your arms toward your body while keeping them at waist level.

3. Vary your practice of this posture by increasing the distance between your feet, by changing the degree to

which you flex your knees, by varying the level of your arms, and by using different breathing patterns.

Lunge and Lean

The following are the steps for performing this posture (Figure 6-65):

1. Begin by performing the steps in the **lunge** movement previously described.

2. Rather than keeping your torso upright throughout the movement, incline it forward (lean) as you shift your weight onto the forward leg. At the forward portion of the motion, there should be a straight line from the top of your head, through your torso, to the heel of your back leg. The movement of this posture is from upright with your weight on your back leg, to leaning with the weight on your front leg, and back again.

3. Once you have mastered the performance of the lean during the weight shift, add the arm movement previously described in the lunge and reach posture.

Wide-Stance Knee Bend

This position is also known as the horse or warrior stance. The following are the steps for performing this posture (Figures 6-66, 6-67A, and 6-67B):

FIGURE 6-64 A, B. Lunge and reach. Arms extend from an upright torso as you shift your weight to the forward leg. This exact movement is used for superficial effleurage.

FIGURE 6-65 Lunge and lean. The therapist is shifting his weight over the front leg as he leans forward; extending his back knee slightly will complete the forward movement. Using exactly this movement, the therapist transfers pressure to the client during various neuromuscular and connective tissue techniques.

FIGURE 6-66 First, practice the wide stance (horse stance) without movement (the "upper bent-knee position").

FIGURE 6-67 A. Knee bend in the wide stance. As the therapist bends his knees, he simultaneously executes a posterior pelvic tilt so that the lumbar region lengthens. Use this type of leg movement for some neuromuscular techniques like wringing. **B.** A common error of movement is to increase the lumbar lordosis as the knees are bending.

1. Stand with your feet placed more than shoulder-width apart and your feet pointed straight forward or in a small degree of external rotation.
2. While keeping your upper body upright, flex your hips and knees a few degrees. Hold this position. This is the "upper bent-knee position."
3. Adjust the distance (width) between your feet until you are in a position that you can comfortably hold for 2 to 3 minutes.
4. Slowly increase the degree of knee flexion so that you lower your body 6 to 8 in. This is the "lower bent-knee position."
5. While keeping your torso upright, perform a posterior pelvic tilt (using the steps previously described) so that your lower spine lengthens as you lower your body. Place a hand on your lumbar spine to monitor its position during this movement.
6. Slowly extend your knees and return to the upper bent-knee position without hyperextending your lumbar spine or your knees.
7. Repeat.
8. Gradually work up to 100 repetitions of this sequence of movements from neutral to the upper and lower bent-knee positions.
9. Vary your practice of this posture in one of several ways:

a. Change the distance (width) between your feet.
b. Flex your knees more.
c. Rotate your upright torso in one direction as you go down and rotate to the original position as you come up.
d. Perform the knee bend beside a massage table while transferring a portion of your upper body weight to the table through your bent arms.

Standing Controlled Lean

The following are the steps for performing this posture (Figure 6-68):

1. You need a massage table or any other stable object against which you can lean to perform this. The table should be within reach of your partially extended arms.
2. Begin by performing the steps of the **lunge and lean** posture previously described.
3. As you shift weight onto your forward leg, lean forward and extend your arms. Allow your hands to contact the table and slowly transfer some of your weight to the table. As you do this, you should feel a shift of weight onto your extended back leg.

FIGURE 6-68 Use a standing controlled lean to apply pressure during many neuromuscular and connective tissue techniques.

A

4. Slowly return your arms to their original position and shift your upper body back over your back leg.
5. Repeat this back-and-forth movement and transfer some of your body weight to the table at the appropriate point in each movement. The compression and release should be slow and controlled.

Seated Controlled Lean

The following are the steps for performing this posture (Figures 6-69 and 6-70):

1. Begin in the **seated aligned posture** facing a massage table or any other stable object against which you can lean.
2. Place your hands on the supporting surface.
3. Gradually lean forward from your waist and apply pressure to the supporting surface so that you feel balanced as you do so.
4. Alternatively, sit upright on the edge of a firm bed or massage table and face one end of it. If you are on a massage table, the leg closest to the table will be off the ground and the other foot will have a secure contact with the floor.
5. Slowly lean forward to transfer your body weight in the manner described above.
6. Vary your practice of this posture by changing the amount of weight you transfer to the supporting surface, the height of contact, and the compression time (without losing continuous control and relaxed shoulders).

B

FIGURE 6-69 A. A seated controlled lean using a chair. This is often used when treating the client's shoulders. **B.** A seated controlled lean sitting on the edge of the table. When treating clients, it is acceptable to sit on the edge of the table as long as the therapist only contacts the client with his hands or forearms, not his thigh or pelvis.

FIGURE 6-70 The therapist is obviously not using the client to support his body. He demonstrates flawless control of the amount of body weight that he could transfer to a client in this position.

TAKEAWAYS

1. The taxonomy for massage techniques for Outcome-Based Massage™ is based on anatomy, operational requirements, and outcomes. In this taxonomy the order is techniques that affect superficial tissues, those techniques that affect deeper tissues, those techniques that affect multiple tissue layers, methods that require the clinician to palpate and observe similar phenomena together, and those techniques that require clinicians to acquire simpler skills before those techniques that require complex skills.

2. The categories of massage techniques for Outcome-Based Massage™ are superficial reflex techniques, superficial fluid techniques, neuromuscular techniques, connective tissue techniques, passive movement techniques, and percussive techniques.

3. Intelligent touch has six skills that clinicians must master before they can use massage techniques successfully: attention, concentration, discrimination, identification, inquiry, and intention.

4. Intelligent practice of massage involves the integration of knowledge of anatomy and physiology with palpation skills and attention to the patient's response.

5. Therapy students need the repeated receipt of massage or other manual techniques from competent, experienced professionals in order to grasp the overall flow, pacing, and rhythm of an effective treatment.

6. Clinicians need to prepare themselves physically before they begin to interact with the patient by following a comprehensive exercise program that includes aerobic, flexibility, resistance, and balance training in order to maintain a trouble-free level of function and to prevent ongoing damage.

7. Clinicians need to prepare themselves physically and mentally prior to patient interactions by using appropriate time management and stress control techniques.

8. When selecting and preparing the treatment materials, clinicians need to consider which tables, lubricants, and linen are appropriate for their treatment setting and patients' needs.

9. During the intervention, clinicians need to ensure that they have positioned the patient appropriately and draped the patient both prior to and during the massage.

10. During the intervention, clinicians need to ensure that they have positioned themselves well and use correct body mechanics during the intervention.

Clinical Case: *Preparation and Positioning for Massage*

Clinician's Profile

A healthy 30-year-old clinician in good physical condition began to experience frequent tightness and aching in his lower back after doubling his weekly workload of massage. His pain level has been increasing each week and is now affecting his ability to work.

Clinical Findings

Subjective Findings:

The clinician reports that his symptoms appear after a couple of hours of work, get progressively worse until the end of the workday, and then disappear after an hour of rest. Stretching, especially stretching his spinal extensors, relieves his symptoms. He cannot identify which actions are contributing to his symptoms while he works and reports that both standing and seated positions seem to be at fault.

Objective Findings:

The clinician is right-hand dominant. His posture shows a minor **upper-crossed** pattern. Active lumbar range of motion is within normal limits. Abdominal strength is grade 5/5. He has hamstring tightness based on the sit-and-reach test. On palpation, there is **elevated resting tension** in the thoracic and lumbar erector spinae and related **latent trigger points** that reproduce his pain.

Treatment Approach:

The clinician's profile and findings suggest that his back pain is biomechanical. A likely mechanism is that he is overusing his spinal extensors—a common result of trying too hard to maintain an upright posture.

He has several options:

- He can have a colleague monitor his posture during work to look for signs of lumbar hyperextension. He can then correct this with feedback.
- While working, he can periodically place a hand in the small of his back to monitor his lumbar extensors for signs of excessive contraction or tightness.

- In order to refine his awareness of pelvic position and related extensor contraction, he can practice pelvic tilt daily in lying, seated, and standing aligned positions.
- He can follow a daily program of lumbar stretching.
- When working, he can train himself to stop at the first sign of tightness or pain, stand back briefly, relax, take a breath, and adjust his posture before continuing.
- He can adjust the **ergonomic** load while he is working by modifying his posture during treatments.
- He can decide whether these symptoms stem from general fatigue secondary to overwork and reduce his workload.

Critical Thinking Questions

1. How is the taxonomy of massage techniques for Outcome-Based Massage™ different from the traditional approach to organizing and naming massage techniques?
2. Describe the six skills within the framework of intelligent touch. Based on your self-assessment of your ability to perform massage techniques, identify which of these six skills you wish to improve.
3. Describe the ways in which receiving skilled massage from an experienced clinician has influenced your ability to perform massage techniques. Outline a plan for receiving skilled massage on an ongoing basis.
4. Some systems of exercise such as **Hatha Yoga** teach physical conditioning and physical awareness together. Which other systems teach both physical conditioning and physical awareness together? Choose one system of exercise and describe how the conditioning and awareness involved in that system will help you to perform massage.
5. Identify two factors within your treatment environment and personal life that may put you at risk for

burnout. List some strategies that you can use to prevent burnout.
6. Compare and contrast the characteristics of portable treatment tables versus portable treatment chairs and identify appropriate treatment settings for both.
7. Assemble a group of different lubricants. Spread them on a variety of body parts in differing amounts. What do you perceive to be the advantages and disadvantages of each type of lubricant?
8. How would you adapt the positioning and draping procedures illustrated in this chapter for use at a public hospital ward, a private home, an office, and a sports competition in an arena?
9. Describe the legal, ethical, and practical aspects of draping. Identify a situation in which your professional code of conduct will permit you to undrape a patient's pelvis.
10. Which of the described postures do you find hardest to perform? Why? Use your understanding of your body structures to explain this difficulty.

References for Chapter 6 are on p. 461.

CHAPTER 7

Superficial Reflex Techniques

After studying this chapter, you will have the information that you need to do the following:

1. Describe how the massage techniques in this category affect different types of tissues.
2. Describe each massage technique in terms of the contact surface, pressure, tissues engaged, amplitude, direction, and rate.
3. Demonstrate how to perform each massage technique and how to apply it in the context of a practice sequence.
4. Speculate about the mechanisms by which massage techniques achieve their effects.
5. Describe the outcomes of care, indications, contraindications, and common uses associated with each massage technique.

Superficial reflex techniques are those massage techniques that engage only the skin and primarily affect the level of arousal, autonomic balance, and perception of pain. These techniques include static contact, superficial stroking, and fine vibration. This chapter describes these techniques, how to perform them, and how to apply them in a practice sequence. It also discusses relevant outcomes and evidence, cautions and contraindications, and how to use the technique in treatment. Finally, Table 7-1 summarizes those outcomes for superficial reflex techniques that are related to body structures and functions. Therapists are advised to review the cautions and contraindications for these techniques and to use them as their scope of practice and skill level permit.

Static Contact: Evidence

DEFINITION

Static contact: Motionless contact of the therapist's hands with the client's body performed with minimal force.[1-7]

NAMES AND ORIGINS

Static contact is probably the simplest, oldest, and most universal of massage techniques. In other texts or massage-related systems, the technique that we call static contact is also known as "resting position," "passive touch," "superficial touch," "light touch," "static touch," "maintained touch," or "stationary holding."[1-3,7] It is used extensively in **energetic approaches**, such as Therapeutic Touch, Reiki, and Polarity Therapy, that attempt to regulate the magnetic or energy field of the body.

USES

Therapists use static contact to establish rapport, to promote **relaxation**, and to assist with client education. They often use it when they must avoid more forceful techniques.

OUTCOMES AND EVIDENCE

Static contact is the least mechanically stimulating of the massage techniques. It has a variety of physiological and psychological effects.[8-29] Therapists can use it to enhance the flow of interventions, to achieve **outcomes** related to clients' psychological and physiological impairments, and to clarify client education. Therapists can use static contact to facilitate the flow and **coherence** of interventions in two ways: to establish a **therapeutic rapport** with the client[30-34] and to reduce **anxiety** and induce sedation[35-37] at the beginning and end of massage interventions that incorporate other techniques.[38-41] Static contact has many psychological

effects. Therapists can use it by itself to decrease anxiety and the perception of pain in conditions in which the use of movement or force is contraindicated or poorly tolerated. For example, it can be used in situations of trauma, acute conditions, extreme or **intractable** pain, illness, dying, postsurgery, systemic weakness, convalescence, emotional distress, hypersensitivity, and posttraumatic stress and when there is a history of violence, sexual abuse, or poor physical self-image.[1,3,4] Static contact is also indispensable when teaching a client breathing techniques (see Figures 7-2 and 7-3) or when cueing a client to become aware of any body segment.[42-49] Furthermore, therapists can use it to facilitate movement. Finally, static contact is integrated into therapeutic approaches such as Therapeutic Touch, Reiki, and Polarity, which conceptualize the philosophy of treatment in terms of energy or life force.[50] Table 7-1 summarizes the main outcomes for body structures and functions for static contact.

HOW STATIC CONTACT MIGHT WORK

Researchers are uncertain how this very simple technique achieves its therapeutic effects. In other words: How do cutaneous nerves generate a relaxation effect? It is possible that gentle stimulation of the skin boosts the activity of the **parasympathetic** nervous system.[40,41,46-48,51-59] This parasympathetic activity may result in changes in the neuroendocrine system such as reduced **cortisol** and increased **serotonin**.[38-41] Practitioners of **Reiki**, **Healing Touch**, and **Therapeutic Touch** propose that it is possible to use the simplest form of touch to manipulate the energy field or magnetic field of the client's body. The questions this position raises are: Do humans actually have a biomagnetic field? Can a skilled therapist project a magnetic field from his or her hands? Can this in turn affect the magnetic field of the client? Oschman reviews the scientific evidence for these ideas at length in the book *Energy Medicine: The Scientific Basis* and related articles.[61-69]

EXAMINING THE EVIDENCE

The Center for Complementary Care in the United Kingdom performed an uncontrolled, preliminary evaluation of "healing by gentle touch" in 35 clients with cancer.[61-69] Therapists used "a simple repeating pattern" of "non-invasive touch on the head, chest, arms, legs, and feet for approximately 40 minutes" that would be difficult to replicate without reviewing the references cited in the study. Outcome measures included reasonable pre- and posttreatment measures of physical and psychological function. The most pronounced improvements were seen in the clients' subjective ratings of perceived stress and relaxation, severe pain/discomfort, and depression/anxiety. This was particularly evident in those clients who had the most severe symptoms on entry. This research study was conceptually clear, relevant, and well reported. The study's primary drawback was its lack of a control group for its pretest, posttest design. The authors concluded that a more rigorous evaluation using a randomized pretest, posttest design with a control group was warranted.[49]

Weze C, Leathard HL, Grange J, Tiplady P, Stevens G. Evaluation of healing by gentle touch in 35 clients with cancer. *Eur J Oncol Nurs.* 2004;8:40–49.

Static Contact: Practice

COMPONENTS OF STATIC CONTACT

Static contact has the following components:

Contact: Whole hand, fingertip(s), and thumb

Pressure: Minimal

Engages: Skin

Direction: N/A

Amplitude/length: N/A

Rate: N/A

Duration: 60 seconds to 15 minutes or more

Intergrades with: Compression and vibration

Context: May be used alone. It is often used as a "framing technique," performed at the beginning and end of regional or full-body sequences that use other techniques to engage deeper tissues

PALPATION PRACTICE

The following palpation exercises will help you develop the manual skill and focus you need to perform static contact well:

1. Mold the entire palmar surface of your hand to household objects of varying sizes and shapes. The aim is to maximize hand contact without tensing your hand or compressing the object.
2. Chaitow[70] suggests palpating household objects made of different materials (e.g., metal, glass, and plastic) that you perceive to be warm or cold when they are at normal room temperature. What would explain the perceived differences in temperature? Are different parts of your hand more sensitive to temperature?
3. With your eyes closed and hands placed lightly on a practice partner's ribcage, monitor the breathing rhythm. Try this with your hands more distant from the ribcage. Can you detect the breathing rhythm when contacting the pelvis, the knees, or the feet?
4. With your forearms supported on the table, cradle the client's occiput in both hands for 10 minutes. What rhythmical movements can you detect?

MANUAL TECHNIQUE

In Figures 7-1 to 7-7, static contact is applied to the various regions of the body. Figures are ordered from head to foot in supine and then prone. Each figure illustrates most of the guidelines for manual technique:

1. Use relaxed, full-hand contact that conforms evenly to the surface contours of the client's body.
2. In general, you place your hands on the client's body in a symmetrical position. This allows you to maintain contact with the left and right sides of the client's body simultaneously (Figures 7-1A and 7-1B, 7-3, and 7-6).

3. Do not attempt to apply force or to manipulate the client's tissues physically in any way. The partial weight of your hands may rest on the client's body if the client finds this tolerable.
4. Make and break contact with the surface of the client's body gradually and gently. To a large degree, the manner in which you make and break contact contributes to the client's level of **relaxation**. Changing contact frequently may decrease the **sedative** effect of this technique.
5. Hold your hands steady when they are in contact with the client's body. Your hands should not shake from fatigue, even during prolonged application.
6. The author's clinical observation suggests that you are more likely to achieve the effect of deep relaxation when you apply static contact for longer periods (5 minutes or longer) at the midsacrum and/or occiput (Figures 7-1B and 7-7).[70] Contact with the client's hands, feet, and face may also be more likely to produce relaxation than other areas of the body.[3] This may be because of the density of nervous innervation in these areas (Figures 7-5 and 7-6).

FIGURE 7-1 A. Hand position for applying static contact to the occiput with the client in supine. Note that the forearms are supported on the table. **B**. Static contact applied to the occiput. This nonthreatening approach to reducing spasm or hypertonicity in the client's neck can also produce sedative effects.

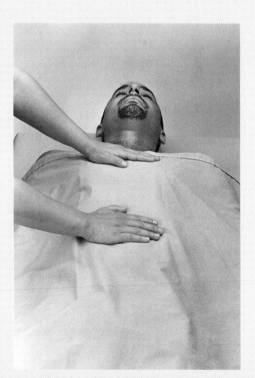

FIGURE 7-2 Static contact used to draw the client's awareness to the movement of the upper ribs and abdomen during breathing.

FIGURE 7-3 Static contact used to facilitate instruction of the client in lateral costal breathing.

FIGURE 7-4 Simultaneous contact to the forehead and abdomen.

FIGURE 7-5 Appropriate contact to the hand(s) can be both intimate and comforting.

FIGURE 7-6 Bilateral static contact to the soles of the feet.

FIGURE 7-7 Prolonged simultaneous contact at occiput and sacrum can produce relaxation in the client.

THERAPIST'S POSITION AND MOVEMENT

1. Use the basic positions described in Chapter 6, in the sections **Standing Aligned**, Seated Aligned, **Lunge**, and **Lunge and Reach** postures.
2. Select a posture that is comfortable and stable to minimize inadvertent shaking of your hands when you must sustain contact for longer periods.
3. You may prefer to sit when working on the client's feet and head or when working unilaterally. Sitting allows you to support your forearms on the edge of the table, providing increased stability and reducing the likelihood of arm fatigue during the technique (Figures 7-1A and 7-1B).

PALPATE

As you perform the technique, palpate the client's skin for the following:

1. Skin texture
2. Skin temperature
3. Presence of perspiration and moisture

OBSERVE

As you perform the technique, observe the client for changes in the **level of arousal** and **autonomic balance** that reflect increasing relaxation. The signs listed below may indicate increased relaxation:

1. Decrease in rate and depth of breathing
2. Deeper voice tone
3. Changes in skin color such as flushing. Pallor may indicate an undesirable **sympathetic response**
4. Systemic reduction of **resting muscle tension**, as evidenced by softening of the tissue contours or broadening and flattening of body segments
5. Muscle twitches and jerks
6. Increases in peristaltic noises
7. Decreases in heart rate, as evidenced by change in pulses that are visible at the neck, wrist, and foot
8. Agitation or sweating, which may indicate an undesirable sympathetic response

COMMUNICATION WITH THE CLIENT

Communicate to encourage general relaxation, to guide the client's awareness of areas of the body, or to facilitate the client's breathing pattern. Here are some examples of statements that you can use:

1. "Let your … relax, as much as you're able."
2. "Feel the weight of your body" or "Let your body sink into the table."
3. "Notice what's occurring in your body. It's not unusual to experience sensations some distance from the location of my hands."
4. "Let your awareness move to …"
5. "It's not unusual to have emotions or feelings arise in response to touch. Just observe them and express them if you need to."
6. "Deepen your breathing without forcing it in any way."
7. "Notice how your ribs move here when you inhale."
8. "What is happening with your pain?" You can use this statement when you are applying the technique to reduce pain. It allows you to check how the client perceives that the intervention is affecting her pain at intervals during the application of the technique.

A Practice Sequence for Static Contact

Practice time: 30 or 60 minutes per person.

Hold each position bilaterally for about 1 minute for a 30-minute session or 2 minutes for a 1-hour session. Therapists who use static contact extensively often recommend a sequence that proceeds in a direction from head to toe as is described here. We suggest that students try different orders and draw their own conclusions.

SUPINE	PRONE
Vertex	Vertex
Occiput	Parietal bone
Eyes/frontal bone	Temporal bone
Cheeks/jaw	Occiput
Anterior neck	Posterior neck
Anterior shoulders	Upper trapezius
Upper ribs	Mid- and upper thorax
Lower ribs	Lower thorax
Elbows	Elbows
Dorsum of hands	Palms
Upper abdomen	Lumbar area
Lower abdomen	Sacrum
Hips	Gluteal area
Knees	Knees
Ankles	Ankles
Dorsum of feet	Plantar surface of feet

> **Home study:** Devise comparable sequences that
>
> 1. Move in a toe-to-head direction
> 2. Incorporate more contact between joints
> 3. Spend half of the allotted time on a specified region such as the legs

CAUTIONS AND CONTRAINDICATIONS

Therapists need clinical training and supervised practice when learning static contact. Advanced training may be advisable when dealing with pathological conditions. Static contact is a **reflex technique**; consequently, the contraindications for the use of **mechanical techniques** do not generally apply (see Chapter 5).[3,35,71] The primary exception to this rule is that the use of static contact may be contraindicated locally in areas of acute inflammation because of pain. Furthermore, clients who are experiencing considerable pain or distress or who are dying may not tolerate touch at all.

There are several cautions for the use of static contact.[1] Because therapists can use it with frail clients, high-risk infants, or terminally ill clients, they need to be sensitive to the emotional and physical needs of these clients. Static contact looks deceptively simple and causes minimal mechanical effects. Nevertheless, like all massage techniques, it can give rise to very complex physical and emotional responses, including **touch-triggered memory**.[1] As with all massage techniques, therapists must obtain **informed consent** from the client prior to using this technique. When the client's condition results in an impairment of the client's cognitive function or level of consciousness, the therapist may have difficulty obtaining informed consent to treat. In addition, the therapist must maintain clear and consistent communication with the client throughout the intervention when she is applying the technique for long periods or over large areas of the client's body.

USING STATIC CONTACT IN TREATMENT

Before considering the use of static contact for treatment, you should be able to perform **diaphragmatic breathing** while standing and sitting. You should also know how to assess and track autonomic function in a client.

Relaxation

There are several modalities that you can use in a complementary manner with static contact to promote relaxation.

1. You can use **progressive relaxation or diaphragmatic breathing**[72] prior to, or simultaneously with, static contact to enhance sedative effects. For example, you can combine prolonged contact with the client's occiput, ribcage, or abdomen with instruction on diaphragmatic breathing.
2. Moist **hot packs** can enhance sedation and analgesia, if the use of heat is appropriate for the client's condition.[50]
3. Some **craniosacral** therapy techniques may have a calming effect on the client.[73]
4. Instruct the client to rest from 10 to 30 minutes and to resume activity slowly if experiencing the sedative effects of static contact.

Superficial Stroking: Evidence

DEFINITION

Superficial stroking: Gliding over the client's skin with minimal **deformation** of subcutaneous tissues. Therapists usually apply this stroke unidirectionally over large areas of the client's body.

NAMES AND ORIGINS

In other texts or massage-related systems, the technique that we call superficial effleurage is known as "light stroking," "feather stroking," "nerve stroking," or "reflex stroking."[74] Some authors do not distinguish between stroking and **effleurage**[7,75] or consider stroking to be similar to effleurage without the restriction of the direction of the stroke.[1,6] This is discussed further in Chapter 8. This book uses **Mennell's**[7,76] definition, which considers superficial stroking to be a distinct reflex technique that is performed with a lighter pressure than that used with effleurage.

USES

Therapists can use superficial stroking to reduce pain and to relax or stimulate clients depending on the contact, direction, and rate of application. It may also have effects on resting muscle tension and neuromuscular tone.

OUTCOMES AND EVIDENCE

Superficial stroking has a variety of physiological and psychological effects.[76] Therapists can use superficial stroking to change the client's level of arousal, for pain reduction, and to facilitate changes in resting muscle tension and **neuromuscular tone**. Since superficial stroking can result in sedation or stimulation, depending on the contact, direction, and rate of application,[77-79] therapists often use it at the beginning or end of an intervention session to adjust the client's **level of arousal**. Like static contact, this technique is well suited to difficult situations in which the use of pressure is contraindicated. Frequently, superficial stroking has been incorporated into interventions, such as the "**slow-stroke back rub**" described in the nursing literature,[7,75] that are used to improve mood and relieve anxiety in the critically ill.[80-88] Superficial stroking that can stimulate the client's level of arousal,[81-84] when judiciously applied, may temporarily ameliorate some symptoms of debility, convalescence, lethargy, and depression. Superficial stroking may have a role in treating pain when **mechanical techniques** are contraindicated. In this case, pain relief may occur because light touch and vibration increase large-diameter afferent nerve input and may reduce the transmission of "slow" pain impulses through the spinal gate of the segment being touched.[7,75] It may also occur because stroking boosts the levels of oxytocin.[5,7]

Superficial stroking may minimally facilitate or inhibit local muscle tone via musculocutaneous reflexes and may reduce **spasm**. Finally, therapists can use it locally and over the posterior primary rami to decrease limb **spasticity**.[89-92]

Research also suggests that superficial stroking and gentle passive movement (infant massage) can have a positive effect on the physiological and psychological development of premature infants,[3,93] ill infants,[94-110] and full-term infants,[111,112] while enhancing maternal health and mother–child interaction.[113-120] Leading researchers[112,121-125] suggest that "light" (superficial) pressure is less effective in promoting weight gain than "moderate" pressure for normal infants.

Table 7-1 summarizes the main outcomes for body structures and functions for superficial stroking.

HOW SUPERFICIAL STROKING MIGHT WORK

The "**gate theory of pain**" first proposed by Melzack and Wall provides an explanation for the use of superficial stroking to reduce pain. Superficial stroking supplies a barrage of sensory information carried on large-fiber cutaneous afferents that may reduce the transmission of pain impulses through the same level of the spinal cord to the higher centers of the central nervous system. Researchers have recently questioned whether the gate theory is the mechanism for analgesic effects of massage.[118] Nonetheless, stroking may reduce pain[60] by boosting levels of **oxytocin**.[89-92,126]

Superficial stroking adds components of rate and rhythm to the light touch of static contact. Could the element of periodicity cause a relaxing effect beyond that of the touch itself? Consider the idea of **entrainment**—the alteration of a biological rhythm in response to an external stimulus.[89-92] Research suggests that listening closely to music or sounds of specific frequencies can alter biological rhythms of the body such as breathing and heart rate.[127-130] Perhaps a rhythmical kinesthetic stimulus such as superficial stroking induces effects comparable to a rhythmical auditory stimulus, entraining the autonomic system toward a state of relaxation.

EXAMINING THE EVIDENCE

In a randomized controlled trial, researchers at the University of Georgia and the University of Miami's **Touch Research Institute** examined the effects of 5 days of massage therapy on stable preterm infants who averaged 30 weeks at delivery.[1,129,130] The 15-minute intervention consisted of 5 minutes of "moderate pressure stroking with the flats of the fingers of both hands" that covered the whole body, 5 minutes of passive flexion/extension movements of the limbs, and 5 more minutes of stroking. The intervention was performed three times a day. The 16 massaged infants gained 53% more weight and slept less than the 16 infants in the control group. No placebo treatment is described for the control; presumably, the researchers had a "no massage" control group. The small sample size was nonetheless large enough to show statistical significance in daily weight gain between the massage and nonmassage groups. Overall, this study is succinct, complete, and rigorous.

Dieter JN, Field T, Hernandez-Reif M, Emory EK, Redzepi M. Stable preterm infants gain more weight and sleep less after five days of massage therapy. *J Pediatr Psychol.* 2003;28:403–411.

Superficial Stroking: Practice

COMPONENTS OF SUPERFICIAL STROKING

Superficial stroking has the following components:

Contact: Palmar surface of your hand or fingertips

Pressure: Minimal

Engages: Skin only

Direction: Usually parallel to the long axis of the body segment being stroked

Amplitude: The full length of the body segment

Rate: 5 to 100 cm/s

Duration: 10 seconds to 10 minutes or more, depending on the therapist's intention

Intergrades with: Superficial effleurage

Combines with: May be combined with fine vibration or shaking

Context: May be used alone. Therapists often use it as a "framing technique," performed at the beginning and end of regional or full-body sequences that incorporate deeper techniques

PALPATION PRACTICE

The following palpation exercises will help you develop the manual skill and focus you need to perform superficial stroking well:

1. Stroke a carpet or broadloom and determine the direction of the nap. Stroke textured woven fabrics and attempt to describe the pattern of the weave by palpation alone.
2. With closed eyes and constantly moving palmar contact, run your hand over large objects maintaining constant light pressure: car bodies, furniture, and wood and metal sculptures. Form a mental image of the shape. How much detail can you discern about the surface finish without using your eyes?
3. Stroke the bare limb of a practice partner in one direction. Try to perceive variations in temperature and texture between areas. Do you come to the same judgments if the stroke goes in the opposite direction?

MANUAL TECHNIQUE

In Figures 7-8 to 7-15, superficial stroking is applied to the various regions of the body. The order of figures is from head to foot in supine and then in prone. Each figure illustrates most of the guidelines for manual technique outlined below:

1. Lubricant is not usually required to achieve glide without binding.
2. Relax your hands when you use the full palmar surface to perform the stroke. Use only enough hand weight to ensure good contact with the client's skin.
3. Perform superficial stroking in one direction, unless the desired outcome of the intervention is stimulation, since the reflex effects of superficial stroking are dependent on direction.
4. Return your hands to the starting position in the air for the **return stroke**. Use the same speed for the return stroke as for the stroke itself because this encourages a stable rhythm, which is necessary to achieve systemic sedation.
5. Although responses vary from person to person and with the context of treatment, you can achieve different effects by adjusting the type of contact, rate, and direction of the stroke.[95] Palmar contact, slow steady rate, **centrifugal** direction on the limbs, and caudal direction on the back tend to produce sedation (Figure 7-13A). Conversely, fingertip contact, fast or irregular rate, **centripetal** direction on the limbs, and cephalad direction on the back tend to

FIGURE 7-9 Fingertip superficial stroking of the face and scalp can provide a refreshing end to a massage sequence.

produce arousal (Figure 7-14). Fingertip stroking is usually stimulating and may sometimes be irritating (Figures 7-9, 7-13B, and 7-14).

6. You can substitute a succession of overlapping short strokes for a single long stroke (Figure 7-15). The technique of breaking up a long stroke into overlapping shorter ones is called "layering," "shingling," or

FIGURE 7-8 Slow, bilateral superficial stroking of the face with palmar contact can produce sedative effects.

FIGURE 7-10 Dorsal and palmar contact surfaces alternate during transverse, bidirectional superficial stroking of the abdomen.

FIGURE 7-11 Continuous hand-over-hand palmar superficial stroking of the abdomen in the direction of colonic flow.

"thousand hands."[1,3-7,75] This technique enables you to cover a large area with less reaching for each stroke, and it creates a sensory experience that may help some clients to relax.

7. On the abdomen, you may perform the stroke across the abdomen or in the direction of colonic flow (Figures 7-10 and 7-11).[7,75]

8. Contact with the spinal column from occiput to sacrum, hands, feet, and face may produce stronger clinical effects than that with other areas of the body, possibly because of the density of nervous innervation in these areas (Figures 7-8, 7-9, and 7-13A).

FIGURE 7-13 A. Slow, regular palmar stroking down the spine produces sedative effects. The return stroke in the air (dotted line) is made at the same rate as the stroke. **B**. Fingertip contact can yield a more stimulating effect than palmar contact, with other components being the same.

ONLINE VIDEO

FIGURE 7-12 Superficial stroking can be applied through fabric, and the therapist may choose a seated aligned posture.

FIGURE 7-14 Fast, multidirectional, superficial fingertip stroking can be very stimulating and may be used judiciously to produce increased arousal in sedated clients.

FIGURE 7-15 For long regions such as the posterior leg, the therapist may use overlapping short strokes instead of one long stroke.

ONLINE VIDEO

9. You should use superficial stroking with caution on the plantar surface of the feet.
10. You can apply superficial stroking effectively through the client's clothes or a sheet (Figure 7-12). In this situation, take steps to prevent bunching of the fabric over the skin, since this will detract from the regularity of the sensory input that the client receives during the stroke. You may tuck the drape securely or use one hand to tighten the intervening fabric while your other hand performs the technique.

THERAPIST'S POSITION AND MOVEMENT

1. Use the basic positions described in Chapter 6, in the sections Standing **Aligned**, Seated Aligned, **Lunge**, and Lunge and Reach positions.
2. Keep your shoulders and arms relaxed during the stroke, without straining to reach at the end; never extend your elbows fully.
3. It is easier to perform long strokes by using a relatively wide foot placement and shifting the weight of your upright torso from one leg to the other as the stroke proceeds.

PALPATE

As you perform the technique, palpate the client's skin for the following:

1. Skin texture
2. Skin temperature
3. Presence of perspiration and moisture
4. Slight horizontal stretch of the skin that occurs in the direction of movement. Because of the light pressure and relatively fast rate, this stretch does not approach the **elastic barrier** of the skin.

OBSERVE

As you perform the technique, observe the client for increases or decreases in the client's level of arousal and autonomic balance. The following signs may indicate increased relaxation:

1. Change of rate and depth of breathing
2. Changes in voice tone
3. Changes in skin color such as flushing or pallor
4. Systemic reduction of **resting muscle tension**, as evidenced by softening of the tissue contours or settling of body segments
5. Muscle twitches and jerks
6. Peristaltic noises
7. Change in heart rate as evidenced by change in pulses that are visible at the neck, wrist, and foot
8. Agitation or sweating may indicate an undesirable sympathetic response

COMMUNICATION WITH THE CLIENT

Communicate to encourage general relaxation or guide the client's awareness of areas of the body. Here are some examples of statements that you can use:

1. "Let your … relax, as much as you're able."
2. "Feel the weight of your body" or "Let your body sink into the table."
3. "Notice what's occurring in your body. It's not unusual to experience sensations some distance from the location of my hands."
4. "Let your awareness move to …"
5. "It's not unusual to have emotions or feelings arise in response to touch. Just observe them and express them if you need to."

6. "What is happening with your pain?" You can use this statement when you are applying the technique to reduce pain. It allows you to check how the client perceives that the intervention is affecting her pain at intervals during the application of the technique.

A Practice Sequence for Superficial Stroking

Practice time: 30 to 45 minutes per person.

Begin with palmar stroking down the spine from the crown to the sacrum. Begin at a fast rate (100 cm/s) and decrease the rate gradually over a period of 10 minutes until it is very slow (5–10 cm/s). Follow with 5 minutes of static contact at both the sacrum and occiput.

After communicating changes in your intentions to your client, experiment with a variety of combinations of contact, rate, and direction that include different regions of the body in any orderly sequence. Examples of these combinations are as follows:

- Moderate rate, palmar, layered from occiput to sacrum
- Fast, palmar, across the back
- Fast and irregular, fingertip, on the back
- Slow, fingertip, down one limb
- Fast, palmar, up the opposite limb
- Moderate rate, palmar, across the abdomen
- Slow, palmar or fingertip, up the face and scalp

Finish with palmar stroking down the spine and static contact at the sacrum and occiput. Ask the client for feedback.

Note: It takes time and repetition to produce sedative effects; it takes neither to achieve increased arousal.

CAUTIONS AND CONTRAINDICATIONS

Therapists need clinical training and supervised practice when learning superficial stroking. Advanced training may be advisable when dealing with pathological conditions. Superficial stroking is a reflex technique; consequently, the contraindications for the use of mechanical techniques do not generally apply (see Chapter 5).[75] The primary exception to this rule is that the use of superficial stroking may be contraindicated locally in areas of acute inflammation because of pain. In this situation, treat the client's pain by performing the technique on adjacent areas as tolerated by the client. Furthermore, clients who are experiencing considerable pain or distress or who are dying may not tolerate touch at all.

There are several cautions for the use of superficial stroking.[1] When the client's condition results in an impairment of the client's cognitive function or level of consciousness, the therapist may have difficulty obtaining informed consent to treat. Because therapists can use superficial stroking with frail clients, high-risk infants, or terminally ill clients, they need to be sensitive to the emotional and physical needs of these clients. Although recent myocardial infarction was once considered to be a contraindication for massage, light massage is now considered to be permissible. A further cardiac-related caution is that a 48-hour wait is advisable after coronary artery bypass surgery.[1] Finally, if superficial stroking is being used for reflex stimulation, the therapist needs to ensure that the application of the technique does not become irritating. Ticklishness frequently occurs in areas where there is underlying muscular tension. If the application of superficial stroking tickles the client, the therapist should try the following strategies: switch to a broader contact, add lubricant, check that the stroke direction does not run against the grain of the client's body hair, or change to a technique that uses more pressure.

USING SUPERFICIAL STROKING IN TREATMENT

Before considering the use of superficial stroking for treatment, you should be able to perform diaphragmatic breathing while standing and sitting, and you should know how to assess and track autonomic function in a client.

Relaxation

There are several modalities that you can use in a complementary manner with superficial stroking to promote relaxation:

1. You can use progressive relaxation or diaphragmatic breathing[131] prior to, or simultaneously with, superficial stroking to enhance sedative effects.
2. Moist hot packs can enhance sedation and analgesia, if the use of heat is appropriate for the client's condition.[50]
3. Some craniosacral techniques may have a calming effect on the client.[73]
4. Instruct your client to rest from 10 to 30 minutes and to resume activity slowly if experiencing the sedative effects of superficial stroking.

Fine Vibration: Evidence

DEFINITION

Fine vibration: A fast, oscillating or trembling movement that is produced on the client's skin and that results in minimal deformation of subcutaneous tissues.[74,132-153]

NAMES AND ORIGINS

In other texts or massage-related systems, the technique that we call fine vibration is known as "vibration," "mechanical vibration," "cutaneous vibration," "transcutaneous vibration," or "vibratory stimulation."[132-156] The term "vibration" has been used by some authors[154-158] to denote markedly differing techniques that involve shaking, compressing, or percussing the client's subcutaneous tissues with considerable force, as illustrated in Figure 7-21. This text distinguishes between fine vibration and the more vigorous forms of vibration, which have mechanical effects and are described in Chapters 9, 11, and 12. Recent research addresses fine vibration produced by small portable devices operating at frequencies varying from 20 to 200 Hz, with 100 Hz being the most commonly used.[3,5,132-153] The documented effects of machine-produced vibration, often referred to as mechanical vibration, cannot be extrapolated to manually produced fine vibration except with caution.

USES

Therapists can use fine vibration to achieve pain relief and produce changes in neuromuscular tone.

OUTCOMES AND EVIDENCE

Fine vibration has a variety of physiological and psychological outcomes.[154-157] Therapists can use machine-produced vibration to achieve pain relief and changes in neuromuscular tone. Machine-produced vibration can be an effective analgesic for acute and **chronic pain** of various causes such as dental pain, phantom limb pain, **myofascial pain**, tendinous pain, neurogenic pain, and idiopathic pain.[132-151,159] Although the mechanism of **analgesia** is not well understood, researchers have noted that the reduction of pain and accompanying elevation of the pain threshold can persist for some time after the intervention.[157] Analgesic effects are increased with sustained application of machine-produced vibration for 15 to 30 minutes or longer.[143,149,150] In addition, therapists can obtain analgesic effects when they apply machine-produced vibration to different regions of the client's body in relation to the site of pain, including direct application to the site of pain over a large area, distal to the site of pain, to the antagonist muscle group, to adjacent **dermatomes**, or even contralateral to the site of pain.[135,139] Combining the vibration with moderate pressure, if the client's condition permits, may enhance the analgesic effects of the vibration.

Machine-produced vibration can result in an elevation of resting tone of the muscles under the site of application.[136,141,142,144,151,157] This effect may be used, when treating clients with neurological conditions, to promote more balanced movement and to prepare the client to perform functional activity.[152-154] Other effects ascribed to fine vibration are reflex relaxation, especially when it is applied to the feet,[153,154] healing of chronic peripheral nerve lesions,[155] and reduction in frequency of postsurgical complications.[156] Table 7-1 summarizes the main outcomes for body structures and functions for fine vibration.

Effective application of manual fine vibration, using the technique described in this chapter, takes much practice. In addition, it requires considerable skill on the part of the therapist to perform sustained application of manual fine vibration for more than a few minutes, hence the frequent use of machine vibration. The light touch of superficial stroking is a less taxing manual alternative to manual fine vibration that also produces large-fiber afferent input.[158] Consequently, therapists may alternate superficial stroking with, or substitute it for, fine vibration. In this situation, they may obtain similar analgesic effects if the duration of application is comparable.

HOW FINE VIBRATION MIGHT WORK

The **gate theory of pain** first proposed by Melzack and Wall provides an explanation for the use of machine-produced fine vibration to reduce pain. Fine vibration supplies a

EXAMINING THE EVIDENCE

A small (n = 17) uncontrolled study compared the ability of machine-produced 20-Hz vibration, 100-Hz vibration, and control treatment to reduce pain (both "magnitude" and "unpleasantness") in subjects with temporomandibular disorders.[142,147-150] **Visual analog scale** ratings and drawings both showed that pain was reduced by 100-Hz vibration but not by 20-Hz vibration. The results and analysis of spatial and temporal patterns of analgesia hint at the complexity of both the phenomena of pain and of its measurement. Spatial analysis showed that ipsilateral and contralateral effects of vibration were statistically equivalent for subjects with chronic temporomandibular joint pain. This suggests that vibratory analgesia for chronic pain relies, in part, on central nervous system mechanisms. Analgesic effects were statistically significant but judged to be too modest to be of clinical significance. However, this study used 10-minute applications of vibration, a much shorter time than previous researchers have recommended for maximizing analgesia using this technique.[157] It would be worthwhile to repeat this study using longer vibration times and including a separate control group.[135,140]

Roy EA, Hollins M, Maixner W. Reduction of TMD pain by high-frequency vibration: a spatial and temporal analysis. *Pain.* 2003;101:267-274. Erratum in: *Pain.* 2003;104:717.

barrage of sensory information that is carried on large-fiber cutaneous afferents and reduces the transmission of pain impulses through the same level of the spinal cord to the higher centers of the central nervous system. Researchers have recently questioned whether the gate theory is the mechanism of massage's analgesic effects.[160] However, one recent study found that ipsilateral and contralateral applications of 100-Hz vibration produced equally significant changes in pain associated with temporomandibular joint dysfunction. This finding suggests that some type of central nervous system mechanism is at work[60] other than **endorphins** or another endogenous opioid.[157]

Fine Vibration: Practice

COMPONENTS OF FINE VIBRATION

Fine vibration has the following components:

Contact: Palmar surface or fingertips are most common
Pressure: Minimal
Engages: Skin
Direction: N/A

Amplitude/length: Less than 1 to 5 mm
Rate: 4 to 10 Hz or more for manual vibration; 100 Hz is common for machine-produced vibration
Duration: 5 to 40 minutes for analgesia
Intergrades with: Shaking
Combines with: Superficial stroking or compression
Context: Machine-produced vibration can be used alone. Manual fine vibration is often alternated with superficial stroking and/or static contact in situations in which the indications for treatment are similar.

MANUAL TECHNIQUE

In Figures 7-16 to 7-21, fine vibration is applied to the various regions of the body. The order of figures is from head to foot in supine and then in prone. Each figure illustrates most of the guidelines for manual technique outlined here:

1. The amplitude of fine vibration is scarcely visible and is generally less than 1 to 5 mm. Fine vibration exerts minimal mechanical effects beyond the surface of the client's skin.
2. Use your forearm and wrist to produce the motion, with as little recruitment of your shoulder muscles as possible. One efficient method of generating fine vibration is to use a rapid, low-amplitude, alternating pronation and supination of the forearm—a "flutter" (Figures 7-16A and 7-16B). Do not attempt to compress and release the client's tissues with the whole contact surface during the application of fine vibration.

This action will usually recruit your shoulder muscles and result in a more vigorous and fatiguing manipulation that has mechanical effects on the client's subcutaneous tissues.

3. Your two hands are rarely even in ability. You can improve the ability of the less competent hand by practicing the application of fine vibration with both hands together in mirror image. Some therapists choose to use only their dominant hand for fine vibration.
4. If you cannot produce an even vibration, try reducing the speed of the oscillation. It is preferable to produce a slow, controlled vibration than a fast, uncontrolled one. Control and speed of application come with practice.
5. You can combine fine vibration with superficial stroking to yield a "running" vibration whose reflex effects will also depend on the contact, rate, and direction of the stroking (Figure 7-18).

FIGURE 7-16 A. To create a fine vibration, the therapist may use low-amplitude alternating pronation and supination of the forearm. **B**. Or the therapist may use alternating radial and ulnar deviation of the wrist or forearm.

FIGURE 7-17 Fine vibration with stabilized fingertip contact applied to the abdomen.

FIGURE 7-20 A handheld device for producing fine vibration.

FIGURE 7-18 Fine vibration may be combined with stroking to produce a "running vibration," here shown on the quadriceps and anterior leg.

THERAPIST'S POSITION AND MOVEMENT

1. Use the basic positions described in Chapter 6, in the sections Basic Standing Aligned and Seated Aligned Postures. See also Figure 7-19.
2. Relax your shoulders (down) and flex your elbows. You will experience less fatigue if you engage your shoulder muscles as little as possible.

FIGURE 7-19 Whatever the manual method, posture must be aligned (standing or seated), and particular care must be taken to let the shoulders relax.

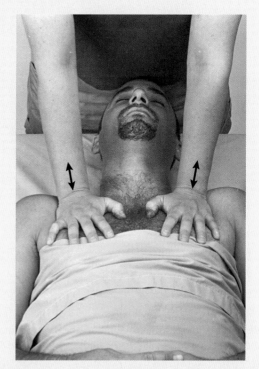

FIGURE 7-21 Coarser types of vibration that move subcutaneous tissue—such as the repeated rapid pumping of the ribcage shown here—have significant mechanical and proprioceptive effects and are discussed in later chapters.

3. You may find it helpful to sit with your elbow or part of your forearm resting on the edge of the table.
4. Your body position must be stable, since inadvertent postural shifts will detract from the intended effects of fine vibration.

PALPATE

As you perform the technique, palpate the client's skin for the following:

1. Skin texture
2. Skin temperature
3. Presence of perspiration and moisture

OBSERVE

As you perform the technique, observe the client for decreases in the level of pain or general signs of relaxation. The following signs may signal this:

1. Decrease in rate and depth of breathing
2. Deeper voice tone
3. Changes in skin color such as flushing. Pallor may indicate an undesirable sympathetic response.
4. Systemic reduction of resting muscle tension (see Observe sections in previous parts of this chapter), as evidenced by softening of the tissue contours or broadening and flattening of body segments
5. Muscle twitches and jerks
6. Increases in peristaltic noises
7. Decreases in heart rate as evidenced by change in pulses that are visible at the neck, wrist, and foot
8. Agitation or sweating, which may indicate an undesirable sympathetic response

COMMUNICATION WITH THE CLIENT

Communicate to monitor the client's pain and to encourage general relaxation. Here are some examples of statements that you can use.

1. "What is happening with your pain?" You can use this statement when you are applying the technique to reduce pain. It allows you to check how the client perceives that the intervention is affecting her pain at intervals during the application of the technique.
2. "Deepen your breathing without forcing," "Let your body sink into the table," "Let yourself relax completely" can be used to facilitate relaxation. Altered autonomic functioning may, in turn, affect the perception of pain.

A Practice Sequence for Fine Vibration

Practice time: 15 minutes per day for several days.

1. Stand with your shoulders down and elbows flexed to 90°. Breathe deeply. Try to make an even vibration of only your hand of less than 1 cm in the air. The wrist and forearm will move slightly, too. Continue for 1 minute, and then rest for a minute.
2. Begin again. Try to generate an equal movement of the two hands. Continue for a minute and then rest again.
3. Begin again. Slightly flex and extend your shoulders, then your elbows, and then your wrists. Move through various combinations of shoulder, elbow, and wrist flexion while continuing the vibration. Rest.
4. Place one hand on the opposite posterior deltoid. While vibrating with the free hand, can you tell if you are recruiting any shoulder girdle muscles to produce the vibration? Gradually increase the amplitude of the vibration to discover when your shoulder muscles begin to tense. Decrease the amplitude of the vibration and find the position and manual technique that recruits your shoulder muscles the least. Switch arms. Practice this sequence once a day, gradually extending the time for which you can perform the fine vibration continuously without fatigue until you have reached 5 minutes. Then begin practice on clients, alternating periods of fine vibrations with superficial stroking.

Note: Remember to relax, breathe, and let your shoulders drop.

CAUTIONS AND CONTRAINDICATIONS

Therapists need clinical training and supervised practice when learning fine vibration. Advanced training may be advisable when dealing with pathological conditions. Fine vibration is a reflex technique; consequently, the contraindications for the use of mechanical techniques do not generally apply (see Chapter 5). If, however, the therapist is using fine vibration to treat pain in a client with an acute condition, the client may find the weight of the therapist's hand or a mechanical device intolerable. In this situation, the therapist should administer fine vibration in adjacent areas as tolerated by the client.

USING FINE VIBRATION IN TREATMENT

Analgesia

Before considering the use of fine vibration for treatment of pain you must perform a basic pain assessment and attempt to discover the cause of the client's pain. It is important to distinguish between acute nociceptive pain, chronic pain, and chronic pain syndrome. There are several modalities that you can use in a complementary manner to enhance pain relief while using fine vibration:

1. Application of transcutaneous electrical nerve stimulation increases the analgesic effect of fine vibration.[157]
2. A variety of applications of heat, such as moist hot pack, **fluidotherapy**, and whirlpool, can enhance sedation and analgesia in the client.[147,148] Applications of cold, including cold packs, **ice massage**, and cold baths, can enhance analgesia in the client.[74,161] You must ensure that the selected modality is appropriate for the client's condition.
3. You can instruct the client in the home use of a vibrating massage device and in appropriate hydrotherapy for analgesia.

IN CONCLUSION

Superficial reflex techniques have a variety of uses, therapeutic effects, and outcomes. Table 7-1 summarizes those outcomes for superficial reflex techniques that are related to body structures and functions.

Table 7-1	Summary of Outcomes for Body Structures and Functions for Superficial Reflex Techniques

	Technique		
Impairment-Level Outcome of Care	**Static Contact**	**Superficial Stroking**	**Fine Vibration**
Increased sedation	✓	✓	✓
Decreased anxiety	✓	✓	P
Increased arousal	?	✓	?
Counterirritant analgesia	P	P	✓
Increased local resting muscle tension or neuromuscular tone	?	?	✓
Decreased local resting muscle tension or neuromuscular tone	✓	✓	?
Stimulated peristalsis	P	P	P

✓, the outcome is supported by research summarized in this chapter; P, the outcome is possible; ?, the outcome is debatable (research results are absent or inconsistent).

REVIEW SECTION

TAKEAWAYS

1. Superficial reflex techniques are those massage techniques that engage only the skin and primarily affect the level of arousal, autonomic balance, and the perception of pain.

2. Static contact is motionless contact of the clinician's hands with the patient's body performed with minimal force.

3. Clinicians use static contact to establish rapport, to promote relaxation, and to assist with patient education. They often use it when they must avoid more forceful techniques.

4. Researchers are uncertain how static contact achieves its therapeutic effects. It is possible that gentle stimulation of the skin boosts the activity of the parasympathetic nervous system

5. Superficial stroking is gliding over the patient's skin with minimal deformation of subcutaneous tissues.

6. Clinicians can use superficial stroking to reduce pain and to relax or stimulate patients depending on the contact, direction, and rate of application. It may also have effects on resting muscle tension and neuromuscular tone.

7. The "gate theory of pain" first proposed by Melzack and Wall provided an initial explanation for the use of superficial stroking to reduce pain. Researchers have recently questioned whether the gate theory is the mechanism for massage's analgesic effects.

8. Fine vibration is a fast, oscillating, or trembling movement that is produced on the patient's skin and that results in minimal deformation of subcutaneous tissues.

9. Clinicians can use fine vibration to achieve pain relief and produce changes in neuromuscular tone.

10. Fine vibration supplies a barrage of sensory information that is carried on large-fiber cutaneous afferents and reduces the transmission of pain impulses through the same level of the spinal cord to the higher centers of the central nervous system.

Clinical Case: *Superficial Reflex Techniques*

Patient Profile

Your patient is a 35-year-old recently separated mother of two adolescents. The psychologist who is treating her for issues related to self-esteem, **body image**, and a history of physical abuse has referred her for treatment.

Clinical Findings

Subjective Findings:

Her medical history is unremarkable, other than having had one cesarean delivery. She requests help to cope with **stress**, learn how stress affects her body, and alleviate occasional neck pain and stiffness.

Objective Findings:

- Observation: Postural analysis shows a moderate kyphosis.
- Range of motion: She has mildly limited range of motion in her cervical spine secondary to elevated resting tension and muscle tightness.

Treatment Approach

- Initial outcomes include developing good rapport (trust), fostering relaxation, and improving body awareness.
- The patient's history of physical abuse necessitates that you pay special attention to the process of obtaining informed consent. As you obtain **informed consent**, communicate clearly and carefully and explain the intervention protocol fully. Offer her the option of doing the work fully clothed. In addition, ask her which areas of her body she does not want you to touch, or about which she has concerns. Finally, discuss the possibility of **touch-triggered memory** and **somato-emotional release** with her.

- Once the patient is on the table, remind her where you will be beginning. Gently apply static contact, and sustain it for a couple of minutes or until the patient indicates that you can proceed to an adjacent area. (The Practice Sequence in this section gives one example of how you can proceed from place to place.) Communicate with the patient to encourage breathing and general relaxation, or guide her awareness of the areas of her body that you are treating. Allow the patient the freedom to talk about her experiences as the need arises. Once you have covered one region with static contact, apply superficial stroking to it for a minute or so. Remind her which region you will be treating next. Proceed through the regions of the body using the allotted treatment time.

- As this patient's episode of care proceeds, you will likely introduce other techniques, presented in later chapters, in order to address the kyphosis and muscle tension. At that time, continue to begin each subsequent **intervention** with several minutes of static contact and superficial stroking to establish safety and relaxation. End each session with static contact and superficial stroking to allow the patient time to reflect and to obtain closure.

Critical Thinking Questions

1. Which layers of tissues are engaged by superficial reflex techniques?
2. What are the primary effects of superficial reflex techniques?
3. What characteristics of static contact make it well suited to the treatment of seriously ill people?
4. List three potential uses of static contact and identify a clinical condition for which these uses would be appropriate.
5. How does superficial stroking differ from static contact?
6. Why is stroking usually performed *down* the limbs?
7. List three potential uses of superficial stroking and identify a clinical condition for which these uses would be appropriate.
8. List two potential uses of fine vibration and identify a clinical condition for which these uses would be appropriate.
9. How could you use a fine vibration device during an intervention without reducing the time you have available to perform other hands-on techniques?
10. What are the similarities and differences between the physiological mechanisms for pain relief using superficial stroking and fine vibration?

References for Chapter 7 begin on p. 461; see Further Reading list on p. 464.

CHAPTER **8**

Superficial Fluid Techniques

OBJECTIVES | After studying this chapter, you will have the information that you need to do the following:

1. Describe how the massage techniques in this category affect different types of tissues.
2. Describe each massage technique in terms of the contact surface, pressure, tissues engaged, amplitude, direction, and rate.
3. Demonstrate how to perform each massage technique and how to apply it in the context of a practice sequence.
4. Speculate about the mechanisms by which massage techniques achieve their effects.
5. Describe the outcomes of care, indications, contraindications, and common uses associated with each massage technique.

Superficial fluid techniques are massage techniques that therapists apply to tissues superficial to muscle to increase the return flow of blood or lymph. These techniques include superficial effleurage and superficial lymph drainage. This chapter describes these techniques, how to perform them, and how to apply them in a practice sequence. It also discusses relevant outcomes and evidence, cautions and contraindications, and how to use the technique in treatment. Finally, Table 8-1 summarizes those outcomes for superficial fluid techniques that are related to body structures and functions. Therapists are advised to review the cautions and contraindications for these techniques and to use them as their scope of practice and skill level permit.

Superficial Effleurage: Evidence

DEFINITION

Superficial effleurage: A gliding technique performed with light pressure in the direction of venous and lymphatic flow that deforms tissue down to the investing layer of the deep fascia.[1-8]

NAMES AND ORIGINS

In other texts and massage-related systems, the technique that we call superficial effleurage is known as "effleurage," "gliding," "stroking," and "deep stroking."[1-8] The use of the word "effleurage" in current texts is (alas) highly variable with respect to the type and depth of tissues engaged by the stroke being described. Some authors use the terms "effleurage" and "stroking" interchangeably.[1-5] This book follows the convention used in many texts, including *Beard's Massage*,[6] which distinguishes between effleurage and stroking on the basis of the pressure, direction, tissues engaged, and clinical effects of the strokes.[6-8] Although superficial effleurage may be used to produce **reflex effects** similar to those produced with superficial stroking (discussed in Chapter 7), it has additional effects on fluid dynamics. Additionally, this book makes a further distinction between superficial effleurage and the similarly patterned deep effleurage, which uses sufficient pressure to engage and **deform** muscle (see Chapter 9). The precedent and clinical rationale for making this distinction is that therapists must learn to discriminate clearly among the various tissue layers—skin, subcutaneous fascia and fat, and muscle.[1,3,5,7] This ability will enable the therapist to selectively direct the force of a massage stroke toward each tissue layer, as required to achieve the desired treatment **outcomes**.

USES

Therapists use superficial effleurage to increase **venous return** and **lymphatic return**, to spread oil at the start of regional massage, and to relax patients. They often use it at intervals during **classical massage** to give clients a "break" from deeper or more aggressive techniques.

OUTCOMES AND EVIDENCE

Therapists can use this light, flowing technique to improve the flow of interventions and to achieve circulatory effects, psychological effects, and a variety of physiological effects. Superficial effleurage is ideal for spreading lubricant, and therapists often use it as an introductory stroke in regional massage and **general massage**. They can also use it as a transitional stroke and between deeper techniques that engage the client's muscles (see Chapter 9).

Superficial effleurage has a variety of physiological and psychological effects.[9-16] It is best known for its circulatory effects. Numerous sources state that effleurage (in some form) increases **lymphatic and venous return** from the region to which it is applied.[1-8] One possible mechanism for this effect on lymphatic flow is that the gentle mechanical stresses of the technique cause a contraction of small lymphatic vessels, thereby increasing the formation and return of lymph.[17] Furthermore, superficial effleurage may produce direct movement of lymph when the pressure of the stroke is light and the rate of glide is slow. Notwithstanding its **mechanical effect** on lymphatic vessels, superficial effleurage does not appear to affect local arterial or venous flow, at least in healthy tissues.[18-20] Effects on lymphatic flow make superficial effleurage an indicated treatment for conditions of lymphatic congestion, including dependent **edema**; edema or effusion associated with the acute and subacute phases of common musculoskeletal injuries such as bursitis, sprains, strains, contusions, dislocations, separations, and fractures; **reflex sympathetic dystrophy**; and congestion of the breast associated with menses or lactation. It may also be of use when treating venous stasis[20] and related conditions such as varicosities and venous ulcers. Finally, superficial effleurage is useful in the treatment of **lymphedema** following surgical excision of lymphatics.[21] Because of its range of effects on lymphatic flow, superficial effleurage is a component of some systems of **manual lymph drainage** (MLD).

Its other effects include both physiological and psychological outcomes. As with superficial stroking, superficial effleurage can be used to decrease anxiety, induce relaxation[22,23] (with one dissent[24]), temporarily decrease lower motor neuron excitability,[25,26] and stimulate peristalsis.[27,28] Because of its mild mechanical effects, therapists can use superficial effleurage with superficial reflex techniques to induce **sedation**, increase general comfort, and reduce the perception of pain in postoperative situations. Finally, it is also indicated for infant colic.[28] Table 8-1 summarizes the main outcomes for superficial effleurage.

HOW SUPERFICIAL EFFLEURAGE MIGHT WORK

Superficial effleurage compresses veins and lymph vessels, mechanically pushing blood and lymph forward through these vessels, which contain valves to prevent backflow.[1-8,29] Once a section of a vessel has emptied, a suction effect also draws distal fluid proximally.[7] The resulting increase in venous return may increase cardiac stroke volume,[29] although not overall systemic flow,[17,18,29] in healthy subjects.[18] In addition, light pressure on terminal lymphatics may stimulate the smooth muscle of these vessels to contract, pushing lymph forward.[18] Finally, repetitive rhythmic pressure may entrain a relaxation response.[19] (See the discussion of entrainment in the section titled How Superficial Stroking Might Work in Chapter 7.)

EXAMINING THE EVIDENCE

Meta-analyses are uncommon in the massage literature, and those that examine the effects of a single massage technique are rare. In 1997, nursing researchers Labyak and Metzger[23] conducted a **meta-analysis** of nine studies that applied from 3 to 10 minutes of effleurage ("**slow-stroke backrub**") to various groups of hospitalized clients. They concluded that massage caused a drop in heart rate and respiration rate for all subjects, while only male subjects achieved an overall reduction of systolic and diastolic blood pressure. Clients in all studies consistently reported feeling more relaxed and comfortable after the backrubs.

This study had several problems that make these conclusions suspect. The authors did not describe their procedure for searching databases to find articles clearly. Five of nine papers included in the meta-analysis were unpublished dissertations. Beyond stating the inclusion criteria, the authors did not include descriptions of the studies they selected, and they did not evaluate the methods in those studies. Some of the studies were pre-test, posttest designs but lacked control groups. Furthermore, treatment lengths in the studies were varied and brief. Finally, potentially confounding variables included: the presence of cardiovascular disease in clients, clients' age, and the gender of the therapist.

Labyak SE, Metzger BL. The effects of effleurage backrub on the physiological components of relaxation: a meta-analysis. *Nurs Res.* 1997;46:59-62.

Superficial Effleurage: Practice

COMPONENTS OF SUPERFICIAL EFFLEURAGE

Superficial effleurage has the following components:

Contact: Whole relaxed palmar surface of hand
Pressure: Light
Engages: Skin, superficial fascia, and fat
Direction: On limbs, **centripetal**; on torso, toward axillary or inguinal lymph nodes
Amplitude: Length of the region
Rate: 5 to 50 cm/s
Duration: 2 minutes or longer
Intergrades with: Petrissage and superficial stroking
Context: Used for extended periods alone or alternating with superficial lymph drainage technique to facilitate return of lymph and possibly blood. Often used as a prelude and follow-up to extended application of neuromuscular techniques.

PALPATION PRACTICE

The following palpation exercises will help you develop the manual skill and focus you need to perform superficial effleurage well:

1. On a practice partner, estimate the thickness of the layer of fat (and associated **superficial fascia**) that lies on top of the most superficial muscle layer. Be sure to do this in several regions since fat is not evenly distributed. Compare several people. Compare men and women.
2. Palpate the superficial veins and arteries embedded in the superficial fat and fascia.
3. Try to locate and palpate the **investing layer of deep fascia**. This layer is harder than the fat above it and is often harder than the muscle beneath it. If you are palpating muscle fibers then you are too deep. Be sure to explore the following areas where this layer is thicker and easier to find: over the scapula, in the lumbar area, lateral to the shin, and on the palms of the hand and soles of the feet. It will be helpful to have a photographic atlas of anatomy at hand that shows this layer.

MANUAL TECHNIQUE

In Figures 8-1 to 8-9, superficial effleurage is applied to the various regions of the body. The order of figures is from head to foot in supine and then in prone. Each figure illustrates most of the guidelines for manual technique outlined in this section.

1. Therapists prefer to use **lubricant** when performing superficial effleurage. Nevertheless, unless the skin is moist or very hairy, you can perform superficial effleurage effectively without lubricant.

2. Let your hands be as soft and relaxed as possible while gliding over the client's skin. Continuously mold the entire palmar surface of your hand to the changing contours of the client's body, like water flowing over substrate. You may spread your fingers apart, but not so widely that your hand becomes tense. You may abduct your thumb and use your thumb, fingers, and web space to encircle a limb.

3. Point your hand in the general direction of the pressure stroke. Small deviations of the wrist allow your hand to conform to local body contours. Avoid large wrist movements in order to prevent **repetitive strain injury**.

4. Pressure of the stroke is toward axillary or inguinal lymph nodes when you are working on the trunk (Figure 8-3) and toward the heart when you are working on the limbs (Figures 8-4A and 8-4B, 8-5, 8-7, 8-10, and 8-11). When you apply this technique to the client's back, the stroke typically begins at the

FIGURE 8-1 Bilateral superficial effleurage of the neck and shoulders. The stroke moves down the neck, over the clavicles toward the axilla, finishing at the deltoid, and settling the shoulders with a gentle downward pressure.

FIGURE 8-2 A. Unilateral superficial effleurage of the rotated neck. The stroke may end at the root of the neck or continue over the clavicle toward the axilla. **B**. A light return stroke may be added at the end of the stroke. To perform this, the forearm supinates while the hand maintains contact with the client's skin. **C**. And the hand draws lightly back toward the occiput.

FIGURE 8-5 Medial and lateral surfaces of the client's leg can often be included in the same stroke. Note the therapist's upright posture.

FIGURE 8-3 On the chest, for both men and women, strokes are directed toward the axilla while avoiding the region of the client's nipple. (For concepts related to the ethics of touching the breast, see Chapters 5 and 6.)

sacrum and moves toward the axilla (Figure 8-6), although it can also be applied from the head down.

5. Engage progressively deeper layers of tissue with each repetition of the **centripetal** pressure stroke, advancing as deep as the investing layer of the deep fascia. Repeat strokes 5 to 10 times or more to overcome the **inertial resistance** of fluid. Using the same pattern of movement, you can gradually increase the amount of pressure you apply and engage underlying muscle, if this is indicated (see Chapter 9).

6. Some authors suggest that the pressure of each stroke can be increased with increasing proximity of the hand(s) to the heart.[6,8] You can also use a distinct pause with slight **overpressure** at the proximal end of the stroke, preferably over a set of lymph nodes.

7. The rate of the stroke can vary from 5 to 50 cm/s. One author specifies a rate of 15 cm/s or 6 to 7 in./s.[6]

8. There are varying opinions on the use of the **return stroke**. You may omit the return stroke, since the production of even a slight centrifugal pressure conflicts with the aim of assisting fluid return (Figures 8-1 and 8-2A). Alternatively, you may allow your hand(s) to remain in contact with the client's body for the return stroke but use minimal pressure while performing dragless superficial stroking with either palmar or fingertip contact (Figures 8-2B and 8-2C). If you choose

FIGURE 8-4 During superficial effleurage of the arm, the therapist alternates application of the stroke to the lateral and medial surfaces of the client's arm. **A.** The lateral surface. **B.** The medial surface. Note the change in the therapist's stance.

FIGURE 8-6 A, B. Bilateral superficial effleurage of the back begins at the sacrum and can follow different paths. The therapist may alternate these different paths on consecutive strokes.

FIGURE 8-7 A. Superficial effleurage of the posterior leg, including the gluteals. **B.** For this technique, which requires light pressure, the therapist should achieve the stroke length primarily through leg movement while maintaining an upright torso. Here, on the other hand, the therapist is reaching and leaning; if repeated, this action will place unnecessary strain on the lower back.

to use a return stroke, you must make the transition from one direction to the other smooth.

9. Alternating, two-handed superficial effleurage, with the return strokes performed in the air, is a useful variation.

10. Use thumb or finger contact on smaller parts or around the periphery of swelling with the same general intention (Figures 8-8 and 8-9). Encircle forelimbs and digits with a "bracelet" or "ring" contact.

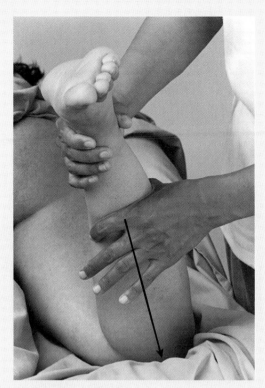

FIGURE 8-8 Superficial effleurage applied to the ankle with an encircling "bracelet" contact.

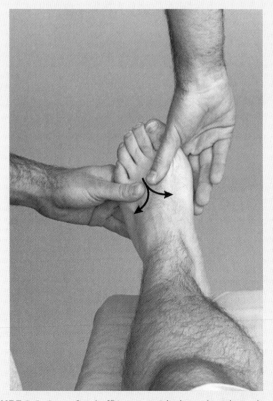

FIGURE 8-9 Superficial effleurage with short thumb strokes will increase lymphatic return from the foot. Similar short strokes can be used to drain posttraumatic edema in a centrifugal direction, away from the periphery of swelling.

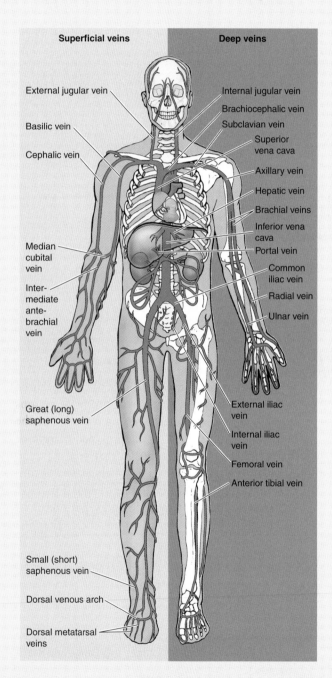

Superficial veins   Deep veins

External jugular vein
Internal jugular vein
Brachiocephalic vein
Basilic vein
Subclavian vein
Cephalic vein
Superior vena cava
Axillary vein
Hepatic vein
Brachial veins
Inferior vena cava
Median cubital vein
Portal vein
Intermediate antebrachial vein
Common iliac vein
Radial vein
Ulnar vein
Great (long) saphenous vein
External iliac vein
Internal iliac vein
Femoral vein
Anterior tibial vein
Small (short) saphenous vein
Dorsal venous arch
Dorsal metatarsal veins

Principal veins

FIGURE 8-10 Venous return to the heart. (Reprinted with permission from Moore K. *Clinically Oriented Anatomy.* 4th ed. Philadelphia, PA: Lippincott Williams & Wilkins; 1999:33.)

FIGURE 8-11 Lymphatic watersheds with indication of the direction of flow of lymph. (Redrawn from Tappan FM, Benjamin PJ. *Tappan's Handbook of Healing Massage Techniques.* 3rd ed. Upper Saddle River, NJ: Prentice-Hall; 1998:227. Copyright 1998. Adapted with permission from Prentice-Hall, Inc., Upper Saddle River, NJ.)

11. When you use superficial effleurage to treat localized swelling, it is preferable to treat proximal regions first. When you work near swelling, ensure that the individual strokes begin at the proximal margin or the periphery of the swelling so that you make no attempt to push fluid into or through an area of congestion. Later chapters discuss the design of massage sequences to increase lymphatic and venous return.

THERAPIST'S POSITION AND MOVEMENT

1. Use the basic positions described in Chapter 6, in the sections **Standing Aligned**, **Lunge**, and **Lunge and Reach** postures.
2. When applying superficial effleurage to a large region such as the back or the legs, you achieve the full length of the strokes through correct movement of your legs, rather than through overreaching with your arms. Throughout the stroke, keep your torso upright to reduce repetitive flexion and extension of your lumbar spine (Figures 8-5 and 8-7B).

PALPATE

As you perform the technique, palpate the client for the following:

1. Skin texture
2. Skin temperature
3. Presence of perspiration and moisture
4. Horizontal stretch of the skin and subcutaneous **superficial fascia**, which occurs in the direction of movement. Because lubricant reduces drag, these superficial tissues are not stretched to their elastic limit.
5. Subcutaneous fatty lipomas, which are common on the back,[20] and floating, hard fibrositic nodules, which are common around the iliac crest and occiput. Both of these can be tender on palpation.
6. Surface contours

7. Pliability of superficial subcutaneous tissues. This normally increases as these tissues become less viscous with continued application.
8. Inertial resistance of the subcutaneous tissue, which reflects its fluid content (i.e., interstitial fluid pressure)
9. Resorption of fluid from edematous tissue, which is accompanied by changes in surface contours and the **viscosity** and inertial resistance of the subcutaneous tissues

OBSERVE

As you perform the technique, observe the client for signs of reduction of swelling or of relaxation. These signs are listed in the following sections.

Reduction of Swelling

1. Normalization of skin color and texture
2. Change of surface contours
3. Visible reduction of swelling, which may often occur within 15 to 45 minutes. Cumulative reduction of swelling will occur during the course of the intervention, with resolution of an inflammatory process, or with resolution of circulatory and lymphatic dysfunction.

Relaxation

1. Decrease in rate and depth of breathing
2. Deeper voice tone
3. Changes in skin color such as flushing. Pallor may indicate an undesirable **sympathetic response**.
4. Systemic reduction of **resting muscle tension**, as evidenced by softening of the tissue contours or broadening and flattening of body segments
5. Muscle twitches and jerks
6. Increases in peristaltic noises
7. Decreases in heart rate, as evidenced by change in pulses that are visible at the neck, wrist, and foot
8. Agitation or sweating, which may indicate an undesirable sympathetic response

COMMUNICATION WITH THE CLIENT

Get feedback on the client's level of comfort during the technique. Here are some examples of statements that you can use:

1. "Let me know if this pressure becomes uncomfortable." When you are treating close to the areas of acute or

---

A Practice Sequence for Superficial Effleurage

The following sequence of body regions, which you can complete in 30 minutes, proceeds from proximal to distal. Apply superficial effleurage to each region in succession. Begin the strokes distally within each region and cover the entire region with centripetal strokes that run the full length of the region. Repeat strokes several times.

- Supine: Neck, face, chest, arm, abdomen, and anterior legs
- Prone: Back, gluteals, and posterior legs

Try variations that

- Use only the centripetal pressure stroke
- Use superficial stroking to return to the starting position
- Use constant pressure
- Increase pressure slightly as the strokes move proximally
- Pause over lymph nodes at the proximal end of the stroke
- Use different rates (5 to 50 cm/s)

How you would apply the technique using only side-lying positions while working from proximal to distal regions?

---

subacute inflammation, ensure that the pressure of the technique does not increase the client's level of pain.
2. "What is happening with your pain?" You can use this statement when you are applying the technique to reduce pain. It allows you to check how the client perceives that the intervention is affecting her pain at intervals during the application of the technique.
3. Encourage the client to perform deep diaphragmatic breathing during the intervention to assist lymphatic drainage and relaxation.

CAUTIONS AND CONTRAINDICATIONS

Therapists need clinical training and supervised practice to master the proper application of superficial effleurage. Advanced training may be advisable in certain situations, particularly when dealing with pathological conditions. Although superficial effleurage only uses enough pressure to deform superficial fat and fascia, with their associated vessels, the therapist should consider all contraindications and cautions to massage (see Chapter 5).[1] There are several contraindications for clients with cardiac, orthopedic, and metabolic conditions. Critically ill clients typically tolerate superficial effleurage well.[23,30,31] Acute cardiac conditions are the exception to this rule. Although light massage is beneficial after myocardial infarction, there is a caution to allow a 48-hour wait after coronary artery bypass surgery before using massage.[30] Furthermore, the therapist must exercise caution when the client presents with cardiac insufficiency or congestive heart failure because an increase in venous return can compromise cardiac or pulmonary function. Clients with acute orthopedic injuries or reflex sympathetic dystrophy may not tolerate local application of superficial effleurage. It may also be a contraindication for clients with these conditions. In these situations, the therapist should apply the technique proximal to the site of the injury to enhance drainage. In general, the therapist should not apply superficial effleurage over newly forming scars,[32] areas of confirmed or suspected infection, cellulitis, and thrombus. The use of superficial effleurage may increase the rate of kidney filtration in clients with serious kidney pathology or nutritional deficiency and lead to complications. Finally, even the use of light massage may reduce the duration of effectiveness of epidural anesthesia.[33]

USING SUPERFICIAL EFFLEURAGE IN TREATMENT

Before you consider using superficial effleurage for treatment, you should be able to recognize the signs and symptoms of major vascular disease and major lymphatic dysfunction and understand their implications.

Orthopedic Injuries

To treat **edema** secondary to trauma, apply extended, repetitive superficial effleurage proximal to the site of trauma. Combine this with ice or the application of cold, elevation of the limbs to 30° or 45°, and passive movements and gentle joint mobilization techniques to reduce pain. Encourage the client to perform deep diaphragmatic breathing to assist lymphatic return. The postintervention self-care intervention for orthopedic injuries includes rest, ice or the application of cold, compression, and elevation of the limbs to 30° or 45° (RICE).

Lymphedema

The comprehensive treatment of **lymphedema** requires detailed, expert instruction on hygiene and skin care, regular use of compression bandages and garments, and specialized active exercises. Depending on the nature and extent of lymphedema, any of the following direct interventions may be indicated: gait, locomotion, balance, and **postural awareness** training; **strengthening**; and functional training in self-care and home management, including the use of assistive and adaptive devices.[34] Neuromuscular and connective tissue massage techniques may be useful for fibrosed edema.

Venous Stasis

To treat edema associated with venous stasis, ensure that thrombus or thrombophlebitis are absent and then apply the technique proximal to the site of stasis, avoiding the immediate area of ulcers or varicosities. Elevation of a limb during the intervention and raised leg exercises for home care may be helpful.[35]

Superficial Lymph Drainage Technique: Evidence

DEFINITION

Superficial lymph drainage technique: A nongliding technique performed in the direction of lymphatic flow, using short, rhythmical strokes with minimal to light pressure, that deforms subcutaneous tissue without engaging muscle.[36-46]

NAMES AND ORIGINS

Superficial lymph drainage technique is a variant of superficial effleurage that was developed in the 20th century by Emil **Vodder** and subsequently elaborated on by several schools of **MLD**.[36-44,46] Superficial lymph drainage and superficial effleurage have in common the application of light pressure directed centripetally through the same tissue layer. During superficial effleurage, however, the therapist's hands glide over the skin—it is a faster and more general manipulation. Conversely, during superficial lymph drainage technique, the therapist very gently stretches the client's skin, superficial fascia, and accompanying lymphatics to their elastic limit in the direction of lymphatic flow, without compressing deeper structures, and then carefully releases the stretched tissues.

Superficial lymph drainage technique is a principal technique of the various schools of MLD, which may also use superficial effleurage, compression, and other massage techniques in their interventions. It is used as part of a comprehensive intervention known as **complex** or **complete decongestive therapy** or **physiotherapy** (CDT, CDP, or CDMT). This intervention includes bandaging or **compression garments**, specific exercises, and education on hygiene.[42-44]

USES

Therapists use superficial lymph drainage technique to increase lymphatic return. When they perform it correctly, this technique also has a secondary sedative effect.

OUTCOMES AND EVIDENCE

Superficial lymph drainage technique has a variety of physiological and psychological effects.[47-51] Local use of superficial lymph drainage technique can increase lymphatic return from the region to which therapists apply it. When the therapist applies this technique to larger areas of the client's body, it can produce an increase in the volume of lymph that is returning to the venous system. The proposed mechanism for these effects is that the slow, delicate, rhythmic stretching of the tissues promotes the formation of lymph,[46] stimulates contraction of the lymphatic vessels,[19,36,40,46] propels lymph through the collapsible superficial lymphatics,[36,40,46,52] increases local blood flow,[53] and reduces the time required for alternative lymphatic pathways (anastomoses) to form after lymphatic pathways have been interrupted by damage. When therapists perform this technique skillfully, it can result in **sedation** (parasympathetic activity), reduced pain (counterirritant analgesia), and improvement in general immune function.[36,46,54]

CDT is a well-documented intervention that extensive research suggests is effective in the treatment of lymphedema,[55-73] particularly lymphedema that arises after surgical intervention in breast cancer.[43,57,64,74-87] There is currently debate about how much MLD contributes to the effectiveness of this intervention.[58,77,88-92] Superficial lymph drainage is effective for traumatic edema,[93-96] venous insufficiency,[97,98] acne,[36,40] and a variety of other conditions,[99-106] but is not more effective than exercise for complex regional pain syndrome.[107] Table 8-1 summarizes the main outcomes for superficial lymph drainage.

HOW SUPERFICIAL LYMPH DRAINAGE TECHNIQUE MIGHT WORK

The light rhythmical pumping of superficial lymph drainage causes repeated pressure changes in the interstitium that stimulate the formation of lymph.[46] As with superficial effleurage, the light pressure deforms the most distal lymph vessels, mechanically pushing lymph forward through these vessels, which contain valves to prevent backflow.[7,29] Once a section of a vessel has been emptied, a suction effect also draws the fluid in the distal interstitial spaces proximally.[7,46] Light pressure also stimulates contraction of the smooth muscle of the collecting vessel segments called lymphangions,[46] which pumps lymph forward.[7,19,46] Finally, repetitive rhythmic pressure may entrain a relaxation response. (See the discussion of entrainment in the section titled How Superficial Stroking Might Work in Chapter 7.)

EXAMINING THE EVIDENCE

In 2004, the **Cochrane Database of Systematic Reviews** examined physical methods used to treat lymphedema, including bandaging, compression sleeves, hosiery, and MLD.[108] The research team selected for review **randomized clinical trials** indexed in major medical databases that had a follow-up period of more than 6 months. The three papers that met these criteria did not study the same intervention. In the single trial that considered massage, the effect of MLD on lymphedema was no greater than that achieved with compression bandages. The review's major conclusion was that there is a clear need for well-designed, randomized trials of the whole range of therapeutic interventions in order to determine the best approach to managing lymphedema.

This study was rigorous and well documented. Search strategies, selection criteria, and review procedures were detailed at length. The authors described 10 studies that initially met the inclusion criteria in detail and provided reasons for excluding seven of them. The end product of this rigor was that the authors were left with too few studies to perform a meta-analysis and could only conclude that more and better research is required.[88]

Badger C, Preston N, Seers K, Mortimer P. Physical therapies for reducing and controlling lymphoedema of the limbs. *Cochrane Database Syst Rev.* 2004;4:CD00314183.

Superficial Lymph Drainage Technique: Practice

COMPONENTS OF SUPERFICIAL LYMPH DRAINAGE TECHNIQUE

Superficial lymph drainage technique has the following components:

Contact: The entire relaxed palmar surface of the hand, heel of the hand, and grouped fingers

Pressure: Minimal to light (5 mm Hg, "the weight of a nickel")

Engages: Skin, superficial fascia, and fat only

Direction: Centripetal, in the direction of lymphatic pathways

Amplitude/length: Short, less than 2.5 cm (1 in.)

Rate: Slow, about 2.5 cm/s

Duration: 5 to 60 minutes or longer

Intergrades with: Superficial effleurage

Combines with: May be combined with varying amounts of compression (for fibrosed edema)

Context: Used alone for extended periods or alternated with superficial effleurage.

PALPATION PRACTICE

The following palpation exercises will help you develop the manual skill you need to perform superficial lymph drainage technique well:

1. Estimate the thickness of the layer of fat (and associated superficial fascia) that lies on top of the most superficial muscle layer. Be sure to do this in several regions because fat is not evenly distributed. Compare several people. Compare men and women.
2. Try to palpate the actual investing layer of deep fascia. This layer is harder than the fat above it and is often harder than the muscle beneath it. If you are palpating muscle fibers, then you are too deep. Be sure to explore the areas over the scapula, the lumbar area, the area lateral to the shin, the palms of the hand, and the soles of the feet.
3. Find the **elastic barrier** of the skin and superficial fat and fascia. How far can you stretch this tissue layer before your hand begins to slide over the skin? How far can you stretch this tissue layer without putting any pressure on the investing layer of deep fascia? Try this exercise in several regions, including those listed in the previous exercise.

MANUAL TECHNIQUE

In Figures 8-12 to 8-20, superficial lymph drainage technique is applied to the various regions of the body. The order of figures is from head to foot in supine and then in prone. Each figure illustrates most of the guidelines for manual technique outlined in this section:

1. Do not use oil. If either your skin or your client's skin is moist, you may apply enough unscented fine talc, cornstarch, or chalk to your hands to prevent sticking.

2. This technique demands supreme relaxation of your hands, which only comes from extensive practice. You can use any part of your hand, as long as the manual contact is soft and evenly distributed (Figures 8-15, 8-16, and 8-19). You may abduct your thumb so that the web space becomes a part of the contact surface (Figure 8-15). Fingerpad or thumb contact is useful when you are treating smaller parts of the body (Figures 8-12, 8-13, and 8-20).

3. Placing two hands side by side can create a larger contact, which is more suitable for broad areas such as the torso or thigh (Figure 8-16).

4. Use minimal pressure to engage the skin and sink slightly into the subcutaneous fat; little or no indentation should be visible. Then gently stretch the skin and superficial fascia in the general direction of

A

B

FIGURE 8-13 A. Fingerpad contact can be used for superficial lymph drainage of the face. **B**. Fingerpad contact can also be used for the submandibular region.

FIGURE 8-12 A series of strokes down the neck ends near the junction of the venous and lymphatic systems. Direct pressure inferiorly under the clavicle and medially toward the "terminus." This sequence clears the most proximal portion of the lymphatic system and begins any intervention. The therapist should repeat this stroke several times.

lymphatic flow (see Figure 8-11), without engaging underlying muscle, by applying pressure in a direction that is parallel to the surface. You can obtain better results if the stroke shape is semielliptical or semicircular. In this way, stretch of the tissues occurs in two directions on the plane of the surface of the client's skin, while you maintain a general centripetal orientation.[36,40]

5. The working surface of your hand does not glide over the client's skin. Areas of the hand that are adjacent to the working surface may glide in small amounts.

6. Pause at the end of each slow, short stroke, when you have stretched the skin and superficial fascia in a manner that takes the slack out of these tissues. Then gradually release the pressure you exerted and allow the skin to return to its original position.

FIGURE 8-14 Axillary and inguinal areas are treated prior to work on the related limb, and the therapist returns frequently to these areas during work on the client's limb. The hand directs pressure toward the midline of the arm and superiorly.

7. You may keep your hands in one place and perform several strokes on the same location. In that situation, take care to ensure that you do not exert any **centrifugal** pressure when your hand follows the skin back to its original position (Figures 8-12, 8-14, 8-16, and 8-18). Alternatively, you may gently break contact

FIGURE 8-15 The index finger, abducted thumb, and adjacent palm form a surface that can fit the arm well. The hands alternate and move proximally with each stroke. The sequence from elbow to axilla may be repeated several times. (A similar sequence uses the ulnar border of the palm to make contact.)

FIGURE 8-16 Stationary ellipses on the anterior thigh. The return stroke (dotted line) must be applied without centrifugal pressure. Instead, the therapist's hand should follow the elastic recoil of the skin.

with the client's body and move your hand(s) slightly proximally with each successive stroke, essentially "walking" your hands along the client's body segment (Figures 8-15 and 8-17). In either case, repeat strokes or series of strokes several times to overcome the inertial resistance of the fluid. Bear in mind that you must practice many, many hours to develop the fine control of pressure required by this technique.

8. The order of the intervention is important when you are using superficial lymphatic drainage techniques. Begin the intervention at the proximal junction between the lymphatic and venous systems (Figure 8-12), treat the client's neck, and drain the client's related trunk quadrant before proceeding to an affected limb. If time for the session is constrained, reduce the amount of time you spend treating the affected area, rather than the time you spend on the proximal areas.[42] Begin work on the

FIGURE 8-17 The two hands can work together: one moving the lymph forward and the second holding the lymph as the first hand moves more proximally in preparation for the next stroke.

FIGURE 8-18 The popliteal nodes are treated with the client in supine.

FIGURE 8-20 Fingerpad technique along the intercostal spaces; pressure is gently directed into the rib spaces and toward the spine to access deeper intrathoracic lymphatics.

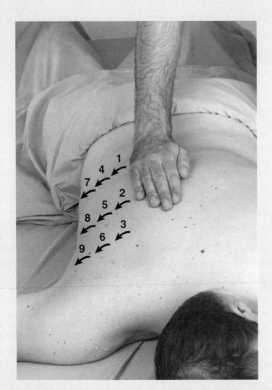

FIGURE 8-19 A series of strokes on the back directs pressure toward the axilla.

limb by opening axillary or inguinal areas, whether or not the associated lymph nodes are intact (Figure 8-14). Furthermore, treat proximal portions of an affected region before distal portions. Finally, make frequent returns to the proximal areas that you cleared earlier in the intervention, thus making frequent movement back and forth from proximal areas to distal areas.

9. If the client's lymphatic vessels have been obstructed or recently irradiated, direct your strokes across normal lymphatic watersheds to the nearest group of nodes that have intact drainage. These are often the contralateral axillary or inguinal nodes or the ipsilateral abdominal nodes. First, drain these areas thoroughly in order to prepare them to receive lymph.[42]

10. Once you are familiar with the delicate contact required for performing superficial lymphatic drainage, strive to attain regularity of stroke rhythm to enhance the technique's sedative effect.

11. Superficial lymphatic drainage technique and its related complementary modalities are time-consuming to deliver. During the initial stages of treatment, daily interventions of up to 45 to 90 minutes are often desirable, depending on the client's condition and the severity of his or her edema.[40,42]

THERAPIST'S POSITION AND MOVEMENT

1. Use the basic positions described in Chapter 6, in the sections Standing Aligned, Seated Aligned, and Lunge Postures. Because superficial lymph drainage technique strokes are short, relatively little reaching is required.
2. Adjusting the manual contact to the contours of the client and the region of application requires flexibility in the movement of your shoulders and elbows. Consequently, you may use relatively large movements of the arm to achieve small manual movements.

PALPATE

As you perform the technique, palpate the client for the following:

1. Skin texture
2. Skin temperature
3. Presence of perspiration and moisture
4. Stretch in skin and subcutaneous fascia. Because the rate of movement is slow, you can palpate the **end feel** of this gentle stretch of the superficial tissues. Work up to, but not through, this barrier.
5. Subcutaneous fatty lipomas, which are common on the back,[29] and floating, hard fibrositic nodules, which are common around the iliac crest and occiput. Both of these can be tender on palpation.
6. Surface contours
7. Increased pliability that reflects the reduction of viscosity of healthy superficial subcutaneous tissues, which normally occurs with continued application of the technique
8. Inertial resistance of the subcutaneous tissue that reflects its fluid content (interstitial fluid pressure)
9. Density of edematous tissue related to its degree of fibrosis
10. Resorption of fluid from edematous tissue, which is accompanied by changes in surface contours, tissue stretch, tissue density, and the viscosity and inertial resistance of the subcutaneous tissues

OBSERVE

As you perform the technique, observe the client for the following signs of reduction of swelling:

1. Normalization of skin color and texture

2. Reduction of **trophic changes**
3. Reduction of surface contours
4. Visible reduction of swelling, which may often occur within 15 to 45 minutes. Cumulative reduction of swelling will occur during the course of the intervention, with resolution of an inflammatory process, or with resolution of circulatory and lymphatic dysfunction.

COMMUNICATION WITH THE CLIENT

Get feedback on the client's level of comfort during the technique. Here are some issues that you need to address and examples of statements you can use:

1. "Let me know if this pressure becomes uncomfortable." When you are treating near areas of acute or subacute inflammation, ensure that the client finds the mechanical stimulus of the technique tolerable. This technique should be painless at all times.
2. Advise the client to urinate before the intervention, and inform her that she may still need to urinate during the intervention or soon after its conclusion.[45]
3. Explain to the client that it is not uncommon to experience fatigue after the first intervention. In addition, ask the client to report the occurrence of other sequelae such as more than mild nausea, shivering, or postintervention pain, which suggest overtreatment.

 A Practice Sequence for Superficial Lymph Drainage Technique

As with superficial effleurage, the best sequence of regions to facilitate return of lymph is to begin with proximal regions and proceed to distal ones. Because superficial lymph drainage technique is slow, a complete full-body sequence like the one below will take anywhere from 1.5 to 3 hours, depending on the amount of repetition that you use.

Apply the technique to each region in succession. Begin the strokes distally within each region and cover the entire region several times with short centripetal strokes, which gradually move proximally. For shorter practice periods, you can cover any region, preceded by the neck, within half an hour:

- Supine: Neck, face, chest, arm, abdomen, and anterior legs
- Prone: Back, gluteals, and posterior legs

Finding soft, comfortable, and relaxed hand contacts that best conform to the regional contours of the client's body can take some experimentation. Try variations that use

- The full palmar surface
- The ulnar border of your hand
- The thumb, index, and included web space
- Flat hands, including the fingers

How would you apply the technique using only side-lying positions and working from proximal to distal regions?

CAUTIONS AND CONTRAINDICATIONS

Therapists need clinical training and supervised practice to master the proper application of superficial lymph drainage technique. Advanced training may be advisable in certain situations, particularly when dealing with pathological conditions. The contraindications to the use of techniques with mechanical effects apply to the use of superficial lymph drainage (see Chapter 5).

The contraindications to the use of superficial lymph drainage technique include acute systemic or local inflammation due to bacterial or viral infection, untreated metastatic disease, allergic reactions, recent thrombosis, and edema due to right-sided heart failure (the client may be massaged outside the area of the edema).[36-38,40,109,110] There are several cautions to the use of superficial lymph drainage technique. The therapist must exercise caution when the client presents with cardiac insufficiency or congestive heart failure, since an increase in venous return can compromise cardiac or pulmonary function. When the client presents with thyroid hyperactivity, avoid local application in the area of the thyroid. If the client has asthma, then treat between attacks, use shorter interventions, and avoid applying around the area of the sternum.

The therapist should avoid the client's abdomen during menstruation and reduce or omit treatment during pregnancy. If the client has low blood pressure, use

caution and shorten interventions in early stages of treatment.[37,40,111] When treating traumatic edema, as with any condition, ensure that the application of superficial lymph drainage is painless and pleasant. If the client is unable to tolerate a local application of this technique, only apply it proximally. Using superficial lymph drainage technique on chronic inflammation may stimulate a transient acute inflammation.[38] Finally, the client may experience slight nausea or fatigue following full-body sessions.[40]

USING SUPERFICIAL LYMPH DRAINAGE TECHNIQUE IN TREATMENT

Before you consider using superficial lymph drainage technique (MLD) for treatment, you should be able to recognize the signs and symptoms of major vascular disease and major lymphatic dysfunction and understand their implications.

Orthopedic Injuries

To treat edema secondary to trauma, use extended repetitive superficial lymph drainage technique proximal to the site of trauma. You can combine this with ice or the application of cold, elevation of the limbs to 30° or 45°, and passive movements and gentle **joint mobilization** techniques to reduce pain. Encourage the client to perform deep diaphragmatic breathing to assist lymphatic return. The postintervention self-care intervention for orthopedic injuries includes rest, ice or the application of cold, compression, and elevation of injured limbs to 30° or 45° (RICE).

Lymphedema

The comprehensive treatment of lymphedema requires detailed, expert instruction on hygiene and skin care, regular use of compression bandages and garments, and specialized active exercises. Depending on the nature and extent of lymphedema, any of the following direct interventions may be indicated: gait, locomotion, balance, and posture awareness training; strengthening; and functional training in self-care and home management, including the use of assistive and adaptive devices.[34] Neuromuscular and connective tissue massage techniques may be useful for fibrosed edema.

Venous Stasis

To treat edema associated with venous stasis, ensure that thrombus or thrombophlebitis are absent, and then apply the technique proximal to the site of stasis, avoiding ulcers or varicosities. Elevation of a limb during the intervention and raised leg exercises for home care may be helpful.[35]

IN CONCLUSION

Superficial lymphatic drainage techniques have a variety of uses, therapeutic effects, and outcomes. Table 8-1 summarizes those outcomes for superficial lymphatic drainage techniques that are related to body structures and functions.

Table 8-1	**Summary of Outcomes for Superficial Fluid Techniques**	
	Technique	
Outcome of Care	**Superficial Effleurage**	**Superficial Lymph Drainage**
Systemic sedation	✓	✓
Decreased anxiety	✓	✓
Counterirritant analgesia	P	P
Increased venous return	?	✓
Decreased edema	P	✓
Increased lymphatic return	P	✓

✓, the outcome is supported by research summarized in this chapter; P, the outcome is possible; ?, the outcome is debatable (research results are absent or inconsistent).

REVIEW SECTION

TAKEAWAYS

1. Superficial fluid techniques are massage techniques that clinicians apply to tissues superficial to the muscle to increase the return flow of blood or lymph.
2. Superficial effleurage: A gliding technique performed with light pressure in the direction of venous and lymphatic flow that deforms tissue down to the investing layer of the deep fascia.
3. Clinicians use superficial effleurage to increase venous return and lymphatic return, to spread oil at the start of regional massage, and to relax patients. They often use it at intervals during classical massage to give patients a "break" from deeper or more aggressive techniques.

4. Superficial effleurage is best known for its circulatory effects. Numerous sources state that effleurage (in some form) increases **lymphatic and venous return** from the region to which it is applied. Superficial effleurage compresses veins and lymph vessels, mechanically pushing blood and lymph forward through these vessels, which contain valves to prevent backflow.
5. Superficial effleurage can be used to decrease anxiety, induce relaxation, temporarily decrease lower motor neuron excitability, and stimulate peristalsis.
6. Superficial lymph drainage technique: A nongliding technique performed in the direction of lymphatic flow, using short, rhythmical strokes with minimal to light pressure that deforms subcutaneous tissue without engaging muscle.

7. Clinicians use superficial lymph drainage technique to increase lymphatic return. When they perform it correctly, this technique also has a secondary sedative effect.

8. Local use of superficial lymph drainage technique can increase lymphatic return from the region to which clinicians apply it. When the clinician applies this technique to larger areas of the patient's body, it can produce an increase in the volume of lymph that is returning to the venous system.

9. The light rhythmical pumping of superficial lymph drainage causes repeated pressure changes in the interstitium that stimulate the formation of lymph. As with superficial effleurage, the light pressure deforms the most distal lymph vessels, mechanically pushing lymph forward through these vessels, which contain valves to prevent backflow.

10. The contraindications to the use of superficial lymph drainage technique include acute systemic or local inflammation due to bacterial or viral infection, untreated metastatic disease, allergic reactions, recent thrombosis, and edema due to right-sided heart failure.

Clinical Case: *Superficial Fluid Techniques*

Patient Profile

Your patient is an 18-year-old recreational runner who rolled over on his right ankle 2 days ago during a cross-country run. He had increasing pain and swelling of the ankle after the injury. Twelve hours later, he went to the emergency department, where a doctor gave him the diagnosis of grade 2 ankle sprain after taking X-rays to rule out a fracture. This injury is a repeat of a similar one that he had about 10 years ago.

Subjective Findings:

- Complaint of constant right ankle pain that is "on the outer side" of his ankle
- Reports swelling of his right ankle
- Complaint of reduced ability to weightbear on the affected ankle. He walks with a limp and cannot run.

Objective Findings:

Impairments in Body Structures or Function

- Gait: **Antalgic** gait and an inability to bear weight on the right foot in standing.
- Requires crutches for ambulation.
- Edema: **Non-pitting edema** on his right foot extends from the metatarsal heads to several inches above the malleoli. The skin is discolored in the region of the edema.
- Pain: There is exquisite point tenderness in the location of the anterior talofibular ligament.
- Range of motion: Right ankle active and passive inversion and plantarflexion are limited by 50%, with pain at the end of range.
- Special tests: Anterior drawer and varus stress tests reproduce his pain.

Activity Limitations:

- Difficulty climbing stairs and walking for greater than 10 feet without crutches.
- Unable to participate in running and other sport activities.

Treatment Approach

- Explain that the course of recovery will be several weeks and that forcing himself to bear weight on his ankle when it is not ready will only compound problems.
- Place the patient on the table in supine, elevate the leg to 30° with several pillows, and apply ice to the ankle for 10 minutes. Instruct the patient on how to perform **diaphragmatic breathing**. Apply superficial effleurage to the proximal portion of the affected leg and then to the distal portion, only working as far distally as the proximal margin of swelling in the lower leg. Alternate back and forth from proximal to distal portions of the leg. Use contact that encircles the leg as much as possible and be sure to include the medial surface. Continue to apply superficial effleurage in this manner for as long as the treatment time allows. You can also apply **reflex** techniques, such as static contact and superficial stroking, on the site of injury as the patient tolerates.
- As the patient's **episode of care** proceeds, you will introduce other massage techniques, to facilitate tendon healing and treat muscle tension in both legs.
- Instruction in RICE; hydrotherapy; electrotherapeutic modalities; ankle strengthening, stretching, and balance exercises; ankle taping; and return to activity program are relevant complementary treatments.

Critical Thinking Questions

1. Which layers of tissues are engaged by superficial fluid techniques?
2. What are the primary effects of superficial fluid techniques?
3. List two potential uses of superficial effleurage and identify a clinical condition for which these uses would be appropriate.
4. Why is superficial effleurage performed with centripetal pressure? Why not with centrifugal pressure?
5. List two potential uses of superficial lymph drainage and identify a clinical condition for which these uses would be appropriate.
6. In what ways are the components of superficial effleurage and superficial lymph drainage technique similar and different?
7. What are the differences between superficial lymph drainage technique, MLD, and complex decongestive therapy?
8. Which types of edema can clinicians treat successfully with massage techniques? Which types of edema will not respond as well to massage techniques?
9. Describe the physiological mechanism for how superficial lymph drainage techniques increase lymphatic return. Compare and contrast this with how superficial effleurage achieves its circulatory effects.
10. There are a variety of cautions and contraindications for the use of superficial fluid techniques. List two of these that are common to both superficial effleurage and superficial lymph drainage techniques.

References for Chapter 8 begin on p. 465; see Further Reading list on p. 467.

CHAPTER 9

Neuromuscular Techniques

OBJECTIVES

After studying this chapter, you will have the information that you need to do the following:

1. Describe how the massage techniques in this category affect different types of tissues.
2. Describe each massage technique in terms of the contact surface, pressure, tissues engaged, amplitude, direction, and rate.
3. Demonstrate how to perform each massage technique and how to apply it in the context of a practice sequence.
4. Speculate about the mechanisms by which massage techniques achieve their effects.
5. Describe the outcomes of care, indications, contraindications, and common uses associated with each massage technique.

Neuromuscular techniques are those massage techniques that palpate muscle, affect the level of resting tension of muscles, and have additional psychoneuroimmunological effects. These techniques include broad-contact compression, petrissage, muscle stripping, and specific compression. This chapter describes these techniques, how to perform them, and how to apply them in a practice sequence. It also includes a discussion of relevant outcomes and evidence, cautions and contraindications, and how to use the technique in treatment. Finally, Table 9-3 summarizes those outcomes for neuromuscular techniques that are related to body structures and functions. Therapists are advised to review the cautions and contraindications for these techniques and to use them as their scope of practice and skill level permit.

Broad-Contact Compression: Evidence

DEFINITION

Broad-contact compression: A **nongliding** technique that therapists deliver with a broad-contact surface such as the palm or a loose fist. This technique engages the client's muscle, and the pressure and release of the stroke are perpendicular to the surface of the client's body.[1-7]

NAMES AND ORIGINS

In other texts or massage-related systems, the technique that we call broad-contact compression is also known as "compression," "pressure," and "pressing."[1-7] Broad-contact compression owes its current classification as an independent technique largely to its applications in athletics.[1-3,5,8] The technique is not usually discussed in older texts[9-11] and is still omitted from some modern ones.[6,12] Nevertheless, this stroke is the technical foundation and prerequisite for many classical gliding techniques that **knead** muscle (see the section on petrissage). Although broad-contact compression lacks the component of "**drag**" (horizontal tension) that characterizes petrissage, it is an extremely versatile technique in its own right.

USES

Therapists can use broad-contact compression to assess the general quality and level of **resting muscle tension** of larger skeletal muscles, to increase venous and lymphatic return, and to assist the client's expiration. Since it can be **sedating** or **stimulating**, therapists often use it in **sports massage** to prepare athletes for competition and after an event to help the athlete cool down while maintaining high levels of oxygen to help with the oxygen debt.

OUTCOMES AND EVIDENCE

Broad-contact compression is a useful introductory stroke that therapists can use to assess the general quality and the level of resting tension of larger skeletal muscles. They can also use this technique to achieve effects on circulation, resting muscle tension, and rib cage mobility. Table 9-3 summarizes the main outcomes for broad-contact compression. Broad-contact compression has a variety of physiological and psychological effects that are outlined in this section.

Cardiopulmonary Effects

Although various texts state that the repetitive, rhythmic nature of broad-contact compression results in "increased circulation,"[1-7] this postulated direct **mechanical effect** may be an increase in **perfusion**, arterial supply, **lymphatic return**, or **venous return**. For example, broad-contact compression applied to the rib cage may assist systemic lymphatic return.[13] This is especially true in the region of the upper anterior and posterior ribs and over the junctions of the right lymphatic and thoracic ducts with the venous circulation.[13-15] In addition, when therapists perform it on clients' soles or palms, it may assist lymphatic return from the limb.[14,15] The circulatory effects of broad-contact compression have not, however, been evaluated systematically in the research on massage. Furthermore, research on the effect of the similar compressive **petrissage** technique on fluid flow is inconclusive (discussed in this chapter).[16]

Nevertheless, there are two extensive areas of related research that support circulatory effects of broad-contact compression that warrant consideration: closed-chest cardiac massage (CPR) and pneumatic devices that apply compression. Vigorous compression of the rib cage in the context of CPR produces forward blood flow.[17-19] Pneumatic devices that apply compression ("intermittent pneumatic compression," or "impulse compression") to clients' limbs increase venous return and are useful in the treatment of a variety of circulatory conditions.[20-25] Research also suggests that applying a moderate circumferential pressure on the limbs using a pneumatic cuff can increase circulatory supply[25] and lymphatic return.[26,27] In one study, the rate of lymphatic return increased with the pressure applied (up to 320 mm Hg), and a wait of at least 8 seconds was required after each local compression to permit refilling of terminal lymphatics.[12] Compression of the rib cage is used in a variety of ways in cardiopulmonary rehabilitation. Rib cage compression is incorporated into breathing retraining techniques that improve breathing patterns and promote increased respiratory volume during inspiration and expiration.[28] When therapists perform broad-contact compression vigorously and repetitively on the client's rib cage ("shaking" or "rib springing"), it facilitates the movement of secretions through the bronchial tree.[12,29,30] This technique can be used alone or combined with **postural drainage** (see Chapter 12).

Effects on Resting Muscle Tension

Texts are inconsistent on whether broad-contact compression increases or decreases resting muscle tension.[1-3,5] It is possible that broad-contact compression may result in a transient and marginal increase or decrease in resting muscle tension, depending on the rate and vigor of the application of the technique. Therapists often use broad-contact compression in pre/postcompetition sports massage for several reasons: it has a possible effect on tone, it does not require a lubricant or the removal of clothing, and it can be adapted to be either sedative or stimulating.[1-3,8] It is possible to perform effective full-body massage sequences that have specific effects on several of the clients' systems with the skillful use of only broad-contact compression.

HOW BROAD-CONTACT COMPRESSION MIGHT WORK

The mechanisms for cutaneous reflexes, **entrainment** to rhythm, and forward movement of fluid in valved vessels discussed for more superficial techniques in the earlier chapters also apply to broad-contact compression.[1,7]

In addition, broad-contact compression spreads muscle fibers apart.[1,7] This spreading causes **proprioceptive** input that may reduce **neuromuscular tone**.[7,12] Furthermore, sustained pressure may produce connective tissue effects[12] by reducing **collagen** cross-linking and increasing hydration of the **connective tissue matrix**.

EXAMINING THE EVIDENCE

Clinical trials that evaluate the use of manual compression alone are difficult to find. A small (*n* = 36) **randomized controlled** study examined the effects of compression with a mechanical pneumatic compression device on the circulation of clients with occlusive arterial disease.[25] Researchers applied circumferential pressure to the proximal third of the clients' thigh and synchronized it with the systolic pressure wave. The results showed that mechanical compression produced significant increases in walking distances and lower extremity circulatory volume compared with a control group, which received only medication. These conclusions warrant further clinical trials to test various techniques of manual compression to see whether researchers can obtain comparable results.

Allegra C, Bartolo M, Martocchia R. Therapeutic effects of Vascupump treatment in patients with Fontaine stage IIB arteriopathy. *Minerva Cardioangiol.* 2001;49:189-195.

Broad-Contact Compression: Practice

COMPONENTS OF BROAD-CONTACT COMPRESSION

Broad-contact compression has the following components:

Contact: Whole palmar surface of the hand, heel of the hand, dorsal surface of proximal phalanges together (fist), or forearm

Pressure: Light to heavy

Tissues engaged: Muscle, associated tissues, and the underlying structures, such as the rib cage, that therapists reach through muscle. Therapists engage connective tissue elements when they sustain compression

Direction: Perpendicular to surface of the client's body

Amplitude/length: NA

Rate: 5 to 10, or more, seconds per cycle of compression/release

Duration: 20 to 60 seconds or longer

Intergrades with: Petrissage, specific compression

Combines with: Can be combined with **rocking**, although neither technique is improved by this combination

Context: Can be used by itself extensively. Therapists often use it as an initial assessment tool, after effleurage, and/or as a prelude to more specific **neuromuscular techniques**.

PALPATION PRACTICE

1. With full palmar contact, slowly apply light and then moderate pressure to regions of your practice partner's body that have substantial muscle mass such as the chest; front of the shoulder; anterior and posterior arm and forearm; the back adjacent to the spine; anterior, posterior, and medial thighs; and calves. How much does the tissue **deform** with pressure? Do tissues tend to displace one way or another when you direct pressure into the body?

2. With full palmar contact, slowly apply light and then moderate pressure to major bony prominences of your practice partner's body such as the acromion, clavicles, rib cage, iliac crest, ischial tuberosity, lateral femur, and anterior tibia. How do related joints move during each compression?

3. Rest your hands on your supine partner's upper ribs and describe the movement of this part of the rib cage during relaxed breathing. Now, have your partner perform full forced inspiration and expiration. Note the difference. Repeat both parts of this exercise with your hands placed on your partner's lateral ribs and then on your partner's lower ribs.

MANUAL TECHNIQUE

Figures 9-1 to 9-8 show therapists applying broad-contact compression to the various regions of the body. The order of the figures is from head to foot in supine and then in prone. Each figure illustrates several of the guidelines for manual technique outlined in this section.

1. Therapists can best perform broad-contact compression with little or no lubricant.
2. Therapists usually apply this technique to areas where there is muscle tissue (Figures 9-4 to 9-7). Nevertheless, they can also apply it over bone to achieve specialized effects (Figures 9-1 and 9-3).
3. Relax your hands to facilitate palpation and distribute pressure evenly over the entire contact surface. When using the palmar surface, spread your fingers apart slightly to increase the size of the contact surface (Figure 9-4). When you apply the stroke with significant force, avoid loading your wrist while it is extended or hyperextended by using your fist or your proximal forearm as the contact surface (Figures 9-5A and 9-5B, 9-6, and 9-7).
4. Compress and release gradually and smoothly when the rate of application is slow. You should still perform this technique smoothly when you increase the speed of the stroke.
5. The initial direction of application of pressure is perpendicular to the surface of the client's body. Do not direct the stroke in a horizontal direction or parallel to the surface of the client's body. Applying pressure

in this manner will cause the individual muscle fibers to spread apart. As the pressure of application increases, the tissues in large muscle groups, such as the gluteals, may tend to roll and produce some horizontal movement (Figures 9-5A and 9-5B).

6. (Tempo) will vary with the clinical use of the technique. Therapists often use a fast rhythmic rate (1 to 2 strokes per second) in **pre/postcompetition sports massage**. Alternatively, you can sustain a single compression for 10 to 20 seconds, allowing time to gradually apply and release the pressure (Figure 9-7). You will often achieve a more sedative effect and may more readily affect connective tissue elements of the muscle if you take the compression to the end of the tissues' available range of motion.
7. You can lift the client's tissues between each stroke when you are applying faster rhythmic compression to large muscle groups such as the hamstrings or quadriceps.
8. Rhythmic compression can produce a rocking motion that has its own clinical effects, particularly when you apply it around the pelvis (see Chapter 11).

FIGURE 9-1 Gentle bilateral palmar compression of the head can assist sinus drainage.

FIGURE 9-2 Compression of the upper thorax to assist expiration.

FIGURE 9-3 Broad-contact compression to the distal extremity promotes general mobility.

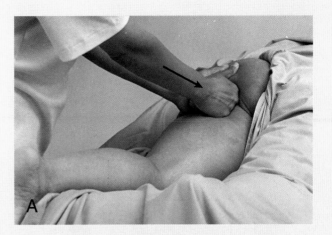

9. To enhance **venous and lymphatic return** from a limb, begin compression proximally at the junction between the limb and the limb girdle. Then apply a series of compression strokes that move from distal to proximal. From that point, begin each successive series of compressions distal to the previous series (Figure 9-8). When you are performing the technique to increase lymphatic return, consider waiting at least 8 seconds before compressing the same local area again.[31]

FIGURE 9-5 A. Broad-contact compression of the glutei to produce sedation can be done either directly on the client's skin or through fabric. The therapist has a choice of contact surfaces: reinforced or doubled fists or palms. **B.** Gluteal compression using the forearm in a lunge-and-lean posture. The therapist uses her free hand to make the posture more stable.

ONLINE VIDEO

THERAPIST'S POSITION AND MOVEMENT

1. Use the basic positions described in Chapter 6 in the sections on standing **aligned** posture, standing controlled lean, **lunge**-and-lean, and **wide-stance knee bend** postures. You can increase the pressure you apply by shifting or rocking a stable **center of gravity**

FIGURE 9-4 Bilateral palmar compression of the shoulders using a standing controlled lean. The heels of the hands are in contact with the acromial portion of the upper trapezius muscle.

FIGURE 9-6 Compression with the forearm or elbow is one of the few techniques that gives the therapist enough leverage to produce a mechanical effect on the superior attachment of the hamstring muscle. The technique must be executed carefully and should be done bilaterally to avoid producing a pelvic rotation in the client.

FIGURE 9-7 Elbow or forearm compression with the client seated is an effective approach to soften a chronically indurated upper trapezius muscle. The therapist bends his knees, inclines his trunk slightly, and maintains relaxed shoulders to transfer his body weight to the client's body in a controlled manner.

forward over the compressed segment of the client's body. Alternatively, you can bend both your knees to lower your upper body weight onto the client (Figures 9-4, 9-5B, 9-6, and 9-7).

2. Regardless of the working posture that you select, ensure that both of your feet remain flat on the floor with your toes pointing toward your work, your hands and forearms remain as relaxed as possible, your elbows are flexed, and your shoulders are as relaxed as possible. Avoid standing statically when applying this technique; instead shift from foot to foot as you work.

3. Use contact surfaces other than your hands for applying large amounts of pressure. When you do so, gauge how the client's compressed tissues are deforming under your body weight (Figures 9-4 to 9-7). This type of palpation might be termed "proprioceptive palpation," as opposed to strict manual palpation, since you are using proprioceptive sense to judge the movement of the client's tissues. The development of this "proprioceptive palpation" skill is essential to learning how to apply higher force neuromuscular and connective tissue techniques.

FIGURE 9-8 The numbers indicate the sequence in which compressions are performed to enhance fluid return from the limb. (See Manual Technique, item #9, page 269, for description.)

PALPATE

When performing the technique, palpate the client's tissues for the following:

1. General resistance or resilience of soft tissues
2. Localized areas of hardness or tautness that may require the use of a more specific technique
3. Increased pliability that reflects the reduction in **viscosity** of healthy superficial subcutaneous tissues, which normally occurs with continued application of the technique
4. Resorption of fluid from edematous tissue, which accompanies changes in surface contours, and the **viscosity** and **inertial resistance** of the subcutaneous tissues
5. Change in resting muscle tension with continued application of the technique
6. Change in the mobility of the rib cage when you apply the technique locally

OBSERVE

When performing the technique, observe the client for changes in muscular tension, circulation, or breathing pattern. The signs listed below may signal this.

1. Reduction of **resting muscle tension**, as evidenced by softening of the tissue contours or broadening and flattening of body segments.
2. If you are using the technique to treat respiratory conditions, note abnormalities in the client's usual breathing pattern and changes in these patterns with your application of the technique.
3. If you use the technique to treat **edema** and apply it proximal to the site of edema, visible reduction of swelling may often occur within 15 to 45 minutes. Cumulative reduction of **swelling** will occur during the course of the intervention, with resolution of an inflammatory process or with resolution of circulatory and lymphatic dysfunction.
4. Normalizing of skin color and texture that reflects circulatory changes.

COMMUNICATION WITH THE CLIENT

Communicate to obtain feedback on the client's comfort during the application of techniques. Here are some examples of statements that you can use.

1. "Let me know if this starts to feel uncomfortable." Ensure that the client finds the depth of the compression comfortable.
2. "Can you feel this pressure on your rib cage? Now breathe into my hand(s)." If you are applying the technique to the client's rib cage (Figures 9-2 and 9-4), ensure that the resistance that you are providing with the compression stroke does not impede the client's breathing.

A Practice Sequence for Broad-Contact Compression

Allow 30 minutes per person.

Allow 4 to 5 seconds per stroke, including the phases of gradual compression, hold, and gradual release. Synchronize the strokes with your breathing to achieve an even, relaxing tempo. Bend your knees and slowly rock your body weight over the contact surface to produce a deep, even compressive force. Use relaxed, broad contact.

Supine

Partially rotate the client's head away from the side that you will be working on and gently apply techniques in the following manner:

1. Down the sides of his neck from the mastoid process to the clavicle. Note that this is a sensitive area on many people.
2. Across the upper chest from the sternum to the axilla inferior to the clavicle.
3. From the anterior deltoid down each arm. Then compress the hand as a unit.
4. Down the sternum. Use a narrower contact surface, such as the ulnar border of your hand, to avoid the client's breast tissue.
5. Across the lower ribs from midline toward the axilla. Avoid direct pressure on the xiphoid process when doing so.
6. Gently, with soft hands, around the abdomen in clockwise circles.
7. From the inguinal crease to just above the client's knee. Repeat to cover the anteromedial and anterolateral surfaces of the thigh.

(Continued)

8. Rotate the leg medially to perform this along the tibialis anterior and extensor digitorum longus muscles working from just below the knee to the lateral ankle.

Prone

Gently apply techniques in the following manner:

1. Bilaterally along upper trapezius to the acromion process. Perform this while you are standing at the head of the table. *Note:* You can use considerable pressure here.
2. From the posterior deltoid, move down each arm.
3. Down either side of the spine from the occiput to the sacrum. Repeat, moving slightly more laterally on the back with each new series of compressive strokes.
4. Unilaterally and bilaterally on the lumbar musculature with broad palmar contact.
5. From the iliac crest on one side, down the gluteals, and distally to the knee. Repeat to cover the posteromedial and posterolateral surfaces of the thigh. If pressure on the posterior surface causes the client to report knee pain, place additional pillows under his ankles or lower legs from his knees to his feet.
6. From just below the knee to the ankle, and then on the plantar surface of the feet. Try using loose fists for the feet.

CAUTIONS AND CONTRAINDICATIONS

Therapists need clinical training and supervised practice to master the proper application of broad-contact compression. Advanced training may be advisable when dealing with pathological conditions. All of the general and local contraindications noted for massage techniques apply to the use of broad-contact compression (see Chapter 5). There are also specific contraindications to the use of this technique, including clients with hemophilia and local sites of acute inflammation and infection and clients with confirmed or suspected thrombus, thrombophlebitis, or malignancy. If the therapist is applying broad-contact compression to the client's rib cage to mobilize the chest wall or to mobilize bronchial

secretions and enhance airway clearance, some contraindications include a flail chest, an immobile rib cage, fractured or brittle ribs, and recent chest or spinal surgery.[12] The therapist should perform a careful examination and moderate her use of pressure with clients who have confirmed or suspected osteoporosis, clients with wounds that are in the early stages of healing, and clients who are taking anticoagulants. The therapist should also exercise caution when treating areas of **spasm**; areas of **hypotonia**; **active trigger points**; and the rib cage when there is potential for bronchospasm.

USING BROAD-CONTACT COMPRESSION IN TREATMENT

Stress

Broad-contact compression is useful in general massage to address the effects of **stress**, whether therapists use it alone or combine it with other techniques. It is probably most effective for **relaxation** when therapists apply each stroke slowly and with considerable pressure, which they sustain for 2 seconds or more. In situations in which the client presents with a generalized elevation of resting muscle tension because of stress, use moist heat and **diaphragmatic breathing** or **progressive relaxation** as adjuncts to the intervention.

Chest Wall Mobility

Broad-contact compression, especially when sustained, helps to improve chest wall mobility. Ensure that there are no contraindications, such as osteoporosis, especially in the elderly. Complementary methods that can be included during massage include the following:

1. Myofascial release applied to the upper body (see Chapter 10)
2. Direct fascial technique applied to the rib cage (see Chapter 10)
3. Breathing exercises that encourage full inspiration and expiration
4. Conventional upper body stretching

The client can also receive the latter two techniques as home care activities.

Petrissage: Evidence

DEFINITION

Petrissage: A group of related techniques that repetitively **compress**, **shear**, and release soft tissue—primarily muscle—with varying amounts of **drag**, **lift**, and glide.[1-7]

NAMES AND ORIGINS

Petrissage (from the French *pétrir*, to knead)[3,12] is one of two techniques that are predominantly used in **classical** or **Swedish massage** (the other is effleurage). It is indispensable when the therapist is treating muscle. In other texts, the technique that we call petrissage is sometimes known as "kneading."[1-7] The term petrissage was formerly used to refer to techniques that repetitively grasp, lift, shear, and release muscle tissue between the hands (see sections on wringing, muscle squeezing, and picking-up in this chapter). Other texts also defined related techniques that repetitively compress, shear, and release muscle against underlying muscle and bone separately as "kneading," although sometimes these definitions were reversed. It is common now for both lifting and compressive forms of these techniques to be grouped under the single term of petrissage,[1,2,6,7,12] although slightly differing usages persist (one recent text drops the French term entirely).

Authors generally agree that petrissage, in either **lifting** or **kneading** forms, repetitively compresses and releases muscle. Some authors,[3] however, follow **Kellogg's** usage[11] and classify other techniques that compress and release muscle as forms of "**friction**." We prefer to reserve the term friction for a precise, specific technique directed toward connective tissue (see Chapter 10).

Contemporary authors' opinions differ as to how much skin **glide** should occur when applying compressive or kneading forms of this technique.[2,6,7,12] Varying the amount of glide, rate, and pressure produces many varieties of petrissage that intergrade. Slowing the rate of application and using less lubricant will increase the amount of drag, or sustained horizontal force, that results and may produce greater effects on connective tissue.

A regrettable drawback of a lot of massage research is that researchers often give the most cursory descriptions of the **interventions** that they performed. Although this is changing, the word "petrissage" does not often show up in methodological descriptions, although it is often the predominant technique of classical (Swedish) massage and sometimes the only technique that is used. For this text, in situations in which the techniques performed in the intervention were not specifically mentioned or were characterized broadly as "massage," "standard massage," "Swedish massage," or "classical massage," we have assumed that therapists have used petrissage (which, in our view, includes "deep effleurage" and "kneading") directed toward skeletal muscle. As a result, the discussion of the research base for petrissage and the list of related outcomes are larger for this technique than those for the other massage techniques. Note that some of the following discussion may be applicable to other techniques, especially the other **neuromuscular techniques** described in this chapter.

USES

Petrissage is the workhorse of the **classical massage** techniques. Therapists use it to promote relaxation, reduce resting tension of skeletal muscle, and improve connective tissue **extensibility**. They can use it to treat many causes of musculoskeletal pain. Through its general relaxing effect, it also helps to reduce the perception of many other types of pain. Although the literature often states that petrissage increases local circulation, it is more accurate to say that it changes **perfusion** and, possibly, increases venous and lymphatic return. This may also refer to the hyperemia produced. Its reflex effects on visceral function are less certain.

OUTCOMES AND EVIDENCE

Much of the research on massage focuses on the **psychoneuroimmunological** effects of classical massage. Nevertheless, petrissage may also have physical effects on musculoskeletal, cardiopulmonary, and neurological systems and function.[32] In addition, it may also affect **pain**, athletic performance, and specific clinical conditions. Finally, the effects of petrissage on circulation and reflex effects on visceral function are less certain. Table 9-3 summarizes the main outcomes for petrissage.

Psychoneuroimmunological Effects

Mood

Classical massage may reduce **anxiety** (measured by state-trait questionnaires and salivary **cortisol** levels), reduce stress, and improve relaxation.[33-43] Researchers have observed this anxiolytic effect in a wide variety of clinical settings and clinical conditions. In addition, petrissage may be useful in alleviating the behavioral symptoms of depression,[35,39,43-46] hyperactivity,[47] and other conditions with affective components.[42,47,48] Furthermore, the positive effects of petrissage on rehabilitation and mood have been consistently demonstrated in other contexts.[33-43,45,46,49-58]

Immune Function

Several studies have shown improved immune function and positively altered allergic responses following the application of petrissage.[41,59,60]

Musculoskeletal Effects

Resting Muscle Tension

One cannot separate the effect of petrissage on the level of resting muscle tension from its psychological effects.[4] Anxiety has a well-documented generalized effect of increasing the level of resting tension of skeletal muscle.[61-63] As a result, interventions that reduce anxiety may have indirect effects on the level of resting tension. Furthermore, some authors state that petrissage can reduce the level of resting muscle tension in the area to which therapists apply it as a result of mechanical stress on proprioceptors.[1,3,5,12] Other researchers are equivocal about this effect or do not mention it at all.[2,6]

Range of Motion

Research notes that increases in joint range of motion may occur after the application of petrissage[49,64,65] (with one dissent[66]).

Position Sense

One study notes an increase in **joint position sense** after massage that included petrissage.[67]

Tissue Extensibility

Texts[1,3,6,12] and research studies[50,51,68] list increased extensibility and mobility of connective tissue as effects of petrissage. Increased extensibility may be responsible for the ability of perineal massage to reduce the incidence of tears during labor.[68-72] However, it is unlikely that petrissage will lengthen connective tissue to the same degree as connective tissue techniques, which apply more sustained tensional load or drag (see Chapter 10).

Neurological Effects

Tone

Research suggests that petrissage decreases **motoneuron excitability** but only during the application of the technique.[73-80] This may be of limited clinical usefulness,[81,82] except when treating patterns of abnormal movement and abnormal neuromuscular tone (**spasticity**) that are associated with lesions of the brain or spinal cord.[75]

Cardiovascular and Pulmonary Effects

Pulmonary Function

The observed positive effects of petrissage on pulmonary conditions, such as asthma, chronic obstructive pulmonary disease (COPD), and cystic fibrosis, may be a result of the combined effects of decreased anxiety and increased **chest wall mobility**.[83-85]

Circulation and Visceral Function

Although most texts state that petrissage increases venous return,[2,3,6,12] research suggests otherwise. This technique may have marginal effects on blood chemistry and local blood flow.[86-88] Furthermore, its effect on regional and systemic flow is likely to be both small and transient.[89-94] Consistent with the finding of a marginal effect of petrissage on blood flow is the observation that "**sports massage**" (including petrissage) does not always increase the rate of removal of **lactate** from muscle after exercise above the rate for passive rest.[95-100] Some research suggests that petrissage may have cardiac effects.[101,102] A more likely effect is an increase in lymphatic return. Most studies documenting this effect have, however, used repetitive compressive techniques produced by machines.[103-106] This may be the mechanism that explains the reduction of edema, which is a possible effect when the technique is applied proximal to the edema and around the periphery of swelling (if tolerable).

Finally, foreign studies intriguingly suggest that therapists can use classical massage (including petrissage) to achieve reflex effects on circulation and visceral function that are absent in the English literature.[102,107-115]

Multisystem Effects

Pain

Clients who received petrissage reported a significant reduction in their perception of pain during labor,[116-118] after surgery,[119] with cancer,[120,121] with migraine,[122] and with chronic orthopedic conditions.[123-125] Petrissage may also be of value in the reduction of low back pain.[126,127] To date, the mechanisms of the analgesia that might result from the application of petrissage are not fully understood. Current theories include the **gating** of pain impulses, increased **serotonin** levels, improved **restorative sleep**, and reduction of **substance P**.[16,125,128,129]

Athletic Performance

Although massage has experienced much recent popularity among athletes, reviews are generally skeptical about its ability to enhance many types of function in a sports context.[130-132] For example, research has not shown that petrissage before athletic activity can greatly enhance performance[133-135]; its effects on **delayed-onset muscle soreness** are equivocal[136-141]; and postperformance reports on repair of damage and recovery of function are mixed.[99,100,142-150] Conversely, reports on mood and perception of fatigue after exercise are more positive.[99,145,147,151]

Use in Multimodal Interventions

Petrissage has been used in conjunction with a variety of other techniques in multimodal interventions for clinical conditions such as headaches, **trigger point syndromes**, low back pain, **fibromyalgia**, and emphysema.[52-58,127] In these situations, the positive effects of petrissage appear to be enhanced in programs that include the use of **modalities** and client participation.[53,54,127]

HOW PETRISSAGE MIGHT WORK

The mechanisms for cutaneous reflexes, **entrainment** to rhythm, and forward movement of fluid in valved vessels discussed for more superficial techniques in the earlier chapters also apply to petrissage. In addition, petrissage spreads muscle fibers apart, **shears** muscle layers between the contact surfaces, and applies **tension** (drag and stretch) to connective tissue in the muscle.[1-7] Spreading and shearing of muscle causes proprioceptive input that may reduce **neuromuscular tone**.[1,4,7,12] Finally, slow rates of glide that maximize tension forces may produce connective tissue effects[4,7] by reducing **collagen** cross-linking and increasing hydration of the **connective tissue matrix**.

EXAMINING THE EVIDENCE

The following elegant study[73] is unusual on a couple of counts: it studies petrissage alone, and it tests the mechanism by which petrissage reduces the **H-reflex**, which is a measure of spinal reflex excitability. Researchers monitored neurologically normal subjects (who acted as their own controls) at rest, during the application of petrissage, and during the application of petrissage with their skin anesthetized. Reporting of the interrupted repeated-measures study protocol was very detailed and included a precise description of massage technique. The H-reflex was lower during petrissage, whether or not the skin was anesthetized, compared with the level during rest periods. This suggests that deep mechanoreceptors, not superficial ones, mediate the inhibitory effect of petrissage on the H-reflex. We suggest that this finding may have clinical significance for the treatment of spasm. However, researchers would have to repeat the protocol with subjects with spasm to test this hypothesis. Additionally, clinical significance may be limited because the H-reflex returned to normal as soon as massage stopped.

Morelli M, Chapman CE, Sullivan SJ. Do cutaneous receptors contribute to the changes in the amplitude of the H-reflex during massage? *Electromyogr Clin Neurophysiol.* 1999;39: 441-447.

Petrissage: Practice

COMPONENTS OF PETRISSAGE

Components of Petrissage 1, Muscle Squeezing

Muscle squeezing has the following components:

Contact: The entire palmar surface, the thumb and index finger, and the included web space

Pressure: Light to moderate

Engages: Muscle and associated **fascia**

Direction: Applied around the (partial) circumference of the muscle belly or limbs

Amplitude/length: N/A

Rate: 1 to 3 seconds or more per cycle of compression/release

Duration: 10 to 20 seconds or more

Intergrades with: Other forms of petrissage

Context: Usually used as an introductory muscular technique that is preceded by **superficial effleurage** and followed by more specific forms of petrissage. Can be used as a finishing stroke or by itself to address a region in a short time

Components of Petrissage 2, Wringing

Wringing has the following components:

Contact: Palmar surface of both hands

Pressure: Light to heavy

Engages: Muscle, associated fascia, and contained tissues

Direction: Across the long axis of the body segment

Amplitude/length: Half circumference of the body segment to which wringing is being applied

Rate: 1 to 3 seconds per cycle of compress/release

Duration: 20 to 60 seconds or more

Intergrades with: Other forms of general petrissage

Context: Usually used as an introductory muscular technique that is preceded by **superficial effleurage** and followed by more specific forms of petrissage

Components of Petrissage 3, Picking-Up ("C-Kneading")

Picking-up ("C-kneading") has the following components:

Contact: Palmar surface, especially the web space between the thumb and index finger

Pressure: Light to moderate

Engages: Muscle and associated fascia

Direction: Parallel to the long axis of the body segment

Amplitude/length: 5 to 20 cm or more

Rate: 1 to 3 seconds per cycle of compression/release

Duration: 20 to 60 seconds or more

Intergrades with: Other forms of general petrissage

Context: Usually preceded by superficial effleurage and more general forms of petrissage and followed by more specific forms of petrissage

Components of Petrissage 4, Broad-Contact Kneading and Deep Effleurage

Broad-contact kneading and deep effleurage have the following components:

Contact: Full palmar surface of the hand, often reinforced on the wrist and/or metacarpals, fist/knuckles, or proximal forearm

Pressure: Light to heavy

Engages: Muscle and associated tissues. Slower strokes and greater **drag** (horizontal tension) will lengthen connective tissue elements of the muscle more

Direction: Circular or elliptical. The long axis of the ellipses is often oriented parallel to the long axis of the muscles or muscle groups

Amplitude/length: 10 cm or more

Rate: 10 to 25 cm/s

Duration: 20 to 60 seconds or more

Intergrades with: Superficial effleurage and other forms of petrissage. A notable, commonly used variation, sometimes called "deep effleurage" or "deep stroking," has the same long, gliding template of superficial effleurage but engages muscle with a considerable amount of pressure. This is not a superficial maneuver and has much in common with the broad-contact kneading described here. Nongliding forms using fingertip contact intergrade with **friction** (see Chapter 10)

Context: Usually preceded and followed by superficial effleurage, alternated with other general forms of petrissage and followed by more specific forms of petrissage.

Components of Petrissage 5, Specific Kneading (Thumbs, Fingerpads, Fingertips)

Specific kneading has the following components:

Contact: Fingertips, fingerpads, or thumbs form the working surface. In any case, the heel of the hand remains in contact to stabilize the hand

Pressure: Light to moderate

Engages: Muscle and associated tissues. Slower strokes and greater drag (horizontal tension) will likely lengthen connective tissue elements of the muscle more than faster strokes

Direction: Circular or elliptical. The long axis of ellipses is often oriented parallel to the long axis of muscles or muscle groups

Amplitude/length: Up to 10 cm (determined by size of therapist's hand)

Rate: 0.5 to 2 seconds per cycle of compression/release

Duration: Up to 20 seconds at one time, provided the therapist does not experience hand fatigue

Intergrades with: Stripping

Context: Usually preceded by, alternated with, and followed by superficial effleurage and more general forms of petrissage such as wringing or palmar kneading.

PALPATION PRACTICE

Over a period of weeks, perform the following for each major skeletal muscle in the body:

1. Locate the attachments and borders of the chosen muscle on a practice partner, using an atlas as reference. Using your fingertips, palpate across the muscle fibers to confirm their direction.
2. With a washable marker, draw the muscle in place on one side of the body. Mark the fiber directions.
3. Observe your partner. How do the anatomical structures you have drawn influence the surface contours of the body?
4. Grasp the muscle and attempt to lift it off the underlying tissues. How easily does it lift? Does it lift away by itself, or do other muscles lift with it?
5. With the muscle lifted, attempt to bow it between your two hands. How easily does it bend?
6. Lastly, compress the muscle onto the underlying tissues. How much resistance do the tissues offer to the compression? What underlying structures provide the resistance to compression?

MANUAL TECHNIQUE: PETRISSAGE 1, MUSCLE SQUEEZING

Figures 9-9 to 9-15 show therapists applying muscle squeezing to the various regions of the body. The order of the figures is from head to foot in supine and then in prone. Each figure illustrates most of the guidelines for manual technique outlined in this section.

1. Therapists can perform this **nongliding** technique best without lubricant, and they can apply it effectively through fabric (Figure 9-12).
2. Use one or both hands to grasp, lift, and squeeze a muscle, muscle group, or body segment, with minimal glide. It is easiest to perform on mid-sized body segments such as the calf (Figure 9-15), upper arm, upper trapezius (Figure 9-13), hand, and foot (Figure 9-12).
3. Therapists can squeeze smaller muscles, such as the sternocleidomastoid, between their thumb and index finger (Figures 9-9 and 9-10).
4. If you use two hands, you can add a bowing action to **shear** the muscle further.
5. Because this technique uses mostly hand and forearm strength, we do not recommend extended application. This is especially true if you are treating large muscle groups such as the quadriceps (Figure 9-11).

FIGURE 9-10 Squeezing either head of the sternocleidomastoid between thumb and index may elicit pain from latent myofascial trigger points (see other sections in this chapter). The therapist must be able to distinguish between the two divisions of the muscle.

FIGURE 9-11 Two-handed squeezing of bulky muscle groups, such as the quadriceps, taxes the hands and should not be done for long periods.

FIGURE 9-9 Gentle squeezing of facial muscles and superficial tissues between index and thumb.

FIGURE 9-12 Squeezing the whole foot through the sheet or a towel often gives the therapist a better grip and thus yields a deeper application of technique than working directly on the skin.

FIGURE 9-13 Squeezing of the upper trapezius muscle can be done with the client prone, supine, side-lying, or seated. An additional bowing force can be added.

FIGURE 9-14 The muscles of the posterior axillary wall (teres major and latissimus dorsi) are easily accessible for squeezing when the client is in side-lying. One hand squeezes while the other hand positions the scapula, as desired, to increase accessibility of the muscles.

FIGURE 9-15 Two-handed squeezing of the posterior compartments of the leg can be combined with passive flexion/extension of the knee or with shaking of the ankle and foot.

THERAPIST'S POSITION AND MOVEMENT: PETRISSAGE 1, MUSCLE SQUEEZING

1. Use the basic positions described in Chapter 6 in the sections on standing **aligned** posture and seated aligned posture.
2. Your position can be quite variable. When you are treating larger body segments, face the long axis of the muscle(s) you are going to squeeze (Figures 9-12 to 9-15).

MANUAL TECHNIQUE: PETRISSAGE 2, WRINGING

Figures 9-16 to 9-22 show therapists applying wringing to the various regions of the body. The order of the figures is from head to foot on the anterior surface and then the posterior surface. Each figure illustrates most of the guidelines for manual technique outlined in this section.

1. For large body segments, rest your hands on opposite sides of the circumference of the body segment you are going to wring and compress them toward each other (Figure 9-18A).
2. Maintaining compression, slide your hands toward each other, lifting and shearing the muscle between them as they pass each other (Figures 9-17, 9-18B, 9-20, and 9-22).
3. Continue to slide your hands, without exerting pressure, until they rest on opposite sides of the body segment on which they began (Figure 9-18C). Then

FIGURE 9-17 Wringing the lower rib cage in prone, supine, or side-lying is an indirect way of loosening the respiratory diaphragm.

initiate a new stroke. After two complete cycles, your hands will be in the positions in which they started.

4. Be careful to apply pressure gradually at the beginning of the strokes in order to avoid jerking.
5. To wring large body segments, such as the torso or quadriceps muscles, adduct your thumbs to avoid strain on your carpometacarpal joints (Figures 9-17, 9-18A–C, and 9-20). For smaller body segments, such as the arms, hands, or feet, you can abduct your thumb so that the entire web space between your thumb and index finger remains in contact during the technique (Figures 9-16 and 9-19). Wringing with abducted thumbs places undue strain on the joints of your thumb and should be avoided except for short treatment periods.
6. As with other forms of petrissage that use the whole hand, begin wringing proximally on the limb and proceed in a distal direction. Return proximally with wringing or with superficial effleurage and repeat. Therapists believe that this will maximize **lymphatic return** by clearing proximal areas first.[82]
7. Areas of elevated resting tension can benefit from extended (5 or more minutes) periods of wringing, although this involves a lot of work on the part of the therapist.
8. *Note*: You need considerable pressure to lift and shear the bulk of large muscle groups between your hands. Do not produce a superficial effleurage that is oriented across the body segment and has no **mechanical effect** on the muscle itself.

FIGURE 9-16 On small body segments, such as the upper arm, wringing can be done with thumbs abducted. In this position, the client's arm must be completely relaxed.

FIGURE 9-18 A. For bulky regions, such as the quadriceps, the hamstrings, and the back, effective wringing requires that the therapist use correct body mechanics. At the start of the stroke, the hands are diametrically opposed. They then begin to compress together. The therapist's posture is wide-stance ("horse stance") with bent knees. **B.** The therapist's legs straighten, adding force to the lift and shear produced by the passing hands. **C.** The relaxation phase: the hands pass each other, release tissue, and move to a position opposite the starting position. Simultaneously, the knees bend again in preparation for the next stroke.

THERAPIST'S POSITION AND MOVEMENT: PETRISSAGE 2, WRINGING

For large body segments, such as the torso or thighs, you must perform wringing with correct leg movements in order to generate sufficient force to compress, lift, and shear large masses between your hands. You can achieve this leg movement with the following steps:

1. Stand facing the long axis of the body segment you are going to wring (Figure 9-18A).
2. Begin in the wide-stance knee bend posture with your knees flexed between 30° and 45°. The lowered position allows some palmar contact of your near hand while reducing extension of your wrist (Figure 9-18A).

FIGURE 9-19 Wringing an entire foot or hand engages many structures with each stroke and is a good choice of technique when time is limited.

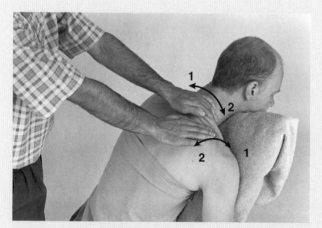

FIGURE 9-20 Wringing the upper trapezius with the client seated.

FIGURE 9-21 A variation of wringing involves one- or two-handed lifting of the torso in prone or supine. Gravity provides the opposing force.

FIGURE 9-22 Wringing the calf.

3. During the **power stroke**, as your hands compress and slide toward each other, straighten your legs without hyperextending your knees (Figure 9-18B). During the **return stroke**, as your hands slide apart, flex your knees again (Figure 9-18C). Thus, for each stroke, you flex and extend your knees so that you generate most of the power for the application of the technique from the extension of your knees.
4. Coordination of your leg and arm movements takes practice. The reward is a secure, smooth, very deep, and effective technique.
5. Initially, your legs may fatigue or become sore. This will pass as the strength and endurance of your leg muscles increases.

When wringing smaller body segments, you can use a variety of aligned postures that are described in Chapter 6.

MANUAL TECHNIQUE: PETRISSAGE 3, PICKING-UP ("C-KNEADING")

Figures 9-23 to 9-28 show therapists applying picking-up to the various regions of the body. The order of the figures is from head to foot in supine and then in prone. Each figure illustrates most of the guidelines for manual technique outlined in this section.

A. One-handed technique for smaller body segments such as the arms, forearms, and calves (Figures 9-23 to 9-24C):
1. Abduct your thumb so that your hand forms a "C" shape, with the four fingers grouped together in adduction.
2. Grasp and squeeze while gliding your hand in a **centripetal** direction. Most of your hand remains in contact with the client's body, with the focus on your thumb, index finger, and web space. Squeeze the client's tissues through the closing web space for the power stroke, and abduct your thumb progressively toward the end of the stroke ("squeezing off the stroke").
3. During the power stroke, make an effort to lift the tissues off the underlying bone (Figures 9-24A–C).
4. Reopen your hand to a "C" shape as it glides back to its original position with minimal pressure (return stroke).
5. One author suggests using a four count as follows: compress on one, grasp and lift on two, release on three, and move/glide on four.[7]

A

B

C

FIGURE 9-23 Unilateral picking-up of upper trapezius muscle in supine.

FIGURE 9-24 Upper arms are an ideal size for one-handed picking-up. **A.** The biceps brachii. **B.** The triceps brachii (with the glenohumeral joint in the loose-packed position). **C.** The triceps with the shoulder and elbow flexed. Apply pressure in a centripetal direction and lift the tissues away from the underlying bone.

ONLINE VIDEO

FIGURE 9-25 Two-handed picking-up of rectus abdominis. Return stroke is shown in a dotted line. Practice is required to attain good contact during two-handed picking-up on flat surfaces like the abdomen or the back.

FIGURE 9-26 One-handed picking-up of the adductors of the hip.

FIGURE 9-27 Two-handed picking-up is a good technique for the lateral edge of the latissimus dorsi. The therapist can work her way down to the iliac crest. Placing the client's arm overhead also improves access to the abdominal obliques and quadratus lumborum muscles.

ONLINE VIDEO

FIGURE 9-28 Hand position to begin two-handed picking-up of the glutei.

B. Alternate two-handed technique for larger or flatter body segments such as the thighs and back (Figures 9-26, 9-27, and 9-28):

1. Place your two hands facing each other in an open "C" position as described in Step A4 (Figure 9-28).

2. The individual motion of each of your hands is similar to the one-handed technique described in section A. The difference is that your hands work in contrary motion: one hand performs a short power stroke, while the other is performing a short return stroke. Deliver power strokes toward the opposing hand; with return strokes, move away from the opposing hand.

3. For optimal effectiveness, you should sustain some compression between your hands throughout the application of this technique. This results in a continuous lifting of the tissue between your hands.

4. On limbs, begin the sequence of strokes proximally, and gradually move the focus of the strokes distally.[82]

5. Coordination between your hands takes practice. Once you master it, it yields a technique that clients perceive to be very pleasant.

6. Picking-up (one- or two-handed) for more than a couple of minutes at a time is not advisable because of wear on the therapist's hands and forearms.

THERAPIST'S POSITION AND MOVEMENT: PETRISSAGE 3, PICKING-UP ("C-KNEADING")

1. Use the basic positions described in Chapter 6 in the sections on standing aligned posture, **wide-stance knee bend**, and wide-stance knee bend with trunk rotation.
2. To generate more force during the application of one-handed forms, shift or lean forward into the client's body during the compression and lift portion of the stroke. Then shift or lean back during the release-and-move portion.
3. For the application of two-handed forms, face the long axis of the client's body segment in the wide-stance knee bend, as for wringing. Flexing your knees in this position may reduce hyperextension of your wrists by bringing you closer to the level of the client (Figure 9-27).
4. To generate more power for two-handed forms, rotate your ipsilateral shoulder to lean slightly into each power stroke (wide-stance knee bend with trunk rotation). This increases the force and effectiveness of the technique, minimizes hand and forearm fatigue, and results in a smooth upper body rhythm.
5. Do not let your shoulders elevate when applying the technique.

MANUAL TECHNIQUE: PETRISSAGE 4, BROAD-CONTACT KNEADING AND DEEP EFFLEURAGE

Figures 9-29 to 9-36 show therapists applying broad-contact kneading to the various regions of the body. The order of the figures is from head to foot in supine and then in prone. Each figure illustrates most of the guidelines for manual technique outlined in this section.

1. As with wringing and picking-up, there is a pressure stroke and a return stroke. Combine the pressure stroke and return stroke to form circles or ellipses that are oriented along or across the fibers in the different muscle layers (Figures 9-30A and 9-30B and 9-33). Most often, the long axis of the stroke runs parallel to the long axis of the body segment or muscle to which you are applying the technique, especially when significant pressure is required (Figures 9-30A and 9-33). Elongating the ellipse results in "**deep effleurage**," provided the pressure is centripetal (Figures 9-33 and 9-34).
2. Maintain your wrist in neutral (no radial or ulnar deviation). This is critical to reduce joint stress during high-pressure applications of broad-contact kneading (Figures 9-29, 9-30A and 9-30B, 9-33, 9-35, and 9-36).

FIGURE 9-30 A. Reinforced palmar kneading of the anterior thigh. Return stroke is shown in a dotted line. **B.** One version of "box kneading." The hands can work in opposition, lifting tissue and/or pushing it proximally.

FIGURE 9-29 Kneading the posterior triangle of the neck with the heel of the hand.

3. You may reinforce the dorsal surface of your hand or wrist with your other hand (Figures 9-30A and 9-33) or bring your hands together so that they reinforce each other (Figure 9-35).

FIGURE 9-33 Reinforced palmar kneading to the erector spinae muscles performed with a slightly arched hand. The strokes may take the form of smaller circles or of one long ellipse that covers the erector spinae muscles in a single stroke ("deep stroking" or "deep effleurage").

ONLINE VIDEO

FIGURE 9-31 Effective kneading requires correct application of the therapist's body weight. This is especially true when kneading the iliotibial band, which is composed of dense connective tissue. The therapist stabilizes his elbow against his iliac crest and carefully shifts his body weight toward the client.

4. More specific contact can be obtained by bridging or arching your hand slightly (flexing the metacarpophalangeal and interphalangeal joints). This produces two contact surfaces—broader at the heel and more specific at your fingertips (Figure 9-33).

5. As with the application of all types of petrissage, begin proximally and proceed in a distal direction while maintaining **centripetal** pressure to maximize lymphatic return.

6. Variations: Some authors describe a form of circular **kneading** in which no glide occurs over the skin.[6] This technique engages muscle and is, in its effects, probably the same as kneading that glides over the skin.

FIGURE 9-32 This therapist is committing at least five common errors of body mechanics while attempting a forceful kneading of trapezius. Common errors of body mechanics are detailed in Chapter 6.

FIGURE 9-34 Using the forearm along the erector spinae muscles. The therapist must be careful to avoid compressing the spinous processes. The return stroke is often omitted.

ONLINE VIDEO

FIGURE 9-35 Reinforced fist kneading of the superior gluteal attachments is most effective when tissue is moved away from the sacrum or iliac crest.

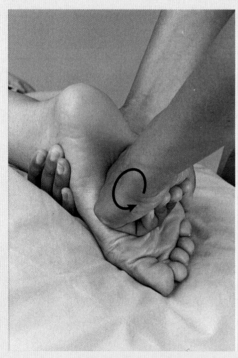

FIGURE 9-36 Fist kneading to the sole of the foot is easier to control if the fist is rotated during the stroke. A deeper but less comfortable technique is obtained if the foot is passively dorsiflexed.

7. Other variations: Some authors describe a two-handed form of kneading, termed **fulling** or broadening, in which your hands compress down and away from each other to spread or broaden the muscle belly and then lift the muscle up on the return stroke.[3,5]

8. Other variations: Some authors describe a two-handed form of kneading, termed **box kneading**, in which you position your hands so that they are diametrically opposed on the client's limb. You then compress them toward each other and finally move them proximally. This stroke is recommended to increase fluid return (Figure 9-30B).[6]

THERAPIST'S POSITION AND MOVEMENT: PETRISSAGE 4, BROAD-CONTACT KNEADING AND DEEP EFFLEURAGE

1. Use the basic positions described in Chapter 6 in the sections on **lunge**, lunge and reach, lunge and lean, and standing **controlled lean**. In these positions, point your torso toward the point of contact (Figures 9-31 and 9-35). Your feet should also be pointed toward the point of contact. If your back foot is rotated laterally, you may be tightening/shortening your deep lateral hip rotators and piriformis.

2. To create the power portion of the stroke, hold your elbows partly extended, and drive forward with your legs during the lunge, or incline your body toward the contact point during the lunge and lean (Figures 9-31 and 9-35).

3. Use your shoulders and arms to transmit the force from the correct lower body movement, not to generate the force. You can generate much greater force for kneading through correct use of the lunge-and-lean posture.

4. Common errors that occur, especially when you are trying to generate more pressure, are as follows:

    a. Hyperextension of your elbows ("straight-arming")
    b. Excessive elevation and/or protraction of your shoulders
    c. Tilting of your head
    d. Excessive leaning forward at your waist (Figure 9-32)

All of these errors are more likely to occur if the table is too high.

MANUAL TECHNIQUE: PETRISSAGE 5, SPECIFIC KNEADING (THUMBS, FINGERPADS, FINGERTIPS)

Figures 9-37 to 9-44 show therapists applying specific kneading to the various regions of the body. The order of the figures is from head to foot in supine and then in prone. Each figure illustrates most of the guidelines for manual technique outlined in this section.

A. Fingertip and fingerpad technique (Figures 9-37, 9-39, 9-42, and 9-43):

1. Unless the surface you are kneading is relatively small (Figure 9-37), hold the fingers of your hand together (Figures 9-42 and 9-43). The heel or the entire rest of your hand may remain in contact with the client's body to provide stability (Figure 9-42). When you require light pressure, as when you are kneading the face, you can omit this stabilization.
2. Perform repetitive circles, applying the pressure during the portion of the stroke that pushes away from your body. This potentially allows you to use your body weight to increase force.
3. You may use the other hand to reinforce across the carpals and metacarpals of your working hand in order to stabilize your wrist and enhance the force of the technique (Figure 9-43).

FIGURE 9-38 Alternate thumb-kneading to the belly of the frontalis muscle.

FIGURE 9-39 Fingertip kneading of the scalp can be performed lightly with glide over the skin and through the hair or with more pressure and no glide.

FIGURE 9-37 Fingertips and fingerpads are ideal for petrissage of the face, which is usually done without applying lubricant. Fingerpad kneading of the masseter muscle.

FIGURE 9-40 Alternate thumb-kneading is a technique that fits onto forelimbs beautifully. Begin proximally, proceed distally, and return with a long centripetal stroke to the starting position. On the calf, the return stroke will "split" the heads of the gastrocnemius muscle.

FIGURE 9-41 Slow, rhythmic thumb-kneading of the thenar and hypothenar eminences is deeply relaxing. Because of the large number of structures in the hand (or the foot), thorough petrissage can take 30 minutes or longer.

A

FIGURE 9-42 Fingerpad kneading to the lateral border of rectus abdominis.

B

FIGURE 9-44 **A.** The therapist kneels at the foot of the table to perform alternate thumb-kneading to the sole of the foot in supine. **B.** The same technique in prone.

FIGURE 9-43 Reinforced fingertip kneading of the quadriceps muscle.

B. Thumb technique (Figures 9-38, 9-40, 9-41, 9-44A, and 9-44B):

1. Place your hand close to or flat on the surface of the client's body, with your fingers parallel (Figure 9-38). Your fingertips remain loosely in contact with the client's body. Depending on the shape of the region you are kneading, the heel of your hand may also remain in partial contact (Figure 9-40).

2. Use the ventral surface of the distal thumb phalanx to deliver pressure in small ellipses. The long axes of these ellipses will be parallel to the long axis of your thumb. Do not abduct your thumbs widely during this motion (Figures 9-41 and 9-44A).

3. Ensure that you exert the pressure along, rather than across, the long axis of your thumb.

4. Usually, you use both thumbs in a technique known as alternate thumb-kneading. One thumb performs a pressure stroke while the other performs a return stroke (Figures 9-38, 9-41, and 9-44A and 9-44B).

5. The technique described in Steps 1 to 3 may seem awkward at first, but it places a minimum amount of stress on the mobile, vulnerable joints of your thumb.

6. Perform specific kneading sparingly for short periods and alternate it frequently with other techniques that place different stresses on the joints of your hand.

THERAPIST'S POSITION AND MOVEMENT: PETRISSAGE 5, SPECIFIC KNEADING (THUMBS, FINGERPADS, FINGERTIPS)

1. Use the basic positions described in Chapter 6 in the sections on standing, seated, or kneeling **aligned** posture. Face the body segment you are going to treat.

2. During thumb-kneading, the movement of your thumbs is quite constrained, as described under Thumb Technique. Small movements at the carpometacarpal, carpal, and elbow joints create the force of the technique, which brings the weight of your forearm and upper arm into play.

3. During fingertip kneading, you can increase force by leaning slightly into the power stroke.

PALPATE: ALL FORMS OF PETRISSAGE

Palpate the client's skin and tissues for the following:

1. General resistance and resilience of soft tissues
2. Mobility of the interfaces between the muscles and muscle layers
3. Resistance to further stretch toward the end of the excursion of each stroke
4. Localized areas of hardness that may require use of more specific techniques

5. **Taut bands** in muscle, which may reflect **trigger point** activity (see other sections in this chapter)
6. **Fibrosis**, **adhesions**, and **indurations** within and between muscle layers, which can indicate **chronic inflammation**
7. Decrease in local fluid **viscosity** with continued application of the technique
8. The palpable softening of muscle tissue, which often results when the therapist applies petrissage for several minutes. This may reflect a decrease in the viscosity of superficial tissues caused by increased temperature; an increase in the hydration of the connective tissue matrix; a softening of taut bands, which is consistent with reduced activity of trigger points; and a marginal systemic decrease in the level of resting tension of skeletal muscle, if the massage is relaxing.

In addition, slow the rate of petrissage when working in deep layers to facilitate palpation and to allow superficial tissues to move aside with each stroke.

OBSERVE: ALL FORMS OF PETRISSAGE

As you perform petrissage, observe the client for changes in the level of **resting muscle tension** and **edema**. Following are some of these signs:

1. Systemic reduction of muscle tension, as evidenced by softening of the tissue contours or broadening and flattening of body segments.
2. General consistency and resting level of tone. How fluid does the tissue appear as you move it?
3. Taut, visible bands in resting muscle. A muscle that has a visibly well-defined anatomical form when it is not in use is probably hypertonic.
4. Hyperemia. A **reactive hyperemia** may accompany the application of this technique.
5. If you are using petrissage to treat edema (proximal to the edema) or fibrosed edema (on-site), note the following signs of resorption of fluid from edematous tissue: changes in surface contours, reduction in size or hardness of edema, and changes in the viscosity and inertial resistance of the subcutaneous tissues.
6. The depth of the penetration of the stroke. As the client's muscles relax and the fluid viscosity of the tissues decreases, the same force will produce effects deeper into the client's tissues. Consequently, you do not always require greater force to achieve a greater penetration of effects; instead, the appropriate application of the technique for longer periods is required.

COMMUNICATION WITH THE CLIENT: ALL FORMS OF PETRISSAGE

Communicate to ensure the client's comfort during the application of the technique. Here are some examples of statements that you can use.

1. "Is this pressure okay?" "Would you like it deeper?" "Would you like less pressure?" "Which feels better, this (adjust depth) or this?" Ensure that the depth of technique is comfortable for the client.
2. "Is it tender here?" "When I work here, do you feel this or other sensations anywhere else?" In cases in which the client examination suggests that there is elevated resting muscle tension, slowly increase the depth of application of the technique while inquiring about tenderness and possible **referral** of pain/sensation.

Regional Modifications

- Back: You can designate proximal and distal as being at either end of the client's back.
- Abdomen: Where possible, for example, with effleurage and kneading, apply the techniques in a generally clockwise direction and sequence.
- Face: Use light pressure and no lubricant. You can apply most of the techniques as described with slight adaptations. Use only two fingers or finger and thumb for "smaller" versions of wringing, picking-up, and squeezing where you can lift the tissues. Fingertip kneading is the most useful technique.
- Hands and feet: You can address many small muscles, ends of tendons, and fascial sheaths individually with excellent results. As with the face, the amplitude of the techniques is smaller. You can, however, use considerable amounts of pressure because of the density of connective tissue in these regions.

A Practice Sequence for Petrissage

First, attempt each technique individually until you are confident about the basics of the manual technique and body movement. You can then apply the following basic sequence, initially allowing 15 to 20 minutes for any region. You can adapt the same sequence, with minor variations, for all regions.

1. Apply a small amount of lubricant to the client's body using superficial effleurage.
2. Begin by applying **wringing** proximally on the region and then move distally.
3. Once you reach the most distal part of the region, either apply wringing on the way back up or return with superficial effleurage.
4. Using a similar pattern, which begins proximally and proceeds distally, introduce in turn

   a. Muscle squeezing
   b. Picking-up
   c. Broad-contact kneading
   d. Specific kneading

Whenever possible, maximize **centripetal** pressure. At the end, finish with wringing and then superficial effleurage.

CAUTIONS AND CONTRAINDICATIONS: ALL FORMS OF PETRISSAGE

Therapists need clinical training and supervised practice to master the proper application of petrissage. Advanced training may be advisable when dealing with pathological conditions. All of the general and local contraindications noted for massage techniques apply to the use of petrissage (see Chapter 5). In addition, there are several specific contraindications to the application of petrissage: clients with hemophilia, local sites of acute inflammation and infection, confirmed or suspected thrombus,[115] thrombophlebitis, and potentially metastatic malignancy. Therapists must conduct a careful examination and moderate the pressure with which they apply petrissage for clients who have confirmed or suspected osteoporosis, who have wounds in the early stages of healing, or who are taking anticoagulants. Furthermore, therapists must exercise care when treating areas of **spasm**, **hypotonia**, and **active trigger points**. The use of excessive pressure may damage delicate terminal lymphatics, although this damage may facilitate the drainage of edema.[152] Finally, difficulties may arise with the application of any massage techniques to clients who have profound learning disabilities or dementia.[153,154]

USING PETRISSAGE IN TREATMENT

Psychosocial Stress

Therapists can use petrissage by itself or in combination with other techniques in general massage to address the effects of psychosocial **stress**. It is often effective for relaxation when therapists apply it slowly and rhythmically, gradually building up to short periods of higher pressure, which they alternate with periods of less pressure. In situations in which the client presents with a generalized elevation of resting muscle tension because of stress, therapists can use moist heat and **diaphragmatic breathing** or **progressive relaxation** as adjuncts to petrissage.

Orthopedic Injuries

Local application of petrissage is useful for treating orthopedic injuries in the subacute and chronic states. Depending on the severity and stage of the injury, therapists can complement this technique with **superficial fluid techniques**, other neuromuscular techniques, **connective tissue techniques**, and **passive movement techniques**. Furthermore, petrissage is an excellent prelude to passive stretching, **proprioceptive neuromuscular facilitation** techniques, and **joint mobilization**.

Postintervention Self-Care Instructions

1. Extensive deep petrissage may occasionally produce mild local soreness during a 24- to 48-hour period after treatment. A warm bath, a warm Epsom salts bath, or the application of moist heat may reduce this soreness.
2. Pain of increasing severity, persistent postintervention pain, or pain that arises in adjacent areas during or following treatment may indicate activation of a **latent** or **satellite trigger point** (see other sections in this chapter) or the generalized **reactive tightening** of antagonist muscle groups. Always instruct clients to contact you when more than mild, transient pain results from any massage intervention.
3. Depending on the clinical situation, use therapeutic exercise, **self-mobilization** techniques, diaphragmatic breathing, or progressive relaxation exercises.
4. You can teach clients self-massage of accessible areas.

Family members can be taught to perform basic petrissage and the cautions involved in applying this within a home program.[85]

Stripping: Evidence

DEFINITION

Stripping: A very slow and specific gliding technique that therapists apply from one attachment of a muscle to the other for the purpose of reducing the activity of myofascial trigger points. A trigger point is a hyperirritable area in skeletal muscle that is associated with a hypersensitive and palpable nodule located in a taut band. The area is painful on compression and can give rise to a variety of symptoms including referred sensations such as pain and tenderness, motor dysfunction, and autonomic phenomena.[1-7,155]

NAMES AND ORIGINS

In other texts and massage-related systems, the technique that we call stripping is called "stripping massage," "deep stroking," "deep stroking massage," and "muscle stripping."[155] Travell and Simons[156] first coined the term stripping massage. Technically, it is related to specific petrissage (see relevant sections in this chapter), because it involves the compression and release of muscle fibers, and to direct fascial technique (see Chapter 10), because of the slow rate of glide. In this text, we consider it separately because of its well-defined method and excellent effect on trigger point activity.

As defined by Chaitow[157] and others, "neuromuscular therapy" or "neuromuscular technique" is a complex system of techniques that includes, among other techniques, finger and thumb strokes that resemble stripping, which we defined in other sections.

"Strumming" or "cross-fiber stripping" is a form of direct fascial technique that is directed along[158] or, more often, across[155,158] muscle fibers. This may sometimes resemble stripping and may have effects on trigger point activity.

USES

Therapists use stripping to reduce the activity, pain, and other symptoms of trigger points and to help restore the length and strength of the affected muscle.[155]

OUTCOMES AND EVIDENCE

Stripping

Stripping has a variety of physiological and psychological effects.[159] Therapists can use stripping to reduce the activity, pain, and other symptoms of trigger points and to help restore the length and strength of the affected muscle.[155] It can be the preferred manual technique when trigger points are located near the center of a muscle. Since stripping applies similar forces to the same tissue layer as petrissage, stripping may have many of the effects of petrissage when therapists systematically apply it to a region (see sections on petrissage in this chapter). Stripping may also share some effects with direct fascial technique (see Chapter 10). Table 9-3 summarizes the main outcomes for stripping.

Myofascial Trigger Points

A myofascial trigger point is a hyperirritable area in skeletal muscle that is associated with a hypersensitive and palpable nodule located in a taut band. The area is painful on compression and can give rise to a variety of symptoms such as referred pain, referred tenderness, motor dysfunction, and autonomic phenomena.[155] A trigger point has a characteristic response to palpation: a local twitch response of the taut muscle fibers and referred sensation (pain, tenderness, etc.) in a specific pattern for that muscle, which occurs or increases on direct compression of the trigger point.[155,158] There are two questions to answer when categorizing trigger points: (1) Is the trigger point active or latent? and (2) Is the trigger point primary (key) or a satellite? An active trigger point in a muscle will refer sensations (pain, tenderness, etc.) whether the muscle is working or at rest, can weaken a muscle, and can prevent it from lengthening fully. By contrast, a latent trigger point gives rise to sensation only when you palpate it. The application of trigger point pressure release to a latent trigger point will evoke the characteristic referral pattern for that trigger point. A muscle containing a latent trigger point can also be shortened and weakened. Primary trigger points arise in response to trauma, acute and chronic

overload (**tendinopathies** and **repetitive strain injuries**), **postural imbalance**, fatigue, and emotional stress. These trigger points are exacerbated by a variety of factors.[155,158] Satellite trigger points may develop in response to altered biomechanics, in the referral area of a primary trigger point, or in the synergist and antagonist muscle groups of the muscle that contains the primary trigger point.[155] Finally, key trigger points are responsible for activating satellites. Consequently, inactivation of a key trigger point will inactivate its associated satellites.[155]

Trigger points may also occur in connective tissue, such as fascia, ligaments, and periosteum, and produce a variety of symptoms.[155,158] Trigger points located in muscle are frequently the cause or the consequence of common musculoskeletal complaints such as tension headache, temporomandibular joint problems, spinal pain, chronic low back pain, disk herniation, chronic pelvic pain, painful rib syndrome, nonarticular pain, and other myofascial pain syndromes.[155,157,158,160-175] In addition, trigger points in muscle can cause **nerve entrapments**[155,160,172,174] and may also mimic nerve entrapments, radiculopathies, and visceral pathology.[155,160,171]

HOW STRIPPING MIGHT WORK

An integrated hypothesis for the etiology of trigger points suggests that dysfunction at motor endplates causes sustained depolarization of the postsynaptic membrane, continuous release of calcium from the sarcoplasmic reticulum, and sustained shortening of sarcomeres in the region of the trigger point.[124,155,172-176] In addition, locally reduced blood flow and hypoxia sensitize nociceptors to produce the characteristic pain referrals.[155] Furthermore, two studies have shown that repeated deep massage of **fibrositic nodules** (trigger points) causes them to release myoglobin.[124,176] Simons and Travell support this theory by suggesting that the shortened sarcomeres of a trigger point "contraction knot" may be more susceptible to rupture by the pressure of a technique like stripping. They propose that the therapist's application of massage results in cell rupture. Following this rupture, the cell spills myoglobin, which probably destroys the involved neuromuscular junction as a functional structure, thus effectively terminating the contracture and associated energy crisis. As the technique eliminates more and more contraction knots within a nodule, the client will experience an increasing relief of symptoms.[155] Finally, stripping along the length of the muscle may apply a lengthening tension that restores the normal length of the sarcomere, the taut band, and the muscle as a whole.[155]

EXAMINING THE EVIDENCE

There are no clinical trials in the literature for stripping or for equivalent techniques such as "deep stroking" or "deep tissue massage." One case report[177] documents the use of **Active Release** techniques for the treatment of shoulder pain, reduced range, and weakness in a client 2 years after surgical repair of a Bankart lesion. The Active Release system combines soft tissue techniques similar to stripping, as described in this chapter, with active and passive movement into specific protocols for particular muscles. In this case, researchers provided "treatment directed to the muscles of the rotator cuff, with an emphasis on the subscapularis" twice a week for 2 weeks. The client's function, as measured by the BIODEX isokinetic testing of shoulder rotation, improved significantly. This otherwise quite thorough case report contains no description of the protocols used for treatment, and it is probable that these are not readily available except by taking Active Release workshops. This begs the question, Can we assess evidence properly when critical information is withheld from the public domain?

Buchberger DJ. Use of Active Release techniques in the postoperative shoulder: a case report. *J Sports Chiropract Rehabil.* 1999;13:60-66.

Stripping: Practice

COMPONENTS OF STRIPPING

Stripping has the following components:

Contact: Reinforced finger(s) and/or thumb(s), proximal interphalangeal joints (knuckles), olecranon process

Pressure: Light to heavy. Pressure varies with the muscle layer engaged and the sensitivity of that layer. The range of pressure can range from (a) scarcely more than the weight of the hand, when stripping a taut band harboring an active trigger point in a superficial muscle, to (b) controlled upper body weight reinforced with pressure from the legs, when stripping deep hamstring fibers

Tissues engaged: Muscle and related fascia

Direction: Along or parallel to fibers

Amplitude: Length of muscle

Rate: Very slow. **Travell** and **Simons**[155,156,172-175] give the rate as 0.8 cm/s, or slow enough to obtain a palpable release[155]

Duration: 10 seconds to several minutes

Intergrades with: Specific petrissage and direct fascial technique

Context: Follow inactivation of a trigger point with passive stretch for 30 seconds and then with active range of motion to produce an isotonic contraction of the involved muscle. With severe or long-standing trigger points or those in deeper muscles, it is advantageous to apply regional **petrissage** before and after stripping.

PALPATION PRACTICE

The following muscles often harbor **active or latent trigger points**: upper trapezius, sternocleidomastoid, erector spinae, pectoralis minor, extensor digitorum, opponens pollicis, gluteus medius, the hamstrings, and tibialis anterior.

1. Review the attachments and fiber direction for these muscles.
2. Palpate some of the trigger point areas. Begin lightly, using digital contact, and work slowly across the fibers. Can you find a **taut band**? Taut bands run parallel to the muscle fiber direction, are often visible, and are often clearly palpable. The area will feel "hard," "hypertonic," "tight," "wiry," or "ropy." Do you notice any **twitch responses**?
3. Have an instructor confirm the taut bands that you find.

MANUAL TECHNIQUE

Figures 9-45 to 9-52 show therapists applying stripping to the various regions of the body. The order of the figures is from head to foot in supine and then in prone. Each figure illustrates most of the guidelines for manual technique outlined in this section. The manual technique presented largely follows Simons et al.[155,156,172-175]

1. Place the client in a position that will comfortably allow full stretch of the target muscle. The target muscle should be neither slack nor tautly stretched.
2. If lubricant is not already present, apply a small amount (a drop or two) either to your hands or to the client's skin.
3. **Reinforce** your fingers or thumbs whenever possible by placing your hands together (Figures 9-46, 9-48, and 9-50) or using your fingers as a group, rather than individually (Figures 9-47 and 9-52). Whenever possible, use pushing strokes because they place less stress on the muscles of your hands, are easier to control than pulling strokes, and allow you to use more force when you need it (Figures 9-45 to 9-52). When stripping larger or deeper muscles, using your elbow as the contact surface allows you to use body weight to increase pressure (Figures 9-49 and 9-51). Your selected hand and body positions must be stable.

FIGURE 9-46 Reinforced fingertip stripping of the sternal head of pectoralis major muscle in a cross body position. If the client finds the pulling of hair uncomfortable, the therapist can add more lubricant or break the longer stroke into a series of shorter strokes, which follow the same line, at a comparable rate. Avoid curling fingers since this will make it difficult to push across the muscle.

FIGURE 9-47 This stroke—very much like stripping except in its orientation to the intercostal muscle fibers—follows the intercostal spaces and will improve chest wall mobility.

FIGURE 9-45 Fingertip stripping of the temporalis muscle, a common contributor to temporal headaches.

FIGURE 9-48 Stripping of extensor digitorum with reinforced fingertips.

FIGURE 9-49 The upper trapezius muscle, the most common cause of myofascial pain felt in the temple, is best addressed with the client seated. The client maintains an upright seated posture and pushes with his feet against the floor for support.

FIGURE 9-51 The elbow, a side-lying position, and considerable pressure may be needed when stripping the gluteus medius or minimus muscles. When trigger points are located near the iliac attachment (as with most gluteus medius trigger points), a superior-to-inferior path of application avoids pinching superficial tissue against the iliac crest.

4. Beginning on one side of the trigger point, apply enough pressure to engage the taut band. Then, in one continuous motion, glide slowly and with equal pressure along the band, across the trigger point, and all the way to the attachment of the muscle.[155,156,172-175] The next stroke glides in the opposite direction, across the trigger point, and toward the other attachment. If

FIGURE 9-50 Stripping the infraspinatus muscle. With this contact, the thumbs are doubly reinforced against each other and against the flexed index fingers.

FIGURE 9-52 Stripping the tibialis anterior muscle with the knuckles. In addition to its effects on trigger point activity, stripping will likely lengthen the anterior fascial wall of the anterior compartment.

the taut band softens and the tenderness and pain referral diminish, you can repeat this procedure again with the same pressure. Alternatively, increase the pressure incrementally with each application of the technique.

5. The suggested rate of glide in the literature is 8 mm/s[155,156,172-175] or slowly enough to allow the nodule in the taut band to palpably release or soften beneath the advancing finger(s).[155] In either case, the rate of glide is much slower than that of standard petrissage.

6. You must maintain flawless control over the depth and pressure of this technique. During the initial pass along the taut band, you may find it necessary to reduce pressure quickly and smoothly as your contact surface passes over the trigger point so that you maintain a level of pressure that the client can tolerate.

7. Do not persist with the application of this technique if the taut band and referral are unchanged after two or three passes. Lack of response to treatment means that the trigger point may respond better to another technique or that the trigger point is a **satellite** and you need to treat the **key trigger point**.

8. Follow successful deactivation of a trigger point, as shown by an absence of pain referral on compression, right away with careful passive stretch for 30 seconds or more. Then, as soon as possible, ask the client to perform careful active movement through the full range of motion in order to produce an isotonic contraction of the muscle you have treated.[155] If it is not possible to have the client perform active movement while he is on the treatment table, then he should perform it at the end of the intervention. Finally, apply moist heat for several minutes.

9. When you treat several trigger points in an area, it may help to precede and follow stripping with petrissage and superficial effleurage. You can use a regional approach for a **myotactic unit** with multiple trigger points, especially if these trigger points are chronic or highly symptomatic.

THERAPIST'S POSITION AND MOVEMENT

1. Your posture must be very stable, especially when stripping an active trigger point, since inadvertent small deviations in pressure may produce large increases in pain referral from the trigger point. Figures 9-49 and 9-51 show two variations of a standing **controlled lean** that allow the therapist to

transfer his body weight to the client in a controlled manner. Whatever position you choose, you must remain in perfect control of pressure, especially high pressure, at all times.[178]

2. Slight shifts in the direction of pressure can make a critical difference in whether you can access a trigger point. For example, stripping of iliocostalis lumborum trigger points may yield no increase in referred pain (or therapeutic effect) when you apply the pressure in a strictly anterior direction. On the other hand, a large increase in referred pain may occur when you direct the same amount of pressure along the same taut band in an anteromedial direction (see Figure 9-61).

PALPATE

As you perform the technique, palpate the client's tissues to assess the following:

1. Taut bands. The direction of muscle fibers and the referral pattern will enable you to identify the involved muscle. The taut band will often show approximately even levels of tension along its length. Therefore, the therapist must develop an ability to identify layers of equal tension during palpation.

2. Local hardness. The trigger point itself may present as a very small area of local hardness (palpable nodule) in the taut band.

3. Twitch responses. As you palpate, note whether you can detect twitch responses in superficial muscles.

4. Jump sign. A client may produce a large involuntary contraction and other gross affective signs of pain when you palpate the trigger point.

5. Generalized hardness. If there are adjacent trigger points in overlapping layers as, for example, often occurs between the scapulae, you may find it difficult to palpate anything other than a generalized hardness.

6. Softening of tissues. Softening of taut bands and regional hardness should occur with continued application of the technique.

As with petrissage, you also palpate for the following:

1. Tissue resistance. General resistance or resilience of soft tissues.

2. Tissue mobility. Mobility of the interfaces between muscles and muscle layers.

3. Signs of inflammation. Fibrosis, adhesions, and indurations within and between muscle layers, which are associated with chronic inflammation.

OBSERVE

As you perform the technique, observe the client for signs of trigger point activity. The signs listed below may indicate trigger point activity or a positive response to treatment.

1. Taut bands in superficial muscles are often easily visible.
2. Twitch responses are transient events (1/4 second) that are often more easily seen than felt. They may occasionally appear as a "flutter" that cascades into adjacent muscles.
3. Softening of the contour of the taut band with continued application of the technique. Sometimes the contour of an entire muscle will soften and, more rarely, relaxation of the muscles throughout an entire region occurs as the activity of one trigger point diminishes.

As with petrissage, you may also observe the following:

1. Systemic reduction of muscle tension, as evidenced by softening of the tissue contours or broadening and flattening of body segments.
2. General consistency and resting level of tone.
3. Local hyperemia. A reactive hyperemia (caused by release of substance P)[179] may accompany the application of this technique.

COMMUNICATION WITH THE CLIENT

Communicate to ensure the client's comfort during the application of the technique. Here are some examples of statements that you can use.

1. "As I pass over the trigger point, you may notice that it intensifies the sensation you've been feeling in your …." Explain to the client what a trigger point is, what the sensation being referred means, and that his symptoms may be temporarily reproduced or intensified as you pass over the trigger point. It is very important for the client to understand that the discomfort of the technique has a therapeutic purpose.
2. "The pressure may feel somewhat uncomfortable, but it shouldn't be really painful. It should be tolerable. Tell me if at any time the discomfort is too great." Ensure that the pressure you apply is tolerable to the client. Although client discomfort is acceptable, outright pain is counterproductive. Recheck the client's tolerance with every increase in pressure.

Obvious pain behavior indicates that you must reduce pressure. In addition, you can explain the use of a 10-point pain scale and ask that the client not let the pain of stripping exceed level 4. If the resting pain of an active trigger point already exceeds level 4, then the application of the technique should not increase the client's pain more than a point and should only do so if the client shows no obvious pain behavior and clearly agrees to the procedure.

3. "Does this bring back the exact pattern of pain you've been feeling in your …?" When you locate a trigger point, you may pause over it briefly and allow the client to compare the pattern of pain referral of the trigger point with the presenting symptoms.

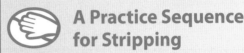

A Practice Sequence for Stripping

Allow at least 30 minutes per person.

Many people have latent trigger points in the fibers of the upper and middle trapezius and the rhomboids. If your client does not happen to have these, you can still practice stripping in this regional exercise.

Before you start, assess the range and ease of motion of glenohumeral and scapular movements.

Prone
1. Apply a small amount of oil to the client's back, using superficial effleurage.
2. Perform regional petrissage to all of the muscles of the upper back and posterior shoulder girdle using a sequence similar to that described in the section titled "A Practice Sequence for Petrissage." Begin with broad-contact techniques that cover a wide area and gradually proceed to more localized techniques such as fingertip kneading. Gradually progress deeper.
3. During this part of the massage, observe closely for muscles that appear to contain hard taut bands, twitch responses, and spots that are tender or produce sensation referrals.
4. If you think you have found a trigger point, confirm this using palpation.
5. Progressively strip all of the fibers of the trapezius muscle, being attentive to the fiber directions. The muscle should be slightly stretched but not taut during this procedure. To strip the upper trapezius effectively in prone, you may have to sit at the head

(Continued)

of the table and apply substantial, reinforced pressure in a caudal direction on the cervical portion where the fibers are vertical. Strip from medial to lateral across the superior aspect of the shoulders to complete the upper trapezius.

6. Periodically intersperse stripping with broader strokes like palmar kneading or picking-up.

7. On any active or latent trigger points, strip the taut band in alternating directions until the client's level of sensitivity decreases.

8. Repeat Steps 5 and 6, focusing on the rhomboids. You will have to use marginally more pressure for this. The fiber direction and the pain referral patterns will help you identify which layer you are on.

9. Conclude with regional petrissage and then superficial effleurage.

10. Get feedback on how your client feels. If your client has begun to experience a temporal headache, you have likely activated a latent trigger point in the upper trapezius muscle. In this case, return to Step 5. If your client has begun to experience a supraorbital headache, then the sternocleidomastoid is implicated and needs more treatment.

11. Reassess range and ease of movement of the scapular movements.

Many people also have latent trigger points in the pectoral muscles on the anterior surface. How would you adapt this sequence to address those?

CAUTIONS AND CONTRAINDICATIONS

Therapists need clinical training and supervised practice to master the proper application of stripping. Advanced training may be advisable when dealing with pathological conditions. All of the general and local contraindications noted for massage techniques apply to the use of stripping (see Chapter 5).[1] Specific contraindications to the use of stripping include clients with hemophilia, local sites of acute inflammation and infection, confirmed or suspected thrombus,[115] thrombophlebitis, and potentially metastatic malignancies. Therapists who are treating clients who have confirmed or suspected osteoporosis, who have wounds in early stages of healing, or who use anticoagulants may choose to use a noncompressive manual method of inactivating trigger points, such as the combination of ice and stretching.[155] In addition,

therapists should use care when treating muscles that are adjacent to areas of spasm or acute inflammation.

Travell and Simons[155,156,172-175] state that therapists must locate trigger points using palpation. Conversely, research suggests that therapists may not reliably locate latent trigger points using palpation.[180] Consequently, therapists must make every effort to locate the points with precision. In addition, because trigger points can cause entrapments[155,156,172-175] and may mimic entrapments, radiculopathies, and visceral pathology,[155,160,169] therapists must take particular care with their differential examination and promptly refer the client to his physician if they suspect a more serious clinical condition.

Active trigger points can cause excruciating, debilitating pain and can be exquisitely sensitive to touch. In these cases, it is particularly important for therapists to apply stripping with absolute respect for the client's pain tolerance. With long-standing or recurrent trigger points, therapists must be careful to treat agonist, antagonist, and synergist muscle groups. Therapists may want to also address the area of referral in addition to looking for satellites. They should also address the factors that may perpetuate the trigger points, such as structural asymmetry and repetitive ergonomic loading.[155-157,160,172-175,181] If an active trigger point remains after the correct application of treatment techniques, this may indicate that the trigger point is actually a satellite and that therapists must treat the key trigger point first. Extensive application of massage techniques to one muscle or muscle group around a joint may cause **reactive tightening** (reactive cramping) in the antagonist or synergist muscle groups or on the opposite side during, or soon after, the intervention.[155] Postintervention pain or tenderness, which differs markedly from the client's presenting symptoms, is often a result of the activation of a latent or satellite trigger point and may indicate a need for therapists to treat the client's referral area and synergist and antagonist muscle groups more comprehensively.

USING STRIPPING IN TREATMENT

Trigger Points

There are several modalities that therapists can use in a complementary manner to decrease trigger point activity. When treating acute trauma, apply cold packs to assist resolution of the acute inflammation, regardless of the effect that this has on the trigger points.[155,156,172-174]

Once the clinically acute stage has passed, the following massage techniques may also be useful:

1. Petrissage
2. Specific compression: trigger point pressure release[155,156,172-175]
3. **Connective tissue techniques** such as **skin rolling**,[155] **myofascial release**,[155,160] and **direct fascial technique**

Therapists can also use the following related techniques to treat trigger points effectively. Ensure that you use those techniques that are within your scope of practice.[155,156,172-175]

1. Sustained gentle passive stretch (required after trigger point inactivation)
2. Active range of motion to produce an isotonic contraction of the affected muscle (required after trigger point inactivation)
3. **Post-isometric relaxation**
4. Contract-relax, hold-relax, and related muscle energy techniques
5. Moist heat application
6. Ice (or vapocoolant spray) and simultaneous passive stretch. Readers are referred to *Myofascial Pain and Dysfunction*[155,156] for the necessary comprehensive instructions.

7. **Therapeutic ultrasound**
8. High-voltage **galvanic stimulation**
9. **Transcutaneous electrical nerve stimulation**. While this is not a specific intervention for trigger points, it may provide temporary relief of pain.

A multidisciplinary approach to treatment that includes appropriate medical management is most effective for the treatment of myofascial pain syndromes and trigger points.[15,155,156,172-175] Therapists can instruct clients in many of the aforementioned complementary modalities for home use. Of particular importance are the following:

1. Correct self-stretch techniques and post-isometric relaxation
2. Gentle active range of motion through the full range of motion to produce an isotonic contraction of the affected muscle
3. Moist heat application to the trigger point (not the area of referral)
4. How to apply stripping in accessible areas, as appropriate
5. Ergonomic education related to posture or repetitive activity

Specific Compression: Evidence

DEFINITION

Specific compression: A nongliding technique that therapists apply with a specific contact surface to muscle, tendon, or connective tissue. Therapists apply compression and release in a direction that is perpendicular to the target tissue, and they often sustain the compression.

NAMES AND ORIGINS

In other texts and massage-related systems, the technique that we call specific compression and trigger point pressure release is called "focal compression," "digital compression," "digital pressure," "sustained digital pressure," "direct pressure," "direct inhibitory pressure," "direct static pressure," "static friction," and "deep touch."[1-3,5-7,12,155,156,158] Along with static contact, specific compression is probably the most widespread of all massage techniques. It is either used alone or as a component of more elaborate methods and systems including **positional release**,[182] **myotherapy**,[183,184] **trigger point pressure release**,[155] **neuromuscular technique**,[157] **Shiatsu**,[185,186] **acupressure**,[187,188] and **reflexology**.[1-3,6,12] Specific compression and trigger point pressure release has been applied with a bewildering variety of rationales and names.

USES

Specific compression is an effective manual technique for reducing the activity and symptoms of **myofascial trigger points**, where it is used as a trigger point pressure release. It may also be a means of inhibiting the tone of the related muscle for a short time in conditions such as spasticity. In addition, it may be effective in softening adhesions and fibrosis in muscle, tendon, and fascia when therapists apply it in a slow and sustained manner. Finally, foot **reflexology**[3,5,6,12,181,189,190] and **Eastern-influenced massage systems**[185-188] use specific compression to influence pain and physiological function at sites that are remote from application of the technique. Table 9-3 summarizes the main outcomes for specific compression.

OUTCOMES AND EVIDENCE

Musculoskeletal Effects

Specific compression has a variety of physiological and psychological effects.[191,192] Specific compression can be an effective manual technique for reducing the activity and symptoms of myofascial trigger points, especially for thin muscles that overlie bone.[155,156,160,172-175] For detailed definitions and descriptions relating to trigger points, see the section on stripping or Table 9-1. During a "manual trigger point pressure release,"[155,156,172-175] therapists apply trigger point pressure release to the trigger point itself (not to the area of referral) and follow it with passive stretch and active movement. Because therapists can use it to reduce the activity of trigger points, trigger point pressure release has wide applicability when treating the effects of a variety of conditions. These conditions include trauma; acute and chronic overload such as tendinopathies and repetitive strain injuries; postural imbalance; fatigue; emotional stress; common musculoskeletal complaints such as tension headache, temporomandibular joint problems, spinal pain, chronic low back pain, disk herniation, chronic pelvic pain, painful rib syndrome, and nonarticular pain; and other myofascial

pain syndromes.[155,156,160,171,172,177,180-190,193,194] Our clinical observations suggest that specific compression may also be effective in softening adhesions and fibrosis in muscle, tendon, and fascia when therapists apply it in a slow and sustained manner.

Neurological Effects

Specific compression can also be used as a proprioceptive stimulation technique.[195-199] In addition, therapists can also apply firm and moderate specific compression (inhibitory pressure) to tendons as a means of inhibiting the tone of the related muscle for a short time.[195] Furthermore, intermittent or sustained application of specific compression to tendons, but not muscle, will also cause a reduction of motor neuron excitability (H-reflex), but only during the application of the stimulus.[196-199] This application of specific compression for the purpose of inhibiting muscle contraction has been integrated into many therapeutic techniques that seek to facilitate movement in conditions associated with abnormal neuromuscular tone such as **spasticity**.

Other Effects

Finally, foot reflexology[1-3,5,6,12,189,190,200] and Eastern-influenced massage systems[185-187] use specific compression extensively to influence pain and physiological function at sites that are remote from application of the technique. These systems suggest that the effects of treatment occur through postulated, complex somatovisceral reflexes. Table 9-3 summarizes the main outcomes for specific compression.

HOW SPECIFIC COMPRESSION MIGHT WORK

Trigger point pressure release may reduce the activity of trigger points through the same mechanism as stripping (see the discussion of stripping in this chapter). This involves rupturing the shortened sarcomeres in the trigger point and destroying the dysfunctional neuromuscular junction, thereby terminating the trigger point and its symptoms.[155] It is important to follow specific compression for trigger points with a full passive stretch of the involved muscle to restore the normal length of the sarcomere, the taut band, and the muscle as a whole.[155] The mechanisms by which specific compression and trigger point pressure release might produce reflex effects and effects distant to the site of its application are less clear and are discussed at length in Key Points 9-1 and 9-2.

Table 9-1	Types of Trigger Points[195]
Trigger Point Type	**Description**
Active	Produces pain in a characteristic pattern at rest
Latent	Produces pain in a characteristic pattern only when palpated
Primary	Arises in response to trauma or acute or chronic overload
Key	Is responsible for activating (and inactivating) satellites
Satellite	Is activated by a key trigger point, by being in its area of referral, or by being its antagonist or synergist
Central	Is located near the center of muscle fibers
Attachment	Is located in a muscle's tendon or aponeurosis

EXAMINING THE EVIDENCE

A **randomized clinical trial** with controls and a placebo, or **sham**, treatment examined the effects of foot **reflexology** on the symptoms of multiple sclerosis.[200] Once a week for 11 weeks, subjects (*n* = 53) received either 45 minutes of "full reflexology treatment" with calf massage or the placebo treatment of 45 minutes of "nonspecific calf massage." Significant improvement in paresthesias, urinary symptoms, and spasticity occurred in the reflexology group, and the improvement in paresthesia remained significant 3 months after treatment. The placebo that the researchers selected seems to be a reasonable control for **nonspecific treatment effects**.

Unfortunately, the researchers only describe the treatment and placebo protocols very briefly in a single sentence. This raises questions such as, Were the two treatments applied with comparable pressure? The researchers sought to reduce the confounding variable of the skill of the therapists by having each therapist treat one client in the treatment group and one in the control group. For the most part, this study is thoughtful and convincing.

Siev-Ner I, Gamus D, Lerner-Geva L, Achiron A. Reflexology treatment relieves symptoms of multiple sclerosis: a randomized controlled study. *Mult Scler.* 2003:9:356-361.

Reflex Effects of Specific Compression: Foot Reflexology

Key Points:

9-1

Foot reflexology is based on the premise that specific points on the feet (and hands) are reflexly related to other body segments or organs of the body (Figure 9-53).[2,3,6,12,189,190] In reflexology, pain, tenderness, or soft tissue hardening in particular areas of the foot is thought to reflect acute or chronic dysfunction of the related body segment or organ. On this basis, specific compression is applied to the reflex points on the foot to normalize function in the corresponding body segments or organs by "restoring lost balance" or "activating the movement of energy."[2]

The mechanisms for the effects of reflexology are unknown. Research and review on the subject are not common and often appear in untranslated European journals.[201-219] Results and opinions on the methods and effects of reflexology are not always positive,[211-217] but some research does support the possibility of specific effects on organ function.[203,205,209,218,219] Specific positive outcomes have been noted for infant colic,[220] multiple sclerosis,[200] and nausea and vomiting.[221] More general outcomes that may result from the application of foot reflexology include reduced anxiety; increased relaxation; and improved mood, energy, and quality of life.[2,3,12,201,222-224] Foot reflexology is logistically simple to perform and requires no oil, towels, or significant disrobing of the client. Contraindications and cautions to the application of reflexology are relatively few. They are mostly local contraindications such as gout, peripheral vascular disease, and contagious or infectious foot conditions.[3] In addition, therapists may have to shorten interventions for weak, convalescent, or elderly clients. A full intervention that consists only of the application of foot reflexology may take from 30 to 60 minutes. Alternatively, therapists may use foot reflexology for 5 or 10 minutes to precede or follow a massage sequence that addresses another area of the body.

Following the client examination, a typical intervention might proceed in the following manner. After a brief foot bath, therapists position clients comfortably in supine, sitting, or lying. Therapists apply general, broad neuromuscular techniques such as wringing, compression, and passive joint movements of the ankles, metatarsals, and toes for several minutes.[2,12] Beginning with the toes and proceeding proximally,[12] therapists apply specific compression systematically and thoroughly to all surfaces of the foot, using a slow, stable rhythm. Therapists usually use their thumbs or knuckles for the plantar surface of the foot and their fingers for the dorsal surface.[2,3] They sustain pressure for several seconds on each point and can prolong it for an additional 15 to 30 seconds if a point is tender or hard. The pressure is usually deep, but as with any massage technique, therapists should moderate the pressure of application so that it feels pleasant or causes only mild discomfort, as opposed to pain.[3] Therapists can also use a short gliding stroke, similar to stripping or direct fascial technique.[2,3,12] More detailed descriptions of the technique of foot reflexology are offered in books that address this subject exclusively.[189,190]

Clinical Significance

At the very least, reflexology provides a method for performing a thorough foot massage with associated general benefits.[33,201] Therapists who perform extended specific compression on the feet, hands, or ears should be mindful of its possible effects. Applying this type of massage technique on the client's feet, hands, or ears can produce systemic effects, which are far greater than the area of the feet, hands, or ears they are treating might suggest. This occurs because altering patterns of tension and tenderness in the feet and hands may affect physiological processes elsewhere in the body.

(Continued)

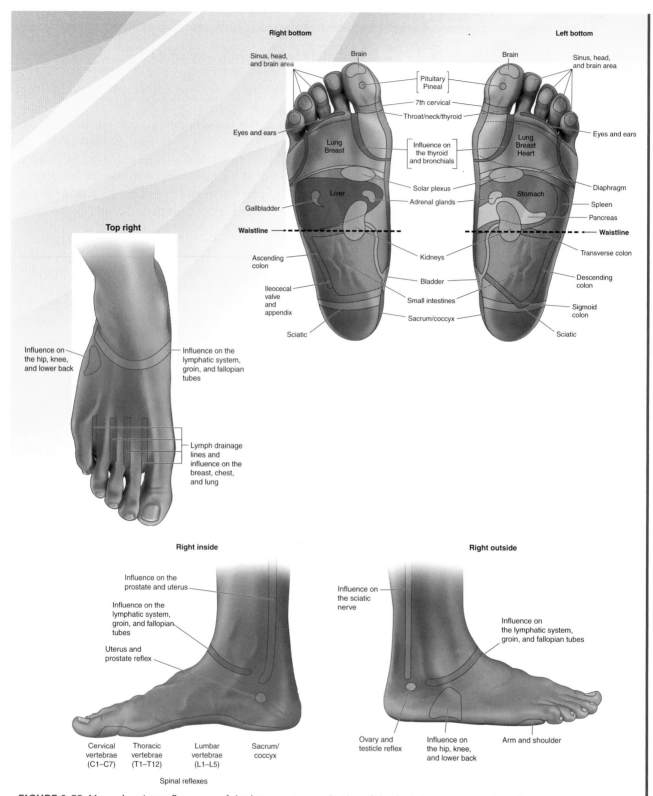

FIGURE 9-53 Maps showing reflex areas of the bottom, top, and sides of the foot that correspond to distant body segments or organs. (From Williams A. *Spa Bodywork*. Philadelphia, PA: Lippincott Williams & Wilkins; 2007:159-160. Reprinted by permission of the publisher Lippincott Williams & Wilkins.)

Reflex Effects of Specific Compression: Meridian Theory and Acupoints

Traditional Chinese medicine is an ancient, vast, and sophisticated system of philosophy, clinical theory, and practice that has come to the attention of the West in recent decades primarily because of the evidence for the analgesic effects of **acupuncture**.[1-3,6,12,225,226] Fundamental to the system of Chinese medicine are several interrelated concepts that have no parallel concepts in Western medicine. In Chinese medicine, energy (qi, chi, ch'i) circulates through the body in well-defined cycles through conduits or channels called meridians.[2,227] There are 12 bilateral paired meridians and 2 median sagittal meridians.[1,2,225] Each meridian is associated with an "organ," for which it is named, and has associated physiological functions that do not correspond exactly to organ functions as defined in Western medicine. Each meridian also has a basic quality of energy that is characterized as being yin or yang.[1,2,227] Yin energy, metaphorically described as "female" and "negative," is ascending and is associated with hollow organs such as the stomach. Yang energy, metaphorically characterized as "male" and "positive," is descending and is associated with solid organs such as the liver.[1,2,227] Health is conceptualized as a dynamic balance between yin and yang energy flowing in precise diurnal patterns through the various meridians.[2,227] Pathways of the meridians do not consistently correspond to any material anatomical structure, although they sometimes follow intermuscular depressions and paths of major nerves.[2,6]

Strung along each meridian, at depths ranging from immediately below the surface up to 1 inch (2.5 cm), are dozens of small points, or **acupoints**, which have lower electrical resistance and higher overlying skin temperature and show altered sensitivity during states of imbalance or disease (Figure 9-54).[2,227] While the position of most acupoints coincides with locations of nerves, trigger points, or motor points,[2,6] there is debate as to how these various entities might correspond to each other.[182,228,229] Acupoints can be activated by a variety of precise approaches to achieve remote effects on the meridian, its associated organ, and related physiological processes.[2,227] Each meridian has several points of unusual clinical importance including activating points, soothing points, and stabilizing points.[2,182,227] Activating and soothing points stimulate and sedate, respectively, the meridian and its related organ and functions. Stabilizing points link the functions of one meridian with those of others. Finally, a variety of other points show sensitivity or tenderness when there is a dysfunction in the related meridian.

Methods of stimulating acupoints include needling (acupuncture), massage, electrical current, laser, and moxibustion.[6] Manual systems that stimulate acupoints, such as acupressure and Shiatsu, rely extensively on deep, sustained specific compression on the points themselves and may include small nongliding circular movements, tapping, and stretching.[185-188] Recent research suggests a variety of clinical effects of stimulation of acupoints with pressure. Most evidence suggests that sustained specific compression on individual acupoints (the pericardium-6 point, located in the middle of the ventral wrist crease) is an effective intervention for nausea, gagging, and vomiting associated with surgery, chemotherapy, pregnancy, or motion sickness[230-251] (with several dissents[252]). Acupressure may also be useful for anxiety,[253-256] various types of pain[257] (though possibly not postsurgical pain[258-263]), sleep disorders,[253] constipation,[264-267] COPD,[268,269] and women's reproductive disorders[270,271] and in palliative care.[272-274] Interventions aimed at restoring the harmonious flow of energy in the presence of imbalance or disease often involve the stimulation of multiple acupoints and the use of other interventions and complex diagnostic procedures. Acupuncture, acupressure, and related modalities rely on elaborate, sophisticated, and radically different conceptual **models** of body processes than those used in Western medicine.

Understanding the rationale of how to stimulate acupoints requires extensive study of these conceptual models and is beyond the scope of this book. The interested reader can consult comprehensive texts.[275]

Clinical Significance

Therapists who use trigger point pressure release extensively to treat trigger points should be aware of the following issues. Remote analgesic effects from specific compression may arise in patterns that do not always correspond to those suggested by trigger points. This may occur because therapists are treating an acupoint, rather than a trigger point. In addition, patterns of pain and tension in the musculature, especially if they are recurrent, may reflect remote physiological and pathological processes. Always apply specific compression within the client's pain tolerance and expect a palpable tissue response to the application of the technique to occur quickly. Therapists should avoid applying the technique if the client's tissues are extremely sensitive and should not persist with application if it fails to produce a quickly palpable tissue change. If the application of specific compression causes symptoms to abate for a short period followed by a recurrence of the symptoms, therapists should identify the underlying causes of the symptoms before reapplying the technique.

(Continued)

FIGURE 9-54 A map showing meridians with acupoints strung along it. (From Tappan FM, Benjamin PJ. *Tappan's Handbook of Healing Massage Techniques.* 3rd ed. Upper Saddle River, NJ: Prentice-Hall; 1998. Copyright 1998. Reprinted by permission of Prentice-Hall, Inc.)

Stomach | ST
Gallbladder | GB
Kidney | KI
Spleen | SP

Governing vessel | GV
Heart | HT
Small intestine | SI
Large intestine | LI
Lung | LU

Bladder | BL
Liver | LV
Triple warmer | TW
Pericardium | PC
Conception vessel | CV

FIGURE 9-54 (*Continued*)

Specific Compression: Practice

COMPONENTS OF SPECIFIC COMPRESSION

Specific compression has the following components:

Contact: Reinforced fingers or thumbs, reinforced proximal interphalangeal joints, olecranon process

Pressure: Light to heavy

Engages: Muscle and/or connective tissue

Direction: Perpendicular to the target tissue layer. This is often, but not always, perpendicular to the surface of the body. Slight shifts in direction may facilitate access of individual trigger points

Amplitude/length: N/A

Rate: 5 to 30 seconds or more per compression

Duration: 5 minutes or more for a series of compressions applied to a muscle belly or region

Intergrades with: Broad-contact compression, specific petrissage, stripping

Context: Follow inactivation of a trigger point with passive stretch for 30 seconds and then an active range of motion to produce an isotonic contraction of the involved muscle. If therapists apply this technique repetitively in a small area or to a deep muscle, they should apply regional petrissage before and after their application of the technique. They should also follow specific compression, which they are using to inhibit abnormal neuromuscular tone, with the desired movement or functional activity. Key Points 9-1 and 9-2 describe contexts for **reflexology** and **acupressure**.

PALPATION PRACTICE

1. Begin by reviewing locations of some common trigger points.
2. With your instructor's help, locate one or more taut bands.
3. With fingers or thumbs, strip along the taut band very slowly. Look for twitch responses and/or jump signs.
4. Try to locate a trigger point precisely. The trigger point itself is not always distinctly palpable. You can identify it as a taut band by local tenderness, by a twitch response or jump sign, and by the production of referred sensation. Can you elicit a clear referral pattern? If not, then increase the pressure carefully and try again. When you find a trigger point, have your client give as clear a description of the referral as possible. Match the description with points shown in a larger text like *Myofascial Pain and Dysfunction*[155,156] or *Neuromuscular Therapy Manual.*[174]
5. Alternatively, you may try grasping and squeezing the taut band between your finger and thumb ("pincer palpation"). This method works well with muscles that are easy to pick up, like the sternocleidomastoid. Using a pincer grip on the upper trapezius requires considerable hand strength to elicit referral.
6. Passively stretch any muscle in which you found a trigger point for 30 seconds.

MANUAL TECHNIQUE

Figures 9-55 to 9-62 show therapists applying specific compression or trigger point pressure release to the various regions of the body. The order of the figures is from head to foot in supine and then in prone. Each figure illustrates most of the guidelines for manual technique outlined in this section.

For all applications of specific compression:

1. The contact you choose depends on the relative size of the therapist and the client, the area to be treated, and the hardness of the tissue. It is important to choose a contact surface that fits the local "topography" of the client's body easily. Your thumb and fingers are better suited to working smaller muscles such as those in the rotator cuff, neck, and calves, and you should reinforce them as needed (Figures 9-55A and 9-55B, 9-56, 9-57, and 9-60). Your elbow is a good contact when the client's tissues are very hard and on

FIGURE 9-56 The lateral pterygoid muscle may be implicated in temporomandibular joint dysfunction. Intraoral specific compression of this muscle demands excellent communication skills and great sensitivity of execution. An alternate to the photograph shown is to work on the same side of the body as you stand so that your fingernails are not facing the cheek.

FIGURE 9-57 Effective direct access to trigger points in the pectoralis minor muscle: slide under pectoralis major muscle, across the ribs, toward either the coracoid process or rib attachment. The approach must often be very slow because of tenderness. Your other hand stabilizes the arm (and scapula) laterally. You can also perform this technique with the client in supine.

FIGURE 9-55 Digital compression of occipital attachments is an effective nonspecific technique for tension headaches and neck tension. This can be done (**A**) using the thumb with the neck rotated or (**B**) on lined-up fingertips with the neck in neutral.

ONLINE VIDEO

FIGURE 9-58 Specific compression of tensor fascia lata using the elbow in a seated controlled lean.

FIGURE 9-61 Angle of approach is often important when applying specific compression to trigger points. Here the therapist directs pressure anteromedially onto the iliocostalis lumborum muscle. A single thumb and light pressure may be adequate to accentuate pain referral from an active trigger point; reinforced thumbs or an elbow and some body weight might be required to elicit pain referral from latent trigger points.

FIGURE 9-59 While applying specific compression with the elbow to the upper trapezius muscle, ask the client to adjust the head position to obtain the strongest pain referral. The therapist is using his left hand to stabilize the point of contact and to palpate for softening of the taut band.

FIGURE 9-60 Specific compression applied to the rhomboids/mid trapezius muscle area with reinforced double-thumb contact.

FIGURE 9-62 The lateral edge of the quadratus lumborum is accessible to specific compression in side-lying only with correct positioning. The client's ipsilateral arm is fully abducted, and the ipsilateral leg has been passively stretched downward, to open space at the waist. Doubled thumbs, reinforced fingers, or even the tip of the elbow can be used. Take care to avoid the poorly supported 11th and 12th (floating) ribs.

FIGURE 9-63 Devices that can assist with self-administration of specific compression of trigger points include balls of various sizes and densities and wooden or plastic massage tools.

larger muscles of the back, legs, and pelvis. This contact allows a greater use of upper body weight to sustain pressure and thus minimizes therapist fatigue (Figures 9-58 and 9-59). You may also use wooden or plastic tools (T-bars) that you grip in your hand. Figure 9-63 shows two of these tools.

2. Your chosen contact must be stable, and you must exercise exquisite control of both the direction and depth of pressure of application. For this reason, the client's skin must be free of excess lubricant to reduce slipping of your hands.

3. Apply pressure slowly, increase it gradually to the desired depth, sustain it evenly, and then release it gradually. The duration of compression will vary with the application from a few seconds to more than a minute.

4. When using specific compression in the form of trigger point pressure release to treat a trigger point,[174] the pressure you apply must be enough to reproduce or marginally increase the referred sensation from the trigger point, while remaining tolerable for the client. This amount of pressure will vary from being light, in the case of a highly active trigger point in a superficial muscle, to being heavy, in a less active trigger point in a deep muscle such as the piriformis.

5. Once you have established a tolerable initial depth/pressure in consultation with the client, there are two approaches to initiating and progressing the specific compression of a trigger point:

   ■ *Progression using verbal client feedback:* This approach relies on frequent client feedback, and we recommend it for novice therapists. Maintain the compression at the initial depth of application until the referred pain subsides. For example, "Until you no longer feel pain or tenderness, just the pressure of my thumb." Then increase the depth of application of the compression to a new level that reproduces a tolerable level of referral. Maintain the pressure of compression at that depth until the referral subsides, then repeat the application of the technique as needed. Gradually increase the depth of application in a series of stepwise increments, until the client reports that the symptoms of the referral have disappeared.

   ■ *Progression using feedback from palpation:* Alternatively, you can maintain the pressure of application at a constant level and exclusively use the barrier-release phenomenon to achieve the continuous increase of depth. As the trigger point is alleviated and the tissues soften, the depth of penetration will gradually increase until the client reports that the referred sensation has disappeared. This approach requires that you accurately feel the presence of the tissue barrier to compression and then sense and follow the release of the barrier into the client's tissue. This approach requires more refined palpation skills than the first method and is worth perfecting.[155]

   In the verbal feedback or palpatory feedback method of progression, it may be more practical for you to wait until the client reports that the referral has diminished substantially, rather than waiting for it to disappear completely. When you apply them correctly, both methods can provide clients with a demonstration of a correct and comfortable pressure of application that they can use at home.

6. There are differing opinions about how long to sustain specific compression of a trigger point, with lengths from 10 seconds to more than 1 minute.[155,160,182-184] For less experienced therapists, and especially when treating chronic or highly irritable trigger points, we recommend shorter, more frequent compressions that are sustained from 15 to 30 seconds and are interspersed with the application of petrissage, stripping, passive stretch, and other manual methods. This minimizes the possibility of overtreating the target muscle, activating latent satellites in synergist and antagonist muscle groups, or producing a biomechanical imbalance. Therapists with higher levels of manual skill can use their judgment on the degree to which they extend the period in which they apply compression.

7. It is not always easy to maintain trigger point pressure on the precise spot that reproduces the client's pain referral, even when you have not applied lubricant. Consequently, you must determine whether a client's report of diminished pain referral reflects reduced trigger point activity or the movement of your contact off the trigger point. Stripping pincer grasping or stretching techniques may be better manual approaches for the treatment of "slippery" trigger points. For example, for the upper or mid trapezius, it is much easier to maintain a pincer grasp.

8. Following deactivation of the trigger point, perform a passive stretch of the treated muscle for 30 seconds. As soon as possible after passive stretching, ask the client to perform active range of motion carefully through the available range to produce an isotonic contraction of the affected muscle. Apply moist heat for several minutes.

9. When treating several trigger points within an area, you may find it useful to precede and follow specific compression with petrissage and superficial effleurage. Use a regional approach for a myotactic unit that has multiple trigger points, particularly if these trigger points are chronic or highly symptomatic.

THERAPIST'S POSITION AND MOVEMENT

1. The posture you select must be stable, comfortable, and sustainable.

2. The basic positions are described in Chapter 6 in the sections on lunge and lean (Figure 9-62), standing **controlled lean** (Figure 9-59), and seated controlled lean (Figure 9-58). These positions allow controlled, sustained use of your upper body weight to increase pressure. Note that you should not use the client's body as a support when using these controlled leaning positions. Instead, incline your body toward the client in a controlled manner and apply precisely the desired amount of upper body weight to the contact surface without becoming destabilized or unbalanced.

3. When you use your elbow as a contact (Figures 9-58 and 9-59), assess the degree of release that has occurred by gauging how the client's compressed tissue deforms under your upper body weight.

PALPATE

As you perform the technique, palpate the client's tissues for the following:

1. Taut bands. The fiber direction and the pain referral pattern will enable you to identify the involved muscle.

2. Local hardness. The trigger point itself may present as a very small area of local hardness (palpable nodule) in the taut band. Apply pressure slowly to this nodule until you reach the barrier to further compression.

3. Twitch responses. You can palpate twitch responses in superficial muscles.

4. Jump sign. A client may produce a large involuntary contraction and other gross affective signs of pain if you palpate the trigger point too forcefully.

5. Generalized hardness. If there are adjacent trigger points in overlapping layers as, for example, often occurs between the scapulae, you may find it difficult to palpate anything other than a generalized hardness.

6. As you sustain the pressure of application at the tissue barrier, the palpable nodule or contraction knot associated with the trigger point will soften or release. You may follow this release into the tissue without increasing the pressure of application.

7. Signs of inflammation. Fibrosis, adhesions, and indurations within and between muscle layers are associated with chronic inflammation.

OBSERVE

As you perform the technique, observe the client for signs of trigger point activity. The signs listed below may indicate trigger point activity or a positive response to treatment.

1. Taut bands in superficial muscles are often easily visible.

2. Twitch responses are transient events (1/4 second) that are often more easily seen than felt. They may occasionally appear as a "flutter" that cascades into adjacent muscles.

3. Softening of the contour of the taut band with continued application of the technique. Sometimes the contour of an entire muscle will soften and, more rarely, relaxation of the muscles throughout an entire region can occur as the activity of the key trigger point and its satellites diminishes.

As with petrissage, you also observe the following:

1. Systemic reduction of muscle tension, as evidenced by softening of the tissue contours or broadening and flattening of body segments
2. General consistency and resting tension of muscle
3. Local hyperemia. A reactive hyperemia may accompany the application of this technique.

COMMUNICATION WITH THE CLIENT

Communicate to ensure the client's comfort during the application of the technique. Here are some examples of statements that you can use.

1. "As I press on the trigger point, you may notice that it intensifies what you've been feeling in your …." Explain to the client what a trigger point is, what trigger point referral means, and that his symptoms may be temporarily reproduced or intensified as you pass over the trigger point. It is very important for the client to understand that the discomfort of the technique has a therapeutic purpose.
2. "The pressure may feel somewhat uncomfortable, but it shouldn't be really painful. It should be tolerable. Tell me if, at any time, the discomfort becomes pain and you cannot relax into it." Ensure that the client can tolerate the pressure that you apply. Although client discomfort is acceptable, outright pain is counterproductive. Recheck the client's tolerance with every increase in pressure. Obvious pain behavior indicates that you must reduce pressure. In addition, you can explain the use of a 10-point **pain scale** and ask that the client not let the sensation of stripping exceed level 4. If the resting pain of an active trigger point already exceeds level 4, then your application of the technique should not increase the client's pain by more than a point and should only do so if the client shows no obvious pain behavior and clearly agrees to the procedure.
3. "Does this bring back the exact pattern of sensation you've been feeling in your …?" When you locate a trigger point, you may pause to allow the client to compare the pattern of trigger point referral with her presenting symptoms.
4. "Let me know when the sensation is gone and you can only feel the pressure of my thumb." Instruct the client to report when the referral disappears and she only feels the sensation of pressure.

A Practice Sequence for Specific Compression of Trigger Points (Trigger point pressure release[155,156,172-175]

Allow 30 to 40 minutes.

The following practice sequence begins like the sequence for stripping but substitutes specific compression for stripping at the point in the sequence when the trigger points are treated.

This sequence is for the hamstrings (another fairly common place to find latent trigger points) with the aim of performing the sequence with only one change of the client's position. Before you start, assess the length and strength of the client's hamstrings and consider how to perform the sequence with the minimum number of changes of position for the client.

1. Apply effleurage beginning "superficial" and progressing to "deep."
2. Apply regional petrissage to the posterior thigh with increasing depth and specificity.
3. Using palpation, search for and confirm the presence of trigger points.
4. Place the target muscle on a slight stretch and apply trigger point pressure release for 10 to 30 seconds.
5. Stretch the muscle passively for 30 seconds.
6. Repeat Steps 4 and 5 until the referral declines or disappears and the full length of the muscle is restored.
7. Apply regional petrissage that includes the antagonist and synergist muscle groups.
8. Repeat Steps 3 to 7 on other trigger points. Do not do more than three or four repetitions unless you also do a few minutes of broad-contact petrissage on the lower back, gluteals, and calves. Why do you have to do this?
9. Finish with petrissage and superficial effleurage.
10. You must treat the other leg for an equal time. Why is this?

Retest. Get feedback on how your client feels.

CAUTIONS AND CONTRAINDICATIONS

Therapists need clinical training and supervised practice to master the proper application of trigger point pressure release and specific compression. Advanced training may be advisable when dealing with pathological conditions. As with other compressive neuromuscular techniques, all contraindications for massage techniques apply. (See Chapter 5 for a detailed discussion of contraindications.) Specific contraindications to the use of specific compression include clients with hemophilia; local sites of acute inflammation and infection; and confirmed or suspected thrombus, thrombophlebitis, and malignancy. Specific compression can be very useful when therapists apply it on-site in the subacute stage of trauma, provided that edema has resolved. In this situation, therapists must reduce the force of application and ensure that the technique does not cause the client pain or cause them to brace against pain. Therapists should not perform sustained specific compression directly over superficial nerves, such as the radial or common peroneal nerves, because a compression **neurapraxia** can result.[155,174] Further cautions to

the application of specific compression are osteoporosis, early-stage wounds, anticoagulant therapy, and areas of spasm and hypotonia.[276]

Table 9-2 lists common errors when treating trigger points with specific compression. When therapists use trigger point pressure release to treat trigger points, they must apply this technique with absolute regard for the client's pain tolerance and accompany the application of the technique with careful communication. In the case of long-standing or recurrent trigger points, therapists can minimize the likelihood of recurrence of the trigger points by treating agonist, antagonist, and synergist muscle groups and addressing perpetuating factors such as structural asymmetry and repetitive ergonomic loading.[1,2,6,12] Postintervention pain that differs markedly from the client's presenting symptoms is most often due to the activation of a latent or satellite trigger point and indicates a need to address synergists and antagonists further.[155,156,158,160,172,174,175] Therapists should be aware that specific compression may produce remote reflex effects that are out of proportion to the size of the area they treat and the force they apply.[155]

USING SPECIFIC COMPRESSION IN TREATMENT

Trigger Points

There are several modalities that the therapist can use in a complementary manner to decrease trigger point activity. When treating acute trauma, apply cold packs to assist resolution of the acute inflammation, regardless of the effect that this has on the trigger points.[6,157] Once the clinically **acute stage** has passed, the following massage techniques may also be useful.

1. Petrissage
2. Stripping[155]
3. Connective tissue techniques such as skin rolling,[155,158] myofascial release,[155] and direct fascial technique

The therapist can also use the following related techniques to treat trigger points effectively as long as they take care to work within their scope of practice[155,158]:

1. Sustained gentle passive stretch (required after trigger point inactivation)
2. Active range of motion to produce an isotonic contraction of the affected muscle (required after trigger point inactivation)
3. Post-isometric relaxation

Table 9-2	Common Errors When Treating Trigger Points with Specific Compression
Error	**Result**
Pressure is applied too quickly	Client terminates technique
	Autonomic nervous system/ sympathetic response
Pressure exceeds client's pain tolerance	Client terminates technique
	Autonomic nervous system/ sympathetic response
Pressure is not maintained on the trigger point (sliding off)	No change in symptoms
Insufficient depth achieved	No change in symptoms
Too few repetitions of compression	No change in symptoms
Sustained accurate pressure does not diminish referral	Try a different trigger point
Passive stretch omitted	Recurrence of same trigger point symptoms
Perpetuating factors not addressed	Recurrence of same trigger point symptoms
Satellite and secondary trigger points not addressed	New symptoms appear

4. Contract-relax, hold-relax, and related muscle energy techniques
5. Moist heat application
6. Ice (or vapocoolant spray) and simultaneous passive stretch. Readers should refer to *Myofascial Pain and Dysfunction*[155,156] for comprehensive instructions
7. Therapeutic ultrasound
8. High-voltage galvanic stimulation
9. Transcutaneous electrical nerve stimulation. Although this is not a specific intervention for trigger points, it may provide temporary relief of pain.

A multidisciplinary approach to treatment that includes appropriate medical management may be most effective for the treatment of myofascial pain syndromes and trigger points.[155] Therapists can instruct the client in many of the aforementioned complementary modalities for home use.

Of particular importance in the management of trigger points are the following:

1. Correct self-stretch techniques and post-isometric relaxation.
2. Gentle active range of motion through the full range of motion to produce an isotonic contraction of the affected muscle.
3. Moist heat application to the trigger point (not the area of referral).
4. Self-administration of specific compression. Use balls of varying sizes and hardness or handheld massage devices to demonstrate this (Figure 9-63). Clients must understand basic trigger point concepts prior to performing self-management programs. Advise clients not to repeat compression more than two to three times; to precede the application of compression with some preparation of the muscle, such as superficial stroking; and to follow the application of pressure with an isotonic contraction of the muscle and the appropriate stretching exercise. Above all, advise clients not to compress the same trigger point for minutes at a time even though it may feel good and afford temporary symptomatic relief.
5. An example of a conservative and effective self-management program for a single trigger point that produced significant decreases in trigger point sensitivity

and perceived pain levels and increased frequency of self-care in adults with chronic myofascial neck pain follows.[155,156,158,172-175,181] This program has five primary components that clients perform once a day. The first is gentle superficial stroking of the muscle in which the trigger point occurs for 2 to 3 minutes. The second is the application of trigger point pressure release to the location of the trigger point with a handheld massage device for 15 to 60 seconds. The third is gentle isotonic contraction of the affected muscle for five repetitions. The fourth is stretching of the affected muscle for two repetitions of 30 seconds. The fifth is gentle superficial stroking and kneading of the affected muscle for 2 to 3 minutes. In addition, the client may use the application of moist heat to the site of the trigger point as an adjunct to this self-management program.
6. Ergonomic education related to posture or repetitive activity.

Motor Control

When therapists use specific compression as a proprioceptive stimulation technique, there are several complementary techniques that are available for inhibiting or stimulating neuromuscular tone and facilitating movement responses.

1. Therapists can apply prolonged cold, neutral warmth, and slow **superficial stroking** locally or over the posterior primary rami to inhibit neuromuscular tone and facilitate movement responses (see Chapter 7).[277]
2. Therapists can use **fine vibration**, joint approximation and traction, light brushing, and **static contact** ("maintained touch") with both light and firm contacts to increase neuromuscular tone and facilitate movement responses (see Chapter 7).[195]

IN CONCLUSION

Neuromuscular techniques have a variety of uses, therapeutic effects, and outcomes. Table 9-3 summarizes those outcomes for neuromuscular techniques that are related to body structures and functions.

Table 9-3   Summary of Outcomes for Neuromuscular Techniques

Outcome	Technique			
	Broad-Contact Compression	Petrissage	Stripping	Specific Compression
Increased perceived relaxation and decreased levels of stress hormones	P	√	P	√
Decreased perceived anxiety and levels of stress hormones	P	√	P	√
Stimulated immune function	P	√	P	P
Systemic sedation	P	√	P	√
Sensory arousal	P	√	?	?
Analgesia	P	√	√	√
Increased arterial supply (direct effect)	P	P	?	?
Increased venous return (direct effect)	P	P	?	?
Increased lymphatic return (direct effect)	P	P	?	?
Decreased edema (direct effect)	P	P	?	?
Normalized resting muscle tension and neuromuscular tone	?	P	√	√
Decreased muscle spasm	?	P	P	P
Increased muscle extensibility	?	√	√	√
Enhanced muscle performance (secondary effect)	?	√	√	√
Balance of agonist/antagonist function	?	P	P	P
Improved movement responses	?	P	P	P
Decreased trigger point activity	?	√	√	√
Increased tissue mobility	?	√	√	√
Increased joint mobility	?	√	√	√
Separation and lengthening of fascia	?	P	P	?
Normalized postural alignment	?	P	P	P
Decreased dyspnea	P	P	P	P
Increased rib cage mobility	P	P	P	P
Increased airway clearance/mobilization of secretions	√	?	?	?
Stimulated peristalsis	P	P	P	P

√, the outcome is supported by research summarized in this chapter; P, the outcome is possible; ?, the outcome is debatable (research results are absent or inconsistent).

REVIEW SECTION

TAKEAWAYS

1. Neuromuscular techniques are those massage techniques that palpate muscle, affect the level of resting tension of muscles, and have additional psychoneuroimmunological effects.

2. Broad-contact compression is a nongliding technique that clinicians deliver with a broad-contact surface such as the palm or a loose fist. This technique engages the patient's muscle, and the pressure and release of the stroke are perpendicular to the surface of the patient's body.

3. Clinicians can use broad-contact compression to assess the general quality and level of resting muscle tension of larger skeletal muscles, to increase venous and lymphatic return, and to assist the patient's expiration.

4. Petrissage is a group of related techniques that repetitively compress, shear, and release soft tissue—primarily muscle—with varying amounts of drag, lift, and glide.

5. Petrissage is the workhorse of the classical massage techniques. Clinicians use it to promote relaxation, reduce resting tension of skeletal muscle, and improve connective tissue extensibility. They can use it to treat many causes of musculoskeletal pain.

6. Stripping is a very slow and specific gliding technique that clinicians apply from one attachment of a muscle to the other for the purpose of reducing the activity of myofascial trigger points.

7. Clinicians use stripping to reduce the activity, pain, and other symptoms of trigger points and to help restore the length and strength of the affected muscle.

8. Specific compression is a nongliding technique that clinicians apply with a specific contact surface to muscle, tendons, or connective tissue.

9. Specific compression is an effective manual technique for reducing the activity and symptoms of myofascial trigger points, where it is used as a trigger point pressure release. It may also be a means of inhibiting the tone of the related muscle for a short time in conditions such as spasticity.

10. The mechanisms for cutaneous reflexes, entrainment to rhythm, and forward movement of fluid in valved vessels discussed for more superficial techniques in the earlier chapters also apply to neuromuscular techniques. In addition, the mechanisms for the release of trigger points are common to specific compression, petrissage, and stripping.

Clinical Case: *Neuromuscular Techniques*

Patient Profile

Your patient is a 30-year-old male who is in good physical condition. He complains of persistent right "shoulder joint pain" when playing recreational football (quarterback), especially when he throws the ball. The pain began 2 years ago, during a long game when he passed the ball more than usual. His doctor has ruled out arthritis of the cervical spine and glenohumeral joints.

Clinical Findings

Subjective Findings:

Every time the patient plays football, the same pain reappears after several throws. He feels it deep in his right shoulder and over the entire deltoid. The pain increases in intensity with activity until it limits the force of his throwing and the length of time he is able to play. For a day after playing, his shoulder is stiff, sore, and bothers him if he sleeps on it.

Objective Findings:

- Posture: His right shoulder appears internally rotated. His right scapula is further from the spine than his left scapula.
- Gait: His gait is normal.
- Range of motion: Right active internal rotation is limited by 15°. Other active and passive shoulder motions are within normal limits.
- Strength: Isometric resisted external rotation is weaker than the left.

- Palpation: Light and moderate palpation of the affected rotator cuff muscles produces local tenderness but no familiar referral. The upper fibers of the infraspinatus are extremely tender to deep palpation, and two points reproduce the patient's familiar "joint pain" that he associates with passing the ball.

Treatment Approach:

At the time of the initial injury, the trigger points in the infraspinatus were overloaded during passing by the concentric wind-up and the eccentric contraction required to control the release. They are also reactivated each subsequent game.

The main initial outcomes are

1. To reduce the activity of the key trigger points in the infraspinatus
2. To restore full pain-free range of internal and external rotation
3. To reduce and balance resting tension throughout the affected rotator cuff and shoulder girdle

With the patient in prone, warm up his upper back and shoulders for 10 minutes with broad-contact compression and the broad forms of petrissage and kneading. Then methodically strip the right infraspinatus, increasing the pressure as tolerated with each pass, until the patient reports no referral or tenderness. Stretch the infraspinatus passively while preventing the scapula from winging. Apply regional broad-contact petrissage for several minutes. Apply a hot pack to the area. Perform similar general, broad-contact neuromuscular techniques on the other shoulder for several minutes. Turn the patient supine, and have him perform *full* active movement of his affected shoulder. Finish with 5 to 10 minutes of general neck work.

You may have to repeat this basic intervention once or twice, with additional specific work for the synergists and antagonists of the infraspinatus such as teres minor, the deltoids, subscapularis, and pectoralis major. You may also need to apply other advanced techniques to help alleviate the trigger points. Show the patient how to use heat and how to stretch the infraspinatus properly (which requires preventing the scapula from winging). You may also show him how to perform self-massage of the infraspinatus using a small hard ball such as a squash ball or a golf ball.

Critical Thinking Questions

1. Which layers of tissues are engaged by neuromuscular techniques?
2. What are the primary effects of neuromuscular techniques?
3. List three potential uses of broad-contact compression and identify a clinical condition for which these uses would be appropriate.
4. List three potential uses of petrissage and identify a clinical condition for which these uses would be appropriate.
5. List three potential uses of specific compression and identify a clinical condition for which these uses would be appropriate.
6. How would you apply and sequence the massage techniques described up to this point in this book in order to increase superficial venous and lymphatic return, deep venous and lymphatic return, and arterial supply?
7. Describe the characteristics of trigger points. How do the treatment techniques for myofascial pain developed by Travell and Simons differ from traditional petrissage and broad-contact compression techniques?
8. What are the similarities and differences between how clinicians use specific compression in reflexology and acupressure?
9. What are the important points to remember to be successful at alleviating trigger points when applying specific compression (trigger point pressure release)?
10. What is the relationship between myofascial trigger points and the tender points of fibromyalgia?

References for Chapter 9 begin on p. 468; see Further Reading list on p. 472.

CHAPTER **10**

Connective Tissue Techniques

OBJECTIVES After studying this chapter, you will have the information that you need to do the following:

1. Describe how the massage techniques in this category affect different types of tissues.
2. Describe each massage technique in terms of the contact surface, pressure, tissues engaged, amplitude, direction, and rate.
3. Demonstrate how to perform each massage technique and how to apply it in the context of a practice sequence.
4. Speculate about the mechanisms by which massage techniques achieve their effects.
5. Describe the outcomes of care, indications, contraindications, and common uses associated with each massage technique.

Connective tissue techniques are those massage techniques that palpate, lengthen, and promote remodeling of connective tissue. These techniques include skin rolling, myofascial release, direct fascial technique, and friction. This chapter describes these techniques, how to perform them, and how to apply them in a practice sequence. It also discusses relevant outcomes and evidence, cautions and contraindications, and how to use the technique in treatment. Finally, Table 10-1 summarizes those outcomes for connective tissue techniques that are related to body structures and functions. Therapists are advised to review the cautions and contraindications for these techniques and to use them as their scope of practice and skill level permit.

281

Skin Rolling: Evidence

DEFINITION

Skin rolling: A gliding stroke in which the therapist grasps the tissues superficial to the investing layer of deep fascia and continuously lifts and rolls it over underlying tissues in a wave-like motion.[1-3]

NAMES AND ORIGINS

In other texts or massage-related systems, the technique that we call skin rolling is also known as "rolling" and "tissue rolling."[1-3] "Subcutaneous tissue rolling" would be a more accurate name for this technique; however, the literature consistently uses the term "skin rolling."[1,4-6]

Therapists often classify this unusual technique as a form of petrissage because it grasps and lifts the tissues (see Chapter 9). Skin rolling is, however, fundamentally different from petrissage in that it is not applied to muscle, but rather to the more superficial subcutaneous tissues.[1-12] The resistance to stretch that therapists can palpate during the application of this technique is due to tightness in the skin and superficial fascia. That tightness may, in turn, stem from underlying tension in the fascia and muscle. When therapists apply skin rolling slowly, it produces a **viscoelastic** stretch of the superficial fascia that results in clinical effects and a feel on palpation that is similar to that of other connective tissue techniques described in this chapter (see Key Points 10-1).

USES

Therapists use skin rolling to assess and treat restrictions in the mobility of the client's skin and **superficial fascia**. These superficial restrictions may be the result of burns, wounds, surgery, orthopedic injuries,[3-5] chronically elevated levels of resting muscle tension, **segmental vertebral dysfunction**, or organic pathology.[4,6,7]

OUTCOMES AND EVIDENCE

Skin rolling is a useful technique for both client examination and treatment. It has a variety of physiological and

---

Key Points: 10-1

How Connective Tissue Responds to Stretching Forces

There is extensive research about how dense connective tissue responds to stretching forces.[13-20]
  Some relevant concepts are as follows:

- **Tension/tensile force**: Any force that is oriented in a manner so that its effect is to lengthen a structure.

- **Elastic**: Behaves like a spring. Elastic stretch disappears when one releases the tensile force.

- **Viscous/plastic**: Behaves like putty. Plastic stretch remains once one releases the tensile force.

- **Viscoelastic**: Shows both viscous/plastic and elastic behavior. For a viscoelastic stretch, some of the length that the tissue gains during the stretch will remain when one releases the tensile force.

- **"Creep" (viscoelastic "creep")**: Gradual lengthening of connective tissue that occurs with sustained tensile force and that reflects the viscous or plastic behavior of dense connective tissue under tension. Therapists can palpate "creep" during manipulations that place connective tissue under sustained tension.

The elastic and plastic response of connective tissue to tensile forces can vary with the rate and duration of the force that is applied. The best way to lengthen connective tissue structures permanently, without compromising their structural integrity, is to apply prolonged low-intensity forces.

---

psychological effects that are outlined in this section. The therapist can use skin rolling to assess restrictions in the mobility of the client's skin and superficial fascia, which may be the chronic-stage result of burns, wounds, surgery, and orthopedic injuries (see Key Points 10-2).[3-5] A client's complaints of pain and palpable tissue resistance during skin rolling may indicate an underlying chronic elevation of **resting muscle tension**, segmental vertebral dysfunction, or organic pathology.[4]

As a treatment technique, the therapist can use repetitive applications of skin rolling to improve the mobility of skin and subcutaneous connective tissues and thus to increase joint range of motion.[1-5] When the therapist applies skin rolling slowly and with a greater force, the anatomical continuity of fascial layers may result in the mechanical lengthening effects of this technique penetrating to deeper

How Connective Tissue Responds to Immobility

Key Points: **10-2**

Immobilization of connective tissue, which commonly occurs after orthopedic injury, produces a succession of important biochemical changes.[22-26] These include the following:

- Decreased concentration of **hyaluronic acid** in the **matrix**
- Decreased water-bonding capacity of the matrix
- Decreased water content of the matrix
- Approximation of collagen fibers
- Increased collagen cross-linking

These in turn may contribute to the clinical impairments of

- Increased tissue **stiffness**
- Decreased tissue mobility and extensibility
- Restrictions of joint capsule and ligaments
- Impaired joint mobility
- Pain

Damaged tissue that receives carefully applied stress during the healing process, by appropriate movement or massage, shows improved hydration of the extracellular matrix and more orderly deposition of collagen. This results in stronger, more mobile, and more functional scar tissue.

---

fascial layers. Finally, a common (side) effect of skin rolling is the production of a significant reactive hyperemia.[21]

HOW SKIN ROLLING MIGHT WORK

The mechanical effects of skin rolling are a result of the **tension** that this technique applies to the connective tissue in superficial fascia. In cases of sustained tension, as during slower rates of application, this fascia probably lengthens through a controlled (minor) rupture of **collagen** molecules and **collagen cross-links**.[8] Since superficial and **deep fascia** are continuous,[3-5,8] using a greater, or more sustained force in skin rolling will transmit tension

---

to the deeper layers of fascia and may produce a smaller lengthening effect there.

The mechanisms for the **somatovisceral reflex** effects,[1,4] which some therapists postulate for this technique, are unclear, although Hilton's law[27,28] and Kellogg's[29] and Zabludowski's[29] work are worth considering in this regard.

EXAMINING THE EVIDENCE

There are few references in the literature on the use of skin rolling as a technique for assessment or treatment. In one simple study, chiropractic researchers assessed the usefulness of skin rolling to identify "**segmental spinal dysfunction**."[30] One therapist identified areas in the thoracic paraspinal muscles of 25 chiropractic students that were tender upon skin rolling. The therapist also measured sensitivity to pressure in these tender areas and selected nontender areas using a pressure **algometer**. A second therapist used specific joint challenges, to identify spinal segments that showed reduced mobility, in the same set of subjects. The researchers then correlated tender and nontender areas with mobile and nonmobile areas. They found that dorsal spine skin roll tenderness was a "moderately good indicator" of joint fixation within one vertebrae above or below the level of tenderness. By contrast, areas that showed tenderness during skin rolling were highly correlated with underlying areas that were tender to pressure, as measured by an algometer. The latter finding would be more credible if different therapists had measured the tenderness during skin rolling and performed the algometry testing.

Taylor P, Tole G, Vernon H. Skin rolling technique as an indicator of spinal joint dysfunction. *J Can Chiropr Assoc.* 1990;34:82-86.

Skin Rolling: Practice

COMPONENTS OF SKIN ROLLING

Skin rolling has the following components:

Contact: Distal phalanges of finger(s) plus your thumb, thenar eminence, or heel of your hand

Pressure: Sufficient to allow lifting of the superficial tissues

Tissues engaged: Skin, superficial fascia, and fat; indirectly engages deeper layers of fascia

Amplitude/length: Variable, at the discretion of the therapist

Rate: Slow, less than 1 to 4 cm/s

Duration: 30 seconds or greater

Intergrades with: Direct fascial technique and petrissage

Context: Apply alone to mobilize surface connective tissue restrictions such as **scars**. Apply before and after direct fascial technique or myofascial release to evaluate tissue mobility.

PALPATION PRACTICE

1. For different areas of the body, using fingertips and very light pressure, **drag** the skin in various directions. How far does the skin move before you have taken up all the slack and begin to **glide**? Why is there more skin mobility in some areas than others? If you can, repeat the same exercise with an elderly partner.

2. For all regions of the body, using fingertip palpation, estimate and record the thickness of the tissue layer that is superficial to the **investing layer of deep fascia** and that consists of the skin, superficial fascia, and subcutaneous fat. Compare the thickness in different regions and on different models.

3. Using adducted fingers opposing your thumb, grasp and lift the layer superficial to the investing layer of deep fascia. You can reduce pinching by having 1 to 2 in. between your fingers and thumb before you grasp. How easily does the tissue lift? Once you have lifted a fold or roll of superficial tissue, gently attempt to pull the tissue in various directions without releasing your grasp. How far does it go? Does it go more easily in some directions than others? Compare all the regions and compare several models. For example, what might explain the consistent difference between mobility of the superficial tissues on the dorsal and palmar surfaces of the hand?

MANUAL TECHNIQUE

Figures 10-1 to 10-6 show therapists applying skin rolling to the various regions of the body. The order of the figures is from head to foot in supine and then in prone. Each figure illustrates most of the guidelines for manual technique outlined below:

1. No oil is required. Remove all previously applied oil from the client's skin. You can apply this technique reasonably well through fabric.
2. Grasp the client's skin, superficial fascia, and associated fat between your thumb(s) and fingertips(s). Use as broad a contact surface as possible, except with small body segments (Figure 10-1), to reduce the likelihood

of the client experiencing a pinching sensation. The contact surface can include all the distal phalanges and the entire heel of your hand for areas where the client's skin is looser or where there is more fat (Figure 10-5).
3. Lift the grasped tissues in a direction that is perpendicular to the surface of the client's skin.
4. Simultaneously maintain the stretch on the client's tissues and roll the superficial tissues along the surface in a slow wave. There are two concurrent stretching forces: one perpendicular to the skin and the other parallel to the skin. A gliding motion occurs as you simultaneously gather and release the client's tissues while maintaining the grasping and lifting motion. Glide and roll the tissue toward or away from yourself. Do not release the roll of tissue until the end of the stroke.

FIGURE 10-1 Gentle fingertip skin rolling makes an interesting beginning or ending to a complete face massage.

FIGURE 10-2 Skin rolling over the clavicle and anterior neck engages the superficial fascia with its embedded platysma muscle.

A

B

FIGURE 10-3 A and **B.** Tissue response in the lower back is affected by the underlying lumbar fascia and usually varies with the direction of the strokes.

FIGURE 10-4 Skin and superficial fascia in the region of the sacrum lie over dense fascial attachments and lift less easily.

5. Two-handed and single-handed skin rolling are both possible. Skin rolling is easier to perform two-handed with hands side-by-side and working together.
6. You can perform skin rolling in a variety of different directions. Since skin attaches to superficial fascia differently in the various parts of the body, it may be consistently easier to perform skin rolling in a particular direction in a given region (Figures 10-3, 10-4, and 10-6).
7. In an intervention, perform skin rolling over an entire region once, then return to adherent or sensitive spots for additional passes, performing the technique in different directions, until the client's subcutaneous tissues lift easily and any reported sensitivity has decreased.
8. When applied at a slow rate (<1 cm/s) and with moderate lifting force, skin rolling can produce a **creep** of the client's superficial fascia—an effect that can affect the underlying investing layer of the deep fascia.
9. Even when therapists apply skin rolling with the broadest hand contact, clients may not be able to tolerate it. If clients are very sensitive to the pressure of skin rolling, you can use a superficial **myofascial release** across the client's skin or a **direct fascial technique** applied with a light pressure and a broad contact surface to obtain similar results.

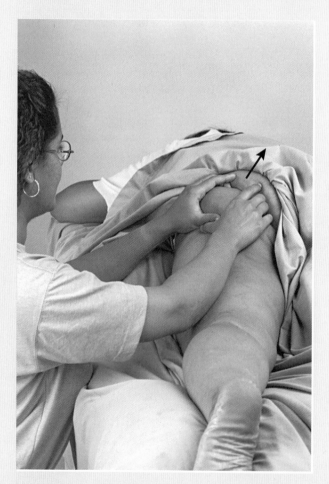

FIGURE 10-5 In fatty areas, such as the glutei, a heel-and-fingers contact will include more tissue.

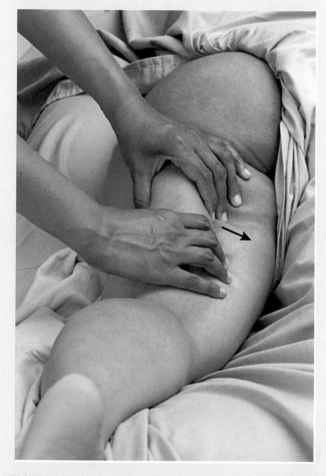

FIGURE 10-6 It is usually easier to perform skin rolling around, rather than along, the limbs.

THERAPIST'S POSITION AND MOVEMENT

1. Use the basic positions described in Chapter 6, in the sections **Aligned** Standing or Sitting Positions.
2. Since your hands produce the entire force of skin rolling, you can use any comfortable aligned standing or seated position.
3. Use of a seated position will reduce wrist hyperextension when you are grasping the client's tissues between your fingers and the heels of your hands (Figure 10-5).

PALPATE

As you perform the technique, palpate the client's skin and tissues for the following:

1. Temperature and texture of the skin.
2. Texture and thickness of superficial fat. **Lipomas** and **fibrositic deposits** are discrete, denser areas of tissue that move readily with the tissue layer. They are common on the back and around the pelvic girdle, but may also be found on the extremities.
3. Tightness of the superficial fascia. You will perceive this as a resistance to stretching the client's tissues perpendicular to the skin surface; resistance to stretching the tissues parallel to the skin surface; or resistance to the ease of rolling the tissues during the stroke.
4. **Viscoelastic** stretch of the tissues. If you perform skin rolling slowly, it may be possible to palpate a slow viscoelastic stretch or "creep" of the client's superficial tissues.

OBSERVE

As you perform the technique, observe the client for the following signs:

1. General appearance of skin, specifically circulatory or **trophic changes**.
2. Visible chronic tension in muscles. This can be associated with tightness of the overlying superficial fascia.
3. Reactive hyperemia. Skin rolling often quickly produces a hyperemia that can last for minutes.

COMMUNICATION WITH THE CLIENT

Obtain feedback on the client's level of comfort and concerns about the effects of the technique. The following are some examples of statements that you can use:

1. "Let me know if you feel a burning sensation as I roll your skin." Initially, skin rolling produces an unpleasant "burning" sensation as you stretch the client's tight superficial fascia. You cannot completely avoid producing this sensation; therefore, moderate the degree of lift you use in response to the client's feedback or change to a broader connective tissue technique.
2. Reassure the client that skin rolling will not produce stretch marks and that it will not temporarily or permanently slacken healthy skin in any visible way.

A Practice Sequence for Skin Rolling

Practice Time: 30 minutes per person.

Prone
Undrape half of the client's posterior torso, from the shoulder down to the gluteal fold. Ensure that spinous processes are accessible:

1. Beginning at the shoulder: Lift the client's skin and as much of the subcutaneous fat as possible and roll the tissue down the back and, if possible, buttock in one long uninterrupted movement.
2. Return to the shoulder: Move laterally or medially and make successive passes in the same direction until you have treated all of the exposed area. During application, mentally note where tissue restrictions occur.
3. Cover the same area with similar long parallel "strokes," this time working in a superior direction. Again, mentally note where tissue restrictions occur.
4. Cover the same area with shorter parallel "strokes," this time working from medial to lateral and then lateral to medial. Note differences in the response of the tissue.
5. Return to the areas that appeared to present with greater restriction. Apply the technique repeatedly in a variety of directions.
6. Reassess the quality of the tissue restrictions. You may wish to have the client stand and actively move before you compare the two sides of the body.

Perform a comparable sequence on the other side of the client's body. At the end, investigate how you can apply skin rolling to other areas of the body such as the scalp, hands, feet, and around joints.

Home study: Devise and apply comparable routines for other regions.

CAUTIONS AND CONTRAINDICATIONS

Clinical training and supervised practice are important when learning skin rolling. Advanced training may be advisable when dealing with pathological conditions. All of the general and local contraindications noted for mechanical techniques apply to the use of skin rolling (see Chapter 5).[5,8,10] As for all of the connective tissue techniques, therapists should not use skin rolling in areas of acute inflammation, around hypermobile or unstable joints, or if the client's skin is fragile due to age or drug use.[5] Therapists can apply skin rolling with reduced force over tissues that are in the subacute **(fibroplastic)** phase of inflammation if swelling has resolved and the client can tolerate treatment. Therapists should use this technique with caution in the presence of **connective tissue diseases**. In addition, in the **osteopathic** tradition, the presence of persistently or recurrently immobile skin overlying a particular spinal segment indicates underlying imbalance, or pathology, in the viscera supplied by that segment.[4,21] In areas of fascial binding, skin rolling can be painful; consequently, therapists must consider the client's pain tolerance when they apply this technique.

USING SKIN ROLLING IN TREATMENT

Mobilizing Chronic-Stage Scars

Skin rolling is the most superficial of the connective tissue techniques. For this reason, therapists use it as a first technique for mobilizing **scars** in skin and subcutaneous fascia in their **chronic stage**. You can also apply myofascial release and direct fascial technique with light force to mobilize scars in these tissues. You can work more vigorously on scars that have matured than on scars in the early chronic stage, as long as you pay close attention to client feedback. Several sources suggest that the clinically chronic stage of scarring usually begins from 2 to 3 weeks after injury[31-33] and continues through **consolidation** and **maturation** phases for up to a year.[31] The determination of the clinical stage of scarring requires a thorough client examination.[31,32] Scars deep to superficial layers are mobilized with myofascial release, direct fascial technique, and friction. Depending on the situation, you can apply other massage techniques locally to damaged tissues earlier in the healing processes to reduce edema and pain and prevent the formation of poorly modeled scar tissue.

For home care, teach the client how to perform self-administered skin rolling in accessible areas and stretching for 30 seconds or longer to help mobilize restrictions in the superficial fascia.

Myofascial Release: Evidence

DEFINITION

Myofascial release: A technique that combines a nongliding fascial traction with varying amounts of orthopedic stretch to produce moderate, sustained tension on the muscle and its associated fascia and that results in palpable viscoelastic lengthening or "creep."[1-3]

NAMES AND ORIGINS

Other texts or massage-related systems, name the technique that we call myofascial release as "myofascial stretching."[34] In addition, other texts use the term "myofascial release" as a synonym for the technique we call

"**direct fascial technique**," which has a component of glide (see the discussion in other sections of this chapter).

Therapists sometimes use myofascial release as part of a wider system of treatment, known by the same name, which may incorporate a variety of craniosacral, osteopathic, and other soft tissue techniques.[34,35] Some authors[7,34] describe both "direct" and "indirect" applications of myofascial release. "Direct," in this sense, means that the therapist directs the force of the technique toward, and then through, the primary tissue restriction. In other words, the therapist applies the motion through and beyond the restrictive fascial barrier. This is in contrast to "indirect" techniques in which therapists apply the force, or move the client, away from the fascial barrier or restriction of motion.[7,36] This book does not cover indirect applications of myofascial release.

Myofascial release is one of several approaches that therapists have developed over the last 50 years to influence structure, as opposed to function, using massage. It owes a large conceptual debt to Ida **Rolf** and shows the influences of osteopathy and traditional stretching techniques.

USES

Therapists use myofascial release to lengthen fascial layers, restore fascial mobility, and decrease the effects of scars and **adhesions** on the locomotor system. They also find it useful for treating postural conditions and the chronic after-effects of trauma.

OUTCOMES AND EVIDENCE

Myofascial release has a variety of physiological and psychological effects that are outlined in this section. Therapists can use myofascial release to lengthen fascial layers, restore mobility between fascial layers, and decrease the effects of adhesions on the locomotor system. Consequently, myofascial release is appropriate for a variety of conditions in which chronic fascial shortening results in limited joint range and ease of movement such as postural conditions (kyphosis, lordosis, scoliosis, elevated shoulders, and anterior head posture), chronic after-effects of trauma, chronic fascial compartment syndromes, and neurological or circulatory compression syndromes such as thoracic outlet syndrome.[35-44] In these situations, myofascial release contributes to improved alignment,[45] balanced muscle function, enhanced quality and quantity of movement, and pain reduction through its direct treatment of the underlying dysfunction.[7,34,35] Myofascial release also has analgesic effects when combined with other modalities.[46-49] This technique may also help resolve trigger point syndromes,[50] counteract the effects of stress,[51] and facilitate athletic performance.

HOW MYOFASCIAL RELEASE MIGHT WORK

The mechanical effects of myofascial release are the result of the sustained tension that this technique exerts on the fascia associated with superficial and deep muscles. This tension probably lengthens fascia by creating minor ruptures of **collagen** molecules and **collagen cross-links**.[3] In addition, it may produce changes in the volume and level of **hydration** of the **ground substance**.[3,34,35] The rebalancing of tension throughout the connected **myofascial network** of the body, which may follow a myofascial release, may cause postural shifts[34,35] and associated changes in the client's awareness and body image.[34] Furthermore, changes in proprioception in the tissues whose length has changed may, in turn, facilitate new patterns of muscular use in the client.

There is no clear explanation for how this manual intervention might alter the function of the autonomic nervous system and increase relaxation.

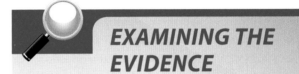

EXAMINING THE EVIDENCE

A randomized controlled trial of 119 subjects, with a complex design, examined the effect of several methods on the immediate reduction of pain caused by active upper trapezius trigger points.[50] Researchers first tested the effect of "ischemic compression" (specific compression in Chapter 9) on trigger point activity by comparing two different pressures and treatments of three different durations. They found that a longer application (90 s) at a higher (but still tolerable) pressure was most effective. In the second stage, researchers tested the effect of various protocols on trigger point activity. The control group received only hot packs and active range of motion exercises. The other treatment groups received the control treatment plus various combinations of specific compression, TENS, stretch and spray, interferential current, and myofascial release. Several multimethod protocols showed a significant reduction of trigger point pain and increase in cervical range of motion. The most effective protocol included hot pack, active range of motion, interferential current, and myofascial release. Unfortunately, the authors' description of the myofascial release procedure was short and did not include even approximate times for its duration. Other than that, this study was unusually thorough in its design, execution, and reporting.

Hou CR, Tsai LC, Cheng KF, Chung KC, Hong CZ. Immediate effects of various physical therapeutic modalities on cervical myofascial pain and trigger-point sensitivity. *Arch Phys Med Rehabil.* 2002;83:1406-1414.

Myofascial Release: Practice

COMPONENTS OF MYOFASCIAL RELEASE

Myofascial release has the following components:

Contact: All or part of both hands or forearms are used.

Pressure: Light to moderate

Tissues engaged: Fascia. The fascial response is the primary object of palpation, although this technique also engages the associated muscle.

Direction: Typically, force is oriented in a direction that is parallel to the long axis of muscles and the muscle fibers. The resulting stretch will occur in the same direction.

Amplitude/length: Length increase for a sustained stretch in a long myofascial unit may approach 3 cm.

Rate: Rate of "creep" is very slow, and region, amount, and health of tissues under stretch will also influence the rate.

Duration: 90 seconds to 5 minutes or greater

Intergrades with: Static contact, direct fascial technique, and conventional orthopedic stretching

Combines with: Combine with specific compression to treat trigger points.

Context: Commonly applied alone or alternated with direct fascial technique. Broad myofascial release can precede or follow specific neuromuscular or connective tissue technique.

PALPATION PRACTICE

1. If necessary, review the anatomy of major skeletal muscles. Palpate the borders, attachments, and fibers, and draw these with a marker on your partner.

2. Select a major muscle or muscle group in the lower limb such as the hamstrings. Test and record its length and observe its appearance with your partner standing. Apply a conventional stretch technique to the muscle on one side for 2 to 3 minutes, while your partner practices diaphragmatic breathing; be sure to increase the stretch as the muscle relaxes. Have your partner stand for observation. What differences do you see and feel between the two sides? Perform the stretch on the other side and repeat the evaluation.

3. Choose a healthy joint on your partner (a single metacarpophalangeal joint or the wrist complex works well for this exercise). Stabilize securely with one hand proximal to the joint and one hand distal. **Distract** the joint with just enough force to take the slack out of the capsule. Maintain the same traction force for up to a minute, while you palpate with your eyes closed. You (and your partner) can usually feel the joint "give" slightly farther as the connective tissue in the capsule begins to **creep** (see Key Points 10-1).

MANUAL TECHNIQUE

Figures 10-7 to 10-14 show therapists applying myofascial release to the various regions of the body.[34,35] The order of the figures is from head to foot in supine and then in[35] prone. Each figure illustrates most of the guidelines for manual technique outlined. Arrows indicate the direction of the applied force. No glide occurs between the therapist's hands and the client's skin:

1. Place the client so that you stretch the tissues you are going to treat, for example, a muscle or an entire limb, to a point just short of tautness or at the point of tautness.
2. Place the chosen contact surfaces at opposite ends of the target tissues that are to be stretched (Figures 10-7, 10-9, and 10-14). Contact surfaces commonly

chosen are the entire palmar surface of your hand, the heel of your hand, or your forearm.
3. Compress the client's tissues enough to engage the investing layer of deep fascia (or deeper), and then exert a light to moderate horizontal drag or traction force in opposite directions. This motion stretches the tissues between your hands in a direction parallel to the line of the muscle fibers. The contact surfaces should not glide over the client's skin.
4. Sustain the horizontal drag or stretching force at a constant level as the client's tissues begin to lengthen slowly.
5. Take up the slack as the tissues lengthen. For example, if you have placed your hands at opposite ends of a muscle, they spread apart very slowly without gliding over the skin (Figures 10-7, 10-9, 10-10, 10-13A, 10-13B, and 10-14). When the client's body weight

FIGURE 10-7 Fingertip contact is used to stretch small muscles such as the masseter.

FIGURE 10-9 Unilateral stretching of upper trapezius from a superior position using crossed hands.

FIGURE 10-8 Stretching of the posterior cervical myofascial units in supine. Caution: Avoid placing fingers on C1–C2 and placing pressure on the atlas.

ONLINE VIDEO

FIGURE 10-10 Crossed-hand stretching of the lower fibers of pectoralis major.

FIGURE 10-11 Sustained traction can be performed with the client's arm (or leg) in almost any position. The therapist maintains traction and moves the client's arm slowly and progressively into full abduction. This maneuver can be done in varying degrees of internal or external rotation.

FIGURE 10-12 Double-arm traction can be performed with the client in prone or supine. Starting from this basic position, the therapist can use small shifts in position to direct the lengthening force to virtually any long muscle group in the upper body. A second therapist can simultaneously provide double-leg traction and thus further expand the effects of the technique.

FIGURE 10-13 A. Unilateral crossed-hand stretching of the lumbar region in prone. Extended gentle application of the technique can be required to address the barriers within the dense, many-layered lumbosacral fascia. Hands can also be positioned centrally and oriented across the body in order to cover the paraspinal musculature on both sides of the client's spine and produce a bilateral stretch. **B.** Unilateral crossed-hand stretching of the lumbar region in side-lying. To facilitate a stretch of the quadratus lumborum, position the client's arm over his head and place a pillow under his opposite side.

stabilizes one end of the stretch, both of your hands will move away from the point that gravity is stabilizing (Figures 10-8, 10-11, and 10-12). One author suggests that a minimum of 90 seconds is necessary for a myofascial release and advises therapists to hold initial releases for 3 to 5 minutes so that lengthening can proceed through a succession of fascial barriers.[35]

6. If you do not observe a palpable or visible stretch after 90 seconds, ask the client to consciously "breathe into" the area being stretched or to cough.[34,35] Adjust the

angle of stretch slightly, lighten the pressure, or change the target tissue entirely to produce an effective release.

7. Crossed-hand positions permit comfortable leverage, especially with large muscles (Figures 10-9, 10-10, 10-13A, and 10-13B). However, when used for prolonged periods of time, these may be stressful on the therapist's wrists.

8. You can exert variable amounts of compression into the client's tissues prior to initiating the lengthening traction; however, it is advisable to begin with a

FIGURE 10-14 Myofascial release of the gluteus maximus. Note: The fibers of gluteus maximus run in an oblique direction; ensure that the stroke follows the direction of the muscle fibers.

light compression. This is necessary because contact that initially appears to engage only superficial tissue layers may affect deeper fascial layers once the myofascial release occurs. It is not primarily the amount of force applied, but the duration of sustained force that results in a stretch of connective tissue (see Key Points 10-1). In addition, the use of greater force is more likely to result in the client experiencing pain, guarding, and apprehension; therefore, do not use more than moderate force.

9. You can sustain the force of the stretch for 3 to 5 minutes, or longer, while the client's tissues release through a series of fascial barriers. Alternatively, you can maintain the stretch for a shorter period, and then reposition the client's body segment in a position of greater stretch and repeat the procedure until the tissues are adequately elongated. With the latter approach, you may alter the force on successive stretches in order to engage different layers and fibers of muscle and fascia.

10. Apply and release pressure gradually.

THERAPIST'S POSITION AND MOVEMENT

1. Use the basic positions described in Chapter 6, in the sections Standing Aligned, Seated Aligned, and Other Postures.
2. Select a posture that is both efficient and comfortable because you may need to sustain it for several

minutes. By using hand and forearm contacts, you can improve body mechanics and avoid prolonged stress to your wrists.

3. Alter the **ergonomic** load on your body by using small shifts of foot position and center of gravity as the release progresses.
4. You can perform whole-limb and full-body releases with the assistance of a second (or even a third) therapist.[34]
5. When you have to sustain a position for a long period with relatively little body movement, breathe using your diaphragm.

PALPATE

As you perform the technique, palpate the client's tissues for the following:

1. Viscoelastic stretch or creep of the tissues. This is relatively easy to palpate during correct performance of myofascial release because the contact surfaces do not move over the client's skin. After you set up the stretch position and carry the initial **elastic** stretch of the tissues to its end point, gradual separation of the contacts will reflect creep. Creep has a slow, soft, "hydraulic" feel (like pulling taffy or putty) that may be due in part to the constrained movement of fluid out of the extracellular matrix under pressure.
2. Location of layers of fascia. Attempt to engage the same fascial layer with both hands so that your hands "communicate." This will enable each hand to sense small changes in the amount and direction of the force that the other hand is exerting, as though they were pulling on opposite ends of a connected sheet. Developing the ability to isolate and palpate layers of fascia is a skill that requires practice.
3. Rhythm and motion of the stretch. Successful application of myofascial release depends on you noting the inherent rhythm and motion of each stretch as it progresses. Closing your eyes can help focus attention on your hands and the results of palpation; this is especially useful when learning the technique.
4. **Cranial rhythm**. Small, palpable shifts in the orientation of the stretch force that seem to occur on their own may reflect the client's cranial rhythm or the untwisting of asymmetrically shortened fascial sheaths. Therapists can perform myofascial release in its simplest form without reference to cranial rhythm. We refer therapists who wish to refine the technique of attending to cranial rhythm during myofascial release to the work of Upledger and Vredevoogd.[52] Even at

earlier stages of learning, however, you should be prepared to palpate the small, three-dimensional movements that can accompany the developing release.

OBSERVE

As you perform the technique, observe the client for changes in muscle tension and tissue lengthening. The following signs may signal this:

1. Local lengthening. During the release, you may observe small amounts (millimeters to 1 or 2 cm) of local tissue lengthening, depending on the size of the area under stretch.

2. Lowered muscle tension. After you release the force of the stretch, local tissue contours may soften and flatten, reflecting lowered muscle tension.

3. **Thixotropic** rehydration. The thixotropic rehydration of the ground substance of tissues may contribute to a further softening of local tissue contours after you release the force of the stretch.

4. Changes in other body segments. Lengthening and positional shifts may appear in proximal, distal, or adjacent segments during the application of myofascial release. You must cultivate the habit of continually evaluating adjacent body segments for changes with the client on and off the table.

5. Structural alignment. Therapists can best assess changes in structural relationships of the client's body segments by the inspection of standing static alignment and gait, both during and at the end of the session.

6. Signs of a shift in autonomic function toward relaxation such as decreased breathing rate, peristaltic noises, and changes in voice tone.

COMMUNICATION WITH THE CLIENT

Encourage general relaxation and an awareness of tissue lengthening. Following are some examples of statements that you can use:

1. "Deepen your breathing without forcing it in any way." Conscious deep diaphragmatic breathing aids release; while lack of it impedes release. Occasionally, coughing can also facilitate the release.

2. "Close your eyes and let your awareness move to…" Ask the client to close her eyes in order to better focus on the sensation of tissue lengthening.

3. "Let me know if you begin to feel uncomfortable." Both the pressure and the sensation of lengthening usually feel pleasant and, at all times, should be tolerable.

4. Ask the client to compare areas that you have treated with areas that you have not treated. For example, ask the client to compare the left and right sides. Clients may find changes more apparent when they are sitting or walking. Giving clients enough time to observe and report, the ongoing effects of the technique is a useful teaching tool, particularly in the case of clients with poor postural habits.

5. "Does anything feel out of place?" "Do your left and right sides match?" "Can you describe the difference between the left and the right sides of your body?" Ensure that the client feels balanced at the end of a session.

6. "It's normal to feel a bit clumsy for a day or so after the treatment." Clients are often aware of altered **proprioception** and biomechanics for a day or two after undergoing a substantial release. While these changes are not painful, the client may find them uncomfortable. Consequently, advise clients that this discomfort may occur and that they can reduce it by simple daily activities such as walking.

7. "Please let me know if you experience anything unusual after the treatment, especially if you have persistent pain." When a significant shift in **agonist/antagonist balance** occurs, the client may experience transient muscle soreness in areas other than those that were treated. This occurs because of an increased loading of antagonists, synergists, or other muscles in the **kinetic chain**. Therefore, advise the client to report any postintervention soreness that is more than mild or that lasts longer than 2 days.

 A Practice Sequence for Myofascial Release

Practice time: 40 minutes per person.

You can extend the following sequence for the more superficial lumbar and pelvic muscles by allowing each stretch to develop for longer than a minute and by pausing more often to take up the slack in the tissues. It is advisable to allocate a comparable amount of time for each of the stretches (90 s or more), so that a balanced intervention results. Before practice, review the fiber directions for the myofascial units to be treated and review static alignment and gait.

Before initiating the intervention, scan the client for static alignment and gait. In particular, pay attention to the relationship between the client's lumbar vertebrae and pelvis:

1. Begin with the client in prone over an abdominal pillow. Apply several crossed-hand stretches across the lumbar portion of the latissimus dorsi.
2. Turn the client to side-lying. Stretch the ipsilateral leg and open the space between the 12th rib and the iliac crest (the lateral fascial portion of the obliques).
3. With the client's leg in the same position, apply myofascial releases between origins and insertions of gluteus medius and minimus.
4. Have the client draw the legs up into a semi-fetal position. In this position, lengthen the lower portion of the erector spinae and then gluteus maximus.
5. Turn client to the other side and repeat steps 2, 3, and 4.
6. Turn the client to supine. Apply myofascial releases to the tensor fascia lata and rectus femoris on both sides. Allow the leg to hang over the side of the table if necessary.
7. Apply a conventional psoas stretch to both sides.
8. To finish, apply gentle sustained traction to each leg. Then apply a gentle sustained spinal traction from the neck and then from the sacrum.

CAUTIONS AND CONTRAINDICATIONS

Therapists need clinical training and supervised practice to master the proper application of myofascial release. Advanced training may be advisable when dealing with pathological conditions. All of the general and local contraindications noted for mechanical techniques apply to the use of myofascial release (see Chapter 5).[5,8,10] As was the case for the connective tissue techniques, there are several cautions and contraindications to the use of myofascial release. These include malignancy,[53] cellulitis, fever, systemic or local infection, acute circulatory conditions, osteomyelitis, aneurysm, obstructive edema, acute rheumatoid arthritis, open wounds, sutures, hematomas, healing fractures, osteoporosis, anticoagulant therapy, advanced diabetes, and hypersensitivity of the skin.[35] In

addition, therapists should use extreme caution when performing myofascial release in the area of flaccid paralysis, lax or unstable joints, or diseased joints that are supported by **fascial "splinting."** Finally, therapists should use myofascial release with caution and only in the nonacute stages of connective tissue diseases.

Therapists need to appreciate the broader impact of myofascial release on the client's system as a whole. Although the force with which the therapist performs myofascial release is not particularly great, significant changes in the client's myofascial balance can occur quickly. Since the client's interwoven myofascial network demonstrates "whole-system" behavior,[3,34,35,54-60] the mechanical effects of myofascial release are not just local or even always predominantly local. Familiarity with fascial anatomy, as described in Myers' book *Anatomy Trains*,[56,61] can help therapists gain an understanding of how fascial work performed in one location may "travel" to affect other locations. Furthermore, this technique can produce strong autonomic effects, reflex effects, and **somatoemotional release**, especially when therapists use it for long periods.[34,62] This necessitates a conservative approach, careful observation, and continuous communication with the client during the application of the technique.

In light of the effects of myofascial release, therapists should ensure that they are able to accurately perform a basic visual postural analysis before they begin to apply myofascial release during an intervention.[54,55,59,60] Furthermore, therapists learning to perform myofascial release should initially limit their use of this technique to less than 10 minutes in any given session and should periodically conduct at least a visual reassessment of the client. In addition, therapists should ensure that the client looks and feels "balanced" at the end of a session, especially if they have performed unilateral work around the client's legs, thighs, or pelvis. Finally, therapists must strive to maintain balanced function of the client's agonist, antagonist, and synergist muscle groups and to use a rigorous analysis of possible treatment effects. Specific strategies for the extensive use of fascial techniques, such as myofascial release, are beyond the scope of this book and are the subject of several recent specialized texts.[56,57]

USING MYOFASCIAL RELEASE IN TREATMENT

To Increase Fascial Extensibility

You can apply myofascial release with specific reference to the **craniosacral rhythm** and integrate it with craniosacral technique and direct fascial technique.[1,34,35] Other massage techniques that increase connective tissue extensibility include skin rolling, **friction**, and probably petrissage, if it is applied slowly and with a high component of drag, as well as conventional stretching that is held for 30 seconds or longer. Self-stretching is particularly useful for client home care. Also of benefit are **muscle energy techniques**, **joint mobilization** and **joint manipulation**, and spinal **traction** performed from the head or pelvis.[35]

In controlled laboratory conditions, the precise heating of tissue facilitates elongation of dense connective tissue without major structural damage.[17,20,63] In clinical practice, however, heating connective tissue prior to any sustained loading can increase the risk of large-scale rupture of collagen. Consequently, the therapist should avoid the application of either heat or cold before performing connective tissue techniques, unless his aim is specifically to rupture or denature collagen.[63] Heat applied after the use of myofascial release can enhance the temporary increase in the pliability of myofascial tissue.

For Postural Conditions

Any of the techniques described in this chapter may be relevant when attempting to lengthen areas of postural shortness. After postural change has occurred, then postural awareness training, neuromuscular education, and movement awareness training may be of benefit.[12] You may use systems of comprehensive postural awareness and movement training, such as the **Alexander technique**,[64] in these situations. Ergonomic retraining related to the client's work environment may be required. Therapists can use strength training and endurance training for areas of **postural weakness**. These may be assisted with electrotherapeutic modalities such as biofeedback and electrical muscle stimulation.[12] Chronic conditions may require correction for bony asymmetry.

Direct Fascial Technique: Evidence

DEFINITION

Direct fascial technique: A slow, gliding technique that applies moderate, sustained tension to the superficial fascia or to the deep fascia and associated muscle. It results in palpable viscoelastic lengthening (creep).[1,3-9,35,57,65]

NAMES AND ORIGINS

In other texts and massage-related systems, the technique we call direct fascial technique is called "fascial technique," "connective tissue technique," "connective tissue massage (CTM)," "myofascial massage," "deep tissue massage," "deep stroking," "myofascial manipulation," "soft tissue mobilization," or "direct release myofascial technique."[1,3-9,12,35,57,57,65]

"Direct," used in relation to fascial technique, means that therapists direct the force of the technique toward, and then through, the tissue restriction. In other words, they apply the motion through, and beyond, the restrictive fascial barrier. This is in contrast to "indirect" techniques, such as counterstrain or positional release, in which therapists apply the force, or move the client, away from the fascial barrier or restriction of motion.[7,36] This book does not cover indirect techniques.

At a glance, direct fascial technique sometimes resembles modern neuromuscular techniques, such as stripping, that engage muscle while producing a sustained unidirectional drag in one plane. When therapists apply direct fascial technique over the client's muscle belly, it may achieve some of the effects of neuromuscular techniques. However, this technique differs substantially from neuromuscular techniques in terms of the focus during palpation, location of application, intention, and effect on connective tissue.

Direct fascial technique is one of the most influential massage innovations of this century, popularized initially through the work of Ida **Rolf** in the United States and Elizabeth **Dicke** in Germany, who both developed and elaborated on the technique for two distinctly different purposes.[55,66,67] Therapists of the various schools of **Structural Integration** or Structural Bodywork, who seek to comprehensively realign bodies, apply direct fascial techniques to superficial and deep fascial layers and throughout the musculature within the framework of a 10-session series. These schools include **Rolfing**[68-71] and its various descendents such as Hellerwork; SOMA (Greek word meaning body and mind); Neuromuscular Integration and Structural Alignment; and Structural Integration and Postural Integration.[5,9,55,72] In Dicke's Bindegewebsmassage (**CTM**), therapists apply direct fascial technique in precise sequences to the skin and superficial fascial layers to elicit specific physiological reflex effects.[1,66,73] The CTM system also uses skin rolling and short strokes, which do not glide but nonetheless exert specific subdermal traction to fascia.[1] This system has a much larger following in Europe than North America.

USES

As was the case for myofascial release, therapists use direct fascial technique to lengthen fascial layers, to restore fascial mobility, and to decrease the effects of scars and adhesions on the locomotor system. Therapists find it particularly useful for treating postural conditions and the chronic after-effects of trauma. In addition, they sometimes use it for analgesia, to balance autonomic function, and, in Europe, for **somatovisceral** effects.

OUTCOMES AND EVIDENCE

Direct fascial technique has a variety of physiological and psychological effects that are outlined in this section. It has general clinical effects that are similar to those of myofascial release, including lengthening and restoring mobility between fascial layers. In addition, therapists can use direct fascial technique within comprehensive systems of treatment, such as Structural Integration or CTM, to address different outcomes. Like myofascial release, therapists can use direct fascial technique in the treatment of conditions in which chronic fascial shortening results in limited joint range and ease of movement. These conditions include postural conditions (kyphosis, lordosis, scoliosis, elevated shoulders, and anterior head posture), chronic after-effects of trauma, chronic fascial

compartment syndromes, repetitive strain injury, neurological or circulatory compression syndromes such as thoracic outlet syndrome, chronic low back dysfunction, and mild spasticity.[35,55,66-77] In these situations, direct fascial technique contributes to normalized structural alignment, balance of agonist/antagonist muscle function, improved quality and quantity of movement between and across body segments, and improved energy consumption.[55,72,76-80] These effects, in combination with the enhanced muscle performance that follows increased muscle extensibility, may make the technique useful for athletic performance. In addition, direct fascial technique has complex direct and indirect effects on pain through endorphin-mediated analgesia, the restoration of mobility, and the reduction of anxiety.[74,78-91] Finally, this technique also often results in a local reactive hyperemia and may indirectly affect local circulation.[1,66]

Within the context of **Structural Integration** interventions, direct fascial technique has other clinical effects. First, it appears to produce an increase in parasympathetic activity,[74] and when applied during a series of sessions, it can result in a lasting reduction in anxiety states.[80-82] Studies on the use of direct fascial technique in CTM interventions have, however, reported less consistent autonomic effects, although the literature on CTM suggests that it is useful for treating autonomic imbalance.[1,66,83,92,93]

When direct fascial technique (or any other massage technique) affects autonomic activity, it can produce generalized, indirect visceral effects. CTM, however, takes this notion further to suggest that therapists can achieve a direct regulating effect on a client's organ function, via **somatovisceral reflexes**, by detecting and freeing tightness in somatic connective tissue.[73,93-100] The scientific basis for this theory is uncertain, although some believe that simply giving more space to organs will facilitate the return of their motility. The literature states that the skin can develop predictable areas of hypersensitivity (Head's zones) and that muscles and related fascia can exhibit predictable areas of increased tone (MacKenzie's zones) in response to specific visceral pathology.[67,93] Unfortunately, there is a scarcity of English language research to support the existence of direct somatovisceral paths of influence on organ function. This is a consequence of the lack of English translations of the potentially substantiating German and Russian literature, even as journal abstracts.[101-104] Review articles in English-speaking journals suggest that there is no empirical evidence for the concept of somatovisceral reflexes.[105] Consequently, advocates of CTM have recently acknowledged that the scientific basis for somatovisceral reflexes requires clarification and research.[93,104] As noted previously, Hilton's law[27-29] and Kellogg's[29] and Zabludowski's[29] work are worth considering in this regard. In addition, perhaps, therapists may look forward to receiving greater clarity on the basic notions about the psyche–soma–viscera relationship in the future.

HOW DIRECT FASCIAL TECHNIQUE MIGHT WORK

The mechanical effects of direct fascial technique are the result of the sustained tension that this technique exerts on the fascia associated with superficial and deep muscle. This tension probably lengthens fascia by creating minor ruptures of collagen molecules and collagen cross-links.[3] In addition, it may produce changes in the volume and level of hydration of the ground substance.[3,34,35,57] It may also affect the activity of contractile cells located within the fascia.[92] The rebalancing of tension throughout the connected **myofascial network** of the body, which may follow a myofascial release, may cause postural shifts and associated changes in the client's awareness and body image.[35,57] Furthermore, changes in proprioception in the tissues whose length has changed may, in turn, facilitate new patterns of muscular use in the client.

There is no clear explanation for how direct fascial technique might alter the function of the autonomic nervous system and increase relaxation. For example, what are the answers to the question: How does working near the vagus nerve at the occiput[57] or near parasympathetic outflow at the sacrum increase activity of the parasympathetic nervous system? Nor is there a suggested mechanism for the **somatovisceral reflex** effects that some therapists attribute to this technique.

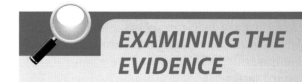

EXAMINING THE EVIDENCE

A pilot study[89] with a **pretest**, **posttest design** examined the effects of a manual therapy program, composed of hot pack, classical massage, and connective tissue manipulation, on 30 female clients with migraine headaches. The researchers evaluated the subjects before and after 20 sessions of treatment that they delivered over a 4-week period. They noted statistically significant decreases in pain intensity, frequency of headache, and frequency of four accompanying symptoms (nausea, vomiting, photophobia, and difficulty concentrating). Decreases in all symptoms were still significant after 6 months. In light of the long follow-up time, these results are promising, but the study lacked a control. In addition, the authors did not describe the massage methods they used in a manner that would permit a therapist to reproduce them. For example, they describe the protocol for the connective tissue manipulation but not for the classical massage; they do not report treatment times for the two massage approaches; and session times varied from 45 to 60 minutes. Finally, this study examined an intensive intervention that is likely to be beyond the means of many clients or facilities to fund.

Akbayrak T, Citak I, Demirturk F, Akarcali I. Manual therapy and pain changes in patients with migraine: an open pilot study. *Adv Physiother.* 2001;3:49-54.

Direct Fascial Technique: Practice

COMPONENTS OF DIRECT FASCIAL TECHNIQUE

Direct fascial technique has the following components:

Contact: Fingers (adducted together, may be reinforced), knuckles, fist, elbow, and ulnar border of your forearm

Pressure: Light to heavy

Tissues engaged: Fascia. Although this technique also engages associated muscle, the fascial response is the primary object of palpation.

Direction: Varies. The force of application is often, but not necessarily, oriented in a direction that is parallel to the long axis of the myofascial units.

Amplitude/length: Less than 5 to 50 cm

Rate: Slow; less than 5 to 15 cm/s

Duration: 5 seconds or greater

Intergrades with: Stripping, frictions, and myofascial release

Combines with: You can enhance the lengthening effects of this technique dramatically by having the client perform simultaneous slow active movement, which further lengthens the treated tissues.

Context: Commonly applied alone or alternated with myofascial release by experienced therapists. It is advisable for the less experienced therapists to precede or follow direct fascial technique with regional broad-contact petrissage (see Chapter 9).

PALPATION PRACTICE

1. Locate, trace on a partner's body, and palpate major superficial fascial structures such as the galea aponeurotica, lumbosacral fascia, retinacula of the wrist and ankle, intermuscular septa of the upper arm and thigh, iliotibial band, anterior compartment, and palmar and plantar aponeuroses. What is the texture and consistency of these tissues?

2. Palpate bones where they underlie the skin with no intervening muscle. How thick is the tissue that covers the bone? In what regions can you follow a fascial layer that overlies bone into adjacent muscle?

3. Attempt to find the **investing layer of the deep fascia** that lies superficial to muscle tissue and below the superficial layer of fat. How well can you distinguish between the investing layer of deep fascia and the muscle fibers that are deep to it?

MANUAL TECHNIQUE

Figures 10-15 to 10-23 show therapists applying direct fascial technique to the various regions of the body. The order of the figures is from head to foot in supine and then in prone. Each figure illustrates most of the guidelines for manual technique outlined here.

1. Fascia is most accessible for treatment at locations where it is exposed and has the least associated muscle bulk, such as at joints, on retinacula, and around bony prominences such as the sacrum and the occipital ridge (Figures 10-15 to 10-18, 10-22, and 10-23). These areas often receive less attention during **classical massage** because they have no muscle bulk, yet they are of great importance when using direct fascial technique. Most systems that use direct fascial technique emphasize the importance of working on the dense lumbosacral fascia at each session, either at the beginning of the session, as in **CTM**, or the conclusion of the session, as in **Structural Integration**[66,67,74] (Figure 10-21, the lower arrow).

2. No oil is required. Remove previously applied oil. To prevent binding, you may need to apply a drop or two of cream or lotion to the working surface of your hands or forearms, but it should be a very small amount. Anything that facilitates glide also reduces your ability to apply tension to the fascia, thereby reducing the effectiveness of the technique. In some areas the application of a very light mist of water to the palm of your hand will help you apply tension to the fascia.

3. There are two basic steps to directing the force. First, compress into the client's tissues to engage the most superficial layer of restriction. Then slowly glide horizontally, while maintaining the same compressive force, to exert traction on the fascial layer you have engaged. The rate of glide is approximately 5 to 15 cm/s.

4. You can produce strokes of any length that freely cross joint lines to follow continuous fascial layers

FIGURE 10-16 A fist usually fits well into the space above the clavicle. Strokes in a posterolateral direction that follow the clavicle can release the scalenes.

FIGURE 10-15 Lifting the scalp aponeurosis with the fingertips. Slow strokes begin at the brow and cross the forehead to the hairline. On the scalp, short interconnected strokes can reduce pulling of the hair. Attempt to generate an equal amount of force with all fingers.

FIGURE 10-17 The entire anterior costal margin is an anchor for fascia from above and below. This costal margin must be treated when lengthening the front of the torso. Avoid the xiphoid process.

FIGURE 10-18 Direct fascial technique applied to the retinacula of the wrist (or ankle) can have a lengthening effect throughout the related girdle. Note the desired neutral position of the therapist's joints.

FIGURE 10-19 Lengthening the fascial sheaths over and between the hamstrings can be done in supine or prone. Individual knuckles can be inserted into the intermuscular septae. On heavier clients, the technique illustrated may require the use of the therapist's elbow.

FIGURE 10-20 The anterior compartment is surprisingly dense and requires the use of body weight. Here, the therapist's body weight is transferred from a controlled kneeling posture.

(Figure 10-18). Shorter strokes may be more tolerable in hairy areas. At the end of the stroke, break contact and pause for several seconds. There is no return stroke.

5. You may direct the horizontal force in any direction in relation to muscle fibers: parallel to them or across

FIGURE 10-21 Fascia associated with the erector spinae can be treated with the client's back in many positions, from neutral to fully flexed in prone, seated, or side-lying. Here, the therapist slides in the spinal groove along the medial surface of longissimus, taking care to avoid the spinous processes.

FIGURE 10-22 The dense iliotibial band requires a forearm or elbow with judicious use of body weight. Include the superior iliac attachments.

FIGURE 10-23 The olecranon and the fist are easily tolerated contact surfaces for applying direct fascial technique to the plantar fascia. The client's foot should be dorsiflexed to at least neutral and further increasing dorsiflexion will expose the fascia to more pressure.

ONLINE VIDEO

them. Experiment with a variety of directions for each location, and evaluate the results of each stroke continuously by inspection and palpation, bearing in mind that the goal of the technique is to achieve an overall increase in tissue length and pliability.

6. Remain in contact with the chosen layer, as far as possible. Since this layer may not always be readily palpable, you can aim to maintain the same compressive force throughout a given stroke, and/or you can stay on the layer of tissue that feels equal in hardness, density, or resistance.

7. Repeat the stroke again, focusing on a less mobile portion of the client's tissues, or cover the original area from a different direction. If you can drag the superficial layer of fascia horizontally in all directions with relative ease, then you can increase compression in order to engage a deeper layer prior to repeating the stroke.

8. The order in which treatment proceeds is important. Work initially with broad surfaces and a general approach to free superficial layers of fascia before working the deeper layers. The benefits of direct fascial technique will accumulate incrementally when you free the fascial layers in an orderly succession from superficial to deep.[67] As a result, it is incorrect to attempt to use great amounts of pressure to move deeper layers of fascia before ensuring that the superficial layers of fascia are thoroughly mobile at least regionally.

9. After two or three strokes, change the location of application regardless of whether or not there is palpable or visible tissue response. There are several actions you can take if shortened tissues do not

seem to respond: change the stroke direction; work on the same layer proximally, distally, or across the midline; or work in a different area, such as the antagonists and synergists, before returning to the area of the unresponsive tissue. Cultivate the habit of thinking about presenting problems in a global manner; because the fascial system is interconnected, what you perceive to be a local problem may be a more generalized issue.

10. When using your hands as contacts, position them so that you avoid hyperextension of any of the joints of your fingers (Figures 10-17 and 10-18). An arched hand position, with the metacarpophalangeal and interphalangeal joints slightly flexed, is acceptable for pushing strokes that require the use of your fingers.

THERAPIST'S POSITION AND MOVEMENT

1. Use the basic positions described in Chapter 6. Since little body movement occurs during the slow strokes, any position that is efficient, stable, and comfortable is appropriate. Standing, seated, and kneeling positions that allow a controlled lean are all useful because they enable you to use your body weight in a controlled manner to engage deeper fascial layers. Figures 10-19, 10-20, 10-22, and 10-23 show good body mechanics in some of these positions.

2. Especially when using body weight to increase the force of the technique, you must use slow and controlled movements. Furthermore, use of body weight must not obstruct your ability to palpate subtle lengthening in the client's fascial sheaths.

3. The treatment of chronic restrictions in soft tissue may require the use of a fair amount of body weight; nevertheless, you must always be relaxed, poised, and alert to signs of overexertion. Common signs of physical and mental overexertion include: elevated shoulders; excessive hand and forearm tension; and uncontrolled leaning. The therapist's posture in Figure 10-21 shows the beginnings of an uncontrolled lean.

PALPATE

As you perform the technique, palpate the client's tissues for the following:

1. Fascial structures. The palpation of the major fascial structures, such as the iliotibial tract, retinacula,

occipitofrontal aponeurosis, clavipectoral fascia, and large intermuscular septae, is relatively easy.[54,66] By contrast, it can be virtually impossible to palpate minor fascial sheaths in areas where there is associated muscle bulk.

2. Fascial texture. Although scarring due to surgery or **consolidated edema** resulting from a major trauma can produce obvious palpable fascial thickening, it requires practice to detect less obvious restrictions in connective tissue. With the application of direct fascial technique, discrete connective tissue structures can become palpably softer and hard and fibrous areas may feel fuller, softer, hydrated, and less fibrous.

3. Fascial "layers." Although you may sometimes clearly palpate the movement of an entire fascial sheath from the point of contact, don't take the term "layer" too literally. In many ways, "layer" is a metaphor to help you focus your attention on a useful object of palpation. As with myofascial release, you must develop the ability to palpate the behavior of an entire layer of connective tissue while it is under sustained horizontal traction and the contact surface is gliding (a very refined skill). In addition, a shift to nonlocal palpation will be challenging if you have much prior practice of classical (Swedish) massage, which focuses attention on the qualities of the tissues that are immediately underhand.

4. Resistance to sustained lengthening. Resistance to a sustained lengthening force may arise from any location in the fascial layer that is under traction. With practice, you may be able to identify resistance to lengthening that comes from a point distant to the point of contact.

5. Viscoelastic stretch or creep. Creep occurs during direct fascial technique, although it is more difficult to identify than when it occurs during myofascial release since the glide of the contact surface occurs at the same time as the creep of the tissue that is under traction.

6. Adhesions or Trigger Points (**TrPs**). During treatment, you may glide over adhesions or trigger points, which may soften with continued application of regional direct fascial technique. If this does not occur, then you may choose to change to a more specific technique such as specific compression or friction.

OBSERVE

As you perform the technique, observe the client for changes in tissue length and quality. The following signs may signal this.

1. Hyperemia. A reactive hyperemia may accompany the application of this technique.

2. Local tissue contours. Observe areas that are drawn in, flattened, elevated, atrophied, or hypertrophied.[66] Tissue contours may change following the application of direct fascial technique.

3. Thixotropic rehydration. The thixotropic rehydration of the ground substance may contribute to a further softening of local tissue contours after you release the force of the technique.

4. Changes in other body segments. Lengthening and positional shifts may appear in proximal, distal, or adjacent segments during the application of myofascial release. You must cultivate the habit of continually evaluating adjacent body segments for changes with the client on and off the table.

5. Structural alignment. You can best assess changes in structural relationships of the client's body segments by inspection of standing static alignment and gait, both during and at the end of the session.

COMMUNICATION WITH THE CLIENT

Encourage general relaxation and an awareness of tissue lengthening. The following are some examples of statements that you can use.

1. "Let me know if you begin to feel uncomfortable." In general, once a client overcomes the initial strangeness of direct fascial technique, it should feel pleasant. You need to inform the client about the different types of sensations that may arise. Clients frequently experience a burning sensation when stretching of superficial fascial layers first occurs. When you use specific contact surfaces, such as the fingers, a cutting or scratching sensation may occur,[66] which is not caused by nails. The client may experience local discomfort when there is a significant local fascial restriction. In general, ensure that the client understands that the amount of pressure used must be tolerable and is under control of the client, not the therapist.

2. "Notice what's occurring in your body. It's not unusual to experience sensations some distance from the location of my hands." Clients frequently report sensations that occur some distance from the therapist's hands and may need to be reassured that this is normal. These sensations are generally of two types: a transient referral from a latent trigger point that you pass over,

or direct mechanical pulling of some distant part of the fascial layer that is currently under traction.

3. "Deepen your breathing without forcing it in any way." "As you breathe in, imagine the breath flowing into your …" Conscious diaphragmatic breathing facilitates fascial release, and lack of it impedes release. It can help to have the client imagine their breath flowing into and out of the area that you are treating.

4. "Can you describe the difference between the left and the right sides of your body?" Ask the client to compare areas that you have treated with areas that you have not treated. For example, ask the client to compare the left side to the right side. Clients may find changes more apparent when they are sitting or walking. Giving clients enough time to observe and report the ongoing effects of the technique is a useful teaching tool, particularly in the case of clients with poor postural habits.

5. "Does anything feel out of place?" "Do your left and right sides match?" "Can you live with this until your next session?" Ensure that the client feels balanced at the end of a session.

6. "It's normal to feel a bit clumsy for a day or so after the treatment." Clients are often aware of altered proprioception and biomechanics for a day or two after undergoing a substantial release. While these changes are not painful, the client may find them uncomfortable. Consequently, you should advise clients that this discomfort may occur and that they can reduce it by simple daily activities such as walking. The rationale for this is that after tissues undergo a change secondary to the application of a connective tissue technique, the body can integrate the changes when the client uses his body. In addition, walking is one of the easiest ways to achieve this integration.

7. "Please let me know if you experience anything unusual after the treatment, especially if you have persistent pain." When a significant shift in agonist/antagonist balance occurs, the client may experience transient muscle soreness in areas other than those that were treated. This occurs because of an increased loading of antagonists, synergists, or other muscles in the kinetic chain. You should advise the client to report any postintervention soreness that is more than mild or that lasts longer than 2 days.

8. When the client presents with a history of past physical or emotional trauma, it is possible, although uncommon, for spontaneous autonomic rebalancing to accompany somatoemotional release. The facilitation of somatoemotional release requires sensitivity and presence on your part. See Chapter 2 for further discussion.

A Practice Sequence for Direct Fascial Technique

Practice Time: 45 minutes per person.

The shoulder girdle, with a focus on the arms, is a good place to begin learning direct fascial technique. Since individuals' forearms and hands are often tense, you can easily observe length changes. In addition, these changes will not affect the dynamics of the weight-bearing lower kinetic chain.

Several factors are important to keep in mind throughout the intervention:

- Use minimal lubricant.
- Contact connective tissue and apply traction to tissue layers in a horizontal direction.
- Work with a slow rate of glide, pause between strokes, and get frequent feedback from your client. Observe tissues for lengthening in addition to using palpation.
- Visually inspect the client's upper body structure.

Supine

1. Apply short fingertip strokes in several directions: over the retinacula of the wrist; repeatedly over the palmar fascia and both thenar and hypothenar eminences; and around the joints and bones of the fingers.
2. Observe the effect that this has on the entire shoulder girdle.
3. Use a broader contact surface such as your forearm, palm, or fist, on both ventral and dorsal surfaces of the client's forearm.
4. Using more specific finger or thumb contact, try to enter the space between the muscles to work on the intermuscular fascial layers. Again, observe the results.
5. Use broad and then more specific contact to treat the client's upper arms, as you did for the treatment of the forearms. Include the fascia over the deltoid, and the lateral and medial intermuscular septae.

Reassess.

Give equal treatment to the client's other arm.

To finish, apply each of the following strokes several times:

- Supine. Reach under the client to the mid-thoracic level, and then drag the tips of your flexed fingers up the erector spinae on either side of the client's spine from the mid-thorax to the occiput.

- Head turned. Use a broad surface like the heel of your hand moving anterior to posterior across the scalenes. Treat one side at a time.
- Seated with trunk flexion. Apply long descending strokes along the erector spinae with your wrist or forearm.

Visually reassess.

CAUTIONS AND CONTRAINDICATIONS

Therapists need clinical training and supervised practice to master the proper application of direct fascial technique. Advanced training may be advisable when dealing with pathological conditions. All of the general and local contraindications noted for mechanical techniques apply to the use of direct fascial technique (see Chapter 5).[5,8,10] As for all of the connective tissue techniques, there are several cautions and contraindications to the use of direct fascial technique. These include malignancy, cellulitis, fever, systemic or local infection, acute circulatory conditions, osteomyelitis, aneurysm, obstructive edema, acute rheumatoid arthritis, open wounds, sutures, hematomas, healing fractures, osteoporosis, anticoagulant therapy, advanced diabetes, and hypersensitivity of the skin.[35] In addition, therapists should use extreme caution when performing direct fascial technique in areas of flaccid paralysis, lax or unstable joints, or diseased joints that are supported by fascial "splinting." Finally, therapists should use direct fascial technique with caution and only in the nonacute stages of systemic connective tissue disorders.

Therapists need to appreciate the broader impact of direct fascial technique on the client's system as a whole. Although the force with which the therapist performs direct fascial technique is not particularly great, significant changes in the client's **myofascial balance** can occur quickly. Since the client's interwoven myofascial network demonstrates "whole-system" behavior,[3,34,35,54-61] the mechanical effects of direct fascial technique are not just local or even always predominantly local. Familiarity with fascial anatomy, as described in Myers' book *Anatomy Trains*,[56,61] can help therapists gain an understanding of how fascial work performed in one location may "travel" to affect other locations. Furthermore, this technique can produce strong autonomic effects, reflex effects, and somatoemotional release, especially when

therapists use it for long periods.[34,62] This necessitates a conservative approach, careful observation, and continuous communication with the client during the application of the technique.

In light of the effects of direct fascial technique, therapists should ensure that they are able to accurately perform a basic visual postural analysis before they begin to apply direct fascial technique during an intervention.[54,55,59,60] Furthermore, therapists learning to perform direct fascial technique should initially limit their use of this technique to less than 10 minutes in any given session and should periodically conduct at least a visual reassessment of the client. In addition, therapists should ensure that the client looks and feels "balanced" at the end of a session, especially if they have performed unilateral work around the client's legs or pelvis. Finally, therapists must strive to maintain balanced function of the client's agonist, antagonist, and synergist muscle groups and to use a rigorous analysis of possible treatment effects. Specific strategies for the extensive use of fascial techniques, such as direct fascial technique, are beyond the scope of this book and are the subject of several recent specialized texts.[56,57]

USING DIRECT FASCIAL TECHNIQUE IN TREATMENT

To Increase Fascial Extensibility

Therapists can integrate direct fascial technique with craniosacral technique and myofascial release.[1,34,35] Other massage techniques that can be used to increase connective tissue extensibility include skin rolling, friction, and probably petrissage, if it is applied slowly and with a high component of drag, as well as conventional stretches that are held for 30 seconds or longer. Self-stretching is particularly useful for client home care. Also of benefit are neuromuscular or muscle energy techniques, joint mobilization and manipulation, and spinal traction performed from the head or pelvis.[35]

In controlled laboratory conditions, the precise heating of tissue facilitates a greater elongation of collagenous structures without resulting in significant structural damage.[17,20,63] In clinical practice, however, the application of heat prior to any sustained loading of connective tissue can increase the risk of large-scale collagenous rupture. Consequently, the therapist should avoid the application of either heat or cold before performing connective tissue techniques, unless the aim is specifically to rupture or denature collagen.[63] Heat applied after the use of direct fascial technique can enhance the temporary increase in the pliability of myofascial tissue.

For Postural Conditions

Any of the techniques described in this chapter may be relevant when attempting to lengthen the areas of postural shortness. When the client experiences significant shifts in posture, postural awareness training, neuromuscular education, and movement awareness training may be of benefit.[12] The therapist may use systems of comprehensive postural awareness and movement training, such as the **Alexander technique**,[64] in these situations. Ergonomic retraining related to the client's work environment may be required. Strength training and/or endurance training is indicated for areas of postural weakness; this may be assisted by electrotherapeutic modalities such as biofeedback and electrical muscle stimulation.[12] Chronic conditions may require correction for bony asymmetry.

Friction: Evidence

DEFINITION

Friction: A repetitive, nongliding technique where a specific contact, such as the fingertips or thumb, is used to penetrate dense connective tissue and produce small movements between its fibers.

NAMES AND ORIGINS

In other massage texts, the technique we call friction is also called "transverse friction," "deep friction," "deep transverse friction," "cross-fiber friction," "Cyriax friction," and "circular friction."

Various forms of this connective tissue technique differ in the direction and the amount of force that is applied. Nevertheless, the treatment aims, clinical effects, focus of palpation, and many aspects of the manual technique are similar, whether the force is directed transverse or parallel to the fiber direction of well-defined structures, such as tendons or ligaments, or to less well-defined dense connective tissue formations such as adhesions and fibrosis.

Historically, the term "friction" has a broad, ambiguous usage that has embraced virtually any manner of rubbing between two surfaces. Some authors describe a "superficial friction" that is a fast chafing of the body's surface.[8,9] Other authors have used the term "friction" to refer to nongliding techniques that repetitively move one layer of muscle over another, which are similar to petrissage in terms of their shearing forces and clinical effects (see Chapter 9). In this text, the term "friction" is reserved for the specific connective tissue technique described in this chapter.

Therapists can apply a much less forceful version of the technique, described in this chapter, to clients with subacute orthopedic injuries as a means of preventing the formation of adhesions.

USES

Therapists use friction to increase the extensibility of connective tissue by promoting the realignment and remodeling of its constituent collagen fibers.[106] This is often required when treating adhesions associated with chronic-stage orthopedic injuries, scars, and repetitive strain injuries.

OUTCOMES AND EVIDENCE

Friction has a variety of physiological effects that are outlined in this section.[107] Friction maintains, or increases, the extensibility of connective tissue by promoting the realignment and remodeling of its constituent collagen fibers.[106] Consequently, therapists can use friction to treat any condition in which mobility may be compromised by irregular tissue remodeling that occurred during the consolidation and maturation stages of connective tissue healing. Use friction for the rehabilitation of virtually all **chronic-stage** orthopedic conditions, including sprains (with one dissenting opinion[108]), strains, fractures, and adhesive capsulitis.[106,108-116] In these situations, friction may result in maintained or increased joint range, capsular mobility, and accessory movement.[106,108,113,116-118] Opinions differ, however, regarding the effectiveness of friction in increasing the extensibility of hypertrophic scar tissue.[119,120] Cross-fiber friction has often been regarded as the manual intervention of choice for **repetitive strain injuries** such as tendinitis, tenosynovitis, bursitis, and plantar fasciitis,[106,108,121-125] in which there is ongoing microtrauma, low-grade inflammation, and tissue remodeling. By contrast, recent reviews[126,127] note a lack of evidence to support its use in the treatment of tendinitis. Finally, like many other massage techniques, application of friction may result in analgesia and transient postintervention hyperemia.[2,106,111]

HOW FRICTION MIGHT WORK

Friction may break some of the cross-links that bind adjacent collagen molecules and adjacent fibers (adhesions and fibrosis), allowing more relative movement between the fibers.[2,106] As a result, these fibers occupy more space and the matrix holds more water (hydrates). Furthermore, the tissues become more pliable, which enables them to better absorb and transmit the tensional loads caused by movement.[106] This, in turn, promotes more orderly modeling of collagen fibers in the long term, as the fibroblasts align along new lines of stress.[33] Finally, friction may also exert a long-term effect on tissue organization by stimulating fibroblast activity.[112]

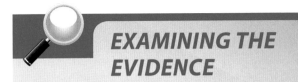

EXAMINING THE EVIDENCE

A **randomized clinical trial** compared clients' early response to two different treatment protocols for adhesive capsulitis.[116] Researchers randomized 40 clients into two treatment groups. One group received hour-long sessions, which included Cyriax deep friction massage, manipulation, active stretching, and pendulum exercises, three times a week. The other group received hour-long sessions, which included hot pack (20 minutes), short-wave diathermy (20 minutes), and similar active stretching and pendular exercises, five times a week. Both groups received the same daily home exercise program of passive range of motion and pendulum exercises. Nineteen clients in the group who received massage and 13 clients in the nonmassage group achieved 80% of full passive range of motion at the end of the second week. However, the improvement in range and decreases in pain with motion were significantly better in the massage group after the first week of treatment. This study focused specifically on early responses to the two methods, so the researchers' lack of follow-up is understandable. One limitation is that the authors give no information, beyond a reference to Cyriax, about the methods they used during the 40-minute treatments of friction and manipulation. While the protocol the authors described for this promising treatment certainly allows for therapist discretion, it is too vague for therapists to reproduce.

Guler-Uysal F, Kozanoglu E. Comparison of the early response to two methods of rehabilitation in adhesive capsulitis. *Swiss Med Wkly.* 2004;134:353-358.

Friction: Practice

COMPONENTS OF FRICTION

Friction has the following components:

Contact: Reinforced finger(s), thumb, knuckle, and olecranon

Pressure: Light to heavy, depending on the location of lesion

Tissues engaged: Dense connective tissue (ligament, tendon, fascia, extraneous deep connective tissue, scar tissue, or fibrosis in muscle)

Direction: Strokes lie in a plane parallel to the body's surface. Currently, therapists most commonly use friction across fibers for ligaments and tendons. Nevertheless, circular friction may be useful, and parallel friction was common in the past.

Amplitude/length: Short; 1 to 2 cm

Rate: Slow; 1 Hz is recommended, 2 Hz is maximum

Duration: 30 seconds, up to a maximum of 15 minutes delivered in shorter segments

Intergrades with: Petrissage, specific compression, and direct fascial technique

Context: May be performed alone. Another option is to precede friction with regional petrissage, myofascial release, or direct fascial technique. You can follow friction with superficial effleurage and passive or active stretches. Apply a cold pack afterward only if overtreatment has occurred.

PALPATION PRACTICE

As time allows

1. Locate and thoroughly palpate from end to end the following ligaments: three lateral and one medial ankle ligaments, and the collateral ligaments of the knee and elbow. Ask your partner if he or she has ever sprained any of these ligaments. If so, compare the texture and sensitivity of the damaged and undamaged ligaments bilaterally, if possible.

2. Fully stretch each ligament listed in step 1. Palpate the ligament again in this stretched position.

3. Locate and thoroughly palpate from end to end the following tendons: Achilles, tendons of biceps femoris and quadriceps femoris, the four tendons that make up the rotator cuff, the two tendons of biceps brachii, the two "common" tendons at the elbow, and the "snuffbox" tendons at the wrist. Ask your partner if he or she has ever had tendinitis at any of these sites. If so, compare the texture and sensitivity of the damaged and undamaged tendons (bilaterally, if possible).

4. Fully stretch each tendon listed in step 3. Palpate the tendon again in this stretched position.

5. Resist a midrange isometric contraction of the muscle(s) attached to each tendon listed in step 3.

MANUAL TECHNIQUE

Figures 10-24 to 10-31 show therapists applying friction to the various regions of the body.[106,108-111] The order of the figures is from head to foot in supine and then in prone. Each figure illustrates most of the guidelines for manual technique outlined here:

1. Prior to performing friction, clip or file your nails so that they are very short (at least 2 mm shorter than the end of your fingertips).
2. No oil is required. If oil is present, remove it using alcohol or witch hazel to prevent slippage.

FIGURE 10-24 To expose the supraspinatus tendon for friction, the client's arm is extended, adducted, and internally rotated. The insertions of the tendons of the rotator cuff muscles lie beneath the thick, coarse-fibered deltoid muscle. Lesions in the rotator cuff muscles are located using the client's response to deep palpation.

3. Position the body segment you will be treating so that there is enough tension in the target tissues for the force of the friction to be isolated to it without affecting the surrounding normal tissues.[99,106,108,110,111] Target tissues are exact portions of the ligament or tendon that are too dense, not the overlying or adjacent tissues. If the target tissues are slack, the contact surface will tend to slide over them, and the force of the friction will fall on adjacent healthy tissue and cause inflammation there. On the other hand, if the target tissues are overstretched, they become hard to penetrate. A useful rule of thumb is that the more superficial the tissue, the more stretch that should be exerted on the body segment. For example, if the lesion is in a synovial sheath, place the related tendon on the fullest tolerable stretch. For ligaments, use a position between neutral and a full stretch, depending on the desired depth for the friction (Figure 10-26). For tendons, use a position between partial and full stretch. If the lesion is deep in the muscle, slacken the superficial tissues to allow access to the lesion. Finally, the degree of stretch that is most effective can also vary with the hardness of the target tissue (Figures 10-24, 10-27, and 10-30).
4. Use focused and specific contact. Usually this involves holding some combination of the first three digits together tightly and reinforcing them. You can reinforce on top of the index finger with the middle finger, or you can reinforce the index finger between your thumb and third digits (Figures 10-26,10-27).

FIGURE 10-25 Lesions in the common extensor tendon ("tennis elbow") can develop anywhere between the tenoperiosteal and musculotendinous junctions. The therapist must pretreat local trigger points and avoid damaging the radial nerve with the friction.

FIGURE 10-26 Friction to the medial collateral ligament of the knee. The knee is positioned to exert a moderate stretch on the ligament. Friction for sprains should be given at the maximum allowable flexion and extension.[77]

ONLINE VIDEO

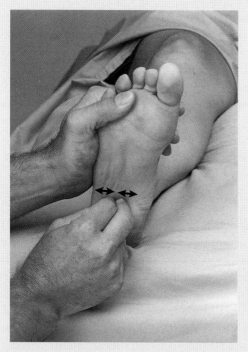

FIGURE 10-27 The foot must be dorsiflexed when applying friction to the dense plantar fascia, particularly when treating plantar fasciitis. If digital contact is difficult for the client to tolerate, precede the use of friction with a more general stroke such as kneading.

FIGURE 10-29 The tendinous slips of iliocostalis thoracis are prone to become "ropy" or "stringy" due to chronic inflammation, especially if a client is hyperkyphotic. This local lack of tissue resilience can be improved with friction.

When the lesion is deep or large and requires the use of body weight to access it, substitute the olecranon process for your fingers (Figure 10-30). When the target tissues are very dense and hard, a wooden or plastic T-bar may be necessary (see Figure 9-63). Regardless of the contact surface that you use,

FIGURE 10-28 The therapist should differentiate the fibrosis commonly found at the lower attachment of the levator scapulae from a trigger point before treating it with friction.

FIGURE 10-30 This friction of the hamstring just distal to its attachment on the ischial tuberosity begins with deep specific compression on the tendon using the therapist's body weight and the elbow. The therapist then uses the client's lower leg to internally and externally rotate the femur in order to control the cross-fiber movement between the contact surface and the target tissue.

FIGURE 10-31 The first two fingers of the therapist's right hand contact the pes anserinus. Controlled movement of the contact surface over the bursa or tendinous insertions can be accomplished easily by flexing and extending the client's knee.

frequent change of contact surfaces will reduce the likelihood of repetitive strain.

5. Do not glide over the client's skin. Your hand does not move in relation to any of the tissues that are superficial to the target tissue because these tissues move with your hand. The aim of friction is to penetrate dense, immobile connective tissue with your fingertips and then to make small motions that move one part of the target tissue with respect to another. This is like using your fingertips to tease apart the fibers of a tightly wound ball of string. It requires good palpation skills and very careful control of pressure.

6. Begin by working on the most superficial layer of the connective tissue that needs remodeling. If the problem is superficial, this may not require much pressure. If, however, the lesion is located beneath the layers of muscle, you may need to use some bodyweight, even after first softening the intervening tissues (Figures 10-29, and 10-30).

7. Use short strokes (<2 cm) to move the superficial part of the target tissues back and forth over the deeper part. Do not slip off or bump over the target tissues since this may damage adjacent healthy tissue. Although Cyriax[110,111] suggests applying friction with

"sufficient sweep," using short strokes will improve your control. If the target tissue is less than 2 cm across, you can cover it with one stroke (Figures 10-24 to 10-26). If it is more than 2 cm across, you will need to use two or more strokes side-by-side.

8. The direction of the stroke is typically across fibers when treating the ligament, tendon, or muscle. When treating fascia or scar tissue where the collagen has a less regular organization, you can alternate directions or use a circular stroke.

9. Therapists typically apply friction at a rate of one to two cycles per second.[106] Two cycles per second is the maximum rate for an experienced therapist working on a superficial lesion. A more modest rate of one cycle per second is effective, facilitates palpation, and reduces the possibility of overtreatment.

10. Maintain contact with the same tissue layer while you perform the friction until a palpable softening of that tissue occurs or for 2 minutes, whichever comes first.

11. Take frequent breaks of several seconds to change the contact surfaces. Take care to locate the lesion accurately and to re-establish a similar depth of friction once you reinitiate treatment.

12. If the client gives positive feedback (see the Communication with the Client section), you can increase pressure to engage a deeper layer of the target tissue or shift very slightly to an adjacent area and then perform another cycle of friction.

13. If the lesion is located on a limb, it may be easier for you to maintain static specific compression on the target tissue with one hand, while moving the client's limb with the other to produce the required motion between the target tissue and your hand (Figures 10-30 and 10-31). This technique is often more tolerable to the client.

14. Depending on the client's feedback about the level of comfort, you can apply friction to one area for a maximum of 6 minutes in the first intervention.[106] You can increase the duration by increments of 2 or 3 minutes per session,[106] with an upper limit (rarely required) of 15 to 20 minutes.[106,108]

THERAPIST'S POSITION AND MOVEMENT

1. Use the basic positions described in Chapter 6.
2. Effective friction demands a careful use of the therapist's body weight. Do not rely on hand and arm strength alone, except when treating small, superficial

lesions. In a standing or seated controlled lean position, you can hold your hand and arm stable and use a slight rocking of the body to produce sufficient force and the required movement of the contact surface.

3. Use of your elbow in standing or seated controlled lean demands skilled **proprioceptive palpation** (Figure 10-30).

PALPATE

As you perform the technique, palpate the client's skin and tissues for the following:

1. Contours. Chronic orthopedic injuries often appear to be "swollen" or enlarged. Soft (fluid-filled) edema cannot, however, be present when you apply friction.
2. Density or hardness of the target tissue. Compare the target tissues with healthy tissue that is adjacent or on the opposite side to form an impression of what normal bulk and texture are for that individual.
3. Fiber direction. Note the fiber direction of discrete structures such as tendon or ligament prior to treatment.
4. Location of target tissue. You must accurately locate the desired target tissue throughout the application of friction.
5. Softening of tissue. Taut bands or hardened slabs of tissue may soften as a result of rehydration of the ground substance or rupture of collagen fibrils. A reduction of tenderness and improvement of the client's key symptoms should accompany this palpable softening.
6. Reduction of hypertrophy. A single session of friction can reduce hypertrophied structures.
7. Resistance to stretch. The resistance to stretch both the contractile and noncontractile tissues should decline as treatment progresses.

OBSERVE

As you perform the technique, observe the quality of the target tissue and for signs of the client's comfort. The following signs may signal this:

1. Surface contours reflect the bulk, tautness, and hardness of the target tissues.
2. Reactive hyperemia. Rapid reddening of the client's skin may indicate an abrasion caused by nails that are too long.
3. Client's facial expression should reflect relaxation and comfort.

COMMUNICATION WITH THE CLIENT

Friction involves the localized application of a repetitive force to a very small area. Consequently, it presents the highest risk for producing local tissue damage of all the massage techniques. If you communicate carefully, you can avoid overtreatment and increasing inflammation. Beyond the production of a transient hyperemia, the point of friction is not to increase inflammation in already damaged tissue, although this may result from overzealous or unskilled application. You can use the following protocol, adapted from Kessler and Hertling,[106] to test the tissues and obtain frequent feedback, thereby reducing the risk of overtreatment:

1. Immediately before applying friction, test the sensitivity of the target tissues in one of two ways: with **contractile tissues**, palpate the tissues while performing resisted isometric movements; with **inert tissues**, palpate the tissues while performing a passive stretch. You can also ask the client to rate current pain on a **10-point scale** to obtain a more objective measure of how sensitive the lesion is to mechanical stress. These **key signs** provide an essential baseline for measuring progress and grading the dosage of friction applied during the session.
2. "Where is it most tender to touch?" You must use orthopedic testing to determine the structure that requires friction. However, you can use client feedback in response to palpation to identify the exact location of the lesion within the implicated structure.
3. Begin the friction at a level that the client finds tolerable, with discomfort rated at no more than 4 on a 10-point scale. The client should not demonstrate signs of pain such as inhibited breathing or grimacing or more subtle signs of sympathetic arousal. Assure the client that the initial discomfort (if any) usually declines as the friction proceeds, and direct the client to speak up right away if discomfort increases during the friction.
4. Friction can be applied for a period from 20 seconds to 2 minutes. During application, the client should report decreasing sensitivity of the target tissue; after application, the key sign should have improved. If so, another equivalent period of friction can be applied to the same (or an adjacent) area, and so on. Pressure and total duration can increase in later sessions.
5. If the tissue becomes more sensitive or reactive, discontinue the use of friction and drain the area with superficial effleurage. Consider applying a cold pack if the tissue is very sore. The next session begins the application with less pressure.

A Practice Sequence for Friction

Practice Time: 30 minutes per person.

To acquire a feel for this technique, practice around large joints where connective tissue is easily accessible. The ankle is a good choice since it is a common location of sprains and is often the site of residual fibrosis. The joint chosen for practice should show no signs of instability.

Connective tissue is remarkably tough, and a stable, healthy joint can certainly withstand up to 5 minutes of properly applied friction without showing the signs of negative effects. Respect your client's pain tolerance; do not apply friction to any given spot (for practice purposes) for more than a minute, and avoid "**endangerment sites**," such as the locations of major nerves (the radial nerve at the elbow).
Ensure that your nails are very short!

1. Begin by applying 5 minutes of petrissage to the major muscles that cross the joint (see Chapter 9). This is particularly useful when treating lesions in contractile tissue.
2. Remove residual lubricant completely.
3. Evaluate for (hypothetical) key signs using passive and/or contractile testing, and thoroughly palpate around the joint for tenderness.
4. Beginning superficially, apply friction for a minute to five or six different locations around the client's joint: on the tendon (also around the tendon), the ligament, and the retinaculum. A minute of friction is generally long enough to detect a palpable change; the tissue to which you applied friction should feel slightly spongy. If you are not sure of tissue change, do a bilateral comparison. If there is no detectable change, increase the pressure slightly and try a different location for a minute.
5. Retest key signs.
6. Have the client stretch the treated area.
7. Drain toward the regional lymph nodes with superficial effleurage or superficial lymph drainage technique.
8. Ensure that the client shows no signs of overtreatment, although it is unlikely to occur with treatment this brief.

Home Study: Superior gluteal insertions are a common site of fibrosis. Devise a comparable sequence for that area that uses knuckle or elbow contact to deliver the friction. Apply this sequence bilaterally.

CAUTIONS AND CONTRAINDICATIONS

Therapists need clinical training and supervised practice to master the proper application of friction. Advanced training may be advisable when dealing with pathological conditions. All of the general and local contraindications noted for mechanical techniques apply to the use of friction (see Chapter 5).[5] As for all of the connective tissue techniques, there are several cautions and contraindications to the use of friction. These include hemophilia, thrombus, malignancy, vascular insufficiency, cellulitis, phlebitis, fever, systemic or local infection, acute circulatory conditions, osteomyelitis, aneurysm, obstructive edema, acute rheumatoid arthritis, open wounds, sutures, hematomas, healing fractures, osteoporosis, advanced diabetes, hypersensitivity of the skin, and client's use of local or systemic analgesic, anti-inflammatory, or anticoagulant drugs (see Chapter 5).[5,8,10,35] All signs of acute inflammation such as spasm, pain at rest, heat, redness, and unconsolidated edema must be absent prior to the use of friction.[106] Therapists should not perform friction in the area of hematomas, calcifications, peripheral nerves, or fragile skin.[108] Therapists should use extreme caution when applying friction around hypermobile or unstable joints such as recurrent sprains or dislocations; in clients with systemic connective tissue disorders; and in clients with osteoporosis. Finally, the therapist should use care when applying friction in hypotonic regions or in the vicinity of active trigger points.

USING FRICTION IN TREATMENT

To Decrease Adhesions and Fibrosis and Increase Connective Tissue Extensibility

The massage techniques for increasing connective tissue extensibility include skin rolling, myofascial release, direct fascial technique, friction, and conventional stretches that are held for 30 seconds or longer. Petrissage may be appropriate when applied slowly and with a high component of drag. Self-stretching is particularly useful for client home care. Neuromuscular or muscle energy techniques, joint mobilization, joint mobilization and manipulation, and spinal traction performed from the head or pelvis may be useful depending on the situation.[35]

In controlled laboratory conditions, the precise heating of tissue facilitates a greater elongation of collagenous structures without resulting in significant structural damage.[17,20,63] In clinical practice, however, the application of heat prior to any sustained loading of connective tissue can increase the risk of large-scale collagenous rupture. Consequently, the therapist should avoid the application of either heat or cold before performing connective tissue techniques, unless his aim is specifically to rupture or denature collagen.[63] This may be the case when using friction to treat a large or dense adhesion. Heat applied after the use of friction can enhance the temporary increase in the pliability of myofascial tissue.

If the client reports increased tenderness after you apply friction, immediately apply a cold pack until vasoconstriction (blanching) occurs. Instruct the client to apply a cold pack to the area for 10 to 14 minutes at intervals for the next 24 hours.

For Contractile Lesions

For repetitive strain injuries involving muscle or tendon and for chronic-stage strains, a local application of myofascial release or direct fascial technique prior to the application of friction may reduce the need for extensive or prolonged use of friction. Preapplication of ultrasound has also been recommended.[108] Gentle pain-free passive stretch of the target tissues for 30 seconds and active movement in the pain-free range of motion can be beneficial following friction.[108] Teach the client to perform these several times a day between interventions. Instruct the client who has a repetitive strain injury to avoid aggravating activities, resistance exercise, and intensive stretching until later in the healing process. At that point, the client may engage in more aggressive stretching and strengthening. Splints, taping, and ergonomic or neuromuscular retraining may be useful in reducing repetitive strain or preventing recurrence of accident.[12]

If the client reports increased tenderness after you apply friction, immediately apply a cold pack until vasoconstriction (blanching) occurs. Instruct the client to apply a cold pack to the area for 10 to 14 minutes at intervals for the next 24 hours.

IN CONCLUSION

Connective tissue techniques have a variety of uses, therapeutic effects, and outcomes. Table 10-1 summarizes those outcomes for connective tissue techniques that are related to body structures and functions.

Table 10-1	Summary of Outcomes for Connective Tissue Techniques			
	Technique			
Outcomes	**Skin Rolling**	**Myofascial Release**	**Direct Fascial Technique**	**Friction**
Decreased resting muscle tension or neuromuscular tone	P	P	P	?
Separation/lengthening of fascia	P	√	P	P
Promotion of dense connective tissue remodeling	P	P	P	P
Increased muscle extensibility	?	√	P	P
Increased joint range of motion	P	√	√	√
Systemic sedation/decreased anxiety	?	P	√	?
Increased rib cage mobility	?	P	P	?
Decreased trigger point activity	P	√	P	P
Pain reduction	P	√	√	√
Normalized structural alignment	?	√	√	?
Balance of agonist/antagonist function	P	P	√	?
Improved quality and quantity of movement	?	P	√	P
Enhanced muscle performance	P	P	√	?

√, the outcome is supported by research summarized in this chapter; P, the outcome is possible; ?, the outcome is debatable (research results are absent or inconsistent).

REVIEW SECTION

TAKEAWAYS

1. Connective tissue techniques are those massage techniques that palpate, lengthen, and promote remodeling of connective tissue.

2. Skin rolling is a gliding stroke in which the therapist grasps the tissues superficial to the investing layer of deep fascia and continuously lifts and rolls it over underlying tissues in a wave-like motion.

3. Therapists use skin rolling to assess and treat restrictions in the mobility of the patient's skin and superficial fascia.

4. Myofascial release is a technique that combines a nongliding fascial traction with varying amounts of orthopedic stretch to produce moderate, sustained tension on the muscle and its associated fascia and that results in palpable viscoelastic lengthening or "creep."

5. Therapists use myofascial release to lengthen fascial layers, restore fascial mobility, and decrease the effects of scars and adhesions on the locomotor system. They also find it useful for treating postural conditions and the chronic after-effects of trauma.

6. Direct fascial technique is a slow, gliding technique that applies moderate, sustained tension to the superficial fascia or to the deep fascia and associated muscle. It results in palpable viscoelastic lengthening (creep).

7. Therapists use direct fascial technique to lengthen fascial layers, to restore fascial mobility, and to decrease the effects of scars and adhesions on the locomotor system. They also find it particularly useful for treating postural conditions and the chronic after-effects of trauma.

8. Friction is a repetitive, nongliding technique where a specific contact, such as the fingertips or thumb, is used to penetrate dense connective tissue and produce small movements between its fibers.

9. Therapists use friction to increase the extensibility of connective tissue by promoting the realignment and remodeling of its constituent collagen fibers.

10. The mechanical effects of connective tissue techniques are a result of the tension that this technique applies to the connective tissue in superficial fascia or the fascia associated with superficial and deep muscles. In cases of sustained tension, as during slower rates of application, this fascia probably lengthens through a controlled (minor) rupture of collagen molecules and collagen cross-links. In addition, friction may break some of the cross-links that bind adjacent collagen molecules and adjacent fibers (adhesions and fibrosis), allowing more relative movement between the fibers.

Clinical Case: *Connective Tissue Techniques*

Patient Profile

Your patient is a 30-year-old avid, accomplished recreational downhill skier who fractured his left lower tibia (a boot top fracture) 2 years ago. The fracture healed to the orthopedist's satisfaction. After cast removal, the patient completed several months of physical therapy that emphasized strength training. He returned to skiing the following season.

Clinical Findings

Subjective Findings:

- Low-grade **pain**, fatigue, and **stiffness** in the left lower leg after skiing for more than 2 hours.
- Reports that the leg "has not felt 100%" since the injury.

Objective Findings:

- Posture: Standing posture is within normal limits. The left lower leg appears to be slightly larger than the right.
- Girth: The left leg is 2 cm larger in circumference than the right leg at the level of the fracture.

- Gait: Gait is within normal limits.
- Palpation: The swelling in the region of the fraction does not feel fluid or watery. There is tenderness to deep palpation throughout the left lower leg.
- Range of Motion: Mild reduction in active and passive motion of the left ankle (10%), with stiffness at the end of range.
- Strength: Grade 5 strength throughout the lower extremities.

Treatment Approach

Despite the time that has elapsed since his injury, this patient presents with signs of chronic inflammation. Patients who have sustained a serious trauma may present with residual impairments that are associated with poor modeling of connective tissue. In this case, the initial treatment outcome is to reduce the connective tissue restriction (**consolidated edema**), which is a likely result of the inflammatory process from 2 years ago.

- You can achieve this treatment goal by using all four connective tissue techniques described in this chapter. In doing so, you will apply them from superficial layers to deep layers and focus on the patient's affected leg. You may also find it beneficial to perform specific and deep direct fascial technique and friction throughout the area of swelling and at the fracture site on the tibia. In addition, you can use deep petrissage, stripping, and specific compression to dense regions, and trigger points pressure release to any trigger points that are found throughout the region.
- If you are able to achieve therapeutic depth for these techniques, then you may need only 1 to 2 hours to restore full mobility to the patient's affected leg. Finally, you must also allot a certain portion of each session to the other leg and the back in order to maintain comparable levels of resting tension, **myofascial balance**, and symmetry.
- The patient's home care should include stretching of lower leg muscles, resumption of his prior strength training program for a couple of weeks, and *careful, incremental* increase of his skiing activity.

Critical Thinking Questions

1. Which layers of tissues are engaged by connective tissue techniques?
2. What are the primary effects of connective tissue techniques?
3. List three potential uses of myofascial release and identify a clinical condition for which these uses would be appropriate.
4. List three potential uses of skin rolling and identify a clinical condition for which these uses would be appropriate.
5. List three potential uses of direct fascial technique and identify a clinical condition for which these uses would be appropriate.
6. List three potential uses of friction and identify a clinical condition for which these uses would be appropriate.
7. Which characteristics and effects of skin rolling result in therapists sometimes classifying it as a form of petrissage?
8. What are the mechanisms for connective tissue "creep" that occurs during connective tissue techniques? Consider possible mechanical and neurological mechanisms in your response.
9. How does direct fascial technique, applied to the lumbar fascia, change the tension of the deeper fascial layers that are adjacent to the viscera?
10. How do friction and myofascial release reduce the negative effects of immobilization on connective tissue?

References for Chapter 10 begin on p. 475; see Further Reading list on p. 477.

Passive Movement Techniques

OBJECTIVES   **After studying this chapter, you will have the information that you need to do the following:**

1. Describe how the massage techniques in this category affect different types of tissues.
2. Describe each massage technique in terms of the contact surface, pressure, tissues engaged, amplitude, direction, and rate.
3. Demonstrate how to perform each massage technique and how to apply it in the context of a practice sequence.
4. Speculate about the mechanisms by which massage techniques achieve their effects.
5. Describe the outcomes of care, indications, contraindications, and common uses associated with each massage technique.

Passive movement techniques are those massage techniques that primarily palpate the movement of tissues and structures, as opposed to palpating their substance or texture. These passive motion techniques, such as shaking, rhythmic mobilization, and rocking, are also used to treat restrictions in tissues and structures. This chapter describes these techniques, how to perform them, and how to apply them in a practice sequence. It also discusses relevant outcomes and evidence, cautions and contraindications, and how to use the technique in treatment. Finally, Table 11-1 summarizes those outcomes for passive movement techniques that are related to body structures and functions. Therapists are advised to review the cautions and contraindications for these techniques and to use them as their scope of practice and skill level permit.

Shaking: Evidence

DEFINITION

Shaking: A technique that moves soft tissue—primarily muscle—back and forth repetitively over the underlying bone, with minimal joint movement.

NAMES AND ORIGINS

In other texts or massage-related systems, the technique that we call shaking is also known as "muscle shaking," "coarse vibration," "rolling friction," or "jostling."[1-8] Shaking is sometimes classified as a form of **petrissage** because both techniques focus force on skeletal muscle.[6,7] In this book, we present shaking in a separate chapter from petrissage because the method, effects, and uses differ from those discussed in Chapter 9. There is also a well-established tradition of presenting shaking as a technique in its own right.[8]

This book makes a distinction between the shaking of tissue over underlying bone, as defined earlier, and the shaking of entire structures such as the rib cage, limbs, and pelvis. The latter techniques involve the movement of joints and thus intergrade with more rigorous joint mobilization techniques (see Rhythmic Mobilization and Rocking later in this chapter). The manual techniques, effects, and uses of these other techniques are different enough to justify this distinction.

USES

Therapists use shaking to reduce "holding," which is what Mense et al.[9] call **unnecessary muscle tension**. Unnecessary muscle tension is an unintentional muscle contraction that is under voluntary control, which is often due to situational stress.[9] They also use shaking to reduce the resting muscle tension of skeletal muscles.[1,2] In addition, they often use shaking in **sports massage** because it may reduce muscle tension while enhancing **arousal** (wakefulness).[3]

OUTCOMES AND EVIDENCE

Shaking has a variety of physiological and psychological effects that are outlined in this section.[10] Traditionally, therapists reported that shaking altered resting muscle tension through the stimulation of complex proprioceptive reflexes.[1-5] They also thought that it had a relaxing effect on skeletal muscle,[1-5] except for vigorous shaking, which might temporarily and marginally increase **muscle tone** via the stretch reflex.[8] Recently, therapists have questioned whether it is possible for any passive technique, such as shaking, to substantially alter muscle tone and suggest that active techniques are far more effective in this regard.[11]

Shaking has a variety of clinical applications. First, it can be an effective approach to reducing "holding," or **unnecessary muscle tension**.[1,2] In this case, reducing "holding" may be the primary goal. On the other hand, therapists can use it as a preparatory technique to reduce unnecessary muscular tension that may interfere with the execution of a technique such as high-grade **joint mobilization**. Second, clients often regard shaking as being pleasurable. Consequently, it is a useful technique for therapists to use when they are seeking to achieve more relaxed skeletal muscle. In addition, shaking is often used in precompetition and intercompetition **sports massage** to achieve systemic arousal and enhanced awareness of the muscle and, possibly, a temporary effect on resting muscle tension.[3,12-14] Finally, shaking has minor **mechanical effects** on connective tissue.[2] When it is applied gently in the fibroplastic stage of connective tissue repair, it may facilitate orderly remodeling of connective tissue. Table 11-1 summarizes the main outcomes for shaking.

HOW SHAKING MIGHT WORK

Shaking may help clients who are holding muscles tensely in response to situational stress to realize that this contraction is unnecessary by rapidly producing changes in muscle position.[1-5] In addition, the spreading and **shearing** of muscle that happens during shaking may cause proprioceptive input that reduces resting tension.[2,3,5] A similar mechanism occurs for petrissage.

EXAMINING THE EVIDENCE

It is difficult to locate studies that evaluate the effects of shaking as an independent technique. Moreover, shaking is not often included in trials of massage that incorporate several techniques. A small study[15] ($n = 14$) examined the effect on **delayed-onset muscle soreness** (DOMS) of a 30-minute sports massage sequence, which included shaking, that therapists performed 2 hours after eccentric exercise. Trend analysis showed significantly less DOMS, lower creatine kinase levels, and a higher neutrophil count for the massage group compared with the control group, who received a treatment consisting of the application of lubricant followed by 30 minutes of rest. The authors make interesting speculations regarding how massage might affect DOMS. This otherwise well-conceived study

is hampered by its small sample. It also illustrates a common methodological quandary in massage research: How much discretion in applying the treatment protocol should researchers give the treating therapists? In this case, researchers specified a fairly rigid sequence that was typical of those used to treat athletes after exercise. This protocol did not allow the therapist much freedom to adapt to each person's presenting issues, as usually happens in practice.

Smith LL, Keating MN, Holbert D, et al. The effects of athletic massage on delayed onset muscle soreness, creatine kinase, and neutrophil count: a preliminary report. *J Orthop Sports Phys Ther.* 1994;19:93–99.

Shaking: Practice

COMPONENTS OF SHAKING

Shaking has the following components:

Contact: Firm but superficial grasp of the muscle or muscles to be shaken. Use variable levels of fingertip contact depending on the depth of the muscle to be shaken and the desired degree of stimulation.

Pressure: Light to moderate. Avoid constant heavy manual pressure since it dampens the wave of motion that is produced through tissues.

Tissues engaged: Hands engage tissues to the depth of the superficial muscle layers. The motion produced by the stroke simultaneously engages all the tissues throughout the muscle group that you are shaking, including muscle, fascia, tendon, ligament, and periosteum.

Direction: Direct your force around the circumference of the long axis of the muscle or muscle group. As a result, the motion produced by the stroke will travel in waves along this long axis.

Amplitude: Depends on the region

Rate: 2 to 5 cycles per second

Duration: 5 seconds or longer

Intergrades with: Fine vibration

Combines with: You can apply broad and specific compression at the same time as shaking. At this point, because of the combination of compression and

(nongliding) movement, it becomes a technique that resembles, although technically is not identical to, **petrissage**, which combines compression and gliding movement.

Context: It can be alternated with other techniques presented in this chapter in interventions that focus solely on movement. You can also alternate this technique with the **neuromuscular techniques** described in Chapter 9.

PALPATION PRACTICE

1. Review regional myology as time permits by drawing the major skeletal muscles on a partner. Palpate the fiber directions, borders, and tendons of all superficial muscles.
2. Assess resting muscle tension through palpation. Attempt to describe the quality of resistance to pressure in detail (see Chapter 4). When the muscle it is at rest, what do muscle, fascia, fat, and fluid contribute to the firmness of each muscle that you feel? Use the discussion in Chapter 4 for assistance.
3. Grasp the long muscle groups of your partner's legs and arms and attempt to roll them around the bones to which they attach. How far do they go? At the limit of each muscle group's excursion, release the limb and watch the resulting motion as the tissues move back to their original position.

MANUAL TECHNIQUE

Figures 11-1 to 11-8 show therapists applying shaking to the various regions of the body. The order of the figures is from head to foot in supine and then in prone. Each figure illustrates most of the guidelines for the manual technique outlined below.

1. Shaking muscle over underlying bone can have a psychologically sedative or **stimulating** effect depending on the contact and rate of application therapists use when they are performing the technique.

   A. For **sedation**: Use an even, relaxed, full palmar contact and a slower rate. Your hand contact is flat on the flatter surfaces of the client's body (Figures 11-1 and 11-4). In this case, a relaxed hand contact that produces minimal tissue compression will produce the greatest tissue excursion. Arch your hand slightly for curved surfaces of the client's body, since this will lift the client's tissues into your palm (Figures 11-3 and 11-5). The client should perceive the pressure as being evenly distributed over the entire contact surface. For each stroke, lift the client's tissues and then allow them to drop under their own weight. Maintain hand contact so that the strokes are connected. It takes practice to perform this technique with the full, comfortable contact that will allow you to apply it for longer periods.

   B. For stimulation: Focus your contact more specifically on your thumb and fingertips (Figure 11-6).

FIGURE 11-1 This superficial shaking of the abdomen does not cause movement of the pelvis or spine (compare with Figure 11-12). All types of abdominal shaking can be useful for constipation.

FIGURE 11-3 When shaking the deltoid, first lift the arm off the table to permit free movement of the client's tissues. If a client involuntary tenses her arm, draw her awareness to the tension and wait until the shoulder relaxes before beginning the shaking.

FIGURE 11-2 Two-handed shaking of the entire thigh with the knee flexed. Hands work together, rolling the tissue around the bone, first one way and then back to, and past, resting position. You can add varying amounts of compression to produce a more forceful and stimulating stroke.

FIGURE 11-4 During shaking of the superficial tissues and muscles of the back, the two hands can be moved in the same, or in opposite, directions.

ONLINE VIDEO

FIGURE 11-7 Shaking the calf.

FIGURE 11-5 Shaking of the gluteals can be done one-handed or two-handed and can simultaneously include the proximal hamstrings. Each hand shakes cross-fiber.

Grasp the client's tissues with more pressure and increase the rate. In addition, make a continuous effort to move the tissues back and forth, rather than allowing gravity or the **elastic recoil** of the tissue to perform the return stroke.

FIGURE 11-8 This two-handed "rolling" technique for the calf is also possible in supine (position as in Figure 11-2).

FIGURE 11-6 One-handed shaking of the adductors of the thigh in prone. You may release and regrasp or you may maintain a loose grasp while shaking the client's limb and gliding distally to the knee (arrow).

2. Let your wrist(s) remain relaxed as you move your hand(s) back and forth rhythmically. When you are on the client's limbs, move your hands perpendicularly to the long axis of the limb to produce waves of

tissue motion that travel along, or parallel to, the long axis of the limb.

3. To achieve movement throughout a region, use a lighter contact and slide your hands along the region as you perform shaking (Figures 11-6 and 11-7). Alternatively, you can release your hand contact every few seconds, move your hands to a new position in the region, and establish a new hand contact. Changing hand positions every few seconds can reduce hand strain. This strategy also results in a stroke that the client may perceive as being more pleasant and less "machine-like."

4. Bear in mind that when you perform shaking with two hands, you will produce differing results when you use different approaches to coordinating the movement of your hands (Figures 11-2, 11-5, and 11-8).

5. "Rolling," or "rolling friction,"[4] is a useful two-handed version of shaking that you can perform on the client's limbs. Begin by resting your hands on opposite sides of the client's limb. Both of your hands will work together to roll the client's tissues around the circumference of the long axis of the limb, using the same motion as you would if you were rolling the cylinder of a rolling pin around its core. Then, reverse the direction of movement of your hands, rolling the tissue back to, and then past, its original position. Repeat these two motions in a rhythmic manner (Figures 11-2 and 11-8).

6. You can combine shaking with neuromuscular techniques by compressing into the client's tissues, or gripping and lifting these tissues, before beginning the shaking motion.

THERAPIST'S POSITION AND MOVEMENT

1. Use **standing aligned posture** and the other basic positions described in Chapter 6. You can avoid producing a choppy, irritating stroke by keeping your wrist, elbows, and shoulders relaxed.

2. When you are performing shaking for longer than 30 seconds, you can maintain a relaxed posture by periodically standing back to shake out your arms and hands briefly.

PALPATE

While performing the technique, palpate the client's skin and tissues for the following:

1. The local skin temperature and texture.

2. The tone of the client's superficial muscles and tissues. Focus shaking strokes on tissues that are tense or hypertonic.

3. The excursion of the tissue that you are shaking. Try to form an impression of how far and how easily the tissues move during the application of the technique. In particular, identify how loose, dense, or tight the tissues feel under your hand and how this relates to the motion of the tissues. Very dense or tight tissues may require more subtle shaking movement in the beginning. Loose tissue may suggest a toning stroke as opposed to one that may reduce tone.

4. Resistance to tissue movement. Note whether there is excessive resistance as you initiate the stroke. In addition, note whether you can relate the resistance to movement to a specific tissue or structure that is involved in producing the motion of the stroke. For example, an adhesion at the proximal hamstring attachment can have a visible and palpable effect on the motion of the entire hamstring muscle during shaking.

5. The rhythmic response or **cadence** of the client's tissues during the stroke. Often, there is a rate and amplitude of shaking that the client finds the most pleasant. This varies with the person, body structure, level of muscle tone, region, and the type of shaking that you are using. It is critical, especially if sedation is the desired effect, to palpate for this optimal cadence and communicate with the client in order to adjust the rate and amplitude of the stroke to the client's needs.

6. The depth of penetration of the effect of the stroke. As the client's muscles relax and the tone and **viscosity** of the tissues decreases, the same force will produce effects deeper into and further along the client's tissues. Consequently, as with petrissage, you will not need to apply greater force to achieve a greater penetration of effects; simply apply the technique for a longer duration.

OBSERVE

As you perform the technique, observe the client to evaluate the degree of muscle movement you have achieved and to ensure that the **draping** maintains privacy. The following signs may signal this.

1. The degree of muscle movement. Movement of the client's muscles will be visibly less within areas of connective tissue hardening and elevated resting muscle

tension. Even in normal tissue, movement will vary with different body shapes, proportions of body fat, and levels of conditioning.

2. Inappropriate draping. Since extended shaking can loosen draping, you may need to adjust or retuck a loosened drape to maintain discreet coverage of the client's body.

COMMUNICATION WITH THE CLIENT

Communicate to ensure the client's comfort during the application of shaking. Here are some examples of statements that you can use.

1. "Is this pressure comfortable?" Alternatively, offer the client a choice: "Which feels better, this … or this?" This will enable you to ensure that your hand contact is comfortable for the client.

2. "Would it feel more relaxing if I slowed down a bit … like this?" Determine whether the rate and rhythm are comfortable for the client.

3. "Is everything okay?" "Are you feeling anything unusual?" When you are applying shaking continuously for longer than 2 minutes, find out whether the client is experiencing unpleasant symptoms of a sympathetic response such as irritation or nausea.

4. "Is this causing pain anywhere?" Use this statement periodically to check whether the client perceives that the intervention is causing pain. When the client presents with spasm or inflammation, the application of shaking to a distant area may result in pain by producing small motions at a distance from the area of spasm or inflammation.

A Practice Sequence for Shaking

Practice time: 15 to 30 minutes per person or longer.

This sequence for anterior and posterior aspects of the legs uses no oil. You can easily perform it through loose clothes or draping, although the techniques are somewhat easier to apply on bare skin.

There are two basic ways of approaching movement sequences. One is to perform each technique in the sequence once for a longer period of time. An alternative, which tends to reduce therapist fatigue and tension, is to introduce all movements quickly, and then alternate frequently from one technique to the next, repeating the sequence as time permits. Strive for smooth continuous motion, without breaks between the various moves. Explore each motion and the infinite number of variations that are possible.

Supine

1. With one-hand contact, shake the quadriceps over the femur. Alternate your hands to reduce fatigue, and focus the technique more to the medial or lateral segment of the quadriceps. Move or slide the point of contact along the full length of the muscle group.

2. With your inner (table-side) hand, shake the adductors from their midpoint and distally.

3. Flex the client's knee to 90°, sit on the foot (wrapped in the bottom sheet), and with two hands, contact the thigh on its medial and lateral surfaces. Shake the tissues of the thigh back and forth repeatedly around the femur.

4. With the leg in the same position, grasp the calf with one hand and shake it while gliding your hand distally. Use whole-hand and fingertip contacts. Repeat.

5. With the leg in the same position, contact the medial and lateral surfaces of the calf with your entire hand. Shake the tissues of the calf back and forth repeatedly around the tibia and fibula. Repeat this sequence two or more times.

Turn the client to prone.

Prone

1. Shake the gluteals over the pelvis with one of your hands, changing your hand positions to cover the entire muscle. Shake the gluteals with two hands, moving your hands toward each other, and then apart, in contrary motion.

2. Flex the client's knee by placing one or two pillows under the ankle. Shake the hamstrings along their length with one hand and with two hands, in contrary motion.

3. With your inner (table-side) hand, shake the adductors from their midpoint and distally.

4. Rest the client's ankle on your toweled shoulder and roll the muscles of the posterior compartment between your palms.

5. Flex the knee to 90°, grasp the heel and ankle, and shake the entire foot.

6. Repeat this sequence two or more times.

Home study: Devise a comparable supine and prone sequence for the arm.

CAUTIONS AND CONTRAINDICATIONS

Therapists need clinical training and supervised practice to master the proper application of shaking. Advanced training may be advisable when dealing with pathological conditions. All of the general and local contraindications noted for massage techniques apply to the use of shaking (see Chapter 5). In particular, therapists should avoid shaking any muscle that contains an acute injury, or crosses an acutely injured bone or joint, even if their hand position is remote from the site of injury. They can introduce less vigorous shaking at later stages, provided they can perform it without causing the client pain. In addition, they should consider shaking a contraindication when the client exhibits spasm, hyperreflexia, or **spasticity**.

USING SHAKING IN TREATMENT

To Reduce Unnecessary Muscle Tension

First, focus the client's attention on an identified area of unnecessary muscle tension. Encourage deep breathing, relaxation, and a feeling of "letting go." Clients may find simple visual images like "melting" or more complex guided imagery scripts[16] useful. Other manual techniques that move the client's body in space, such as rhythmic mobilization, rocking, joint mobilization, and passive relaxed movement, may assist the client in recognizing and releasing patterns of unnecessary muscle tension. Give the client positive feedback when he or she has released tension, since the client may not recognize that this has happened.

For homecare, you can instruct the client to self-administer shaking to accessible areas of the body, such as the arms and legs, and to perform active shaking movements to achieve muscle relaxation and facilitate ease of motion.[17] As an adjunct to the latter, suggest the use of any effective breathing and relaxation methods that are familiar to the client.[16]

To Enhance Arousal (Wakefulness)

You can use shaking with other massage techniques that tend to wake clients quickly such as fast fingertip superficial stroking, fine vibration, and percussion. Commercially available machines can produce the latter two techniques. Brief cold, contrast hydrotherapy, and rubbing the skin with coarse cloth, bristle brushes, or salt also enhance arousal.[18]

In Pre- and Intercompetition Sports Massage

Therapists use this type of massage on the day of competition and, possibly, immediately before the event and vary how they use it depending on the sport and the athlete. In general, they avoid using deeper techniques close to the time of competition.[3] Alternate shaking and rhythmic mobilization with broad-contact compression, light petrissage, percussion, stretching, and a passive range of motion. Keep sessions short (10 to 20 minutes for all included regions), maintain a fast tempo (70 to 90 Hz), and focus on the most important muscle groups the client will be using in the activity.

Rhythmic Mobilization: Evidence

DEFINITION

Rhythmic mobilization: A technique that repetitively moves entire structures, resulting in the movement of soft tissue over bone and the movement of the related joints and internal organs.

NAMES AND ORIGINS

In some texts or massage-related systems, the technique that we call rhythmic mobilization is also known as "shaking." These rhythmic mobilizations are less specific and the contact is determined by comfort of movement, not by the specific tissues being treated. This is in contrast with shaking, where the therapist makes direct contact with the relevant tissues and shakes them manually. Similar relaxed approaches to passive movement are featured prominently in the work of the American physician Milton Trager (**Trager Method of Psychophysical Integration**)[19,20] and the British osteopath **Eyal Lederman** (Harmonic Technique).[21]

Rhythmic mobilization involves the repetitive passive movement of entire structures—usually a limb, a segment of a limb, or the limb girdle—and all of the tissues that the treated body segment contains. At times, rhythmic mobilization may resemble **passive relaxed movements** or **joint play** or **joint mobilization** techniques, both of which other textbooks cover extensively. The techniques of rhythmic mobilization are, however, less specific than joint mobilization or passive relaxed movements. For example, when therapists are treating areas around synovial joints with rhythmic mobilization, they do not attempt to isolate movement to anatomical planes, the joint capsule, or even to a single joint. A single movement by the therapist may result in simultaneous movements from several joints in a **kinetic chain**. Additionally, you can perform the movements in the midrange, rather than through the full osteokinematic range of the joint you are treating.

USES

Therapists use rhythmic mobilization to help a client voluntarily release unnecessary muscle tension, to reduce resting muscle tension, to prepare a client for joint mobilization or **passive range of motion** techniques, and to give precompetition massage to athletes. This technique may also cause passive joint motion that may help to mobilize stiff joints, stimulate joint healing, enhance a client's joint awareness, and mobilize bronchial secretions.[22-28] When therapists apply rhythmic mobilization skillfully, it can have a calming, soothing effect.[21]

OUTCOMES AND EVIDENCE

Rhythmic mobilization has a variety of physiological and psychological effects that are outlined in this section. Some of the clinical indications and **outcomes** for rhythmic mobilization are similar to those for shaking, described earlier in this chapter. Like shaking, therapists can use rhythmic mobilization to reduce holding and muscle tension, to prepare the client for joint mobilization or a passive range of motion techniques, and in precompetition preparation for athletes. Since rhythmic mobilization results in passive joint motion, it may produce some of the effects of more rigorous passive range exercises such as the mobilization of stiff joints, the stimulation of joint healing, and neuromuscular re-education.[22-27] The repeated approximation and distraction of the joint surfaces that occur during the application of this technique may be used to enhance a client's joint awareness.[28] When it is used in the context of **Trager Psychophysical Integration**, rhythmic mobilization may also be of use in the treatment of headache,[29] chronic pain,[30,31] and neurological conditions that alter movement patterns such as cerebral palsy, muscular dystrophy, and multiple sclerosis.[31] Rhythmic mobilization of the rib cage ("shaking"), alternated with rapid repeated compression, percussion ("cupping" or "clapping"), and postural drainage, is a standard intervention for mobilizing bronchial secretions in chest physical therapy (see Chapter 12). Finally, rhythmic mobilization may stimulate vestibular reflexes and result in a generalized decrease in overall postural tone, decreased arousal, and a calming, soothing effect.[11,28] Table 11-1 summarizes the main outcomes for rhythmic mobilization.

HOW RHYTHMIC MOBILIZATION MIGHT WORK

There are multiple mechanisms for the effects of rhythmic mobilization. The compression and release of soft tissue that accompanies rhythmic mobilization may produce modest increases in **lymphatic and venous return** by squeezing vessels with valves. The rhythmic deformation of joint capsules moves synovial fluid through the capsule and facilitates joint nutrition and healing.[1-5] Stimulation of joint afferents[11] enhances joint awareness. In addition, when therapists apply mobilization to the rib cage, it can physically shake and move mucus to a point where the client may be able to cough it out.[8] Sedative effects of mobilization[5] may be due to **entrainment** to rhythm, which is a shift in the autonomic nervous system toward **parasympathetic** function that may occur with certain kinds of rhythmic sensory stimulation (see discussion and references in Chapter 7). Finally, **vestibular reflexes** that are stimulated by rhythmic mobilization may cause a generalized decrease in overall postural tone.[2,5]

EXAMINING THE EVIDENCE

Gentle, unforced, meditative, rhythmic mobilization and rocking are central to the method of Trager Psychophysical Integration. This small clinical trial tested the effect of 20 minutes of Trager on the EMG responses to passive movement in clients with Parkinson's disease, which were considered an indication of **rigidity**.[32] The sample of 30 clients was divided into four subgroups who were assigned to one of four treatment conditions that varied in terms of the treatment position (seated or supine) and the location of treatment (on the more rigid or less rigid side of the body). There was no control group, and the authors did not describe their process for assigning subjects to the groups. The authors observed a decrease in stretch responses immediately after treatment, and this decrease was still evident 11 minutes later. This effect was largest when the researchers applied the intervention with the client in supine and least when it was applied with the client seated. This research is promising. The authors discuss the study's limitations, such as the need for a longer monitoring period after treatment and the need to relate EMG results to a clinical assessment of rigidity. Hopefully, they will complete further studies with greater numbers of subjects and suitable control groups.

Duval C, Lafontaine D, Hèbert J, Leroux A, Panisset M, Boucher JP. The effect of Trager therapy on the level of evoked stretch responses in patients with Parkinson's disease and rigidity. *J Manipulative Physiol Ther.* 2002;25:455–464.

Rhythmic Mobilization: Practice

COMPONENTS OF RHYTHMIC MOBILIZATION

Rhythmic mobilization has the following components:

Contact: Whole palmar surface of one or both hands with your hands as relaxed as possible

Pressure: Moderate. Enough to securely lift or move the body segment.

Tissues engaged: Your hands engage tissues to the depth of the superficial muscle layers. The motion produced by the stroke simultaneously engages all of the joint tissues and soft tissues in the region that you are mobilizing.

Direction: Varies with the region you are treating. Often you repeatedly lift or move a body segment and allow it to drop or settle under the force of gravity.

Amplitude: Depends on the region

Rate: 0.5 to 2 seconds per cycle

Duration: 5 seconds or longer

Intergrades with: Shaking, passive range of motion, joint mobilization, and manual traction

Combines with: Combine with broad-contact compression and muscle squeezing

Context: In interventions that focus solely on movement, you can alternate it with other techniques presented in this chapter. This technique often precedes or follows neuromuscular techniques such as those described in Chapter 9.

PALPATION PRACTICE

1. For each of your partner's extremity joints, perform and measure passive range of motion (the osteokinematic or angular motions at the joint). Explore the quality of the resistance to further movement that you feel at the end of the range.

2. While performing passive range of motion, have your partner alternately tense slightly and relax different muscle groups without warning you. Ensure that you can detect "holding" of skeletal muscles. This exercise works better when you are blindfolded.

3. Attempt to produce pendular motions at extremity joints; the knee and elbow work well. Apply a force in one direction once, and then let your partner's body segment oscillate at its own frequency. Determine the frequency with which the limb oscillates and measure the time for the motion to stop. Compare frequencies and rates of decay at different joints. Compare the frequency and rate of decay at the same joint for different partners. How does your partner's body type influence these parameters?

MANUAL TECHNIQUE

Figures 11-9 to 11-17 show therapists applying rhythmic mobilization to the various regions of the body. The order of the figures is from head to foot in supine and then in prone. Each figure illustrates most of the guidelines for manual technique outlined here.

1. Use a hand contact that is comfortable for both you and your client. Ensure that this contact is relaxed, and use as much of your hand as possible (Figures 11-9 to 11-17). Your hand position for optimal manual

FIGURE 11-11 Shaking of the entire hand can be vigorous. The illustrated contact allows the therapist to control the flexion/extension movement at the client's wrist.

contact will vary with the region you are treating, the size of the client, and your size.

2. Strive to maintain an uninterrupted rhythmic flow of movement, even when you are switching positions and techniques.

3. Since rhythmic mobilization has widely distributed **mechanical effects**, it can easily become too stimulating

FIGURE 11-9 Rhythmic settling of the shoulders. Depress the client's shoulder girdle and then allow the shoulders to rebound passively while maintaining hand contact. If the hands depress the shoulders simultaneously, the shoulders bounce up and down. If the hands alternately depress the shoulders, a lateral rocking results.

FIGURE 11-10 Gentle traction, which the therapist produces by leaning backward, precedes longitudinal shaking of the arm. Perform this technique in the same manner as shaking a rope along its length. Do it gently and do not sustain it beyond one or two movements before releasing traction and reapplying. You can apply a similar technique to the leg.

FIGURE 11-12 Here, the rectus abdominis is gently gathered and lifted off the deeper muscles with a soft, broad contact. The hands maintain this contact, using it to sway the client's abdomen back and forth slowly.

FIGURE 11-13 The thigh is lifted and then allowed to fall rhythmically (dotted line). The hands can slide distally to deliver the lifting force to the lower leg as well.

FIGURE 11-15 "Tossing" the shoulder rhythmically and repetitively. Maintain contact as the client's shoulders are allowed to fall back to the table under their own weight (dotted line). You may use a gentle force to distract the shoulder as it is being lifted.

for the client. Consequently, you should aim to perform the technique with a relaxed tempo that will produce reflex sedation. This requires that you maintain contact throughout the motion, while allowing the freest excursion of movement of the body segment you are treating.

4. The variety of possible rhythmic movements is limited only by your imagination. Here are some examples of these variations.

   A. To mobilize an entire limb from its distal end, with the client in prone or supine: Assume a very comfortable two-handed grip on the client's wrist or ankle. Simultaneously exert a gentle, long-axis **traction** on the client's limb and lift it so that it clears the table. Then, immediately perform one or two gentle whipping motions, using the same motion used to initiate vertical waves along a rope. The client's limb will look and feel like a weighted rope during this maneuver, provided you are using neither too much

FIGURE 11-14 Wrists and hands remain loose while rolling the client's entire foot briskly between the hands (two to three cycles per second). This pleasant stroke is a gentle, effective way to rouse sleeping clients.

FIGURE 11-16 Swinging the dependent arm in prone: rhythmic passive internal and external rotation performed in the midrange of abduction.

FIGURE 11-17 Rolling the dependent forearm between the hands. Hand contact slides proximally and distally on the forearm to focus the movement on different areas.

nor too little traction (Figure 11-10). Release the traction on the limb between repetitions of this technique.

B. For proximal limb segments such as the entire shoulder, with the client in prone or supine, or the thigh, with the client in supine: Position your hands between the client's limb and the table. Lift the client's limb segment and let it drop (Figures 11-13 and 11-15). Repeat this maneuver as needed.

C. To roll the upper arm, with the client in prone, or the thigh, with the client in supine: Roll the client's limb back and forth over the table surface. You may also lift and swing the client's proximal arm from the elbow (Figure 11-16) or roll the client's dependent forearm between your hands (Figure 11-17).

D. To swing the arm, with the client in supine: Grasp the client's wrist and hand, bend the elbow, lift until the upper arm clears the table, and swing the entire arm from the wrist. In this position, you can also bounce the proximal limb segment on the table surface.

E. To swing the leg, with the client in prone: Grasp the client's foot and ankle, bend the knee, lift until the thigh clears the table, and swing the entire leg from the ankle. In this position, you can also bounce the proximal limb segment on the table surface.

F. To shake or roll the client's entire hand or foot. Grasp the client's hand or foot with two hands and briskly shake or roll it (Figures 11-11 and 11-14).

You can shake or roll individual digits using this technique. Shaking of the client's hand or foot is a useful technique for waking sleeping clients.

THERAPIST'S POSITION AND MOVEMENT

1. You must be able to use all of the basic positions described in Chapter 6.

PALPATE

As you perform the technique, palpate the client's skin and tissues for the qualities noted in the following list. In doing so, focus your attention on the qualities of the motion you produce with the technique and on the resistance of the client's tissues to this movement. Strive to palpate, simultaneously and from a distance, the different tissues and structures that influence the movement you produce. Diligent practice is required to refine your awareness of tissue resistance to movement.

1. The local skin temperature and texture of the client's skin.
2. The tone of the client's superficial muscles and tissues.
3. The movement of the joints you are shaking. Try to form an impression of the quality of the motion of the limb, or the body segment as a whole, and its constituent joints. In addition, note how the resistance to movement varies throughout the available range of the induced motion.
4. Resistance to tissue or joint movement. Determine whether you can relate the resistance to movement to a specific tissue or structure that is involved in producing the motion of the stroke. For example, elevated resting tension in pectoralis major or the other internal rotator of the shoulder will have a visible and palpable effect on the upward swing of the arm (as seen in Figure 11-16).
5. The rhythmic response or cadence of the client's tissue during the stroke. Even more so than with shaking, the client will have a rate and amplitude that she perceives to be the most pleasant for any given rhythmic movement.[33] This varies with the person, body structure, **muscle tone**, region, and type of rhythmic mobilization that you are using. As a result, it is critical for you to palpate for this optimal cadence, communicate with the client, and adjust the rate and

amplitude of the stroke to the client's needs in order to ensure sedation and avoid the unpleasant effects of a sympathetic response.

6. The depth of penetration of the effect of the stroke. As the client's muscles relax the same force will produce effects deeper into and further along the client's tissues. Consequently, as with petrissage, you will not need to apply greater force to achieve a greater penetration of the technique. You will simply have to apply it for a longer duration.

OBSERVE

As you perform the technique, observe the client for:

1. The degree of joint movement you achieve and how the stroke moves from the points of contact to adjacent areas of the client's body. This observation can provide you with information about the level of function of intervening tissues and joints. For example, when you are mobilizing the client's entire leg with traction, observe how the lumbar and thoracic spine respond.

2. The degree of muscle movement. Movement of the client's muscles will be visibly less within areas of connective tissue hardening and elevated resting muscle tension. Even in normal tissue, movement will vary substantially with different body shapes and proportions of body fat.

3. Inappropriate draping. Because rhythmic mobilization can loosen draping, you may need to adjust or retuck a loosened drape to maintain discreet coverage of the client's body.

COMMUNICATION WITH THE CLIENT

Communicate to ensure the client's comfort during the application of rhythmic mobilization. Here are some examples of statements that you can use.

1. "Is this hand position comfortable?" Alternatively, offer the client a choice: "Which feels better, this … or this?" Ensure that your hand contact is comfortable for the client.

2. "Would it feel more relaxing if I slowed down a bit … like this?" "Is this motion comfortable, or is the movement too much?" Determine whether the rate and amplitude of motion are comfortable for the client.

3. "Is everything okay?" "Are you feeling anything unusual?" When you are applying rhythmic mobilization continuously for longer than 2 minutes, determine whether the client is experiencing unpleasant symptoms of sympathetic arousal such as irritation or nausea.

4. "Is this causing pain anywhere?" You can use this statement at intervals to check whether the client perceives that the intervention is resulting in pain. When the client presents with spasm or inflammation, the application of rhythmic mobilization to a distant area may produce small motions, at a distance from the point of contact, that result in pain.

A Practice Sequence for Rhythmic Mobilization

Practice time: 15 to 30 minutes per person or longer.

Do not use oil for this sequence for the anterior and posterior aspects of the legs. You can easily perform it through loose clothing or draping, although the techniques are somewhat easier to apply on bare skin.

There are two basic ways of approaching movement sequences. One is to perform each technique in the sequence once for a longer period of time. The other is to introduce all movements quickly, and then alternate frequently from one technique to the next, repeating the sequence as time permits. This alternative tends to reduce therapist fatigue and tension.

Strive for a smooth continuous motion without breaks between the various moves. Explore each motion and the numerous variations that are possible.

Supine

1. Repeatedly lift the client's thigh slightly and let it drop while working down the leg to the heel. Be careful not to hyperextend the knee.

2. Flex and extend the knee rhythmically in the midrange. The hip will also flex and extend. Be careful not to allow the knee to hyperextend. Perform this flexion and extension while gradually internally and externally rotating the hip.

3. With heel-of-hand contacts just proximal to both malleoli, shake the whole foot while the leg rests on the table.

4. Gently circumduct the ankle.

5. Grasp the foot and ankle securely, lift the leg, and apply gentle long-axis traction to the leg. Then gently whip the entire leg briefly, in the sagittal plane, like a rope. Repeat.

6. Hold the posterior ankle above the calcaneus. Lift the leg off the table slightly. Now rhythmically internally and externally rotate the hip joint and the entire leg. Continue this while slowly abducting and adducting the hip joint.

Repeat this supine sequence two or more times.
  Turn client to prone.

Prone

1. Hold the client's ankle with two hands. Flex the knee to 90°, lift the thigh off the table, and swing the entire leg from side to side.

2. With the knee flexed to 90° and the thigh resting on the table, grasp the heel, and shake the entire foot.

3. Grasp the foot and ankle. Lift the leg and apply gentle long-axis traction to the entire leg prior to gently whipping it in the sagittal plane like a rope.

4. Hold the foot and flex the knee to 45°. Passively plantarflex and dorsiflex the ankle joint.

5. Hold the foot and flex the knee to 45°. Make clockwise and counterclockwise circles of various sizes in the air with the heel.

Repeat this prone sequence two or more times.

Home study: Devise a comparable supine and prone sequence for the arm.

CAUTIONS AND CONTRAINDICATIONS

Therapists need clinical training and supervised practice to master the proper application of rhythmic mobilization. Advanced training may be advisable when dealing with pathological conditions. All of the general and local contraindications noted for massage techniques apply to the use of rhythmic mobilization (see Chapter 5). One current list of contraindications for rhythmic mobilization includes metastatic cancer, acute nerve impingement or disk rupture, severe carotid artery disease, use of anticoagulant therapy, and high-risk pregnancies.[19] Therapists should consider a flail chest, fractured or brittle ribs, and recent chest or spinal surgery to be contraindications to

applying this technique to the rib cage for mobilizing bronchial secretions.[8] Avoid performing rhythmic mobilization on, or adjacent to, the site of acute orthopedic injuries.[19] Therapists can introduce this technique at later stages of recovery provided they can perform it without causing the client pain. Apply rhythmic mobilization with reduced force and great sensitivity when clients present with spasm, hyperreflexia, or spasticity. In general, therapists can often move the client's hands and feet quite vigorously. Elsewhere, however, they need to perform rhythmic mobilization at a moderate rate, since it may be too stimulating for the client when they perform it rapidly. Therapists should not use rhythmic mobilization when a client suffers from vertigo or motion sickness.[19]

USING RHYTHMIC MOBILIZATION IN TREATMENT

To Reduce Unnecessary Muscle Tension

First, focus the client's attention on an identified area of unnecessary muscle tension. Encourage deep breathing, relaxation, and a feeling of "letting go." Clients may also find simple visual images such as "melting" or more complex guided imagery scripts useful.[16] Other manual techniques that move the client's body in space, such as shaking, rocking, joint mobilization, and passive relaxed movement, may assist the client in recognizing and releasing patterns of unnecessary muscle tension. Provide positive feedback when the client has released tension because the client may not immediately realize that this has happened. In addition, use rhythmic mobilization as a precursor to traction, joint mobilization, or passive relaxed movement techniques to decrease unnecessary muscle tension that would interfere with your application of those techniques.

For homecare, you can instruct the client to perform active rhythmic mobilization movements to achieve muscle relaxation and facilitate ease of motion. Ensure that you give the client the correct guidance so that active mobilization does not adversely increase unnecessary muscle tension.[17] Encourage clients to use any effective breathing and relaxation methods that they know.[16]

To Enhance Arousal (Wakefulness)

Perform rhythmic mobilization at a faster tempo to wake clients. Other massage techniques that tend to wake clients quickly are fast fingertip superficial stroking, fine vibration, and percussion (use commercially available machines to produce the latter two techniques if your scope of practice, skill level, and comfort with using machines permit). In addition, brief cold, contrast hydrotherapy, and rubbing the skin with coarse cloth, bristle brushes, or salt also enhance arousal.[18]

In Pre- and Intercompetition Sports Massage

Therapists use this type of massage on the day of and immediately before competition. Their application of the technique will vary with the sport and the athlete. In general, they avoid deeper techniques as competition draws near[3] and alternate shaking and rhythmic mobilization with broad-contact compression, light petrissage, percussion, stretching, or passive range of motion. Finally, they use short (15 to 20 minutes for all regions), fast-tempo (70 to 90 Hz) sessions that focus on the most important muscle groups that the athlete will be using in the activity.

To Enhance Airway Clearance

When you are using rhythmic mobilization of the rib cage to mobilize bronchial secretions, use percussion (preferably cupping), postural drainage, steam inhalation, forced expiration, and coughing techniques in a complementary manner. You can also teach clients the last four methods for home use.

Rocking: Evidence

DEFINITION

Rocking: Gentle, repetitive oscillation of the pelvis, torso, or limbs that therapists achieve by pushing the pelvis or torso from a midline resting position into lateral deviation and then allowing it to return to resting position. This repetitive movement results in waves of motion that travel along the body.

NAMES AND ORIGINS

In some texts or massage-related systems, the technique that we call rocking is also known as "pelvic rocking" or "rocking vibration."[1-8,34] This form of rhythmic mobilization results in a lateral motion of the body, especially of the pelvis, lumbar region, and thoracic region. The distinctive elements of the manual technique of rocking and the technique's reflex effects merit an independent description.

Although every mother (and child) has known the effects of repetitive motion since time immemorial,[32,35,36] few people documented a rocking technique prior to the latter part of the 20th century. These relaxed movements figure prominently in the work of the American Milton Trager (Trager Psychophysical Integration)[19,20] and the British osteopath Eyal Lederman (Harmonic Technique).[21]

USES

Rocking has a profoundly **sedative** effect that is useful in the treatment of stress-related autonomic dysfunction, generalized elevation of skeletal muscle tone, unnecessary muscle tension, insomnia, and fatigue. Therapists can also use the sedative effect of rocking to reduce the client's perception of pain indirectly.

OUTCOMES AND EVIDENCE

Rocking has a variety of physiological and psychological effects that are outlined in this section. It may produce a generalized decrease in postural tone and arousal as a result of stimulation of vestibular reflexes.[28] When therapists perform rocking skillfully, it has a profoundly sedative effect. For this reason alone, this technique is worth mastering.[21] As a result of its sedative effect, therapists find rocking useful for treating stress-related autonomic dysfunction; generalized elevation of skeletal muscle tone; "holding" or unnecessary muscle tension; insomnia; and mental, physical, or emotional fatigue. Furthermore, people intuitively use rocking motions to calm infants; consequently, therapists incorporate it into infant massage.[32,35,36] They may also find it valuable for treating a variety of chronic musculoskeletal disorders in which clients present with muscular tension, provided the client is able to tolerate the motion of the technique.[19,29,30] Finally, therapists can use the sedative effect of rocking to indirectly reduce the client's perception of pain.[29,30] Table 11-1 summarizes the main outcomes for rocking.

HOW ROCKING MIGHT WORK

The mechanism for the effects of rocking is similar to that of rhythmic mobilization. Compression and release of soft tissue, and the resulting passive motions, may produce modest increases in lymphatic and venous return by squeezing and stretching vessels with valves. The slight rhythmic deformation of joint capsules may help to propel synovial fluid through the capsule.[2,5] In addition, stimulation of joint afferents enhances joint awareness.[1,12] Sedative effects can be the result of entrainment to rhythm (see discussion and references in Chapter 7). Finally, vestibular reflexes may cause a generalized decrease in postural tone.[2,5,21]

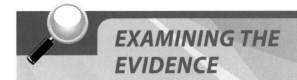

EXAMINING THE EVIDENCE

Several studies have examined the effects of rocking and rhythmic mobilization in the context of Trager Psychophysical Integration[29-31,37] or on children. One text[21] describes many methods of rocking and rhythmic mobilization in detail. This rigorous text also includes chapters about the physics of motion and the effects of motion and passive movement on neurology, tissue and joint repair, fluid flow, and analgesia. It also includes relevant literature, including the theoretical background and related clinical trials, and several clinical examples, which resemble actual case studies.[21]

Lederman E. *Harmonic Technique.* Edinburgh, Scotland: Churchill Livingstone; 2000.

Rocking: Practice

COMPONENTS OF ROCKING

Rocking has the following components:

Contact: Entire palmar surface

Pressure: Light to moderate

Tissues engaged: Hands engage tissues to the depth of the superficial muscle layers. The motion produced by the stroke simultaneously engages all the tissues throughout the body segments that you are rocking. This can include muscle, fascia, tendon, ligament, and periosteum.

Direction: Direct your force so that you produce a lateral deviation of the pelvis and/or spine from the midline. The resulting motion is propagated along the client's body.

Amplitude and length: Lateral deviation may reach 10 cm or more from midline, depending on the duration of application of the technique and the client's body size and type.

Rate: 1 to 2 seconds per cycle

Duration: 60 seconds to 15+ minutes

Intergrades with: Passive range of motion and joint mobilization techniques

Combines with: Combine with compression

Context: May be used alone for sedation. Therapists usually use it at the beginning or end of longer sequences that include other techniques.

PALPATION PRACTICE

1. Using the pads of your index and middle fingers, landmark adjacent spinous processes on your partner's spine. Have your partner perform active lumbar side flexion to the left and right, while you palpate the movement between adjacent vertebrae. Work your way down the spinal column from C2 to S1.

2. The following exercise shows how the natural oscillatory rhythm differs from person to person and suggests how rocking can be synchronized to each individual's body. In prone, move your partner's pelvis laterally 5 to 15 cm (2 to 6 in.) from the midline, then remove your hands, and observe the result. Note how far the body rebounds past midline and how long the motion continues for one or two cycles. Try lateral pushes in several places like the ribs, waist, iliac crest, and greater trochanter, observing the motion in the same way as before. Repeat this palpation exercise on several people who have different body types. How does the natural rocking rate and amplitude compare for **ectomorphs, mesomorphs, and endomorphs**? Repeat the entire exercise again with several partners in supine.

3. Put on a blindfold. Have your partner select an area of the body to consciously tense while you repeat Step 2 above. Can you identify the tensed area without someone telling you?

MANUAL TECHNIQUE

Figures 11-18 to 11-24 show therapists applying rocking to the various regions of the body. The order of the figures is from head to foot in supine and then in prone. Each figure illustrates most of the guidelines for manual technique outlined here.

1. If the client can tolerate lying prone without lumbar support, remove the abdominal pillow, since its presence will significantly dampen the motion that rocking produces. Even clients with back pain, who often require an abdominal pillow when they are prone, may be able to tolerate lying with an increased lordosis as long as the rocking motion continues. You may need to replace the abdominal pillow after application of rocking. This may also be the case for using pillows under the client's knees in supine.

2. Use relaxed whole-hand contact, with your fingers spread, which will evenly distribute the pressure over the contact surface of your hand (Figures 11-18, 11-19, and 11-22 to 11-23B).

3. Gently push the client's pelvis or torso laterally from the midline resting position in supine (Figures 11-18, 11-19) or in prone (Figures 11-22, 11-23); this motion will raise

FIGURE 11-19 As hand contact moves farther from the pelvis, the rocking motion naturally becomes attenuated. In this situation, you can maintain the rocking motion by using upper and lower rib hand contacts.

FIGURE 11-18 Rocking in supine with hand contact on the lower ribs and anterior superior iliac spines.

FIGURE 11-20 Rocking can also be initiated after gently lifting a large muscle mass such as the quadriceps, hamstrings, or gluteals. The cadence at which rocking can be performed will be dictated by the passive response of the pelvis.

FIGURE 11-21 The thigh can be rolled into internal rotation while the rocking motion is maintained from the anterior superior iliac spines.

FIGURE 11-22 Basic hand contact for rocking the back. Hands are placed on the sacrum and the greater trochanter. The therapist directs the force of the motion distally, to produce lumbar traction, and toward the client's contralateral knee. With each stroke, the therapist produces a lateral displacement of the client's pelvis and then allows the pelvis to fall back past the midline without breaking hand contact. The aim is to produce a succession of seamlessly interconnected strokes.

FIGURE 11-23 **A.** Hand contact may be varied to different positions as the rocking motion is maintained. Here, the gluteals are gently stretched distally off their superior iliac attachments with the therapist's left hand. **B.** Here, the gluteals are pushed away from the sacrum with both hands.

the center of gravity of the client's body. Then, allow the client's body to fall back toward the midline passively; momentum will carry the body past its resting position. Precisely at the end of the excursion of the motion of the pelvis or torso, repeat the application of the same pressure, and push the client's pelvis or torso past the midline once more. Ideally, rocking consists of a seamlessly interconnected series of pushes and releases (falls) that produce a continuous oscillation of the client's body. The maximum amplitude of the motion should occur around the client's iliac crest.

4. Although it is preferable for you to maintain contact during the passive **return stroke**, you must do this without impeding the natural "falling" of the body back toward, and through, the resting position.

5. Time the initiation of each push so that the rocking motion you produce is smooth and the client is scarcely aware of your hand pressure and the point at which you apply that motion.

FIGURE 11-24 A. Techniques for the erector spinae. Cross-handed contact permits a gentle traction of the erector spinae (1), while simultaneously performing the rocking motion (2). Hand contact is maintained as the pelvis is allowed to fall back past the midline. **B.** Techniques for the erector spinae. Two hands gather the erector spinae together while producing the rocking motion. **C.** Alternately, one hand draws the opposite innominate bone toward the therapist, and then the other hand gently pushes the erector spinae away from the spinous processes.

6. Change your hand position every 5 to 10 seconds to avoid producing a motion that has a mechanical feel. Slide your hands easily from one contact position to another without interrupting the regular rhythm, so that you are moving your point of contact up and down the client's body.

7. As the application of rocking proceeds and the client relaxes, you will often note an increased amplitude and decreased rate of the rocking motion, with little increase in the amount of force you apply.

8. You may also position your hands on opposite sides of the client's body, so that they can alternately push and pull the client's body to generate the rocking motion (Figure 11-24C). Bear in mind that this approach eliminates the passive return of the client's body to its resting position. Consequently, it is more likely to be inharmonious with the body's natural rhythm and to produce a stroke that is less effective or that the client perceives as being unpleasant.

9. You may find it useful to intersperse rocking with gentle long-axis traction of the client's legs. This enhances the incremental lengthening of the spine that can result from longer applications of rocking.

THERAPIST'S POSITION AND MOVEMENT

1. Use the basic positions described in Chapter 6, in the sections on **standing aligned**, **lunge**, and **lunge-and-lean** postures.

2. Use a standing upright posture when beginning the application of rocking or when the amplitude of the movement is small.

3. Using a standing lunge-and-lean posture, shift your body weight backward and forward from your front leg to your back leg in a gentle rocking motion. Then transfer this motion through your arms to the client. This feels much better to the client than a rocking motion that you generate solely through exertion of your arm and shoulder muscles (Figures 11-19, 11-22, and 11-23A). As with other massage techniques, using your lower body and pelvis to generate the motion of the stroke, rather than your arms alone, will add a perceptible sureness and evenness to the stroke.

4. During the rhythmic lunge-and-lean movement, relax your shoulders and stretch out your arms without locking your elbows in extension ("straight-arming") (Figures 11-22 and 11-23a).

5. The more rhythmic and relaxed the movement of your body is, the more effective the rocking motion you produce.

PALPATE

As you perform the technique, palpate the client's skin and tissues for the qualities noted in the following list. In doing so, focus your attention on the qualities of the motion you produce with the technique and the client's tissues' resistance to movement.

1. The local skin temperature and texture.
2. The tone of the client's superficial muscles and tissues.
3. The weight of the client's body as you set it into motion with rocking.
4. Resistance to tissue or joint movement. The initial resistance to movement from the midline resting position comes from the client's weight. As you push the client's body farther from the midline, additional resistance develops as various tissues are lengthened passively. The goal of rocking is not to achieve the fullest possible passive stretch, but rather to produce a repetitive, pleasurable motion within the inner and midranges of the available range of motion.
5. The inherent rhythm of rocking for the client's body. No two clients' bodies will respond to rocking in the same manner. Several factors can influence the inherent rhythm of the client's body: body type, the amount of body fat, levels of muscular tension, and the client's fascial structure. Muscular tension, especially of the low back, can also reduce the amount of movement that the client can tolerate. You must identify the inherent rhythm of each client's body at the time of treatment, rather than merely imposing the same motion on every client.
6. Changes in ease of application of the technique. As the application of rocking proceeds and the client relaxes, you will note an increased amplitude and a decreased rate of the rocking motion, with little increase in the amount of force you apply.

OBSERVE

As you perform the technique, observe the client for the degree of movement you achieve and signs of relaxation or sedation. The following signs may signal this.

Movement Achieved

1. Observation of the motion throughout the body during rocking. Careful observation can provide information about the client's body, including patterns of muscular tension, the relationship of body segments, and areas of connective tissue tightness due to past trauma. For example, when rocking the pelvis, observe the relative ease of motion of the various spinal segments.
2. Lengthening of the spine, as reflected by a reduction of the client's spinal curves, especially the lumbar lordosis.

Relaxation or Sedation

1. Decrease in rate and depth of breathing.
2. Deeper voice tone.
3. Changes in skin color such as flushing. Pallor may indicate an undesirable sympathetic response.
4. Systemic reduction of muscle tone, as evidenced by softening of the tissue contours or broadening and flattening of body segments.
5. Muscle twitches and jerks.
6. Increases in peristaltic noises.
7. Decreases in heart rate, as evidenced by change in the client's pulses that are visible at the neck, wrist, and foot.
8. Agitation or sweating, which may indicate an undesirable **sympathetic response**.

COMMUNICATION WITH THE CLIENT

Communicate to ensure the client's comfort during the application of rocking. Here are some examples of statements that you can use.

1. "Does this movement bring on the pain that you have been experiencing?" This is a useful measure of whether improvement is occurring with treatment. Ideally, rocking should not reproduce the client's symptoms.
2. "This technique should make you feel very relaxed, even sleepy. It should not feel abrupt." After you establish a motion that you perceive to be consistent with the inherent rhythm of the client's body, check that the motion feels comfortable, rather than forced or excessive in any way.
3. "Do you feel alert enough to drive home?" If you use rocking for long periods during the session or at the end of a session, observe the client's level of function and ensure that he or she is sufficiently alert to resume daily activities safely.

4. The relaxation, sensual pleasure, and motion of rocking may occasionally result in sexual arousal on the part of the client. You must be prepared to maintain clear verbal and physical boundaries with the client in a mature manner.

A Practice Sequence for Rocking

Practice time: Allow 30 minutes per person.

Begin with the client in prone. Establish a stable rocking rhythm that is continuous and does not feel machine-like. Use light soft full palmar contact. Do not remove your hands between each application of pressure ("stroke") because this reduces the sedative effect. Slide your hands from one position to another while maintaining light contact.

Hand positions to try include:

- Trochanter and sacrum
- Trochanter and superior gluteal insertions
- Crossed-hand lumbar traction position
- Both sides of the iliac crest
- Both sides of the waist
- Pelvis and the erector spinae
- Pelvis and rib cage
- Both sides of the rib cage

Initially, check with the client several times to ensure that your hand contact, rate, and rhythm are comfortable. Experiment with moving your hand contacts as far up and down the body as you can, while still maintaining the basic rocking motion. Notice how the client's body responds differently over time: the amplitude of the initial rocking will be smaller until the client's body begins to relax. Periodically intersperse rocking with gentle traction of the client's legs in order to lengthen the client's back as the back muscles begin to relax. Many people will become drowsy or even fall asleep during this sequence. Continue for 15 minutes, and give your client 5 minutes to return to the present before ending the session.

Home study:

- Devise and practice a comparable sequence for rocking in supine, using the trochanter, anterior thigh, iliac crest, anterior superior iliac spines, waist, and lower ribs as contact points. Note whether a supine rocking sequence has effects similar to the ones described earlier for prone.
- Devise a sequence in supine for a person who has had a herniated lumbar disc once you have completed the basic sequences.

CAUTIONS AND CONTRAINDICATIONS

Therapists need clinical training and supervised practice to master the proper application of rocking. Advanced training may be advisable when dealing with pathological conditions. All of the general and local contraindications previously noted for massage techniques and rhythmic mobilization apply to the use of rocking (see Chapter 5). Rocking sets the entire body in motion; therefore, it is contraindicated, or should be used with a reduced amplitude, for any condition in which rocking will increase pain. The effects of rocking vary with the manner in which you perform the technique and the duration for which you use it. If therapists perform rocking abruptly or too quickly, it can quickly produce unpleasant effects such as nausea. Consequently, they should not use rocking when a client suffers from vertigo or motion sickness.[19] When therapists use rocking for more than 10 minutes in the intervention, it can induce a combination of deep relaxation and mild disorientation in the client that may temporarily reduce their competence to perform physical tasks such as driving. In this situation, they must ensure that the client is capable of functioning before allowing him or her to leave. If they have any doubt about the client's capabilities, they should return the client to the table; apply some deep, specific petrissage to the soles of the feet; and then let the client rest for 10 to 20 minutes before reassessing his or her level of mental function.

USING ROCKING IN TREATMENT

For Relaxation or Sedation

There are several modalities that you can use in a complementary manner with rocking to promote relaxation or sedation.

1. Use diaphragmatic breathing[16] prior to, or simultaneously with, rocking to enhance sedative effects.
2. Moist **hot packs** can enhance sedation and analgesia, if heat is appropriate for the client's condition.[18]
3. Some **craniosacral** techniques may have a calming effect on the client.[38]
4. Relaxing massage techniques include superficial stroking and rhythmic petrissage. These may produce greater effects if you apply them to the client's hands, feet, face, occiput, and sacrum.

Instruct the client to rest from 10 to 30 minutes and to resume activity slowly if he or she is experiencing the sedative effects of rocking.

For homecare, you can instruct the client in a form of self-rocking that she can use for relaxation. She will lie in supine, on a cushioned floor or firm bed, with her knees drawn up toward the chest with her hands. She will produce a rocking motion in the sagittal plane by pulling gently on the backs of her knees. During this movement, her thighs, pelvis, and lower back will flex and extend passively, although this differs from the true rocking that therapists perform.

To Reduce Unnecessary Muscle Tension

First, focus the client's attention on an identified area of unnecessary muscle tension. Encourage deep breathing, relaxation, and a feeling of "letting go." The client may find simple visual images like "melting" or more complex guided imagery scripts[16] useful. Other manual techniques that move the client's body in space, such as rhythmic mobilization, shaking, joint mobilization, and passive relaxed movement, may assist the client in recognizing and releasing patterns of unnecessary muscle tension. Give the client positive feedback when he releases tension because he may not realize immediately that this has happened.

For homecare, you can instruct the client to self-administer shaking to accessible areas of the body such as the arms and legs and to perform active shaking movements to achieve muscle relaxation and facilitate ease of motion.[17] You may also suggest the use of any effective breathing and relaxation methods that the client knows.[16]

IN CONCLUSION

Passive movement techniques have a variety of uses, therapeutic effects, and outcomes. Table 11-1 summarizes those outcomes for passive movement techniques that are related to body structures and functions.

	Technique		
Table 11-1	**Summary of Outcomes for Passive Movement Techniques**		
Outcome	**Shaking**	**Rhythmic Mobilization**	**Rocking**
Systemic sedation	P	P	P
Decreased perceived anxiety	P	P	P
Increased arousal	P	P	?
Analgesia	P	√	√
Increased local resting muscle tension or neuromuscular tone	P	?	?
Decreased resting muscle tension	P	P	P
Increased joint mobility	?	P	P
Increased accessory joint motion	?	P	P
Increased rib cage mobility	?	P	P
Increased airway clearance/mobilization of secretions	?	√	?
Decreased dyspnea	?	P	P
Stimulated peristalsis	P	P	P
Alteration of movement responses	?	√	√
Increased ability to perform movement tasks	?	√	√

√, the outcome is supported by research summarized in this chapter; P, the outcome is possible; ?, the outcome is debatable (research results are absent or inconsistent).

REVIEW SECTION

TAKEAWAYS

1. Passive movement techniques are those massage techniques that primarily palpate the movement of tissues and structures, as opposed to palpating their substance or texture.
2. Shaking is a technique that moves soft tissue—primarily muscle—back and forth repetitively over the underlying bone, with minimal joint movement.
3. Clinicians use shaking to reduce "holding," or unnecessary muscle tension, and to reduce the resting muscle tension of skeletal muscles.
4. Shaking may help patients who are holding muscles tensely in response to situational stress to realize that this contraction is unnecessary by rapidly producing changes in muscle position. In addition, the spreading and shearing of muscle that happens during shaking may cause proprioceptive input that reduces resting tension.
5. Rhythmic mobilization is the technique that repetitively moves entire structures, resulting in the movement of soft tissue over bone and the movement of the related joints and internal organs.
6. Clinicians use rhythmic mobilization to help a patient voluntarily release unnecessary muscle tension, to reduce resting muscle tension, to prepare a patient for joint mobilization or passive range of motion techniques, and to give precompetition massage to athletes. This technique may also cause passive joint motion that may help to mobilize stiff joints, stimulate joint healing, enhance a patient's joint awareness, and mobilize bronchial secretions.
7. There are multiple mechanisms for the effects of rhythmic mobilization. The compression and release of soft tissue that accompanies rhythmic mobilization may produce modest increases in lymphatic and venous return by squeezing vessels with valves. The rhythmic deformation of joint capsules moves synovial fluid through the capsule and facilitates joint nutrition and healing.[1-5] Stimulation of joint afferents enhances joint awareness.
8. Rocking is a gentle, repetitive oscillation of the pelvis, torso, or limbs that clinicians achieve by pushing the pelvis or torso from a midline resting position into lateral deviation and then allowing it to return to resting position.
9. The mechanism for the effects of rocking is similar to that of rhythmic mobilization.
10. Clinicians should avoid using passive movement techniques on any muscle that contains an acute injury, or crosses an acutely injured bone or joint, even if their hand position is remote from the site of injury.

Clinical Case: *Passive Movement Techniques*

Patient Profile

Your patient is a middle-aged "type A" manager in a high-stress public relations position who spends 4 to 5 hours per day at a computer and the rest of her time on the phone, in meetings, or giving presentations. She is married and has two teenaged children. Her physician has referred her for treatment of tension headaches. She has no experience with manual therapy.

Clinical Findings

Subjective Findings:

- Constant tightness in her neck and shoulders
- Severe temporal headaches 2 to 3 times a week
- An inability to relax due to her hectic schedule

Objective Findings:

- Posture: Forward head, elevated shoulders bilaterally (left greater than right), and moderate kyphosis.
- Range of motion: Active and passive cervical range of motion is limited by 20% in all directions except extension, with stiffness at the end of range but no pain.

- Resisted tests: Resisted isometric cervical motions do not cause pain.
- Palpation: There is point tenderness throughout the muscles of her neck. Maximal compression of her hard upper trapezius muscles reproduces the temporal headache pattern of **referred pain**.

Treatment Approach

Important initial outcomes include:
- Reducing the resting muscle tension and **trigger point** activity throughout the neck and shoulders, especially in the upper trapezius.
- Increasing her awareness of the posture of her head and shoulders and how it changes in response to stress.

In the first session, perform most of the treatment in supine, focusing on the upper trapezius and the neck. Use rhythmic settling of the patient's shoulders (Figure 11-9) as the **framing general technique**. Begin by applying this technique for a few minutes. Intersperse it with the full range of neuromuscular and fascial techniques to reduce muscle tension, trigger point activity, and fascial shortening in the neck, as tolerated (see Chapters 7 to 9). Every time you palpate or observe palpate softening of tissue or see the shoulders relax downward, return to rhythmic mobilization of the shoulders for a minute. Use rocking and settling of the patient's shoulders as a focus of the treatment because it helps her become aware of her increasing range of motion as it occurs during treatment. Augment the intervention with homecare methods such as stretching, active movement, and postural awareness exercises.

As the patient's intervention proceeds, progress the depth of the neuromuscular and connective tissue techniques; assess and treat other areas of her body such as the chest, jaw, and back; and try approaches like **diaphragmatic breathing** and guided relaxation to encourage general relaxation. Given her personality and lifestyle, she will likely present with elevated shoulders often, and you can incorporate rhythmic mobilization of the shoulders as part of her treatment to help restore her awareness of her posture and muscle tension.

Critical Thinking Questions

1. Which layers of tissues are engaged by passive movement techniques?
2. What are the primary effects of passive movement techniques?
3. What are the physiological mechanisms by which shaking affects resting muscle tension?
4. Discuss how and why a patient with compensating patterns following an injury may benefit from shaking strokes.
5. It seems paradoxical that you can use the same technique to both reduce muscle tension and increase wakefulness in a patient. What are the mechanisms that enable you to achieve both of these effects with shaking?
6. Use clinical reasoning to develop a protocol including the application of rhythmic mobilization techniques for a patient with nonspecific osteoarthritis of the lumbar spine, and a patient in the subacute stage of a 2nd degree ankle sprain.
7. Your patient was unable to tolerate rocking during his first few treatments. You have attempted rocking each time to assess improvement in the tolerance of movement such as rocking. On the fourth session, rocking did not cause pain. Discuss some of the reasons that the patient's tolerance for rocking increased.
8. Explain how you might use passive techniques such as shaking to affect specific, deep tissues. For example, under what circumstances might you choose shaking to affect the vastus intermedius or longissimus thoracis? How will you apply this technique?
9. Would you recommend rocking, shaking or rhythmic mobilizations as self care? Describe how you would instruct clients to use these techniques on their own.
10. Explain why it is preferable to change your hand position every 5 to 10 seconds when rocking to avoid producing movement that feels mechanical. Aside from the general perception of mechanized movement, how might constant repetitive rocking in the same location negatively impact the intended outcome when using rocking techniques? Could this have unintended effects on the surrounding tissues?

References and Further Reading list for Chapter 11 begin on p. 478.

Percussive Techniques

After studying this chapter, you will have the information that you need to do the following:

1. Describe how the massage techniques in this category affect different types of tissues.
2. Describe each massage technique in terms of the contact surface, pressure, tissues engaged, amplitude, direction, and rate.
3. Demonstrate how to perform each massage technique and how to apply it in the context of a practice sequence.
4. Speculate about the mechanisms by which massage techniques achieve their effects.
5. Describe the outcomes of care, indications, contraindications, and common uses associated with each massage technique.

Percussive techniques are those massage techniques that use controlled striking of the body to quickly deform and release tissues. These techniques enhance airway clearance, reduce or increase neuromuscular tone, and increase alertness. This chapter describes the various percussive techniques, how to perform them, and how to apply them in practice sequences. It also includes a discussion of relevant outcomes and evidence, cautions and contraindications, and how to use the techniques in treatment. Finally, Table 12-1 summarizes those outcomes for percussion that are related to body structures and functions. Therapists are advised to review the cautions and contraindications for these techniques and to use them as their scope of practice and skill level permit.

Percussion: Evidence

DEFINITION

Percussion: Repeated rhythmic light striking.[1-11]

NAMES AND ORIGINS

Other texts often call percussion "**tapotement**."[1-11] Although there is unanimous usage of the equivalent terms percussion and tapotement, different names are often applied to some of the forms of percussion. For example, clapping is sometimes known as "cupping."[3,8,10] The section on manual technique earlier in this chapter gives alternate names for the forms of percussion.

USES

Therapists have used the various forms of percussion to improve **airway clearance**, as **proprioceptive stimulation**

techniques, to increase **levels of arousal**, and for **pain** relief. They can also be used to facilitate or inhibit neuromuscular tone. Gentle percussive techniques can also be used to assess the areas of pain and tension when other strokes are uncomfortable or are ticklish. Tapping is used to evaluate potential nerve dysfunction (Tinel's sign) when applied over a superficial nerve and to evaluate sinus congestion when applied on the face. Gentle percussion applied over a vertebral segment may reveal herniation or other injury. Gentle percussion is frequently used to test reflex responses. The use of percussion accompanied by postural drainage for airway clearance is a specialized technique and not appropriate for all therapists to perform.

OUTCOMES AND EVIDENCE

The various forms of percussion have different effects. Therapists can use them for the treatment of **airway clearance**, as **proprioceptive stimulation** techniques, for increasing **levels of arousal**, and for **pain** relief. Therapists use percussion, specifically clapping, to mechanically loosen secretions in the lungs and facilitate airway clearance. They frequently use it in clinical conditions that are associated with the production of copious or viscous mucus.[1,3,12] In traditional cardiopulmonary physical therapy, percussion is combined with **postural drainage** and is followed by, or alternated with, vibration of the rib cage or rapid compression and release of the rib cage (called rib "springing" or "shaking").[1,3,12] Postural drainage has its own indications, contraindications, and outcomes.[1] Research suggests that the entire procedure of postural drainage and percussion (**PDP**) promotes the movement of mucus in a cephalic direction through the bronchial tree and increases the clearance of sputum,[13,13-17] with one dissenting opinion.[18] This effect may be more pronounced in conditions in which there are large volumes of sputum.[19,20] The use of PDP may be declining with the advent of many recently developed techniques for airway clearance that use mechanical motion and ventilation.[14,15,21-29]

There are many issues related to whether the measures used in the research on percussion and postural drainage are relevant. For example, recent reviews question the use of the volume of sputum cleared by the client as a valid outcome measure in research on bronchial conditions,[21,30,31] although sputum clearance has been associated with increased client comfort.[14] Other authors consider blood oxygenation to be a more relevant measure of pulmonary function[12,16,30,32]; however, the relationship between improved oxygenation and the clearance of sputum remains unclear.[12,21,33] In addition, the results of research on the effects of PDP on pulmonary function testing are equivocal for several clinical conditions: postsurgically,[34] in critically ill clients with atelectasis,[12,22,35] in mechanically ventilated children,[36] and in chronic bronchitis and bronchiectasis.[21] Percussion remains valuable in the treatment of cystic fibrosis[14,15,37,38] and some rarer pulmonary conditions,[39] although other methods may be equally effective for clearing sputum.[40]

Several massage texts state that percussion stimulates stretch reflexes that facilitate the contraction and shortening of muscle when it is applied to the muscle belly or tendon.[5,8,10,41]

In addition, traditional physical therapy practice, such as the techniques of Bobath and Rood, has applied various forms of percussion, especially tapping, to muscles or tendons to increase neuromuscular tone and facilitate normalized movement patterns in clients with neurological conditions such as spasticity.[42] Other sources, however, suggest that tapping tendons or muscles may inhibit contraction both locally and in synergist muscle groups by stimulating cutaneous receptors.[43,44]

Therapists consider percussion to have a general stimulating effect that most likely varies with the location, vigor, and duration of its application.[3-6,8-10] This has been the rationale for applying percussion during **precompetition sports massage** or at the end of sedative massage to increase the client's level of arousal.[4] By contrast, Frownfelter[1] notes that the monotonous rhythm and rate of the application of clapping for extended periods may have a relaxing effect.

Applications of percussion may also have a variety of minor effects. It may produce a local hyperemia.[5,10] As with other massage techniques, percussion produces a transient hyperstimulation analgesia, which may make it suitable for pain relief in neuralgia or amputation.[3] Finally, mechanical percussion does not promote recovery from short-term intense muscular activity.[45] Table 12-1 summarizes the main outcomes for percussion.

HOW PERCUSSION MIGHT WORK

The cupped shape of the hand used in chest percussion traps air against the rib cage and sets up a vibration that travels through the chest wall and lung tissue.[3] This vibration dislodges the mucus that is stuck in the bronchial tree.[3,8,11] Percussion used for neuromuscular facilitation may achieve an effect by repeatedly stimulating stretch receptors (spindles) within the muscle.[3,8,11,41] The intense stimulation of percussion may initiate a generalized **sympathetic response** that leads to increased alertness.[8,11] Finally, pain relief may occur through spinal gating.[3,11]

EXAMINING THE EVIDENCE

A crossover study[40] of 24 clients with cystic fibrosis compared the effectiveness of postural drainage and percussion (**PDP**) in enhancing airway clearance with the effectiveness of two mechanized alternatives: interpulmonary percussive ventilation and high-frequency chest wall percussion. The main outcome measure was sputum collected during the 30-minute treatments and for 15 minutes after treatment. The researchers judged PDP, as administered in 12 positions, to be equal with the other methods with respect to its ability to enhance short-term airway clearance. Clients showed no significant preference for any of these treatments. This study is thorough, well described, and repeatable. The authors also discuss the study's limitations, which included a modest sample size and the validity of sputum clearance as an indicator of pulmonary function.

Varekojis SM, Douce FH, Flucke RL, et al. A comparison of the therapeutic effectiveness of and preference for postural drainage and percussion, intrapulmonary percussive ventilation, and high-frequency chest wall compression in hospitalized cystic fibrosis patients. *Respir Care.* 2003;48:24-28.

Percussion: Practice

COMPONENTS OF PERCUSSION

Percussion has the following components:

Contact: Fingers, fingertip(s), ulnar border of hands, palms, heels, and dorsal surface of interphalangeal joints, in various combinations

Pressure: Light to heavy

Engages: Superficial subcutaneous tissues (lighter forms) to deeper muscle and contained viscera such as the lungs (heavier forms)

Direction: The contact and release strokes are perpendicular to the surface of the client's body (except for pounding)

Amplitude/length: N/A

Rate: 2 to 10 or more cycles per second (Hz) using both hands

Duration: 30 seconds to up to 20 minutes when the therapist is treating multiple regions of the lungs

Intergrades with: The various forms of percussion intergrade with each other; however, none of these intergrade with other massage techniques.

Combines with: None of these forms of percussion combine with, or are used simultaneously with, other massage techniques.

Context: Percussion is commonly used in several ways. It is used briefly at the end of a regional or full-body massage for its stimulating effect. It is used immediately prior to the therapeutic exercise to facilitate the performance of exercise. Finally, it is alternated with vibration, rib springing (rapid **compression**), and **rhythmic mobilization** of the rib cage with the client positioned in full or modified **postural drainage** positions.

PALPATION PRACTICE

1. For all regions of the body, using fingertip palpation and graduated pressure, estimate the thickness of the subcutaneous fatty layer and the superficial and deeper layers of muscle.
2. Using a well-illustrated anatomy text as a reference, draw the position of the lungs and their lobes on a partner who is positioned in prone, supine, sidelying, or any of the **postural drainage** positions shown in Figure 12-14.

MANUAL TECHNIQUE: MANUAL CONTACT SURFACES FOR THE FORMS OF PERCUSSION

We organize the forms of percussion described in this section in terms of the amount of force they require for application: from lesser force to greater force. The amount of stimulation that results from each form of percussion will vary with the force of application, the area of the body being treated, and the rate of application. Figures 12-1 to 12-13 show the hand positions and contact surfaces for the various forms of percussion and therapists applying percussion to the various regions of the body.

Pincement (Figures 12-1 and 12-2)[2]

Use the tips of your thumb, index, and middle fingers to gently and lightly pinch and lift or pluck the client's tissues. This is the only percussion stroke in which the tissue is lifted off the surface; the tissues are compressed in all

FIGURE 12-2 Pincement performed on the face.

other forms of percussion. Pincement is at times used on the face.

Tapping (Figures 12-3 and 12-4)[4,6,8-11]

Keep your wrist and forearm still and gently strike the client's tissues with the individual fingertips or finger pads, using the same motion as that for keyboarding. In "point hacking," strike the client's tissues using your fingertips together as a group with a slight accompanying wrist motion.[3] Tapping and point hacking are also suitable for use on the face and are commonly used in **neuromuscular facilitation**.

Hacking (Figures 12-5 and 12-6)

Hold your fingers, wrists, and palms loosely and facing each other in relatively close opposition. Make contact using the ulnar borders of your fifth finger and hands; one author suggested making contact with the posterior surface of the three medial fingers.[6] Alternate hands in order to apply light and rapid strokes.[3] Hacking can be applied to most areas of the body, other than the head, for a mild stimulating effect.

FIGURE 12-1 Hand position and contact surfaces for pincement. The practitioner lifts or plucks the tissue upward.

FIGURE 12-3 Tapping performed one finger at a time on the face.

FIGURE 12-5 Hand position and contact surface for hacking.

FIGURE 12-4 Hand position and contact surface for point hacking.

FIGURE 12-6 Hacking applied to the sole of the foot will gently wake a sleeping client.

Slapping or "Splatting" (Figures 12-7 and 12-8)[4,8,11]

With your hand and fingers held loosely, make contact with the entire open palmar surface. This technique is suitable for large flat areas, such as the back or thighs, when a more stimulating effect is desired.

FIGURE 12-7 Hand position and contact surface for slapping.

FIGURE 12-9 Hand position and contact surface for clapping. Contact occurs only around the rim of the hand.

Clapping (Figures 12-9 and 12-10)[3,5,6,8-10]

Few sources[4] distinguish between "cupping" and clapping; therefore, this text considers the terms to be equivalent. Position your hand so that it forms a hollow "cupped" surface that traps air and does not deform on impact.[1,3] To cup your hand, flex your metacarpophalangeal joints to about 45°, hold your interphalangeal joints in neutral extension, and adduct your fingers and thumb. The degree to which your hand should be cupped will vary with the area of the body that you are treating. For example, your hand should be flatter over flat surfaces, such as the posterior chest, and more cupped to fit curved areas, such as the lateral surfaces of the rib cage.[1] Let your wrist remain as loose as possible and avoid excessive arm movement, since this can cause rapid fatigue. Clapping is the technique of choice when performing **postural drainage** to increase **airway clearance**, and it does not have to be particularly forceful or rapid to be effective for this purpose.[1] You can also use clapping in areas other than the thorax such as over large muscle groups.[3]

FIGURE 12-8 Slapping is very stimulating when applied to bare skin. It is suitable for large, flat areas like the back.

FIGURE 12-10 Clapping applied to the posterior apical segment of the right lung.

ONLINE VIDEO

Beating or "Rapping" (Figures 12-11 and 12-12)[3,4,8]

Position your hand in a loose fist and use the heel of your hand and dorsal surface of the interphalangeal joints to percuss larger muscles or even the sacrum. You can use more force when applying beating than clapping because beating is applied over large muscle groups, while clapping is applied over the rib cage where there is less overlying muscle.[3]

FIGURE 12-13 Hand position, direction of movement, and contact surface for pounding.

FIGURE 12-11 Hand position and contact surface for beating.

Pounding (Figure 12-13)[3,4,8,10]

Position your hand in a loose fist and use the ulnar surface of your hand as the contact surface.[3] Abduct your elbows, hold your hands near your midline, and apply the strokes in circles that move in the sagittal plane away from your chest and return toward your abdomen as you strike the client. This technique is appropriate for large, thick muscle groups such as the glutei and hamstrings.

Note: Some authors consider the compressive vibration and shaking used during PDP to be a form of percussion.[5,6] Chapters 9 and 11 describe coarse vibration and shaking.

MANUAL TECHNIQUE FOR ALL FORMS OF PERCUSSION

1. For all forms of percussion, keep your wrist and hand as relaxed as possible while maintaining the position of the chosen contact surface. Light forms of percussion require only small motions of your fingers or wrist. For the heavier forms, generate force through the combined movement of your wrist and forearm, as well as elbow flexion and extension.
2. Make the contact and release strokes quick, and even. Use both hands and alternate hands while performing the strokes with a fast, stable rhythm. This rhythm can take considerable practice to achieve. Bear in mind that an even rate of application is more important to achieve than increased speed. Consequently, strive to achieve evenness first, and only then increase the tempo of the

FIGURE 12-12 Vigorous beating is suitable for large muscles such as the gluteals.

application. A rate of 3 to 8 Hz is acceptable when the technique is performed with both hands.

3. The form of percussion and the force with which it is applied must be adjusted to the thickness, type, and sensitivity of the target tissue. Use very light force over the face and areas of unprotected bone. Use moderate force over thinner muscle groups, as in the forearm, or where there is dense fascia. Finally, use the heaviest force over large muscles such as the glutei. The force of application of percussion should also be adjusted to the size, age, and general health of the client.

4. Whenever possible, avoid applying percussion over the same area for more than a few seconds, since this can become irritating to the client. Instead, move your hands through the region of focus in a consistent pattern such as a circle or in parallel lines.[1,3]

5. Apply percussion through a gown, a sheet, or a towel as necessary to reduce irritation.

6. Avoid bony prominences such as the clavicles and avoid breast tissue. If the client has large breasts, ask her to use her hand to hold the breast tissue away from the contact area. Another option is to adjust her position on the table so that her breast falls away from the contact area, for example, in side-lying.

THERAPIST'S POSITION AND MOVEMENT

1. When treating the limbs and torso, stand at a right angle to the long axis of the tissues to be treated and use a **standing upright posture** or a **wide-stance knee bend** shown in Chapter 6 (Figures 12-8 and 12-12). Incline or lean toward, or over, the target tissues when applying heavier forms of percussion, such as pounding, or to generate a faster rate of application (Figure 12-6).

2. Hold your elbows partly flexed; the amount of flexion will vary with the form of percussion, area, size of client, and working posture chosen (Figures 12-6, 12-8, 12-12, and 12-13). The power for the strokes of heavier forms of percussion comes from a combination of movements that are performed while the upper arms remain stationary. The primary motion for this stroke is flexion and extension of your wrist, and the secondary motion is a small amount of elbow flexion and extension.

3. Allow your shoulders, elbows, and wrists to remain loose throughout the applications of all percussive techniques.[1,3]

4. During longer applications of percussion (clapping) that address several lung segments and include postural drainage of the lung segments (up to 30 minutes), change positions frequently to minimize the mechanical strain of performing this physically demanding treatment (Figure 12-14).

PALPATE

Since your hands are in contact with the client's tissues for fractions of a second at a time, detailed palpation is impossible. You can, however, form a general impression of the resiliency (springiness) of the tissues being contacted. This resiliency will vary with the amount of subcutaneous fat, level of **resting muscle tension**, and supporting bony structure that are present in the region.

OBSERVE

While performing the technique, observe the client and look and listen for the following signs of correct application of the technique:

1. Each form of percussion makes a characteristic sound on impact. For example, on healthy tissue, cupping makes a hollow resonant sound as the trapped air resonates between the cupped hand and the chest wall. If your hand flattens on impact, this sound will not occur, and more importantly, the effect of the technique may not penetrate as deeply into the lung tissue as needed. Bear in mind that the sound of cupping on impact—dull, resonant, or hyperresonant—may not be a reliable method of assessing the health of the client's underlying tissues.[46]

2. During the application of **PDP**, listen to and observe the client's breathing, coughing, and expectoration.[1]

3. During the application of PDP, periodically check the client's face to monitor the comfort level.[1] When applying any percussion stroke for reflex **stimulation**, watch the client for signs of waking, **arousal**, or irritation.

COMMUNICATION WITH THE CLIENT

Communicate to prepare the client for treatment and to seek feedback on the client's level of comfort during the technique. Following are some examples of statements that you can use.

BRONCHIAL DRAINAGE

UPPER LOBES Apical Segments

Bed or drainage table flat.

Patient leans back on pillow at 30° angle against therapist.

Therapist claps with markedly cupped hand over area between clavicle and top of scapula on each side.

UPPER LOBES Posterior Segments

Bed or drainage table flat.

Patient leans over folder pillow at 30° angle.

Therapist stands behind and claps over upper back on both sides.

UPPER LOBES Anterior Segments

Bed or drainage table flat.

Patient lies on back with pillow under knees.

Therapist claps between clavicle and nipple on each side.

16"

RIGHT MIDDLE LOBE

Foot of table or bed elevated 16 in.

Patient lies head down on left side and rotates ¼ turn backward. Pillow may be placed behind from shoulder to hip. Knees should be flexed.

Therapist claps over right nipple area. In females with breast development or tenderness, use cupped hand with heel of hand under armpit and fingers extending forward beneath the breast.

16"

LEFT UPPER LOBE Lingular Segments

Foot of table or bed elevated 16 in.

Patient lies head down on right side and rotates ¼ turn backward. Pillow may be placed behind from shoulder to hip. Knees should be flexed.

Therapist claps with moderately cupped hand over left nipple area. In females with breast development or tenderness, use cupped hand with heel of hand under armpit and fingers extending forward beneath the breast.

20"

LOWER LOBES Anterior Basal Segments

Foot of table or bed elevated 20 in.

Patient lies on side, head down, pillow under knees.

Therapist claps with slightly cupped hand over lower ribs. (Position shown is for drainage of <u>left</u> anterior basal segment. To drain the right anterior basal segment, patient should lie on his left side in same "posture".)

20"

LOWER LOBES Lateral Basal Segments

Foot of table or bed elevated 20 in.

Patient lies on abdomen, head down, then rotates ¼ turn upward. Upper leg is flexed over a pillow for support.

Therapist claps over uppermost portion of lower ribs. (Position shown is for drainage of right lateral basal segment. To drain the left lateral basal segment, patient should lie on his right side in the same "posture".)

Last Rib

20"

LOWER LOBES Posterior Basal Segments

Foot of table or bed elevated 20 in.

Patient lies on abdomen, head down, with pillow under hips. Therapist claps over lower ribs close to the spine on each side.

LOWER LOBES Superior Segments

Bed or table flat.

Patient lies on abdomen with two pillows under hips.

Therapist claps over middle of back at the tip of scapula on either side of spine.

FIGURE 12-14 Postural drainage positions for adults. (Reprinted from Rothstein J, Roy S, Wolf S. *The Rehabilitation Specialist's Handbook.* 3rd ed. Philadelphia, PA: FA Davis; 2004 with permission of FA Davis.)

In General

1. "I'm going to start the percussion now." Since percussive techniques, even when applied gently, often represent an abrupt change in sensation from other massage techniques, tell the client when you are going to begin percussion. When you select cupping or slapping, you should also prepare the client for the noise of the technique.
2. "Do you feel comfortable?" or "Do you need a break?" Since the application of percussion can be extremely stimulating, ensure that the client is not feeling irritated by the treatment, especially during longer applications.
3. "Does this cause you pain or discomfort anywhere?" The application of percussion should not cause the client pain or discomfort, regardless of the purpose for which it is being applied.[1]

When Clapping Is Used with Postural Drainage to Enhance Airway Clearance

1. Clients may start to cough spontaneously during the application of clapping. Encourage coughing, forced expiration, and expectoration. Also, provide a suitable receptacle for the client's sputum and use appropriate **standard precautions** in the handling of body fluids.
2. A long sequence of PDP (up to 40 minutes) can be a strenuous intervention for the client, as well as the therapist. Assess the client's comfort and level of fatigue every few minutes. Therapists are advised to perform PDP as their scope of practice and skill level permit.
3. Mucus may continue to move for up to an hour following the application of PDP.[1] Encourage the client to cough and expectorate as required after treatment.

A Practice Sequence for Percussion

Practice time: Allow 20 minutes per person.

You will not be able to apply percussion continuously throughout this sequence because it is a demanding technique to perform. Use **broad-contact compression** and coarse vibration in between the different forms of percussion to allow your hands and arms to rest. Note that in practice, longer treatments sessions may also include periods of postural drainage when the therapist is not treating.

Prone

The back and gluteals are a good test area. Undrape one side, and let the other side remain draped. You will treat both sides to determine the effect of the draping on the client's experience of the stroke.

To begin, apply a series of broad-contact palmar compression strokes over the entire area for a minute. Apply pincement for a minute. Return to compression for a minute.

Then apply in turn

- Tapping
- Point hacking
- Hacking
- Slapping
- Cupping
- Beating (apply to gluteals only)
- Pounding (apply to gluteals only)

Alternate palmar compression and the progressively more vigorous forms of percussion. Finish with compression. Solicit feedback from your client about how each form of percussion felt and how the application of percussion differed between the draped and undraped sides.

For additional study: Explore the use of lighter forms of percussion on more densely innervated areas such as the face and hands. How much percussive force is tolerable in each of these areas? Which strokes can and cannot be applied?

A Practice Sequence for PDP of an Adult

Practice time: Allow 30 minutes per person.

You will need an articulated, tilting treatment table or bed to achieve the elevation required for the various postural drainage positions. If this is not available, you can approximate the positions using eight or more standard pillows.[1,47]

Review any factors in your client's history that would require a reduction in force of application of the percussion (see the Cautions and Contraindications section later in this chapter). Note that positioning for pulmonary drainage in tilted positions with the head down will in itself elevate blood pressure, which is a caution for hypertensive clients.[1,3]

(Continued)

Remember to avoid the scapula, clavicle, and breast tissue. If the client has large breasts, ask her to use her hand to hold the breast tissue away from the contact area. Use caution around the floating ribs.

Apply the following cycle of techniques to as many of the segments illustrated in Figure 12-14 as time allows. In a clinical situation, one position should be maintained for 5 or 10 minutes or even longer. You can then apply continuous clapping for 3 to 5 minutes to a small area, followed by vibration and therapeutic breathing exercises. For a practice sequence, you may shorten these times to include a wider selection of positions:

1. Assume a postural drainage position (see Figure 12-14).
2. Apply clapping continuously with a stable rhythm over indicated segment of the lung for 1 or 2 minutes.

   As far as possible, use the cupped hand position and obtain the characteristic resonant sound; this is not always possible for a large-handed therapist. In smaller areas, use only one cupped hand or apply pounding or hacking.
3. Initiate compression and **coarse vibration** at the peak of each deep inspiration and continue them throughout expiration in the following manner. Compress the thorax over the segment as the client begins to exhale. While maintaining this compression, apply coarse vibration throughout the exhalation. Release compression to permit inhalation. In addition, instruct the client to forcibly exhale or vocalize "Ahhh."[8] Instruct the client to expectorate as required.
4. Alternatively, apply repeated rapid compression with a rapid partial release between each compression stroke (rib springing[1]). Instruct the client to forcibly exhale or vocalize "Ahhh" and to expectorate as required.
5. Intersperse rocking using rib contacts, or **rhythmic mobilization** of the rib cage, with the percussion to give both the client and the therapist a break from the more vigorous technique.

Change positions until you have treated several segments of the lung. At the end of this sequence, position the client in prone and finish with 5 minutes of **sedative** massage. Finish by instructing your client to sit up. Then practice giving instruction for appropriate follow-up care.

CAUTIONS AND CONTRAINDICATIONS

Therapists need clinical training and supervised practice to master the proper application of percussive techniques. Advanced training is essential when dealing with pathological conditions and therapists are referred to texts on the use of percussion for pathological conditions for a detailed discussion of cautions and contraindications for these techniques. All of the general and local contraindications noted for massage techniques apply to the use of percussion (see Chapter 5). The application of percussive techniques should not cause the client pain or discomfort. Posttreatment erythema and client reports of discomfort are undesirable effects that indicate incorrect application of the technique or client's intolerance?[1] A thin layer of fabric, such as a sheet or gown, placed between the therapist's hands and the client's skin can reduce skin sensitivity without substantially reducing the force of the technique.[1,3] There are also several specific contraindications to the use of percussion.

Percussion of the thorax is contraindicated in cases of rib fracture, untreated pneumothorax, confirmed or possible coronary thrombosis or pulmonary embolism, unstable cardiac conditions, conditions that are prone to hemorrhage, after chest or spinal surgery, [1,3] and during an acute episode of asthma.[48] The positional changes required for postural drainage may cause increased oxygen demand, carbon dioxide release, blood pressure, and cardiac output.[3,49] Consequently, the head-down position must be used with caution, particularly if clients are hypertensive or have had a head injury. [1,3,50] Percussion used alone can also increase the heart rate and blood pressure.[3,32] Notwithstanding these cautions, PDP can be tolerated by acutely ill clients, provided that the procedure is administered by trained therapists who can perform these techniques within their scope of practice and meet strict guidelines,[211,3,50] such as monitoring critically ill clients for hypoxemia and increasing the administration of oxygen.[17] The procedure should only be applied to clients who have pulmonary conditions that are associated with increased amounts of sputum.[17] Finally, although neither postural drainage nor percussion make gastroesophageal reflux worse,[51] avoid treating clients with these techniques after meals.[1]

There are separate contraindications and cautions for the application of percussion in areas other than the thorax. First, therapists consider even light percussion to be a local contraindication in acute and subacute injuries that are moderate or severe.[3] Therapists are also are advised to avoid muscles with **spasm** and postexercise cramping. In the case of active **trigger points**, or latent trigger points, a few authors have reported performing percussion on trigger points; nevertheless, therapists should use caution in doing so.[3,10,52-54] In addition, use caution when applying percussion over bony prominences such as the clavicles and vertebral spinous processes. Finally, reduce the force of application of percussion, or avoid using this technique, in areas where muscle tone and bulk are less than normal, over the kidneys, or around the floating and lower ribs. Percussion over the kidneys should be avoided completely for clients with a history of kidney stones. Percussion should be avoided when working with clients with a history of physical or other abuse, and wherever there is hypersensitivity.[1,3,4,8,10]

USING PERCUSSION IN TREATMENT

For PDP

Consider the following when using percussion to facilitate airway clearance:

1. There are several approaches to facilitating the thinning and clearance of sputum. If possible, encourage the client to drink water 30 to 60 minutes before the intervention.[1] Steam inhalation (humidification) can reduce the viscosity of the mucus and may also dilate the bronchioles. **Aerosol therapy** using an ultrasonic nebulizer can assist in liquefying and mobilizing mucus.[1] Prior application of warm moist heat to the client's anterior or posterior thorax may facilitate dilation of the bronchioles, if this is appropriate for the client's clinical condition.[55]
2. During PDP, position the client in the sequence of positions for postural drainage (Figure 12-14). Less rigorous, modified postural drainage positions may be as effective as traditional postural drainage positions.[1,35]
3. Intersperse clapping with broad-contact compression and simultaneous vibration of the rib cage.
4. Synchronize vibration with forced expiration, coughing, or audible huffing by the client.[1,3,8]
5. The use of suctioning,[21] methods of modifying mechanical ventilator airflow such as positive expiratory pressure,[15,23,38] and other mechanical devices, such as cyclically inflated pneumatic belts,[23] can be used with clients who have atelectasis or who are critically ill if the therapists' scope of practice and training permit.

After Performing PDP

Consider the following when using percussion to facilitate airway clearance:

1. Encourage the clearance of sputum and rest, as required, for the following hour.[2,24,56]
2. Teach the client techniques for cough stimulation and for effective coughing.[21]
3. The client can benefit from learning exercises for chest wall mobility, training of muscles for respiration. neuromuscular relaxation, and postural training from an appropriately trained therapist.[3,15,56,57]
4. Instruct the client on how to perform self-drainage.[23]
5. Clients may find self-administered chest clapping beneficial, although research has not consistently shown that it enhances the rate of sputum clearance or the level of oxygen saturation.[58]

For Facilitation and Inhibition of Neuromuscular Tone

Therapists using percussion to facilitate or inhibit neuromuscular tone need to consider the following:

1. Use joint traction and approximation, quick stretch, resistance, fine vibration, light touch, and repetitive brushing to increase **neuromuscular tone** and facilitate movement in clients with neurological conditions.[42,59]
2. Specific compression (inhibitory pressure), slow superficial stroking, static contact ("maintained touch"), prolonged cold, and neutral warmth are techniques that can be used to inhibit neuromuscular tone and facilitate movement in clients with neurological conditions.[42,59]

To Increase Arousal

While therapists typically use manual percussion to increase arousal, machines that produce percussion for general use are available and enjoyed by some clients. Since these produce very vigorous percussion, carefully review contraindications and cautions (e.g., the presence of active or latent trigger points) before their use.

IN CONCLUSION

Percussive techniques have a variety of uses, therapeutic effects, and outcomes. Table 12-1 summarizes those outcomes for percussive techniques that are related to body structures and functions.

Table 12-1	Summary of Outcomes for Percussive Techniques		
		Technique	
Outcome	**Clapping**	**Tapping**	**Other Forms of Percussion**
Increased airway clearance/mobilization of secretions	✓	?	?
Increased respiration/gaseous exchange	✓	?	?
Decreased dyspnea due to increased airway clearance	✓	?	?
Pain reduction through hyperstimulation analgesia	P	P	P
Systemic and sensory arousal and enhanced alertness	P	P	P
Normalized neuromuscular tone in patients with some CNS disorders	?	P	P
Alteration of movement responses in patients with some CNS disorders	?	P	P
Balance of agonist/antagonist function in patients with some CNS disorders	?	P	P

✓, the outcome is supported by research summarized in this chapter; P, the outcome is possible; ?, the outcome is debatable (research results are absent or inconsistent); CNS, central nervous system.

REVIEW   SECTION

TAKEAWAYS

1. Percussive techniques use controlled striking of the body to quickly deform and release tissues.
2. Percussive techniques can be used with postural drainage to mechanically loosen secretions in the lungs and facilitate airway clearance, to reduce or increase neuromuscular tone, to increase alertness, and to reduce pain.
3. Pincement is used to gently and lightly pinch and lift or pluck the patient's tissues.
4. Tapping (point hacking) is used to gently strike the tissues, often for neuromuscular facilitation.
5. Hacking involves light and rapid strokes, making contact with the ulnar border of the hand.
6. Slapping, suitable for large flat areas, promotes a stimulating effect.

7. Clapping (cupping) traps air between the cupped hands and the surface treated and is frequently used with postural drainage to increase airway clearance. The cupped shape of the hand used in chest percussion traps air against the rib cage and sets up a vibration that travels through the chest wall and lung tissue and dislodges the mucus that is stuck in the bronchial tree.
8. Beating is applied over large muscle groups with greater force than clapping.
9. Pounding with the ulnar surface of the loose fist is appropriate for large, thick muscle groups.
10. Percussion used for neuromuscular facilitation may achieve an effect by repeatedly stimulating stretch receptors (spindles) within the muscle. In addition, the intense stimulation of percussion may initiate a generalized **sympathetic response** that leads to increased alertness.

Clinical Case: *Percussive Techniques*

Patient Profile

A patient who regularly receives massage presents for a lunch hour massage prior to making an important business presentation later in the afternoon. He usually requests deep neuromuscular and connective tissue techniques and deep moist heat to address elevated resting muscle tension and related shortness in the muscles of his back and neck.

Clinical Findings

Subjective Findings:

- This patient wants the clinician to address the usual issues and areas.
- He does not want to feel drowsy after the massage since he has to perform well later in the afternoon.

Objective Findings:

- Range of motion: Slightly limited cervical range of motion (<10%) related to elevated resting muscle tension.

Treatment Approach

- It is possible to address the elevated resting muscle tension and restrictions of range effectively without resorting to techniques that produce marked sedation. For example, avoid the use of heat, deep pressure, sustained specific compression, direct fascial technique, rocking, and working around the sacrum.
- Your list of techniques might include skin rolling, the full range of neuromuscular techniques, and shaking. Limit the depth to more superficial layers of tissue, and use a somewhat faster pace than you would normally use, with a stroke rate between one and two strokes per second. Use active stretching techniques such as hold-relax to engage the patient.
- Finish each region with a couple of minutes of percussion and with superficial fingertip stroking.

Critical Thinking Questions

1. Percussion is often incorporated as a part of stimulating massage. In what common situations might patients benefit from enhanced alertness?
2. What is the rationale for using percussion to prepare for exercise with patients who have neurological conditions?
3. Discuss the possible reasons for which percussive techniques may be more or less beneficial for a patient preparing for an athletic event versus a patient presenting with chronic tension headaches.
4. Why should clinicians avoid performing percussion over active or latent trigger points?
5. Discuss why percussion may be a better technique than effleurage for ticklish areas.
6. Describe how percussive techniques may lead to the lengthening of a muscle or tendons. Why would not the same technique be used to treat a ligament?
7. Describe signs or symptoms that may be improved by using pincement (pinching and lifting or plucking

tissues) and how this technique might alter the tissues treated.
8. Describe how using percussive techniques in combination with other massage strokes might have different results depending on the order in which they are applied. For example, under what circumstances might it be better to end with percussion versus ending with effleurage?
9. What cautions or contraindications should be considered when planning treatment for an elderly female patient complaining of non-chronic respiratory difficulty in the last stages of a cold who presents with advanced hyperkyphosis and immobility of the thoracic spine?
10. Describe how percussive techniques might benefit a patient recovering from surgery or casting of an injured knee. Consider the progressive phases of healing and explain if and how percussion may promote greater improvements. Would the same techniques be used on the uninjured knee? Why or why not?

References for Chapter 12 begin on p. 479; see Further Reading list on p. 480.

CHAPTER **13**

Sequencing Massage Techniques for Outcome-Based Massage™

OBJECTIVES **After studying this chapter, you will have the information that you need to do the following:**

1. Discuss how to select massage techniques for use in treatment.
2. List the steps in planning a regional massage sequence.
3. List the steps in planning an extensive full-body massage sequence for medical massage or wellness.
4. Describe the concept of coherence and how to achieve it within a massage intervention.
5. Demonstrate how to apply massage techniques in the context of a practice sequence.

This chapter builds on the Outcome-Based Massage™ clinical decision-making model and earlier chapters on techniques by explaining how to create basic sequences of massage techniques. In doing so, it outlines the principles for selecting and ordering massage techniques to achieve specific clinical outcomes. Members of different health care professions will include additional nonmassage techniques with these sequences to create interventions and plans of care that fit their scopes of practice.

Evidence

STEPS IN THE SEQUENCING OF MASSAGE TECHNIQUES

A **sequence** of massage techniques is a structured, outcome-based series of massage techniques that make up an **intervention** or a part of an intervention. We use the term "sequence," instead of the term "routine," because the latter implies the use of massage techniques without the required assessment of the client's needs. Sequences of massage techniques should be highly structured, rather than routine or random. The structure of these sequences should reflect the therapists' understanding of the purpose of the techniques they are using and their clients' needs. It should also be consistent with the **principles of design** that address why therapists combine massage techniques in certain sequences; how interventions begin, proceed, and end; and how the constraints of time and location affect the treatment process. In reality, treatment approaches can vary considerably. When presented with the same situation, 10 experienced therapists will design 10 sequences of massage techniques that will have distinct differences and notable similarities.

The five steps in the design of a sequence of massage techniques are as follows:

1. Summarize the **clinical findings** and **outcomes**
2. Select treatment techniques
3. Specify the scope and duration of the sequence of massage techniques
4. Choose a **framing general massage technique**
5. Sequence the chosen massage techniques according to principles.

We suggest that students initially work in small groups to design sequences of massage techniques and record this design process. Although this is a slow process, the critical thinking that is an integral part of the design process will become second nature with repetition. At that point, students will be able to perform much of the design of sequences of massage techniques mentally during the course of the evaluation and treatment planning phases of the Outcome-Based Massage™ clinical decision-making process.

Summarize the Clinical Findings and Outcomes

The starting point for the design of any sequence of massage techniques is your summary of clinical findings from the client examination and a succinct statement of the desired outcomes (see Chapter 5). You should prioritize this list of outcomes, in consultation with the client, and then decide which **body structures** and **body functions** you can treat.

Select Treatment Techniques

Therapists base their selection of treatment techniques on the outcomes they can achieve with each technique. For that reason, you should familiarize yourself with the outcomes for a variety of massage techniques (see Chapters 7 to 12 and Table 13-1). Clearly, not all massage techniques are useful or indicated for all clinical conditions. You must also go beyond simply matching techniques to outcomes to consider broader questions related to your client and the context of treatment. These questions can include the following: "Has my client indicated an interest in wellness?" "What is his overall energy level and emotional state?" "Is there a problem with the function of a particular tissue or structure?" "Is there any ongoing systemic pathological process?" "Does he have pain, and if so, should I treat it directly or can I treat it by addressing the underlying **impairment**?" "Are there restrictions of positioning or draping that would preclude the use of some massage techniques?" "What are the client's primary treatment goals?" With practice, you can begin to identify a list of potentially useful massage techniques for addressing the client's needs, as answers to these broader questions arise during the course of the evaluation phase. You will also identify other treatment techniques that are appropriate for the client's clinical condition, impairments, and **functional limitations**. You will then refine your list of massage and other treatment techniques during the **treatment planning phase** (see Chapter 5).

Health care professionals who use massage as one of several treatment modalities have to determine how much emphasis to place on massage techniques in an intervention. In these situations, it may help you identify soft tissue dysfunction that can impede your treatment of the client's other impairments. Take, for example, the case of a client who presents with a decreased ability to raise his arm, which appears to be secondary to muscle weakness. During the client examination, the therapist determines that the client has an abnormal **scapulohumeral rhythm** and soft tissue restrictions in the scapular region, in addition to muscle weakness. In this situation, for example both a physical therapist and a massage therapist may consider it more effective to begin by using massage techniques to reduce the soft tissue restrictions in the client's scapular region. Nevertheless, their respective scopes of practice would result in differences in how the intervention would proceed from that point. Both therapists could use some form of **joint play** technique to increase **accessory joint motion**. The massage therapist could have a greater range of massage techniques to use and more focus on massage. In this way, they would address the client's soft tissue dysfunction and decreased accessory joint motion in preparation for exercise used to increase muscular performance and joint mobility. The physical therapist may have a greater range of electrotherapeutic modalities, such as neuromuscular electrical stimulation, and physical agents available to integrate into the intervention. Furthermore, as the client improved, the physical therapist would progress her use of advanced therapeutic exercise techniques and functional training to address the client's functional limitations. Finally, both therapists would ensure that education in self-care was an ongoing component of this intervention.

Table 13-1   Summary of Outcomes for Massage Techniques

Effects/Uses	Category of Technique (Chapter)					
	7	8	9	10	11	12
Decreased capsular restriction	?	?	P	P	P	?
Increased joint mobility	?	P	✓	✓	P	?
Increased joint integrity	?	?	P	P	P	?
Increased muscle extensibility	?	?	✓	✓	P	?
Pain reduction						
Counterirritant analgesia	✓	P	P	P	P	P
Via sedation	✓	✓	✓	P	P	?
Via treatment of dysfunction	?	✓	✓	✓	P	P
Increased venous return (direct)	?	P	P	?	?	?
Increased lymphatic return (direct)	?	✓	P	?	?	?
Decreased joint effusion	?	✓	P	?	?	?
Separation/lengthening of fascia	?	?	P	✓	P	?
Promotion of dense connective tissue remodeling (in chronic stage)	?	?	P	P	?	?
Increased connective tissue mobility	?	?	P	P	?	?
Decreased muscle spasm	P	P	P	?	?	?
Decreased resting tension of skeletal muscle	?	P	P	P	P	?
Decreased trigger point activity	?	?	✓	P	?	?
Increased postural awareness	?	?	P	P	P	?
Normalized structural alignment	?	?	P	P	?	?
Normalized sensation/reduction of nerve compression	?	?	P	P	?	?
Enhanced muscle performance (secondary effect)	?	?	✓	✓	P	?
Balanced agonist/antagonist function	?	?	✓	✓	P	P
Increased rib cage mobility	?	?	P	P	P	?
Increased respiration/gaseous exchange	?	?	?	?	?	✓
Increased airway clearance/mobilization of secretions	?	?	?	?	✓	✓
Decreased dyspnea	?	?	P	P	✓	✓
Increased relaxation	✓	✓	✓	✓	P	?
Decreased level of cortisol	✓	P	✓	P	P	?
Systemic sedation	✓	✓	✓	P	P	?
Normalized neuromuscular tone	✓	✓	P	?	P	?
Alteration of movement responses	✓	✓	✓	✓	✓	P
Stimulated peristalsis	P	✓	P	P	P	✓
Stimulated immune function	P	P	✓	P	P	?
Sensory or systemic arousal and enhanced alertness	P	P	✓	P	P	P
Promoted weight gain/development	✓	?	✓	?	P	?

✓, the outcome is supported by research summarized in this chapter; P, the outcome is possible; ?, the outcome is debatable (research results are absent or inconsistent). This chart shows the effects and outcomes for the categories of techniques discussed in Chapters 7 to 12 on massage techniques.

Specify the Scope and Duration of the Sequence of Massage Techniques

The scope of sequences of massage techniques usually falls into one of two categories: regional sequences or full-body sequences. When you are identifying a region for treatment, treat conventional anatomical regions, as defined by major bony and muscular landmarks, together. In practice, you can make any large adjoining area of a client's body the focus of a regional sequence. Furthermore, you will often treat the client's hands, feet, and face and head as separate regions because of the complexity of those regions. Finally, you can combine regional sequences to address larger areas of the body. Key Points 13-1 lists body segments that therapists often treat together in sequences of massage techniques.

Your decision on whether the scope of the sequence of massage techniques will be a region or a larger area

Key Points: 13-1

Areas Commonly Treated Together as Regions

- Face and head
- Face, head, and neck (all surfaces)
- Head and neck (all surfaces)
- Posterior shoulders and neck
- Arm and hand
- Hand
- Abdomen
- Abdomen and anterior thorax
- Anterior thorax
- Anterior thorax, shoulders, and neck
- Lateral abdomen and thorax (side-lying)
- Back and posterior neck
- Back
- Lumbar and gluteal areas
- Posterior thigh, including gluteals, leg, and foot
- Posterior thigh, leg, and foot
- Posterior leg and foot
- Medial thigh, leg, and foot (side-lying)
- Lateral thigh, leg, and foot (side-lying)
- Foot

depends on the client's clinical condition, the techniques you select, and the amount of time available for the intervention. First, a localized clinical condition, such as a **tendinopathy**, **fasciitis**, and **capsular restriction**, requires a regional focus. You will also have to perform a more localized treatment for inflammation when orthopedic lesions are severe (in either the acute or chronic stage). Nevertheless, as the section on agonist–antagonist balance discusses, the use of certain massage techniques, such as neuromuscular techniques, will sometimes necessitate that you broaden the scope of the regional sequence of massage techniques, regardless of the duration of the intervention. When shorter treatment times are the norm within a clinical setting, it is difficult to address the entire body within an intervention, other than by using very general massage techniques. Short, full-body sequences of 20 minutes or less do not permit much time for local treatment. Consequently, this is advisable only when you seek to achieve general outcomes related to the client's level of arousal such as **sedation** or stimulation. When the time available for treatment is short and the outcomes are general, you and the client may still prefer to focus on a region of choice such as the back. Finally, longer treatment times will often permit the integration of a local treatment into the full-body sequence that you are performing.

It is essential for you to specify and adhere to a time for your application of a given regional or full-body sequence. Some therapists object to this approach on the basis that "clock watching" conflicts with the supportive, nurturing nature of a therapeutic intervention or that it inhibits learning. In practice, the contrary is true. Respect for time boundaries reflects a respect for the client and facilitates a respect for the other boundaries that are required for an appropriate client–therapist relationship. Furthermore, the time available for treatment influences all decisions about the number, type, and ordering of the techniques used, even though it may not change the basic emphasis of the intervention. In other words, it is more difficult to design a good sequence of massage techniques without knowing how much time you have available to execute it.

There are some general guidelines for the timing of sequences of massage techniques. Regional sequences can take from 5 to 45 minutes or more to apply, and full-body sequences can require from 15 to 90 minutes or more. Shorter sequences of massage techniques need to address fewer outcomes with fewer techniques in order to be **coherent** and effective. In addition, the outcomes that you can expect to achieve with treatments of shorter duration will vary with your level of experience,

Table 13-2	Suggested Times for Sequences of Massage Techniques That Seek to Achieve Common Outcomes	

Region	Outcome	Minimum Time (min)[a]
Back	Systemic sedation, decreased anxiety	10–20
Back	Systemic or sensory arousal, enhanced awareness	5–15
Thorax	Increased airway clearance	15–45
Thorax	Increased rib cage mobility	10–30
Limb	Increased lymphatic return	20–60
Limb	Reduced spasticity	10–30
Joint	Increased range (one joint)	5–20
Any	Counterirritant analgesia	15–45
Any	Decreased trigger point activity	3–20
Any	Decreased resting level of tone	5–30
Any	Local fascial lengthening	3–15
Any	Promotion of tendon remodeling	2–15
ALL	Deep systemic sedation	30–60

[a]The first figure represents a minimum duration of treatment (less time than this would make it difficult to achieve the outcome consistently). The second figure represents a comfortable length of time; more time can often be used to good effect. These figures assume treatment by an experienced therapist.

the clinical condition you are treating, and the massage techniques you are using. Table 13-2 provides some suggested minimum times in which experienced therapists can address discrete tasks within the context of a regional sequence of massage techniques. The amount of time that you allocate to using massage techniques, in relation to the other treatment techniques, will also be consistent with the relative impact of the soft tissue dysfunction on the client's functional level and other factors, including your scope of practice and clinical setting. Furthermore, all other factors being equal, when soft tissue dysfunction has a significant impact on the client's functional level, you can justify a greater emphasis on the use of massage techniques.

Choose a Framing General Technique

"**General**" and "**specific**" are useful, if somewhat imprecise, concepts that summarize several of the defining components for massage techniques. General massage techniques[1] engage and provide information about a large area of the body or a large group of tissues. These techniques have a large amplitude, use a broad-contact

surface (sometimes repeatedly over contiguous areas), and are inherently not localized to a particular area. Some examples of general massage techniques include superficial effleurage, direct fascial technique performed with a broad contact, palmar compression done in a series, and rocking. By contrast, specific massage techniques have smaller amplitudes, use small contact surfaces, and are localized to a specific region. Specific compression and cross-fiber friction are examples of specific techniques. It is a worthwhile exercise to attempt to group massage techniques according to whether they are general or specific. The following list suggests an order of selected massage techniques from relatively more general (top) to more specific (bottom):

- Rocking
- Superficial stroking
- Superficial effleurage
- Deep effleurage
- Broad-contact direct fascial technique
- Broad-contact myofascial release
- Shaking
- Wringing
- Picking-up

- Superficial lymph drainage technique
- Static contact
- Broad compression
- Squeezing
- Fingertip and thumb kneading
- Skin rolling
- Friction
- Specific compression

Sequences of massage techniques most often consist of a mix of general and specific massage techniques, although you can use either type of technique by itself. It is unusual to omit a general massage technique in Western systems of massage. On the other hand, Oriental or **Eastern approaches**, such as **Shiatsu**, may consist only of specific compression.[2] Their rationale for massage is very different from that of Western systems (see the discussion of meridian theory in Chapter 9). There are advantages to selecting one general massage technique that you repeat at intervals during the course of the sequence of massage techniques. In this way, this technique becomes the principal palpation tool and serves to frame and connect the other techniques that you use. The repeated use of this general massage technique imparts a sense of structure to the sequence of massage techniques. As Fritz[1] so aptly puts it, this technique can act as the "broth" in which the other, more specific techniques "float." Furthermore, although you can select more than one general massage technique for use in a given sequence, this practice may result in the loss of **coherence** of a sequence of massage techniques. Consequently, you should choose the **framing general massage technique** with the overall outcomes of the intervention in mind. Table 13-3 lists some of the characteristics of general massage techniques that you need to consider before choosing to use them.

Sequence the Chosen Massage Techniques According to Principles

The next step in designing an effective sequence of massage techniques is to organize the massage techniques according to clearly defined principles. The following is a formal summary of sequencing principles that we have implicitly introduced throughout the chapters on techniques (Chapters 7 to 12) in the sections titled Manual Technique and in the Context part of the Descriptions of Components.

Apply General Massage Techniques before Specific Ones[3,4]

You should apply general massage techniques before specific ones for two reasons. First, this approach permits an assessment of the broader manifestations of a local problem. Second, you can use the general massage techniques to affect the client's level of arousal.

When you apply general massage techniques before performing more localized techniques, you obtain a full palpatory scan of the tissues that are mechanically connected to the specific area that may be the focus of your intervention. This allows you to identify imbalances in the tissues adjacent to a local lesion that you may have missed during the client examination. For example, a local lesion can affect antagonist and synergist muscle groups, as well as proximal and distal tissues. This often occurs in predictable patterns that relate to the type of lesion. General treatment over the entire region allows you to assess and address the broader manifestations of the local problem prior to performing a more specific local treatment.

The following example will illustrate this principle. If you are treating a chronic **tendinitis** at the common

---

Table 13-3	**Characteristics of Some General Massage Techniques**

Technique	Requires Oil	Works through Sheet	Advantages/Disadvantages
Broad-contact compression in a series	No	Yes	Takes more time but gives information about deeper tissues
Myofascial release	No	±	Takes minutes
Rocking	No	±	Highly sedative but motion may increase pain
Superficial stroking	No	Yes	Produces only reflex effects
Superficial effleurage	Yes	No	Takes little time

±, the technique may be applied through the fabric, but this may reduce its effectiveness.

extensor origin (tennis elbow), you might use the following progression from general to specific massage techniques. You would first apply the general massage techniques to the client's arm, including regional superficial effleurage and broad neuromuscular techniques to reduce the resting level of tone in the agonist, antagonist, and synergist muscles. You would then apply specific neuromuscular techniques, such as stripping to the agonist muscle, prior to performing cross-fiber friction on the affected tendon. Toward the end of the time you allotted for the sequence, you would reverse the order of massage techniques, from specific to general again. The entire sequence leading up to the friction may take as little as 5 minutes, yet it can still be beneficial.

General massage techniques are ideal for achieving outcomes related to the level of arousal. For example, if **relaxation** or **sedation** is among the desired outcomes, then returning to the long flowing strokes of superficial effleurage or the rhythmic undulations of rocking at intervals will enhance the sedative effects you provide throughout the intervention. You can also use more specific massage techniques to address local restrictions within the same intervention. If you proceed too quickly to treating with specific massage techniques or spend too long on these, it may be more difficult for you to achieve and maintain effective relaxation in your client.

The relative amount of time that you will spend using general and specific massage techniques will vary with the outcomes you seek, the time you have available for the intervention, and the mechanical depth that specific massage techniques must achieve (see the section on the progression from superficial to deeper massage techniques in this chapter). For example, a 20-minute full-body intervention, with relaxation as the desired outcome, might consist only of general massage techniques. On the other hand, a 20-minute regional intervention for a chronic orthopedic lesion, which aims to promote remodeling of dense connective tissue, might include 15 minutes of very specific massage techniques.

Apply Superficial Massage Techniques before Deeper Ones[1-7]

Superficial massage techniques engage structures near the surface of the client's body, whereas deeper massage techniques engage tissue layers that lie deep to the superficial tissues. The appropriate depth of the massage technique you apply will vary with the client's clinical condition. Deeper massage techniques are not necessarily better, and you do not have to engage structures mechanically far below the surface to produce profound or lasting effects.

There are several reasons to begin with the application of superficial massage techniques. Superficial massage techniques allow the client to accommodate to your touch. They also enable you to palpate with your hands in the most relaxed and sensitive position. Finally, some clinical conditions can impede your ability to palpate and treat the client's underlying tissues appropriately. For example, when **edema**, which accompanies acute inflammation, and **fibrosis**, which is associated with chronic conditions, occur at the superficial level, they can limit your ability to palpate deeper structures accurately. In these situations, proceed to the first tissue layer at which you can palpate an abnormality, and then treat that layer until the tissue feels normal. At that point, you may increase your pressure to access deeper structures. A useful analogy for this approach to treatment is peeling the layers of an onion.

When the restriction is in multiple layers of muscle or connective tissue, you may not be able to determine the location of the restriction accurately at the beginning of the intervention. Nevertheless, the basic procedure remains the same: proceed gradually through superficial layers to the first palpable restriction, normalize this restriction, and then treat progressively deeper layers of tissue restriction. Regardless of the massage techniques you use, gradually reduce the pressure and briefly re-engage each layer that you previously addressed as you approach the end of the regional sequence. This allows you to reassess any additional effects that your use of deeper massage techniques may have had on the superficial tissues.

Here are some examples of this progression from superficial to deeper massage techniques. If traumatic edema is present, do not attempt to engage structures underlying the local edema with massage techniques until the edema has resolved. Usually within a day of initiating treatment, you can perform superficial reflex techniques on the site of trauma and then superficial fluid techniques to the proximal margin of swelling, as tolerated by the client. After this, return to superficial reflex techniques. During later interventions, use the same basic pattern of treating from superficial to deep to superficial on the site of the lesion as the edema resolves. With each intervention, you should reach progressively deeper tissue layers.

If the client's subcutaneous tissues are normal but a restriction exists in a superficial layer of muscle, you may progress the depth of the massage techniques within a minute or two to include **neuromuscular techniques** that engage this layer. If the difficulty lies in a deeper muscular layer, begin as noted in the previous example, and then engage progressively deeper layers of muscle before you finally engage the layer in which the restriction lies.

You can use **superficial reflex techniques**, such as static contact, superficial stroking, and fine vibration, at any time in an intervention and for virtually any length of time. Therapists often use these techniques at the beginning and end of full-body or regional sequences. You may omit the use of superficial reflex techniques entirely if muscle or connective tissue is the focus of your intervention.

Coordinate and Repeat the Transitions from General to Specific to General and from Superficial to Deep to Superficial

In practice, you execute the transitions from general to specific to general and from superficial to deep to superficial simultaneously. In other words, begin sequences of massage techniques with general techniques that engage superficial tissues over large areas, and then progress to specific techniques that engage deeper tissues in a succession of smaller areas. You will return to the use of more general and superficial techniques between your treatment of the smaller areas. When time permits, make these transitions in depth and specificity several times during a regional sequence of massage techniques. This strategy permits you to assess the tissue responses continually, and at different depths, throughout the region you are treating. Using these guidelines can reduce the occurrence of agonist–antagonist imbalances that can result from your application of the deep, specific massage techniques needed to treat chronic restrictions in muscle and connective tissue (see other sections in this chapter).

Use Principles Related to Enhancing Fluid Return

The following principles are relevant when you specifically seek to enhance lymphatic or venous return. Although these principles are common in classical sequences that emphasize effleurage and petrissage, you can disregard them if you are not attempting to enhance fluid return.

Use Centripetal Pressure and the Assistance of Gravity When Possible

The use of **centripetal** pressure, with minimal pressure on the return stroke, ensures that the mechanical flow of fluid receives maximal assistance in the direction of its normal return. [1,3-6,8,9]

Begin Proximally, Proceed Distally, Return Proximally, and Repeat [2-4,6,8,9]

When the aim of treatment is to increase **lymphatic return** from a region, begin the massage stroke as proximally (close to the heart) as time allows and progressively move in a distal direction until you approach the region. Ensure that the direction of pressure of each stroke is always centripetal. For the limbs, this requires that you begin at least as proximally as the axillary or inguinal lymph nodes. Repeat this sequence of applying massage techniques from proximal to distal as frequently as the time available for the intervention allows. This approach of beginning the treatment proximally creates a proximal reservoir into which you will direct the fluid that is located in the distal region. [9] If the client's lymphatics in a proximal region are not intact, designate an adjacent proximal body segment as the reservoir to which you will direct the fluid from the distal region. For example, this region may be the contralateral side of the client's trunk or ipsilateral side of her chest.

Maximize the Relaxation of the Proximal Muscle Groups

Mennell[10] noted that deep veins and lymphatics are embedded in skeletal muscle. Consequently, excessive muscular tone can compress the lumen of the deep veins and lymphatics and reduce venous and lymphatic flow. This explains why you reduce the external pressure on the collapsible vessels and passively assist venous and lymphatic return when you ensure that there is maximum pliability of all of the muscles between the heart and the body segment you are draining. If time allows, use neuromuscular and connective tissue techniques to increase the general mobility and muscular relaxation of the muscles of the thorax. In some cases, such as with hand edema secondary to **thoracic outlet syndrome**, addressing mobility and muscular relaxation in the thorax may be your first priority. In practice, you may want to shift your focus quickly to the client's affected limb because of time constraints. Make this decision carefully because addressing proximal regions may be more effective.

The sequencing of massage techniques is often more flexible when you are applying superficial reflex, connective tissue, specific neuromuscular, and passive movement techniques. Note that when circulatory concerns are not the focus of treatment, you may use centrifugal pressure (with the exception of deep centrifugal pressure over incompetent veins or, as some authors suggest, all veins[1,2]), and you may treat distal areas first.

Coordinate All Transitions

Therapists frequently encounter situations in which the tissues in adjacent body segments, which they wish to engage, lie at different depths. For example, with post-traumatic swelling of the wrist, the application of massage techniques on the immediate site of the injury is contraindicated, minimal, or light, depending on the nature and degree of the injury. In this case, begin a regional sequence of massage techniques for the superficial tissue layers on the proximal portion of the client's arm to enhance superficial lymphatic return. Then gradually move your hands in a distal direction toward the proximal edge of the swelling. Progress to using deeper massage techniques for the deeper tissue layers of the upper arm to relax the client's muscles and enhance the deep lymphatic return from his proximal arm. Then alternate between the proximal application of deeper massage techniques and the distal application of superficial massage techniques, moderating the depth of stroke as you move from one body segment to the other. To complete the intervention, apply superficial massage techniques over the entire portion of the client's limb that you are treating.

Apply Massage Techniques from the Periphery to the Center of the Region You Are Treating[4]

When a circumscribed area of local pathology is the focus of your intervention, begin with a general sequence of massage techniques to the region. Then gradually apply massage techniques closer to the periphery of the local area of pathology. This strategy permits you to palpate related tissue changes that may occur in areas that are remote from the local region you are treating. Furthermore, it enables you to gradually introduce massage techniques to an area that may show tenderness and other altered responses to touch.

Use the same principle of applying massage techniques from the periphery to the center of the region when you are treating an area of local swelling. In this case, apply massage techniques in a **centrifugal** direction at the periphery of the area of swelling and gradually move toward the center of the area of swelling as the peripheral fluid is absorbed.

Address Agonist, Antagonist, and Synergist Groups

You must be careful to avoid producing an imbalance in the client's myofascial system when you use neuromuscular or connective tissue techniques. This is particularly important if you are applying these massage techniques in small areas, with a higher force, or for long periods. For example, Simons et al.[11] have noted that releasing trigger points can produce a **reactive tightening**, or cramping, in related muscles and may activate other trigger points. Therapists who use connective tissue techniques also routinely note positional shifts in related body segments in response to the local application of massage techniques.

When you apply deep specific massage techniques locally, without including general massage techniques, clients will commonly experience undesirable responses to the treatment within half an hour to 3 days after the intervention. These responses can include reactive tightening and pain in (a) areas that are immediately proximal or distal to the site that you treated, (b) in antagonist or synergist muscle groups that are located on the same side of an adjacent joint, or (c) in antagonist or synergist muscle groups that lie across a joint. Reactive pain and restrictions can be detrimental to the client's clinical condition. In addition, it may worsen until the imbalance caused by treatment resolves or you treat it. To avoid this situation, you must also address the related areas where reactive tightening may occur whenever you include the application of local, deep, specific massage techniques within an intervention. The less experienced therapist can apply general neuromuscular techniques, such as broad-contact compression or petrissage, for this purpose. A very experienced therapist may use a postural assessment to identify relatively shortened areas that require lengthening in order to maintain adequate myofascial balance. Regardless of your level of expertise, you should alert the client to the possibility of these effects of treatment and ensure that the client understands that it is important to let you know if a troublesome shift in pain or symptoms occurs after the intervention. You may also teach the client appropriate stretching exercises to minimize reactive tightening.

In general, the intensity and duration of the application of massage techniques to balance antagonist and synergist muscle groups will vary in direct proportion to the specificity, depth, and duration of the sequence of massage techniques that you perform on the main area of treatment. This part of the intervention might require from 10% to 50% of your designated treatment time. Your ability to identify which antagonist and synergist muscle groups are the most prone to reactive tightening and to judge how long to spend on addressing this issue will improve with experience and, one hopes, with a minimum of client distress.

Treatment of the Contralateral Side

You may have to treat the client's contralateral side or limb within an intervention that addresses a unilateral lesion. For example, when treating a client with a unilateral **piriformis syndrome**, you may justifiably include petrissage, stripping, and specific compression as the primary massage techniques to lengthen the client's affected piriformis. Nevertheless, you must also treat the client's unaffected gluteals and lateral rotators in order to achieve a balanced bilateral distribution of tension throughout the pelvic musculature. Therapists vary as to whether they apply massage techniques to the contralateral limb before or after their treatment of the client's affected limb. It may be easier for you to judge the depth and intensity of the treatment that is required to achieve balance with the client's contralateral limb after you have treated the affected limb. When you are treating an acute-stage unilateral orthopedic lesion, you may also treat the client's contralateral side as a means of addressing compensations that may arise from altered patterns of muscular use.

Treatment of the Related Axial Skeleton

If you apply deep specific neuromuscular or connective tissue techniques on one of a client's limbs (even the distal limb), you should also treat the related portion of the axial skeleton with general techniques, even if only briefly. For the lower limbs, apply general petrissage to the lumbar musculature bilaterally, and for the upper limbs, apply general petrissage to the cervical musculature bilaterally. For example, when you treat a client with **De Quervain's tenosynovitis**, apply superficial effleurage to the client's entire arm, broad-contact petrissage to his upper arm and then to his lower arm, additional specific neuromuscular techniques to his lower arm, friction to the tendons in the region of the anatomical snuff box, and broad-contact petrissage and superficial effleurage to his entire arm. Furthermore, either precede or follow this sequence of massage techniques with the brief application of broad-contact or general petrissage to the client's contralateral arm and cervical musculature (about 25% of the treatment time).

Sequence Massage Techniques with Other Appropriate Treatment Techniques

You will often use massage techniques in conjunction with other treatment techniques that are relevant to the client's clinical condition. This section contains some examples that illustrate how to sequence massage techniques with physical agents and therapeutic exercise.

Do not alter the sequence of the massage techniques when you are coordinating the application of heat and cold with massage techniques. Instead, apply the selected physical agent either before or after the sequence of massage techniques. Do not routinely apply cryotherapy, such as ice or cold packs, before applying massage techniques that use any amount of force. This application can result in a decrease in the client's sensation in the region that you are treating. This decrease in sensation diminishes the client's ability to provide accurate feedback about the tenderness or pain arising from the involved tissues during the sequence of massage techniques. You can use cryotherapy after these massage techniques to reduce the client's symptoms or the consequences of overtreatment. For example, if you believe that you have overtreated a client with friction (which should happen rarely), then it would be appropriate for you to ice the treatment area after the friction. You may also apply cold packs to another body segment concurrently with the sequence of massage techniques. This would be the case if you were treating an acute orthopedic injury, such as a sprained ankle, and used cold packs on the site of the lesion (as it was elevated) while you applied massage techniques proximally to reduce edema.

If you are treating healthy tissues or chronic lesions, you can apply heat either before or after local sequences of massage techniques. When you are treating muscle, apply heat before sequences of massage techniques to relax the muscle, decrease tissue viscosity, and allow easier access to deep tissue layers.[12] If, however, you are using massage techniques to lengthen or stretch dense connective tissue with greater force, then it is not appropriate to apply heat *immediately* before the sequence of massage techniques because this heating may increase the risk of uncontrolled collagenous rupture.[13]

You often perform sequences of massage techniques before you use therapeutic exercise. In this case, the massage techniques prepare the client's tissue for active or resisted exercise by increasing tissue extensibility, improving the balance of agonist/antagonist function, and enhancing the client's level of alertness. You can also use sequences of massage techniques prior to the application of passive exercise, such as stretching or passive range of motion exercises, to enhance the effects of those techniques. A skillful therapist can alternate between massage techniques and passive exercise so that they blend seamlessly throughout the intervention. Finally, in cases in which the client has abnormal neuromuscular tone, you can use massage techniques as proprioceptive stimulation to normalize neuromuscular tone and the client's movement responses in preparation for therapeutic exercise or functional activity.[14]

DESIGN OF REGIONAL SEQUENCES OF MASSAGE TECHNIQUES

The following are the steps involved in designing a sequence of massage techniques for a region:

1. Summarize findings from the client examination.
2. Identify appropriate functional outcomes.
3. Summarize and prioritize outcomes.
4. Choose relevant massage techniques to address the impairments.
5. Assign time for the regional sequence.
6. Choose the framing technique(s).
7. Sequence the massage techniques, keeping in mind

   - the position of superficial reflex work, if included;
   - general to specific to general;
   - superficial to deep to superficial;
   - proximal to distal, if you are working to enhance fluid return;
   - periphery to center, if you are working with circumscribed local pathology;
   - agonist/antagonist/synergist balance, if you are including neuromuscular or connective tissue techniques to release local restriction;
   - do other regions have to be included? If so, design these sequences and revise the time budget for the intervention.

Using this approach, you can generate a wide variety of sequences of massage techniques that address different outcomes.

Students and novice therapists should not hurry this portion of their training, since the exploration of a variety of different sequences of massage techniques will encourage a flexible, adaptable approach to treatment. Even the design of seemingly simple regional sequences involves considerable reflection and planning on the part of the therapist. Therapists who practice in settings where intervention time is short (10 to 20 minutes) especially need to master the principles of massage design because there is often no extra time in which to address oversights in their planning.

DESIGN OF MORE EXTENSIVE SEQUENCES OF MASSAGE TECHNIQUES

The most common example of a more extensive sequence of massage techniques is the "full-body massage" sequence.

In its simplest form, a full-body sequence of massage techniques is simply a series of regional sequences performed in a chosen order and covering the entire body. These regional sequences are designed using the guidelines outlined in this chapter, employ similar techniques, and are similar in character. The following list expands on the steps required for the design of regional sequences so that you can apply these regional sequences to more extensive sequences:

1. Summarize findings from the client examination.
2. Identify appropriate functional outcomes.
3. Summarize and prioritize outcomes.
4. Choose relevant massage techniques to address the impairments.
5. Assign time for the entire intervention.
6. Choose regions that you will include or exclude.
7. Specify initial times and order for regions.
8. Choose the framing technique(s).
9. Sequence the massage techniques for regional sequences, keeping in mind

   - the placement of superficial reflex work, if included;
   - general to specific to general;
   - superficial to deep to superficial;
   - proximal to distal, if you are working to enhance fluid return;
   - periphery to center, if you are working with circumscribed local pathology;
   - agonist/antagonist/synergist balance, if you are including neuromuscular or connective tissue techniques to release local restriction.

10. If you are including a regional sequence(s) to address a particular condition, do you need to adjust the initial time budget?

When applying these steps, note that if there is a specific condition in one region that requires a different technical approach, then that sequence will differ from the others, and you will need to allocate more time to that sequence. Specifying an order and time for each regional sequence can help you overcome the problem of being unable to complete your treatment in the available amount of time. Furthermore, you must prioritize the outcomes for a given intervention, since you often have more work than you can accomplish. Clear priorities and precise timing will minimize the likelihood that you will lose focus or get sidetracked.

The practice of including all of the regions of the client's body in an intervention is common for "wellness massage" (general full-body relaxation massage).[1,2,5] The regions that you leave out of an intervention will vary with social norms, your training, and the preferences of your client. Within 45 to 60 minutes, it is often possible to address, at least briefly, each region of the client's body. Since many clinical conditions require a more extended local focus, the time constraints of many clinical settings often require that you omit some regions or treat them briefly with general massage techniques. Consequently, it is important that you determine during the initial interview whether the client expects all regions to be included in a longer sequence of massage techniques.

If you practice in a setting where longer interventions (30 to 60 minutes) are possible, you may wish to integrate the specific treatment for a local condition with a more extensive sequence for the entire body. In this situation, you will give the region of focus more time than you would give it in a full-body sequence that has no regional focus. You have two options for allocating treatment time: include all of the remaining regions and shorten the treatment time proportionally or eliminate some regions so that the final sequence addresses less than the full body (e.g., just the upper body). This approach to the design of sequences of massage techniques may seem reasonable if you have first practiced full-body sequence of massage techniques for wellness. *You should not conceptualize the outcome-based interventions that address specified impairments as a full-body sequence for wellness with slight alterations. Often, you must alter a basic full-body sequence so much that the result bears scant resemblance to the general sequences that you perform for relaxation.*

There is no single order in which you must treat regions of the client's body during a full-body sequence of massage techniques.[1-3] You may begin regional sequences at the client's head or feet and then proceed region by region to the other end of the client's body in prone, supine, or side-lying. You will then turn the client and repeat or reverse the order of treatment of the regions. If you have a clear emphasis on one category of technique, then you may face some restrictions to the order in which you can address regions (Table 13-4).

FULL-BODY SEQUENCES OF MASSAGE TECHNIQUES FOR WELLNESS

Approaches to Full-Body Massage for Wellness

If you have performed the practice sequences in Chapters 7 to 12 on massage techniques, then you have already carried out a number of different approaches to full-body sequences of massage techniques to achieve specific outcomes. These "one-technique" sequences have limited scope; however, they can be effective and rewarding for both the client and the therapist. In practice, approaches to full-body massage usually include a greater variety of massage techniques that therapists apply at a consistent rate and rhythm to produce a coherent, structured, sensory experience for the client.

Classical, **or "Swedish," massage**, as it is commonly practiced today, uses mostly superficial fluid and neuromuscular techniques that are applied rhythmically with a broad-contact surface and moderate centripetal pressure.[2,5] (The rate of application is quite slow for

Table 13-4	**Suggestions for Ordering Regions When Emphasis Is Placed on Particular Massage Techniques**
Emphasized Technique	**Suggestions for Ordering Regions**
Connective tissue	If there is extensive connective tissue work, start and/or end with work around the sacrum and iliac crest
Connective tissue, passive movement	Include the axial skeleton (i.e., neck, back, pelvis, and sacrum); if there is deep, specific, or extensive work around the lumbar/pelvic region, include at least briefly the lower legs and feet
Neuromuscular	If there is deep, specific work on limbs, conclude with the related axial skeleton, that is, cervical or lumbar area
Percussive	Rarely if ever emphasized throughout the body; if concentrated in the thorax for an extended period, finish with sedative reflex technique
Superficial fluid	Start on upper thorax and proceed distally to the region of focus; work distally from next major proximal set of lymph nodes
Superficial reflex	Start and finish with sacrum, occiput, face hands, or feet

Note: The chapters on individual techniques (Chapters 7 to 12) discuss the basis for most of these suggestions.

therapists who are trained in North America and faster for therapists who are trained in Europe.) When performed in this way, classical massage increases the return of lymph, reduces the level of resting muscle tension, reduces anxiety, and enhances the client's awareness. This effective approach to the full-body sequence of massage techniques continues to be the archetype for wellness massage in North America.

Increased access to the massage forms of other cultures and the work of modern Western innovators has recently spurred a technical renaissance in the practice of massage. Many of these traditions, or approaches, use a limited spectrum of massage techniques and refine related client examination and palpation skills to a high degree. Table 13-5 summarizes some of these approaches.[1,2,5-8,17] Without trivializing the philosophical differences that exist between these approaches, you can characterize them as the refined application of specialized massage techniques that result in specific effects and different sensory experiences for the client. When appropriate to the clinical situation and executed with skill, any one of these approaches can produce excellent results.

Maximizing Relaxation in Wellness Massage

Repair and regeneration of the body and mind occur more effectively when the nervous system is in a parasympathetic state. A central premise of **wellness massage** is that systemic **relaxation** or **sedation** is a desirable outcome in most situations. Another central premise is that reduction of resting tension of skeletal muscle

is also usually desirable. These facts are also true when you are applying massage techniques to clinical conditions, although other goals related to presenting impairments may be a higher priority for both you and the client.

An important axiom of practice is that *to relax a client, you must be relaxed.* The corollary is equally true: *clients will not relax if you are agitated.* It is as though the physical state of relaxation or tension passes from person to person. Although this axiom is worth remembering, it is very easy to forget in a busy practice. Suggesting that you work from a place of deep calm does not imply that you will show a lack of attention, inquiry, or intention or that you will suspend your capacity for critical thinking. A good therapist is adept at achieving a relaxed, attentive state within herself, while keeping her focus on the objectives of treatment and using precise technique. As discussed in Chapter 6, we advise you to practice gentle stretching, conscious breathing, and some ritual of calming the mind throughout the workday, especially in the few minutes preceding a sequence of massage techniques. Using conscious diaphragmatic breathing and controlled repetitive movement with correct body mechanics can also deepen your relaxation when performing massage.

Students and novice therapists often learn how to perform a general full-body sequence of massage techniques for relaxation in an environment that is relatively free of pressure. When faced with the pressures of completing client examinations, handling complex clinical situations, and managing the time constraints of practice, they commonly fail to relax when performing massage

Table 13-5	Characteristic Massage Techniques of Some Popular Massage-Related Approaches[1,2,4-7,15,16]
Approach, System, or School	**Characteristic Massage Techniques**
Lomi Lomi	Fast, superficial and deep effleurage and fast, broad neuromuscular technique
Manual lymph drainage	Superficial effleurage and superficial lymphatic technique
Myofascial release	Myofascial release, craniosacral techniques
Neuromuscular technique	Specific kneading, stripping, specific direct fascial technique
Polarity	Static contact and compression
Rolfing, Bindegewebsmassage	Direct fascial technique
Shiatsu	Compression, specific (ischemic) compression, stretching
Therapeutic touch, Reiki	Static contact
Trager	Rocking, and sedative rhythmic mobilization and shaking

techniques. Although the resulting sequence of massage techniques may be technically competent, it may feel somewhat disjointed or ineffective to both the therapist and the client because it lacks the critical element of relaxation that contributes so much to the experience of both parties.

Key Points 13-2 summarizes some hints to help you achieve and maintain effective relaxation in your clients. Temper these suggestions with the observation that different techniques will produce deep relaxation from client to client and from day to day. In light of this, you must always monitor the client's subtle body cues and inquire about the client's response to treatment to determine the effectiveness of an intervention to produce deep relaxation.

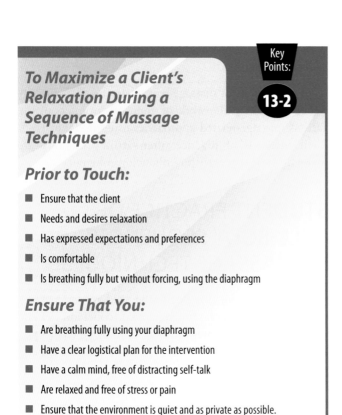

Key Points: 13-2

To Maximize a Client's Relaxation During a Sequence of Massage Techniques

Prior to Touch:

- Ensure that the client
- Needs and desires relaxation
- Has expressed expectations and preferences
- Is comfortable
- Is breathing fully but without forcing, using the diaphragm

Ensure That You:

- Are breathing fully using your diaphragm
- Have a clear logistical plan for the intervention
- Have a calm mind, free of distracting self-talk
- Are relaxed and free of stress or pain
- Ensure that the environment is quiet and as private as possible.

While in Contact, Ensure That:

- The rate and rhythm of similar strokes is constant
- Pressure transitions within each stroke are smooth
- Transitions from one type of stroke to another are smooth
- Contact is made and broken gently and carefully
- Communication is minimal
- The client is comfortable after each change of position

Note that you do not ever rush or hurry. After contact, allow a rest period of 10 to 60 minutes.

Relaxation versus Addressing the Effects of Stress

Although there is no direct link between the autonomic nervous system and skeletal muscle, research suggests that a generalized elevation of resting muscle tension is one of the effects of stress and the activation of the sympathetic nervous system.[18,19] As a result, massage techniques that reduce resting muscle tension are valuable for treating the short-term and long-term effects of stress. Since neuromuscular techniques, connective tissue techniques, and movement techniques can all affect the level of resting tension in skeletal muscle, they are obvious choices for returning a client's body to homeostasis after periods of stress.

Addressing the effects of stress by altering the level of resting muscle tension is not the same as producing relaxation, although you may address them with the same massage techniques. If you want to treat stress in otherwise healthy individuals, try to achieve (at least) the following three outcomes: produce relaxation in the client throughout the sequence of massage techniques, decrease the level of resting tension of skeletal muscle, and improve the quality and quantity of movement, since movement is often restricted by stress-related muscular tension. If you only achieve relaxation with your intervention, the client may soon feel no different than he did before the massage intervention. If, however, you also alter the client's level of resting muscle tension and the movement patterns of the skeletal muscles, then the sedative effect will be more long lasting. A good therapist can seamlessly incorporate massage techniques that alternately, or simultaneously, address all of these outcomes, while addressing the other outcomes for the intervention.

For further details about treatment for stress, see Chapter 14.

THE ART OF COHERENCE

In the context of Outcome-Based Massage™, **coherence** is the consistent order or structure of an intervention. Coherence is the result of clear and consistent intention(s) on the part of the therapist. Maintaining coherence is relevant in all sequences of massage techniques. It is, however, of particular importance in sequences that last longer than 15 minutes and use a wide variety of massage techniques to address multiple outcomes. Coherent sequences can give a client an overall feeling of being in harmony and balance throughout the sequence of massage techniques and after the intervention. It is easy to imagine an incoherent full-body sequence: vigorous fast shaking on one leg, smooth slow superficial effleurage on the other, similarly mismatched massage techniques on the arms, myofascial release on the back, and light percussion on the face. Other examples of strategies that result in lack of coherence are discussed in Key Points 13-3.

In this chapter, we introduced several strategies that can help you to produce coherent massage interventions. The most important of these is your unwavering relaxation around the treatment table. Constant relaxation throughout the sequence conveys a consistency of manner and approach to the client, regardless of the technical content of the intervention. Another strategy for making an intervention coherent is to achieve and maintain a generalized nervous response in the client throughout the intervention. The desired response is usually relaxation. A third way of increasing the coherence of a sequence of massage techniques is to use the same framing **general technique** (palpatory stroke and connecting stroke) to touch all regions of the client's body during the intervention. When you return to the same technique at intervals during the intervention, you give a sense of sensory regularity to the sequence, which can put the client at ease. When you touch all regions of the client's body, even if only briefly with general strokes, you reinforce a client's sense that you are considering his needs as a whole person, not merely as an instance of an illness or disorder. This is often a crucial and unstated concern when the client has experienced long-standing pain or physical disability. Nevertheless, *it is not how much of the client's body that you touch that is critical but the way in which you touch it.* You can unwittingly reduce coherence when you use too many massage techniques, with a large variation in rate, pressure, and palpatory focus. The following list summarizes strategies to enhance the coherence of full-body sequences of massage techniques:

- Let yourself relax thoroughly and continuously during the sequence of massage techniques.
- Choose a small number of outcomes and stick to them.
- Aim for a generalized nervous response in the client (i.e., sedation or arousal).
- Use the same framing general technique in all regions.
- Maintain consistent rhythm in all regions.
- As far as possible, maintain a comparable rhythm in all massage techniques.
- Use similar (not necessarily identical) massage techniques in all regions.
- Be cautious of overloading a sequence with many different sensations.

Practitioners of massage would also be wise to experience or observe the work of good practitioners of the various massage-related approaches listed in Table 13-5. Their methods of practice often artfully demonstrate many of these strategies for enhancing coherence.

STUDENT PRACTICE OF FULL-BODY SEQUENCES OF MASSAGE TECHNIQUES

It is quite common for beginning students of massage to be taught one well-choreographed, coherent, generic routine that incorporates a variety of massage techniques (predominantly neuromuscular) according to the general principles.[5-8] This approach has both good and bad points. In learning the routine, students unconsciously absorb sound principles. By contrast, students often develop a certain rigidity of technical approach that can be detrimental in later clinical practice and that is *very* hard to retrain. It is generally preferable for beginning students and novice therapists to design and practice a variety of coherent full-body sequences that address different outcomes and have differing durations such as 15-, 30-, 45-, and 60-minute sessions. This practice teaches you mental flexibility and prepares you to handle time-consuming clinical problems without sacrificing the emphasis on treating the whole person, which is the hallmark of good treatment.

Thorough training will enable students to perform a large number of different sequences of massage

---

Key Points: 13-3

An Unpleasant Experiment: The Incoherent Sequence of Massage Techniques

Time: Allow about 20 minutes

Prepare for prone or supine.

- Choose massage techniques with conflicting intentions.
- Randomly and rapidly vary rate, rhythm, and pressure.
- Arbitrarily switch back and forth from region to region.
- Ignore your posture: slump or lean in an uncontrolled fashion.
- Talk to the client about whatever crosses your mind.

It usually takes less than 5 minutes to make an unforgettable point to the person on the table. Once the client stops the exercise, help him or her return to homeostasis with some sedative massage techniques.

techniques with a strict observance of the character and duration of each sequence. We caution students against the early development of a particular "style," since this is often a technical limitation in disguise or a projection of personal preference. It is better for you to attempt to master many massage styles and understand how the selected outcomes define the style of any given Outcome-Based Massage™ intervention.

IN CONCLUSION

Mastery of the principles and practice of designing and performing sequences of massage techniques is an essential component of a therapist's education in massage. Whether sequences are regional or full-body, therapists should design them to be structured and outcome-based and reflect the therapists' understanding of the purpose of the techniques they are using and their clients' needs. Sequences should also be consistent with the **principles of design** that address why therapists combine massage techniques in certain sequences; how interventions begin, proceed, and end; and how the constraints of time and location affect the treatment process. In addition, during the performance of sequences of massage, therapists need to incorporate the strategies that enhance coherence and improve the quality of the client's experience of massage.

Practice

Note: This section contains instructions that demonstrate how to use some of the principles of sequencing massage techniques that were introduced in this chapter

DESIGN OF REGIONAL SEQUENCES OF MASSAGE TECHNIQUES

The following sample sequences include some simple examples with questions and instructions to guide students and novice clinicians in the art of designing sequences of massage techniques. These examples are by no means the only possible sequences; they simply illustrate how you can apply the guidelines discussed in this chapter.

A Short Regional Sequence for the Back[2,5]

Purpose

Preparation of the patient's tissues for lumbar joint mobilization techniques and stabilization exercises; this does not require removal of the patient's clothing.

Outcomes

Decreased level of resting tension throughout the muscles of the back and increased muscle extensibility.

Time

10 minutes.

Framing General Technique

Broad-contact compression.

Techniques and Order of Application

1. Beginning prone, apply broad-contact compression with your palms systematically. Work bilaterally from the patient's upper back to his gluteals.
2. Sustain each compression for 30 seconds or until you feel the tissues begin to soften.
3. Encourage the patient to breathe deeply.
4. Apply compression with your forearms to the patient's lumbar area, one side at a time, avoiding direct pressure on his spinous processes.
5. Apply compression with your doubled fists to the gluteus medius, one side at a time.
6. Apply specific compression with your doubled thumbs. Focus on the tightest parts of the lumbar erector spinae and gluteus medius. Sustain this as time permits.
7. Finish with a line of palmar compressions down the patient's back to the gluteals.

A Short Regional Sequence for the Leg[2,5,9]

Purpose

Preparation of a postsurgical (for example, total knee replacement and ligament repair) patient's tissues for joint mobilization techniques, deep stretching of knee musculature, and range of motion exercises; this does not require removal of the patient's clothing.

Outcomes

Increased venous return, decreased edema, increased muscle extensibility, decreased level of resting muscle tension, and reduction of pain.

Time

10 minutes.

Framing General Technique

Broad-contact compression.

Techniques and Order of Application

1. Position the patient supine, with her affected thigh elevated at least to 30° and the knee in a loose-packed position.
2. Encourage diaphragmatic breathing.
3. Apply several palmar compressions to the patient's upper thorax, synchronized with the patient's exhalation.
4. Beginning at the inguinal area, apply broad-contact compression with moderate pressure to the patient's tolerance, following a sequence similar to that illustrated in Figure 9-8.
5. Reduce pressure near the patient's knee. Do not apply the technique over edema or if the patient reports an increase in pain.
6. Repeat the sequence as time allows. Change your emphasis from the central thigh to the lateral thigh and especially to the medial thigh.
7. If the swelling is only on the anterior surface of the patient's knee and not behind the knee, then you may continue with gentle muscle squeezing applied to the calf from proximal to distal in a continuation of the same pattern of proximal to distal to proximal.
8. Finish with superficial stroking down the patient's entire leg.

A Short Regional Sequence for the Neck[2,5]

Purpose

Complementary to joint mobilization techniques, stabilization and postural awareness exercises for a patient with cervical pain and decreased range of motion; this does not require removal of the patient's clothing.

Outcomes

Hyperstimulation analgesia, reduction of trigger point activity, and decreased resting tension of skeletal muscle.

Time

10 minutes.

Framing General Technique

Superficial effleurage.

Techniques and Order of Application

1. With the patient in supine, loosen the patient's collar or bare the neck area as much as possible.
2. Using a small amount of nonstaining lotion, perform superficial effleurage bilaterally and then unilaterally on the posterior and lateral surfaces of the patient's neck. Increase the depth with each repetition of the stroke in order to engage the patient's muscles.
3. Apply several strokes of broad-contact direct fascial technique to the lateral and posterior surfaces of the neck.
4. Use picking-up on the sternocleidomastoid muscles, one side at a time.
5. With your fingertips and thumbs, knead the anterior and posterior muscles of the neck with the patient's cervical spine in neutral and rotated positions.
6. Use stripping or ischemic compression to treat trigger points, as time permits, and follow with the appropriate stretches.
7. Finish with superficial effleurage, gentle traction of the cervical spine, and holding of the occiput.

A Short Regional Sequence for the Arm

Purpose

Complementary to joint mobilization techniques, electrotherapeutic modalities, and therapeutic exercise for patients with lateral or medial epicondylitis; this does not require removal of the patient's clothing.

Outcomes

Hyperstimulation analgesia, increased connective tissue mobility, decreased resting tension of skeletal muscle, and enhanced collagen fiber remodeling.

Time

10 minutes.

Framing General Technique

Myofascial release.

Techniques and Order of Application

1. With the patient in supine, begin with a myofascial release arm pull.
2. Apply more specific myofascial releases to the anterior deltoid, biceps, and entire extensor group of the forearm.
3. Apply broad-contact compression and muscle squeezing to all muscles of the arm and forearm, with as much pressure as the patient can tolerate.
4. Using a small amount of lotion, apply stripping to the patient's wrist extensors. If time allows, apply stripping to the wrist flexors as well.
5. Apply 1 to 2 minutes of friction to the most tender point of the tendon.
6. Apply muscle squeezing and broad-contact compression to both arms.
7. Finish with a bilateral arm pull, followed by cervical traction.

A Regional Sequence for the Abdomen[2,5,20]

ONLINE VIDEO

Caution

When practicing this sequence, keep in mind that deep abdominal pressure is not advisable immediately preceding or during menstruation because of sensitivity and because local congestion limits the clinician's ability to palpate. Even light abdominal massage during menstruation may alter the flow and duration of the menses. See detailed discussion of contraindications and cautions in Chapter 5.

Outcomes

Stimulated peristalsis, relaxation, and decreased resting tension throughout the abdominal musculature.

Time

20 to 30 minutes.

Framing General Technique

Superficial effleurage.

Techniques and Order of Application

1. Static contact applied to navel and occiput.
2. Superficial stroking of the abdomen in clockwise circles.
3. Effleurage progressing from superficial to deep in clockwise circles.
4. Wringing, picking-up, and palmar kneading applied to the entire abdomen.
5. Specific kneading and stripping to abdominal muscle (moderate pressure can be used as long as there is a high horizontal component—high shear—to localize the force to the skeletal muscle).
6. Draw knees up to a crook-lying position to slacken abdominal wall.
7. Deep specific compression applied in **retrograde** sequence from the sigmoid colon to the iliocecal valve.
8. Palmar kneading.
9. Wringing.
10. Large-amplitude sedative shaking.
11. Rocking.
12. Static contact at navel and occiput.

Make the pace slow and the movements rhythmic. Apply each massage technique for 1 to 2 minutes. After you introduce superficial effleurage, return to it for a few strokes before you add each new massage technique. Switch sides as required. The application and release of deep specific digital compression must be very slow, and the clinician must pay close attention to the patient's comfort level. The literature suggests that abdominal massage may have a reflex or mechanical effect on peristalsis.[15,21-29] Clinicians who use massage techniques extensively have a common perception that abdominal massage will promote colonic emptying. Nevertheless, the opinions about the mechanisms by which this might occur vary, since the nervous control of peristalsis itself is complicated. The following techniques may promote peristalsis:

1. Superficial reflex techniques applied over the abdominal wall.
2. Nonspecific neuromuscular techniques that decrease the tone of the skeletal muscle of the abdominal wall and affect intestinal flow via somatovisceral reflexes.
3. Deep massage techniques that mechanically stretch the viscera, causing reflex contractions of the smooth muscle of the intestine.
4. Deep specific massage techniques that mechanically assist movement in the direction of the colonic flow (Mennell[10] doubted that this was possible).

With respect to these four possible mechanisms, the prevalent practice is to perform light massage techniques, such as superficial stroking, in the direction of colonic flow. Neuromuscular techniques and connective tissue techniques, such as wringing, can be oriented according to the direction of the muscle fibers you are treating or in any way that causes an effective stretch of the tissues of the abdomen, as long as strokes do not directly oppose the flow in the colon. Finally, perform deep massage techniques that specifically seek to move intestinal contents over the colon with pressure in the direction of peristaltic flow in a retrograde sequence from the sigmoid colon to the iliocecal valve.[1,2,5] The last mechanism presupposes that the skeletal muscle that forms the abdominal wall has been sufficiently relaxed to allow the pressure of the technique to physically engage the viscera. It is important to remember that promoting a generalized **parasympathetic response** is a nonspecific way of facilitating peristalsis. You can do this when you are working on any region.

Further Exercises

1. Design and practice a 20-minute abdominal sequence with the same aims that you perform through a sheet.
2. Design and practice a similar abdominal sequence that you perform from one or both sides with the patient in side-lying.
3. How might you have accomplished some of the treatment with the patient prone? Consider, for example, what lumbar wringing might achieve.

A Regional Sequence for the Leg[2,5,9]

Outcomes

Increased **lymphatic return** from a leg with an intact lymphatic system and relaxation.

Restrictions

Administer directly on the skin using talc, cornstarch, or chalk as lubricant.

Time

20 to 30 minutes.

Framing General Techniques

Superficial and deep effleurage.

Massage Techniques and Order of Application

1. Position the patient supine with legs elevated 30° to 45°.
2. Instruct patient in deep diaphragmatic breathing.
3. Apply rhythmic palmar compression over the upper ribs for 2 to 3 minutes.
4. Apply superficial effleurage to entire affected leg.
5. Apply superficial lymphatic technique beginning at the proximal thigh and then beginning progressively

more distal with each new series of strokes, until you reach the foot (repeat ad lib).
6. Apply deep effleurage.
7. Use a series of centripetally moving palmar compressions applied in a pattern similar to that used in the lymphatic technique in step 5 (i.e., beginning proximally and starting progressively more distal with each new series until the foot is reached) (repeat ad lib).
8. Use passive relaxed movements for all joints, beginning at the hip and proceeding to the ankle.
9. Apply superficial effleurage.

Although this sequence uses few massage techniques, you must repeat them. Frequent repetition is required when moving fluid. In addition, a repetitive rhythm will assist you in achieving sedation. Note that there are two general massage techniques used here: superficial effleurage is interspersed with the superficial lymphatic technique, whereas deep effleurage is interspersed with the compressions. You could use this sequence to drain a localized traumatic edema anywhere in the leg such as an ankle **sprain**, quadriceps **contusion**, or hamstring **strain**. There are several modifications required for doing so: avoid areas of acute tissue damage, reduce the pressure around these areas, avoid pushing fluid through areas of congestion, and perform passive movements only where they do not recreate the patient's pain.

Further Exercises

1. How would you address the same impairments with massage techniques that use oil as a lubricant? How would you do this without using lubricant?
2. Design and practice a similar sequence that seeks to drain a designated area on the thorax toward the ipsilateral axilla.
3. How would the sequence change if the application of mechanical techniques was a contraindication in the area of the patient's ankle?
4. How would the sequence change to address swelling in the posterior calf (e.g., an acute calf contusion or Achilles tendon rupture)?
5. Should you alter the sequence to include other proximal segments or the contralateral leg?

A Regional Sequence for the Neck, Head, and Face[2,5]

Outcomes

Hyperstimulation analgesia, reduction of trigger point activity, decreased resting tension of skeletal muscle, increased range of motion, and relaxation.

Restrictions

No lubricant.

Time

20 to 30 minutes.

Framing General Technique

Palmar compression.

Massage Techniques and Order of Application

In supine

1. Palmar superficial stroking.
2. Palmar compression done as a series from the top of the neck to the clavicle, unilaterally, then palmar compression to the head (repeat with the head rotated to the other side).
3. Muscle squeezing to neck.
4. Specific compression on either side of spine and to suboccipital muscles, followed by appropriate stretch.
5. Specific compression to sites of upper trapezius and sternocleidomastoid trigger points (use pincer compression for sternocleidomastoid), followed by appropriate stretches.
6. Gentle fingertip kneading to the face and more vigorous fingertip kneading to the scalp.
7. Fingertip fascial technique with short strokes to the scalp.
8. Gentle palmar compression from top of the neck toward the axilla in several series.
9. Superficial stroking throughout with the palms and then fingertips.

Spend from 2 to 4 minutes on each item. Turn the patient's head frequently, and if necessary, ensure that you support the patient's neck with a small pillow for comfort. Return to the application of palmar compression done as a series from the top of the neck to the axilla between each new massage technique. This sequence with slight changes would be valuable in many cases of muscular tension or trigger point headache.

A Regional Sequence for the Back[2,5]

Outcomes

Decreased level of resting tension throughout the muscles of the back, increased muscle extensibility, increased mobility of spinal joints and rib cage, reduction of pain, and relaxation.

Time

20 to 40 minutes.

Framing General Techniques

Superficial and deep effleurage.

Techniques and Order of Application

1. Static contact applied to the sacrum and occiput.
2. Superficial palmar stroking down the spine.
3. Effleurage progressing from superficial to deep.
4. Wringing, picking-up, palmar kneading applied to the whole back.
5. Deep effleurage with forearm; finger and thumb kneading to the erector spinae muscles.
6. Stripping along the erector spinae muscles with elbow.
7. Bilateral specific compression along the erector spinae muscles—10 locations at 20 seconds per location.
8. Palmar kneading.
9. Wringing.
10. Superficial palmar stroking, becoming progressively slower.
11. Static contact at the sacrum and occiput.

Make the pace slow and your movements rhythmic. Apply each massage technique for 1 to 2 minutes. After you introduce superficial effleurage, return to it for a few strokes before you add each new technique. Switch sides every few minutes. It may exacerbate muscular imbalances if you perform all massage techniques on one side of the patient's back before switching. Simply break contact, move around the table, and recommence. Clinicians might use this type of sequence for patients with back pain or tightness associated with prolonged bed rest and in the chronic stage of erector spinae strain or lumbar facet derangement.

Further Exercises

1. Why might you have to address the extensors of the hip after you perform this sequence? How would you alter the sequence to include these?
2. For similar aims and techniques, how would you adapt this routine for other regions? Practice several of these in a similar time interval.
3. For similar outcomes, how would the selected massage techniques differ for a clothed patient? Design and practice a regional back sequence with this restriction in mind.
4. How would you alter this sequence if there were only 15 minutes available for the intervention? If there were only 10 minutes?

A Regional Sequence for the Shoulders

Outcomes

Decreased **resting tension** of skeletal muscle, separation and lengthening of superficial fascial layers, enhanced **muscle performance** (secondary), and increased joint mobility.

Restrictions

Use minimal lubricant.

Time

30+ minutes (to do both the shoulders).

Framing General Technique

Rhythmic mobilization.

Massage Techniques and Order of Application

1. Rhythmic mobilization.
2. General, broad-contact neuromuscular technique (compression and squeezing).
3. Myofascial release arm pull through glenohumeral range from neutral to full abduction.
4. General direct fascial tissue technique applied with a broad contact and combined with slow active arm and shoulder movements.
5. Stripping to rotator cuff muscles, followed by related stretches.
6. Rhythmic mobilization.

Additional

Split the sequence into the application of techniques with the patient in supine and then prone, or perform the entire sequence with the patient in side-lying (both sides). Apply all massage techniques from midthorax to occiput and distal to the elbow. Include all muscles that produce motion at the glenohumeral joint and the scapulothoracic articulation. Use minimal lubricant; otherwise, there will not be enough drag for the connective tissue work. Return to rhythmic mobilization frequently and ensure that it is not too stimulating. Both shoulders should receive equal time, although in different areas. Usually, the patient's dominant shoulder is tighter anteriorly, and his nondominant shoulder is tighter posteriorly. Get the patient off the table after you complete one side and compare the range and ease of movement between the two shoulders. Once you have completed both shoulders, spend at least 5 minutes to address the neck with conventional stretching, myofascial release, and traction.

This would make an acceptable intervention for a **capsular restriction**. If the patient presented with **adhesive capsulitis**, you might add after the stripping: trigger point work (especially to subscapularis[11]), friction to relevant tendons,[30] and joint mobilization.

DESIGN OF MORE EXTENSIVE SEQUENCES OF MASSAGE TECHNIQUES ONLINE VIDEO

The sequences in this section address the same general outcomes in all regions, with about an equal allocation of time between regions.

A Full-Body Sequence for Stress When You Cannot Remove Clothing

Outcomes

Relaxation, decreased perceived anxiety (and **cortisol** levels), improved immune function, and decreased resting tension of the skeletal muscle.

Restrictions

Patient is clothed.

Order of Regions

Prone to supine, head/thorax to feet.

Time

20, 40, or 60 minutes for all regions.

Framing General Techniques

Rocking, broad-contact compression.

Techniques and Order of Application

Beginning prone, apply the following massage techniques in this order in each region:

1. Static contact.
2. Rocking.
3. Broad-contact compression all over the region (you may synchronize its application on the thorax with the patient's exhalations).
4. Alternate between broad-contact compression and specific compression in areas where muscular tension is higher.

5. Intersperse compressions with rocking ad lib.
6. Finish each region by returning to rocking and static contact.

The more you use compression (especially if it is specific), the greater the decreases in the patient's resting muscle tension you will achieve. *It is both possible and useful to learn how to cover all regions in as short an interval as 20 minutes*, although the amount of specific compression that you can include will be very limited. In doing so, ensure that the general character of the sequence remains the same, regardless of the time in which you perform it. Do not increase the speed with which you apply the individual techniques when you have less time for the intervention. Instead, use fewer repetitions and more general techniques. This sequence would be suitable for reducing the effects of stress. You might also incorporate it into longer interventions when anxiety and stress exacerbate primary symptoms in clinical conditions such as asthma (between attacks), fibromyalgia, or chronic whiplash injuries.

Further Exercises

1. Where would you incorporate superficial stroking and muscle squeezing into this sequence?
2. Design and perform a sequence that accomplishes the same aims using lubricant.
3. Design and perform a version of this exercise with the patient in side-lying position (i.e., left side-lying and then right side-lying).

A Full-Body Sequence to Increase the Range of Motion

Outcomes

Generalized increased joint mobility and relaxation.

Restrictions

No lubricant.

Time

30, 45, or 60 minutes for all regions.

Order of Regions

Various orders are possible; finish with at least 15 minutes on the back, neck, and pelvis.

Framing General Technique

All of the techniques used are general, and you could choose any of them to frame the sequence.

Massage Techniques and Order of Application in Each Region

1. Perform one or two strokes of direct fascial technique with a broad contact.
2. Perform one myofascial stretch with wide hand placement.
3. Stretch associated joints (stretch hands and feet as a unit).

You could use this sequence for a healthy individual who complains of generalized stiffness a day after vigorous physical activity. Sixty minutes would allow you to treat 15 to 20 localized areas that you should distribute evenly throughout the body, unless there is an obvious deficit in the range of motion in one joint. Because the chosen massage techniques require time for a viscoelastic response to occur in the patient's tissues, your tempo must be slow, and the pressure should be moderate. The depth of release and the resulting increase of range of motion in any one area will be very small in comparison to what you would achieve if you concentrated the procedure on one or two regions of the body for the entire treatment time. We initially advise students not to concentrate connective tissue techniques around one joint because compensations can arise quickly.

Further Exercises

1. Perform a version of this exercise with the patient in side-lying. Try to foresee and deal with difficulties regarding positioning before you start.

A Stimulating Full-Body Sequence

Outcomes

Systemic **arousal**, enhanced awareness, marginal decrease in resting muscle tension, and increased perceived relaxation.

Restrictions

No lubricant.

Time

20 or 40 minutes for all regions.

Order of Regions

Supine and prone, head to feet.

Framing General Technique

Coarse running vibration.

Massage Techniques and Order of Application in Each Region

1. Coarse running vibration.
2. Shaking.
3. Fast rhythmic palmar compression and muscle squeezing (one to two techniques per second).
4. Light hacking.
5. Superficial fingertip stroking (limit the time spent on this last massage technique, or the effect may be too stimulating for the patient).

This sequence has a character similar to that of some precompetition sports sequences of massage techniques, and you might use it to alleviate lethargy and fatigue temporarily. Because of the brisk tempo and relatively short time, the neuromuscular techniques (step 3) cannot penetrate much below the superficial layers of the muscle.

Further Exercises

1. Outline, and provide a rationale for, a selection of massage techniques and tempo for a precompetition sports situation.
2. For the same outcomes and duration of treatment, how would you alter the sequence if you were to use a lubricant?
3. How short can you make the duration and still have the massage feel **coherent** to the patient?

A Gentle Full-Body Sequence to Relieve Pain and Maintain Joint Range

Outcomes

Maintain joint mobility and integrity, prevention of capsuloligamentous restrictions, increased lymphatic return, analgesia, relaxation, and sensory arousal.

Restrictions

None.

Time

30 to 40 minutes for all regions (full body).

Order of Regions

Supine then prone, head/thorax toward limbs (i.e., proximal to distal).

Framing General Technique

Superficial effleurage

Massage Techniques and Order of Application in Each Region

1. At the outset of the intervention, encourage full breathing using both diaphragmatic and costal segments.
2. Superficial effleurage progressing deeper to engage superficial muscle layers.
3. Gentle wringing and nonspecific kneading.
4. Gentle rhythmic mobilization and rocking.
5. Passive relaxed movements (no overpressure).
6. Return frequently to, and end with, superficial effleurage.

This sequence is similar to the sequence that is traditionally recommended for treating rheumatoid arthritis in the noninflammatory phase.[30] In particular, this sequence is relatively short in order to prevent fatiguing the patient. As in the "Regional Sequence for the Neck, Head, and Face" section the depth of massage techniques is limited because of time constraints.

Further Exercises

1. How might you modify this sequence to address reduced range and complaints of stiffness in the hands?
2. How could you integrate the use of a hot pack into this sequence?
3. If a patient fell asleep during this sequence, what massage techniques—gently applied—could you use to awaken him?

A Full-Body Sequence for General Relaxation

Outcomes

Increased relaxation, improved immune function, and decreased resting tension of skeletal muscle.

Time

60 minutes for all regions (full body).

Order of Regions

Prone to supine, head/thorax to feet.

Framing General Technique

Broad-contact compression, rocking.

Massage Techniques and Order of Application in Each Region

1. Rhythmic rocking.
2. Superficial warming strokes such as effleurage.
3. Petrissage.
4. Specific compression.
5. Gentle passive stretching.
6. Finish each region with tapotement (for gentle stimulation) or rocking and static contact (for relaxation).

Further Exercises

1. Outline the advantages and disadvantages of ending a massage for general relaxation with a stimulating stroke such as tapotement. How can you ensure that the use of this stroke does not adversely detract from the patient's overall level of relaxation?
2. Suggest alternate strokes for finishing each region.

REVIEW   SECTION

TAKEAWAYS

1. A sequence of massage techniques is a structured, outcome-based series of massage techniques that make up an intervention or a part of an intervention.
2. There are five steps in the design of a sequence of massage techniques: Summarizing the clinical findings and outcomes; selecting treatment techniques; specifying the scope and duration of the sequence of massage techniques; choosing a framing general massage technique; and sequencing the chosen massage techniques according to principles.
3. You should apply general massage techniques before specific ones for two reasons. First, this approach permits an assessment of the broader manifestations of a local problem. Second, you can use the general massage techniques to affect the patient's level of arousal.
4. Apply superficial massage techniques before deeper ones. Superficial massage techniques engage structures near the surface of the patient's body, whereas deeper massage techniques engage tissue layers that lie deep to the superficial tissues. The appropriate depth of the massage technique you apply will vary with the patient's clinical condition.
5. In practice, you execute the transitions from general to specific to general and from superficial to deep to superficial simultaneously. In other words, begin sequences of massage techniques with general techniques that engage superficial tissues over large areas, and then progress to specific techniques that engage deeper tissues in a succession of smaller areas.
6. The following principles are relevant when you specifically seek to enhance lymphatic or venous return: use centripetal pressure and the assistance of gravity when possible; begin proximally, proceed distally, return proximally, and repeat; and maximize the relaxation of the proximal muscle groups.
7. Apply massage techniques from the periphery to the center of the region you are treating. This strategy permits you to palpate related tissue changes that may occur in areas that are remote from the local region you are treating.
8. Address agonist, antagonist, and synergist groups to avoid producing an imbalance in the patient's myofascial system when you use neuromuscular or connective tissue techniques.
9. In its simplest form, a full-body sequence of massage techniques is simply a series of regional sequences performed in a chosen order and covering the entire body.
10. The practice of including all of the regions of the patient's body in an intervention is common for "wellness massage" (general full-body relaxation massage). The regions that you leave out of an intervention will vary with social norms, your training, and the preferences of your patient.

Clinical Case: *Juggling Multiple Impairments Within Treatment*

Patient Profile

Your patient is a 55-year-old architect who currently works part-time due to family obligations and health issues. Her family doctor gave her the diagnosis of fibromyalgia 1 year ago after she experienced several years of progressive pain. A neurologist also recently diagnosed carpal tunnel syndrome. She sought treatment for help managing the pain and fatigue associated with **fibromyalgia**.

Clinical Findings

Subjective Findings:

Her main complaints are widespread constant musculoskeletal pain, stiffness, and frequent whole-head headaches.

- Pain: Her baseline VAS (Visual Analog Scale) pain level is about 3/10, and this frequently rises to 6 or 7/10. Pain interrupts her sleep several times a night.
- Paresthesia: She rates the tingling pain in her right wrist as less important; it bothers her only after long periods of computer work and occasionally wakes her up at night.
- Fatigue: She also complains of fatigue, which limits her ability to work and to participate in recreational activities with her family.
- Sleep: She sleeps in the fetal position.

Objective Findings:

- Posture: Hyperkyphosis, an anterior head posture, and an upper-crossed syndrome.
- Observation: There is no obvious swelling anywhere in the upper limbs.
- Range of motion: Cervical range of motion is limited in a capsular pattern; side flexion and rotations are equally limited, extension is limited.
- Neurological tests: Cervical range of motion does not reproduce hand paresthesia. Thoracic outlet tests on both sides show absent pulses without reproducing hand symptoms. Carpal tunnel tests, such as Phalen's, reproduce tingling in the hand on the right side after 15 seconds.
- Palpation: Tender points associated with fibromyalgia. There are numerous trigger points and hard, indurated areas throughout her musculature.

Treatment Approach

The list of this patient's impairments is long and includes stress, interrupted sleep, fatigue, altered body image, acute nociceptive pain, chronic pain, probable deconditioning, elevated resting tension, trigger points, adaptive shortening and lengthening, and decreased postural awareness.

- In developing your plan of care, review the treatment considerations and guidelines for massage techniques associated with these impairments. For example, her potential for fatigue requires an approach that is gentle and not taxing.
- Initially, it may be useful to limit the treatment to 30 minutes and apply massage techniques with light to moderate pressure. Once you learn how she responds to treatment, you will likely be able to increase both the length and depth of treatment. Within this framework, you can attempt the full range of massage techniques, including all neuromuscular and connective tissue techniques.
- Areas of priority include the head, anterior and posterior neck, anterior chest, arms, and back. You will not be able to address all of these in depth in each session. Consequently, you will have to schedule particular areas of focus for the first 5 or 10 sessions, while reserving some time in each session to address areas of concern that arise on the day of treatment. If possible, include the whole body each session, even if briefly. You can accomplish this with the skillful use of rocking and other general techniques.
- Given the likelihood that she has developed a chronic pain syndrome, encourage her to consult service organizations, such as the local Fibromyalgia Society, and other health care professionals.
- For initial home care, teach stretching, especially of the neck and upper body, relaxation techniques such as diaphragmatic breathing, and walking within her tolerance. She may find a nighttime wrist splint helpful.
- You can progress this intervention by increasing the pressure and duration of massage techniques to her tolerance. Progress her home care program by increasing the variety of techniques that you use to address the different impairments.
- Conduct a thorough re-examination of this patient (and of all patients with chronic conditions) at the end of every period for which you have set an outcome, for example, every 6 to 8 weeks. At each re-examination, revisit the outcomes and priorities you have established for this patient and, if necessary, draft a new plan of care (see Chapter 5). Discharge this patient when she has achieved all of the outcomes in her plan of care for that episode of care.

Critical Thinking Questions

1. Describe the reasons why you would design different sequences of massage techniques within the interventions for two patients who have the same clinical condition.

2. What are the arguments for and against using the same sequence of massage techniques at every session within a patient's episode of care?

3. What other order would you suggest to show the continuum from general to specific for the techniques listed in the section titled Choose a Framing General Technique?

4. What is the relationship between the specificity of a technique and the depth at which it is applied?

5. Why is coherence important? List the strategies for achieving coherence and describe how to apply these strategies within a full-body massage sequence for a patient with chronic pain.

6. How would you use the principles for designing sequences of massage techniques to create a sequence to reduce local pain and swelling for a patient with an acute-stage ankle sprain? Which principles are particularly important when you are seeking to enhance fluid return?

7. Why is it necessary to treat other areas of the patient's body when you are treating a local restriction of muscle and connective tissue?

8. What modalities other than massage are within your scope of practice? What are some of the ways in which you can combine massage techniques with these modalities?

9. Identify the differences and similarities between a full-body massage sequence for the treatment of a clinical condition and a full-body massage sequence for wellness.

10. Describe how you would prioritize the treatment of regions and select between multiple regional sequences or a single full-body sequence for a patient with multiple affected regions such as the neck, shoulders, upper back, and lower back.

References for Chapter 13 begin on p. 480; see Further Reading list on p. 481.

Application of Outcome-Based Massage™ to Clinical Conditions and Wellness

OBJECTIVES

After studying this chapter, you will have the information that you need to do the following:

1. Outline the role of impairments in body structures and functions, wellness goals, and outcomes in planning massage interventions using Outcome-Based Massage™.
2. Describe the application of the principles of Outcome-Based Massage™ to treatment planning for specific impairments and wellness goals.
3. Identify possible uses of complementary modalities within massage interventions for clients with clinical conditions and wellness goals.
4. Create and progress plans of care for clients with multiple impairments and wellness goals.
5. Describe the relevant anatomy, impairments, examination techniques, and treatment techniques for common clinical conditions and wellness issues and outline how to apply the principles of Outcome-Based Massage™ to the treatment of these conditions.

The foundation for Outcome-Based Massage™ is the growing body of research that suggests the merits of massage for **wellness** and the treatment of an increasing number of clinical conditions.[1-9] In Outcome-Based Massage™, therapists use the iterative four-phase Outcome-Based Massage™ clinical decision-making process (evaluation, treatment planning, treatment, and discharge phases) to create effective **interventions** that use massage techniques to address each client's individual needs and achieve specified clinical outcomes. The first section of this chapter provides practical guidelines for developing and progressing interventions for wellness and the treatment of

the **impairments in body structures and functions** associated with clinical conditions that use massage techniques to achieve specific clinical outcomes. The other sections outline examples of interventions and progressions that achieve outcomes related to a variety of impairments. The clinical cases in this chapter give additional examples of how to apply the principles of Outcome-Based Massage™ for medical massage (treatment of clinical conditions) and wellness massage. Finally, Quick Treatment Guides for 16 clinical conditions and wellness issues that therapists reported that they commonly treated with massage techniques are included in the insert.

Evidence

THE ROLE OF IMPAIRMENTS AND OUTCOMES IN TREATMENT PLANNING

Historically, in medical massage, the use of massage to treat clinical conditions, therapists have applied standard treatment regimens that are specified for each clinical condition.[1,9] By contrast, Outcome-Based Massage™ suggests that therapists recognize that clients with clinical conditions present with related **impairments** in body structures and functions, secondary to **pathophysiology**, that therapists must assess and treat.[10,11] The central premise of Outcome-Based Massage™ is, therefore, that rather than applying a standard treatment regimen for a clinical condition, therapists using Outcome-Based Massage™ design treatments for each client that vary with the client's presenting impairments in body structures and functions, the **outcomes** that reflect those impairments, and the client's stated treatment goals. In the case of wellness massage, where clients present without impairments in body structures and functions, therapists are guided by the clients' wellness goals. Furthermore, throughout the treatment process, therapists using Outcome-Based Massage™ also use information on the client's impairments in body structures and functions and wellness goals to guide their decisions on massage techniques, treatment progression, **contraindications** to treatment, and special treatment considerations. An additional advantage and characteristic of Outcome-Based Massage™ is that therapists can combine interventions that treat individual impairments and wellness goals within a **plan of care** in order to address each client's unique clinical presentation and goals. To illustrate how to apply the principles of Outcome-Based Massage™ to clinical conditions and wellness, this chapter provides examples of interventions for specific impairments and wellness goals that we developed using this approach.

COMBINING INTERVENTIONS FOR MULTIPLE BODY STRUCTURES AND FUNCTIONS

Few clients present for treatment with a single impairment or wellness goal. Consequently, therapists typically have to address multiple impairments or wellness goals within a single intervention.[1,11] In doing so, they must combine interventions for different impairments, wellness goals, and body structures into a single plan of care. The following guidelines can assist therapists in selecting and combining interventions for differing impairments and body structures. Therapists can incorporate these guidelines into the clinical decision-making steps outlined in Chapters 4 and 5.

Guidelines for Combining Interventions for Different Impairments and Wellness Goals

1. List all of the client's impairments and wellness goals that you plan to address within your plan of care.
2. Consider the **contraindications** and **cautions** to treatment for each impairment, wellness goal, and massage technique.[12-17] You may have to exclude some techniques from the intervention entirely or modify how you apply them locally based on these contraindications and cautions. Each technique you choose for the final list of techniques must be *safe for all* of the client's impairments. Furthermore, each technique you choose must be *effective for at least one* of the client's impairments or wellness goals. At times, the final plan of care may not be the most effective treatment for a given impairment because the preferred treatment technique is contraindicated by one of the client's other impairments or wellness goals.
3. The relative priority of impairments or wellness goals will guide your choice and progression of techniques. Give priority to impairments that are more severe (greater grade) and that cause other impairments. In addition, consider the client's priorities for care. You can give a prioritized impairment or wellness goal more emphasis by
   - Treating it first in the series of interventions
   - Treating it first in each intervention
   - Selecting the majority of treatment techniques in the plan of care to address it
   - Allotting more time to address it during each intervention
4. If you assign impairments or wellness goals equal priority, decide whether you will treat them simultaneously or sequentially within each intervention and within the episode of care as a whole.

PROGRESSION OF INTERVENTIONS

Progression of Interventions for Clinical Conditions

The treatment of a client's clinical condition **progresses** through stages that reflect the clinical course and **prognosis** of that condition and client. Therapists can use information from several sources to guide treatment progression. These sources include practice guidelines, findings from the client examination, and clinical experience.

Professions often establish broad **practice guidelines** for the treatment of clinical conditions to provide therapists with a general framework for planning and progressing interventions. These condition-specific practice guidelines and professional practice guidelines outline a general guide to prognoses, expected numbers of visits per episode of care, **outcome measures**, and relevant types of intervention for a range of clinical conditions. We use the American Physical Therapy Association's *Guide to Physical Therapist Practice*[10] as the example for this chapter. At the time of printing, we were unable to locate a comparable, systematic, national set of practice guidelines for a wide range of clinical conditions written specifically for massage therapists, although the Canadian Consortium of Massage Therapy Regulators has defined practice competencies for massage therapists. Table 14-1 contains an excerpt of the practice guidelines for physical therapy interventions for selected musculoskeletal and neurological disorders.[10] The American Physical Therapy Association did not develop these guidelines for a therapist who uses massage therapy techniques extensively; they assume the use of other clinical techniques as primary modalities. Furthermore, these guidelines are for situations in which therapists are addressing a broader range of impairments and **functional limitations** in their interventions than those that are specific to the use of massage techniques. Consequently, the number of massage-based interventions would be lower for a physical therapist than it would be for a massage therapist who is treating the same condition.

In reality, the appropriate number of interventions using massage techniques will also vary with other factors, including the cause, severity, acuity, and complexity of the client's clinical condition; the use of complementary modalities; and the client's overall health status and age. For this reason, therapists should try to avoid using a standard plan of care for all clients with a given clinical condition. Instead, they need to remain outcome-based in their practices and tailor the progression of massage and other techniques within a given **episode of care** to the client's presenting impairments, functional limitations, and wellness goals. This will involve monitoring the client's progression from one stage of recovery to the next by assessing changes in his impairments and functional limitations, rather than by determining the amount of time that has elapsed since the onset of his clinical condition. At each stage, the therapist should modify the plan of care so that it remains consistent with the client's current impairments and functional limitations.

Therapists' ability to progress interventions effectively can improve with appropriate clinical experience. They can use their observations of clients' responses to treatment and the typical course of clinical conditions as a foundation on which to base their decisions about treatment progression. Furthermore, novice therapists and students can use the consistent application of the clinical decision-making

| Table 14-1 | **Duration of Physical Therapy Regimens and Expected Number of Visits for Selected Orthopedic and Neurological Conditions** |

Condition	Duration of Expected Physical Therapy Regimen	Number of Visits
Tendinitis, bursitis, fasciitis	8–16 wk	6–24
Postural conditions	12 mo	6–20
Sprain/strain/dislocation	2–14 wk	3–6
Uncomplicated joint arthroplasty	6 mo	12–60
Disk herniation	1–6 mo	8–24
Cerebrovascular accident (stroke)	Until maximum independence is achieved	10–60
Peripheral nerve injury	4–8 mo	12–56

Data from American Physical Therapy Association. *Interactive Guide to Physical Therapist Practice.* Alexandria, VA: American Physical Therapy Association; 2003.

process and principles of Outcome-Based Massage™, preferably in collaboration with an experienced therapist, to enhance their skill in progressing interventions.

Progression of Wellness Interventions

The development of interventions that include or focus on wellness-related outcomes follows a similar process to the one outlined for clinical conditions. Prior to embarking on a wellness intervention, it is very important that therapists first identify any impairments in body structures and functions that are present. Often clients who request **wellness interventions** present with impairments, such as **stress**, **altered body image**, **postural conditions**, **elevated resting tension**, **latent trigger points**, and reduced active range of motion. Prior to initiating the wellness intervention, therapists will need to discuss, evaluate, and treat those impairments, as appropriate within their scope of practice, using the guidelines described in this chapter. Once therapists have distinguished between impairments and wellness-related outcomes, they can use the clinical decision-making process (see Chapter 5) to guide their development and progression of the wellness intervention.

During the client examination, therapists identify wellness goals that are of ongoing importance to the client. These wellness goals can include enhancing muscle and general **relaxation**, optimizing **ease of movement**, and achieving optimal mental focus. Based on the examination findings, therapists negotiate reasonable long- and short-term outcomes for each wellness goal through careful dialogue with the client. Through ongoing client re-examination, therapists obtain information on the changes in the client's body structures and functions or functional status that signal the need for progression of the wellness intervention. They also modify or redirect the plan of care so that it remains consistent with the client's current status and moves the client toward the next set of outcomes. In this way, therapists use an iterative clinical decision-making process to facilitate the client's ongoing progress toward his wellness outcomes.

In contrast to the treatment of clinical conditions, there is a lack of practice guidelines for the duration of treatment and the number of visits for wellness goals. Furthermore, the required number of sessions will vary with a variety of factors including the number and nature of identified issues, the complexity of the client's wellness outcomes, the presence and treatment of underlying or related impairments, and the client's overall health status and age. Moreover, wellness interventions often (and should) include a significant educational component.

Consequently, the client's willingness and capacity to learn and implement **lifestyle** changes can affect the duration of treatment.

Therapists should not omit the four-phase Outcome-Based Massage™ clinical decision-making process (evaluation, treatment planning, treatment, and discharge) when they provide wellness interventions. Furthermore, they should not make a wellness plan of care open-ended. As with interventions for clinical conditions, the treatment process should lead to **discharge**. If a wellness client seeks ongoing treatment for legitimate reasons, therapists can follow one plan of care to its completion and then begin another phase of treatment with a formal client re-examination. This enables the client and therapist to consider what they have achieved with each plan of care and avoids the trap of exploiting the client by scheduling an undetermined number of interventions that have an ill-defined purpose.

DISCHARGE

If therapists follow the principles for progressing interventions outlined in this and other chapters, then the transition from the treatment phase to the discharge phase will be gradual and imperceptible. Chapters 2 and 5 outline the steps that therapists follow to prepare their clients physically and psychologically for discharge. Some additional clinical issues are worthy of mention. As therapists identify the resolution of the client's impairments through ongoing re-examinations, they can progress their use of techniques that address the client's functional limitations, such as functional training, as their scope of practice permits. Finally, as discharge approaches, therapists will ensure that they address the client's needs for self-care education, equipment, and referrals to other healthcare professionals and services and other needs that lie within their scope of practice.

Key Points: 14-1

Note about Interventions for Impairments in Chapter 14

The examples of interventions for impairments in Chapter 14 consider both traditional approaches to practice and the growing body of evidence for massage techniques. Although they have undergone peer review by practicing therapists, teachers, and students, we have not subjected them to the extensive review that would lead us to consider them **practice guidelines**. For all of these suggested interventions, bear in mind that clients may present with other impairments or clinical conditions that will have their own set of cautions and contraindications for treatment.

INTERVENTIONS FOR PSYCHONEUROIMMU-NOLOGICAL IMPAIRMENTS

Stress: Impaired Ability to Relax, General Adaptation Syndrome—Early Stages

Relevant Outcomes

- Reduced stress or distress (in a wide variety of situations)[12,18-29]
- Improved ability to relax
- Improved adaptability to stress[30]
- Improved behavior[30-36]
- Improved immune function[3,4,37-48]

Clinical Relevance

The literature suggests that **stress** contributes to a large percentage of clinical conditions.[49-51] In addition, post-traumatic stress and **posttraumatic stress disorder** often follow traumatic experiences.[52-54] Furthermore, many otherwise-healthy clients complain of too much stress or an impaired ability to relax. Reduced stress and associated outcomes are important considerations for clients with depressed immune function.[3,4,38-44,46-48]

Treatment Considerations

At the outset of treatment, determine the stage of the **general adaptation syndrome**[55-57] at which the client presents. This step is important because a client at later stages of the general adaptation syndrome, who is approaching **exhaustion** or "burnout," will involve more cautions and contraindications to treatment than a client at the earlier stages of **alarm** or resistance. Determine whether the client has a diagnosis of **clinical depression**, an **anxiety disorder**, or other psychiatric condition. In addition, ensure that you have a thorough understanding of any physical symptoms associated with his condition, the current management of his condition, and other health care professionals involved in his care. Consult with other treating health care professionals if you have any concerns regarding treatment. Furthermore, regardless of whether or not the client has a psychiatric condition, consider referring him to his physician if his stress levels and physical symptoms

do not improve with treatment. Finally, be conscious and supportive of the fact that a client's habits and thought processes will have a profound influence on their ability to deal with stress.[50]

Guidelines for Using Massage Techniques

- First, prepare yourself so that *you* are fully relaxed.
- Ensure that the treatment area is warm, quiet, and softly lit.
- Speak in a quiet voice.
- Offer the client a choice of several types of relaxing music[58] (yours or his own) or silence.
- Position the client for maximum comfort.
- You can use almost any massage technique for **sedative** or relaxation massage[6] including superficial reflex,[59,60] superficial fluid,[61] neuromuscular, connective tissue, and passive movement techniques.[62] In addition, small amounts of percussion may be appropriate for some clients. Well-performed rocking is possibly the most sedative of all massage techniques.[63]
- Sedative massage is typically fairly slow, rhythmic, and predictable. When performing repetitive petrissage, try using a stroke rate of 50 to 70 cycles/min.[64]
- Many clients who have experienced massage prefer moderate or deep work.[65] They may find superficial work irritating[9] because it does not address their muscular tension. Solicit honest feedback about treatment depth and match the depth of your work to the client's needs.
- Ensure that your application of techniques is not causing pain (around 3/10 to 5/10 maximum on the self-reported pain scale) even when you are performing **neuromuscular** or **connective tissue techniques** on deeper structures.
- There are several key locations for treatment. Since the hands, feet, and head (including face and ears) are high-tension areas, which are highly innervated, include them in treatment unless you are short of time.[32,66-75] The cranium and sacrum contain **parasympathetic** outflow that you can affect manually[76,77] with prolonged holding of these areas or prolonged repetitive palmar stroking from occiput to sacrum. Deep gluteal work, especially around the sacral and iliac attachments, can also be highly effective. Furthermore, any techniques that you perform along the axial skeleton may produce reflex **autonomic** effects as a result of inhibition of **sympathetic** activity[78,79] or facilitation of parasympathetic activity.[3]
- Treatment times that are longer than 30 minutes probably produce much greater sedative responses.[6] Treatment times under 15 minutes may be less effective.[80]

- **Aromatherapy** oils added to the carrier lubricant (at a rate of 5 to 20 drops per 50 mL of carrier)[81] may improve relaxation.[81-85] Sedative oils include melissa, valerian, neroli, passion flower, orange flower, petitgrain, and lavender.[81]
- You can integrate treatment for other impairments into this basic approach for relaxation, and by doing so, you may increase the sedative effects further. For example, you can treat **adaptive shortening** of muscle and connective tissue, trigger points, and elevated resting tension in the shoulder muscles within this treatment framework for relaxation.

Complementary Modalities

You can use the following complementary modalities during an intervention for relaxation:

- **Diaphragmatic breathing** and relaxation techniques, such as **guided awareness**, **progressive muscle relaxation**, autogenic training, imagery, and meditation, make an excellent beginning or end to an intervention.[66,86] You can also use them concurrently with massage techniques depending on the context. If you do not feel confident in your ability to guide clients in these relaxation techniques, you can obtain recorded instructions for clients to use in the clinic or at home.[87,88]
- **Passive movements** and prolonged, gentle **stretching** are appropriate.
- Systemic heat (steam, sauna, whirlpool, or bath) in the range of warm to hot[89] is sedative and is an excellent prelude to the massage if it is available.[89,90] You can also use systemic heat followed by a cool rinse or plunge. Furthermore, a local application of moist heat (hydrocollator or thermophore) is an appropriate alternative to full-body heat.
- Stress management education is also helpful.[30]

Between interventions, clients can use any of the complementary modalities listed above and the following:

- Moderate active exercise such as walking
- Movement systems that emphasize relaxation and awareness such as **Feldenkrais**, **Tai Chi**, or **Hatha yoga**

General Adaptation Syndrome— Later Stages

Relevant Outcomes

- Recovery of autonomic **homeostasis.**
- Reduced stress or distress.[12,18-24]
- Improved ability to relax.

Clinical Relevance

Clients who are approaching the third stage of the general adaptation syndrome, which involves exhaustion, disintegration, or burnout, are a distinct subset of the clients with this condition. They may be experiencing a serious health crisis that requires stress leave from work, medical treatment, or hospitalization.[55]

Treatment Considerations

Ongoing management by a physician and referral to other relevant health care providers is essential.

Guidelines for Using Massage Techniques

- Be conservative in the number and level of stimulation of all techniques.
- Offer shorter treatment sessions, 20 to 30 minutes long, consisting of light, gentle techniques including **reflex techniques**, superficial effleurage, light (at most, moderate depth) neuromuscular techniques.
- Cause no pain.
- Carefully monitor the effects of treatment, both during and after treatment.
- Progress the intervention to include the techniques we described for clients with earlier stages of the general adaptation syndrome as the client shows less **fatigue** and improved tolerance of treatment.

Complementary Modalities

- Suggest simple nonvigorous exercise, such as walking, within the client's tolerance.
- Modify the systemic hydrotherapy procedures that are suggested for early stages of the general adaptation syndrome to techniques of moderate duration that use warmth[89] without contrast or only mild contrast. Local warmth to tolerance is acceptable.

Insomnia, Reduced or Disturbed Sleep

Relevant Outcomes

- Improved pattern and quality of sleep[4,39,83,87,91-104]
- Improved duration of sleep[93,94,97,105-107]

Clinical Relevance

Disturbed sleep is a common symptom of stress. In addition, disturbed sleep often accompanies serious or

EXAMINING THE EVIDENCE

In 2004, a group of psychologists from the University of Illinois published a landmark meta-analysis of massage therapy research.[6] Rigorous search and selection criteria yielded 37 studies with 1,802 participants, including 795 who received massage. The authors examined single-dose effects of massage on **state anxiety**, negative mood, pain, **cortisol level**, blood pressure, and heart rate. They found that massage treatments had statistically significant effects on state anxiety, blood pressure, and heart rate. They also found that massage treatments had statistically significant multiple-dose effects on **trait anxiety**, **depression**, and delayed onset of pain. The authors discussed these results in the context of common theories on the effects of massage techniques. They proposed that some effects of massage techniques may be due to positive expectations of client and therapist and from their interpersonal contact, rather than the particular technique used or the site to which it is applied. This is similar to some of the findings on psychotherapy. This hypothesis may explain general outcomes related to psychoneuroimmunology and pain but may not be valid for the specific effects of massage techniques on physiological impairments such as trigger points or scar tissue.

Moyer CA, Rounds J, Hannum JW. A meta-analysis of massage therapy research. *Psychol Bull.* 2004;130:3-18.

---

terminal diseases, surgery (both before and after), hospitalization,[107] chronic pain, depression, and addiction.[106,108]

Treatment Considerations

Prior to initiating treatment, discuss the cause of the client's sleep disturbance. Stress, clinical depression, addiction, **chronic pain**, and disease all have their own cautions for treatment. Most of these underlying conditions necessitate referral to the client's physician.

Guidelines for Using Massage Techniques

- All of the massage strategies described for the treatment of stress are appropriate.

Complementary Modalities

- All of the complementary techniques described for the treatment of stress are appropriate.
- Clients may need to retrain poor sleep habits by reducing stimulation in the evening, developing a ritual for use prior to retiring, faithfully maintaining a regular sleep time, and avoiding daytime naps.
- Immediately before retiring, the client can use any of the following:
  - Gentle stretching (especially of the posterior surface of the body)
  - Diaphragmatic breathing and relaxation exercises[86,109]
  - A warm, not hot, bath with or without the addition of relaxing essential oils such as lavender,

chamomile, cypress, juniper, neroli, marjoram, and melissa[81,85,89,90,110]
  - A cold abdominal wash[89,90]
  - An abdominal heating compress[89,90]

Fatigue, Lethargy, Suboptimal Arousal

Relevant Outcomes

- Decreased fatigue[19,75,111-117]
- Increased **arousal**
- Preparedness for activity[118]

Clinical Relevance

Uncomplicated fatigue typically results from stress or lack of sleep. Fatigue is also a symptom of clinical conditions such as anemia, thyroid conditions, convalescence, rheumatoid arthritis and related systemic connective tissue diseases, cancer, and depressive psychiatric conditions. At the other end of the clinical continuum, increased arousal is often a requirement for optimal performance in athletic and artistic performance. These related impairments all share a treatment approach that seeks to heighten arousal through physical stimulation.

Treatment Considerations

Prior to initiating treatment for a client who presents with fatigue, ensure that you understand the cause of the client's fatigue. If there is no obvious cause for prolonged fatigue or if you have any concerns about associated systemic or psychiatric conditions, consult with the client's physician. If the client's fatigue is associated with a psychiatric condition, consult with the client's physician or other treating health care professionals and monitor for any signs of self-destructive behavior. Up to a point, therapists can use massage techniques to counteract uncomplicated fatigue. Nevertheless, the best course of action for the client may be to obtain more sleep.

Guidelines for Using Massage Techniques

- Traditionally, massage techniques to counteract fatigue are fast-paced, light, and rhythmic.[1,65] The pace and depth of **stimulating massage** techniques are generally similar to the pace and depth of **precompetition sports massage** techniques.[119] Many studies that reported reduced fatigue after massage techniques did not, however, use this approach. Nonetheless, be cautious when you apply sedative techniques to any client who reports a low energy level.
- Make the treatment duration short. For example, take 20 minutes for all or most of the body.
- Useful techniques for stimulation include superficial stroking, effleurage, broad-contact compression, petrissage, coarse vibration, nonsedative shaking, and percussion. Avoid techniques that require a slower pace, such as fascial work, and techniques that may cause discomfort, such as trigger point release.
- Your depth of penetration will be superficial as a result of the faster pace of treatment.

Complementary Modalities

- You can perform hydrotherapy techniques that use cold, contrast, and friction (rubbing with an abrasive cloth or brush), before or after the treatment. Match the vigor of the technique to the client's tolerance. Some examples of techniques in ascending order of vigor are **dry brushing**, cold wash, **salt glow**, **cold mitten friction**, and high-contrast alternating temperature percussion jet ("blitzguss").[89,90,120] You can modify the strength of the stimulation of a technique by increasing or decreasing the area of the client's body to which you apply it. These techniques may have additional beneficial effects on immune function.[121]
- Instruct the client in the use of brisk, aerobic exercise, within her tolerance, between interventions.

Altered Body Image

Relevant Outcomes

- Improved body image[106,122-126]

Clinical Relevance

Altered body image may be a relevant impairment for clients with eating disorders,[122] depression,[106] serious or life-threatening diseases, cancer,[125,127,128] mastectomy,[124] surgery, amputation, disfigurement through trauma or burns, stroke, aging, history of physical or sexual abuse,[53,126,129,130] and posttraumatic stress disorder.[54,131]

Treatment Considerations

Each condition listed above, with the exception of uncomplicated aging, requires appropriate medical and/or psychiatric management. Refer to and consult with other health care professionals as the client's condition requires.[106]

Guidelines for Using Massage Techniques and Complementary Modalities

- When you are treating clients with altered body image, your approach to the client and her issues are more important than the massage techniques that you use.[54] In particular, provide support, understanding, clear communication with the client, and very careful attention to consent.
- When you apply massage techniques, include as much of the client's body as the relevant contraindications and cautions permit. In addition, treat affected and unaffected areas during the same treatment.
- These clients may have avoided touching an injured or painful area or a surgical site for a long period of time, even years. You may have to treat these areas in stages, beginning with static contact on adjacent areas and gradually moving toward the site.
- Use general massage strokes to cover entire regions and promote relaxation.
- Use guided awareness and static contact to focus the client's attention on areas that are relevant to her presenting issues.
- The relatively rare phenomenon of **somatoemotional release** is more likely to happen when a client has experienced trauma.[52] Key Points 14-2 suggests basic guidelines for working with clients who experience somatoemotional release during interventions.
- Consider structuring interventions in three parts that sequentially aim to establish trust and safety, allow the client to explore sensation, and obtain healthy closure.[54] Consult the details of this process in Chapter 2.

When a Client Experiences Emotional Release

Here are some guidelines for entry-level therapists to use when clients experience emotional release during the intervention.[52,63,131,132]

Do

1. Honor emotional release without encouraging it. Be open to observing it.
2. Let a client who is experiencing a release know that the phenomenon is normal. Briefly explain **tissue memory** and **touch-triggered memory**.
3. Ask him if he wants you to stop working or to take your hands off his body.
4. Relax while you allow the release to take its normal course, often less than 10 minutes.
5. Encourage the client to acknowledge what has happened.
6. Offer the client the opportunity to talk about the experience, without pressuring him to do so.
7. **Ground** the client at the intervention's end with sedative work on the sacrum and feet.
8. Have on hand a pamphlet that explains what touch-triggered memory is. Be prepared to refer to it, if this seems appropriate.
9. Ensure that the client is able to drive or to use public transit before he leaves.

Do Not

1. Move the focus of the intervention to the area where the release is centered.
2. Pressure the client to give details about "what is going on."
3. Engage in or make any attempt to interpret emotional content.
4. Leave the client alone until he indicates that he is ready.

INTERVENTIONS FOR IMPAIRMENTS RELATED TO PAIN

Before Treating Pain

During the evaluation phase, obtain the answers to the following important questions:

1. *Are there any contraindications or cautions that necessitate referral to another health care professional?*
   Pain that is severe, of sudden onset, unfamiliar to the client, and associated with systemic or neurological symptoms or that is unrelated to activity is a "**red flag**" that suggests that you should immediately refer the client to a physician for further investigation.
2. *Is the pain acute or chronic?*
   Acute **nociceptive pain** is usually, but not always, associated with the acute stage of a clinical condition.[133] **Chronic pain** and **chronic pain syndromes** may not be

associated with readily apparent physical signs. You can further distinguish between the categories of pain as summarized in Chapter 4.
3. *What is causing the pain(s)?*
   Surprisingly, therapists often overlook this issue. Use client examination techniques to identify the structure(s) that is the source of pain. Although massage techniques may reduce the perception of pain from an unidentified cause, through **hyperstimulation analgesia** or **sedation**, direct treatment of the cause(s) of pain is preferable, whenever possible.

During the treatment planning phase, try to answer the following questions:

1. *Is any cause of the pain an impairment that you can treat directly with massage techniques?*
   Use appropriate massage techniques to treat the impairments that cause the client's pain, such as **edema**, reduced mobility of connective tissue, elevated resting tension, spasm, and trigger points, directly.
2. *Is hyperstimulation analgesia appropriate?*
   Another strategy for reducing pain is to use massage techniques for hyperstimulation analgesia or counter-irritant analgesia. For example, prolonged mechanical vibration will reduce pain in the same dermatome as the site of application[133] (see information on mechanical vibration in Chapter 7). You can also use heat, cold, and active exercises to achieve this effect.
3. *Is sedation the only strategy for reducing pain when using massage techniques?*
   The least specific approach to managing pain with massage techniques is to use massage techniques to relax or sedate the client in order to change her perception of pain. An example of this is when therapists use massage techniques to modify a client's perception of cancer pain.

   Pain may *contribute* to impairments, such as elevated resting tension and trigger points. Address those associated impairments with massage techniques if this is appropriate.

Acute Nociceptive Pain

Relevant Outcomes

- Reduction of pain[3,12,19,22,23,26,27,29,37,71,73,80,82,84,92,98,107,118,131,134-191]
- Analgesia

Clinical Relevance

This category of pain is relevant to acute injuries, trauma, and a variety of systemic illnesses.

Treatment Considerations

When you are treating acute nociceptive pain, be aware of **red flags** that require immediate referral to a physician. In addition, determine the type of pain your client is reporting: acute nociceptive pain, recurrent episodes of acute nociceptive pain, nociceptive pain associated with the **chronic stage of inflammation**, **chronic pain** due to other causes, pain that is associated with **chronic pain syndrome**, or **myofascial pain**. Communicate with, and refer to, other health professionals as needed to clarify the client's type of pain. Furthermore, if the client's acute nociceptive pain is the result of a systemic illness, then consider the relevant contraindications and cautions listed in Table 5-3.

Guidelines for Using Massage Techniques

If tissues are in the acute stage of inflammation, as a result of a recent orthopedic injury:

- Ensure that the client has received appropriate medical management.
- Treat the impairments that are causing the client's pain, such as edema and muscle spasm, using the approaches discussed in the relevant sections of this chapter.
- Depending on the **grade of injury**, the client may not tolerate touch on or near the site of acute injuries. Do not cause pain or increase the client's pain.
- You may achieve hyperstimulation or counterirritant analgesia by applying superficial reflex or neuromuscular techniques away from the site of injury, on the related dermatome or myotome or on the contralateral side.[19,99,147] Note that a recent **meta-analysis** disputed the mechanism of hyperstimulation analgesia (gate control theory) and concluded that the immediate effects of massage techniques on pain were not significant.[6]
- In addition, techniques to enhance relaxation can decrease the client's perception of pain.

If you cannot address the cause of the client's pain directly with massage techniques, for example, with acute nociceptive pain associated with cancer,[19,37,38,71,75,82,92,95,114-116,134,136,142,147,164,170,173,174,192-204] ensure that the client has appropriate medical management and pay careful attention to the cautions and contraindications related to her particular condition. Once you have done so, use general massage techniques at a tolerable depth to achieve systemic relaxation and hyperstimulation analgesia. Bear in mind that these clients may have other causes of pain, such as trigger points, that you can treat directly with massage techniques.

Complementary Modalities

- Elevate the client's limb and use cold hydrotherapy for acute-stage inflammation in orthopedic conditions.
- You can use heat, cold, and contrast to achieve hyperstimulation analgesia through spinal gating.
- Use systemic or local heat to achieve sedation.
- To produce hyperstimulation analgesia, use passive movements, joint traction, and joint mobilization techniques on, or around, the damaged structures. Base your treatment on the client's tolerance, relevant contraindications, and your scope of practice.

Chronic Pain, Chronic Pain Syndromes

Relevant Outcomes

- Increased functional activity[133,205]
- Analgesia[137,206,207]
- Decreased depression

Treatment Considerations

- *The primary outcome is improved functional activity* when you are treating clients with chronic pain and chronic pain syndromes. While the reduction of pain is desirable, it does not always occur and, consequently, is not always the measure of a successful treatment.
- Be aware of **red flags** that require immediate referral to a physician. In addition, follow the guidelines in this chapter for determining the client's type of pain.
- Chronic pain is a distinct, complex clinical condition that requires an interdisciplinary approach to treatment.[133,208] Treatment, especially of **chronic pain syndrome**, does not depend primarily on the treatment of other impairments, such as edema or muscle tension, although such treatment may be useful.
- Clients with chronic pain may show unusual patterns of pain behavior and are often clinically depressed.[209] Consequently, if a client presents with a diagnosis of chronic pain or you suspect that this may be her diagnosis, communicate with or refer her to a physician for appropriate treatment.
- Be conscious of the client's potential for dependency on your interventions.[210]
- Be aware that the client's expectations about massage techniques may affect their treatment outcomes.[205]

Guidelines for Using Massage Techniques

- *Ensure that you have addressed all treatable causes of pain.*

- Explore the use of *all* massage techniques, since they are potentially useful.
- Progress from superficial to deep massage techniques within the client's tolerance.

Complementary Modalities

- Machines that produce 100 Hz vibration are inexpensive. Therapists can easily incorporate them into massage interventions without sacrificing hands-on time. They are also good for home care.
- **Transcutaneous electrical nerve stimulation (TENS)** relieves many kinds of pain,[211-217] and clients can self-administer this modality.
- Clients may find self-massage useful.
- All hydrotherapy methods are potentially useful, including local hot and cold packs, whirlpool, whirlpool followed by cold shower, percussion douche,[89,90,218] and longer interventions designed to promote autonomic homeostasis.[133,218]
- Encourage aerobic exercise to prevent or reduce deconditioning.
- Use stretching, diaphragmatic breathing, relaxation training, and specific visualization methods for helping clients cope with pain.
- Adapt as many techniques as possible for self-care. Emphasize self-care that improves the client's level of functional activity and independence.

INTERVENTIONS FOR CIRCULATORY IMPAIRMENTS

Impaired Venous Return, Impaired Lymphatic Return, Edema, Lymphedema

Relevant Outcomes

- Improved venous return[219,220]
- Improved lymphatic return
- Reduced edema or lymphedema[95,195,220-228]

Clinical Relevance

This chapter groups impaired venous return, impaired lymphatic return, edema, and lymphedema together because you use a similar treatment approach for these impairments. These impairments can be associated with a variety of clinical conditions, including dependent edema, acute inflammation caused by trauma, varicose veins, chronic venous insufficiency, varicose or venous ulcers, lymphedema secondary to radiation or surgery, cardiomyopathy, and congestive heart failure.

Treatment Considerations

Note that many of the clinical conditions associated with these impairments have their own cautions and contraindications related to the client's medical and pharmaceutical management. In addition to those specific issues, consider the following cautions. Treat traumatic edema according to its stage and clinical presentation[229,230] (see the discussion on inflammation in this chapter). Work gently on or around areas of dystrophic skin. Avoid the immediate vicinity of varicose ulcers and varicose veins.[1,8] *Do not treat clients with congestive heart failure without consulting the supervising physician because increasing fluid return may compromise the client's cardiac function.*[231] Finally, therapists cannot use massage techniques to resolve some forms of lymphedema, such as those due to protein deficiency.[61]

Guidelines for Using Massage Techniques and Complementary Modalities

- Refer Chapters 7 and 13 for details of the principles of increasing fluid return and clinical examples. The general treatment approach is to begin treatment proximally, move contact distally,[62] and then repeat this procedure several times. Use **centripetal** pressure throughout the treatment.
- Interventions to increase fluid return often consist of only modern or only classical technique, and this may be preferable. It is best not to combine modern techniques (superficial lymph drainage technique or **manual lymph drainage**) and classical techniques (superficial effleurage and petrissage) within a given intervention, unless you are experienced in the use of both approaches.
- Therapists who are familiar with both modern and classical techniques may evaluate the effects of the following combination. Instruct the client in deep diaphragmatic breathing, and encourage this throughout the intervention. Begin with the manual lymph drainage **terminus stroke**[61] and follow this with broadcontact compression performed on the client's upper rib cage.[232] Within the region of edema, begin proximally and superficially with one or both superficial techniques, applying them using the basic pattern of proximal to distal to proximal. Then proceed slowly to

the application of deep effleurage and petrissage with the pattern of proximal to distal to proximal. Finally, perform one or both superficial techniques again. Throughout the entire sequence, alternate your contact back and forth from proximal to distal areas repeatedly and then return periodically to either terminus or compression of the rib cage.

■ Elevated resting muscle tension and connective tissue tightness may exert pressure on vessels and restrict fluid return. Therapists may, therefore, consider treating these impairments.

Complementary Modalities

■ Use positioning and passive movement to assist fluid return.[1,220,233]

■ Use joint traction and accessory joint movements to facilitate nutrition of an effused joint.[230,233]

■ Muscle contraction is a major cause of lymphatic return; choose from a variety of active exercises according to the client's condition and level of activity.[234,235] Exercises and compression bandages[220,235] may provide most of the benefit of **complex decongestive therapy** in cases of lymphedema.[195,222,236-238]

■ Clients can use compression pumps[220] and cylindrical rollers[239] for self-massage to promote lymph drainage.

■ Use cold hydrotherapy to treat traumatic edema in the acute stage of injury or inflammation and hot hydrotherapy to treat traumatic edema in the chronic stage of injury or inflammation. In these situations, apply hydrotherapy as baths, compresses, or packs.[89,90]

Impaired Arterial Supply

Relevant Outcomes

■ Improved arterial supply[105,240-243]
■ Improved tissue oxygenation

Treatment Considerations

Clients who present with local impairment of their arterial supply may also have an associated cardiovascular disease that has specific cautions and contraindications. In addition, applying heat to the extremities is often contraindicated in clients with impaired arterial supply (e.g., diabetics) because local heating may increase the metabolic demand of the tissues beyond what the circulatory system can supply[120] and, consequently, result in tissue damage. In this situation, some therapists also believe that **circulatory massage** techniques are contraindicated,[231]

although it is unclear how much massage techniques can increase arterial supply (see the Outcomes and Evidence section for Petrissage in Chapter 9). Finally, both heat and massage techniques may be contraindications for clients with diabetes due to the reduced sensation associated with diabetic neuropathy.

Guidelines for Using Massage Techniques

■ Current research is not consistent about whether any massage technique will significantly increase arterial supply.[3,105,241,242,244-249] It is unlikely that superficial reflex techniques increase arterial supply. The authors suspect that massage techniques, such as broad-contact compression and petrissage, are limited in their ability to produce this effect unless the therapist's manual technique is extremely precise. For example, hyperemia following tapotement may only indicate a change in **perfusion**, rather than an overall increase in the volume of blood going through the tissues.[250]

■ Exponents of European schools of medical massage describe reflex circulatory effects, which can be achieved through precise, studied application of various neuromuscular and connective tissue techniques.[78,79,251]

■ Repetitive mechanical compression devices may increase blood supply[251] as well as return.

Complementary Modalities

■ Exercise, especially aerobic exercise, is the most effective method of increasing arterial supply.

■ Local heat increases arterial supply.[252] Therapists can use it in healthy clients, although it may be contraindicated in those with advanced circulatory disease or diabetes.[231]

■ A short cold wash or a heat treatment applied proximally over a supplying artery may be useful in clients for whom a heat treatment in the affected region is contraindicated.[89,120]

INTERVENTIONS FOR RESPIRATORY IMPAIRMENTS

Impaired Airway Clearance

Relevant Outcomes

■ Improved airway clearance[253-256]
■ Decreased congestion[256]

Clinical Relevance

Impaired **airway clearance** is associated with pulmonary conditions such as chronic obstructive pulmonary disease, chronic bronchitis, emphysema, asthma, cystic fibrosis, pneumonia, recovery from surgery, and the common cold.

Treatment Considerations

All of the conditions listed above, except for the common cold, require medical and pharmaceutical management that makes it important for you to consider cautions and contraindications to treatment.[257] Decreased airway clearance occurs in conjunction with other respiratory impairments discussed elsewhere in this chapter.

Percussion of the thorax is contraindicated in cases of severe rib fracture, untreated tension pneumothorax, confirmed or possible coronary thrombosis or pulmonary embolism, unstable cardiac conditions, and conditions that are prone to hemorrhage; after chest or spinal surgery; and during an acute episode of asthma. The positional changes required for **postural drainage** may cause increased oxygen demand, carbon dioxide release, altered blood pressure, and cardiac output. Consequently, therapists must use the head-down position with caution, particularly if clients are hypertensive or have had a head injury. Percussion used alone can also increase heart rate and blood pressure.[258]

Guidelines for Using Massage Techniques

The standard treatment approach is postural drainage and percussion, although the effectiveness of this procedure is often debated.[253,255,259] Position the client in the relevant postural drainage position. Then apply clapping, rib springing, rhythmic mobilization, and coarse vibration combined with compression to the related portion of the rib cage (see Chapter 11). Encourage the client to exhale forcibly, cough, and expectorate during and following treatment. You may have to teach the client how to initiate a cough.[230] Collect the client's sputum and dispose of it using **standard precautions**.[260] An entire sequence may take 50 to 60 minutes or longer. You may choose to drain only a subset of the client's lobes in one particular session.

Complementary Modalities

- Instruct the client to drink water before and after postural drainage and percussion.
- Immediately precede postural drainage and percussion with a bronchial steam or a bronchial steam with the addition of five drops of eucalyptus or peppermint oil[81] or commercially available products.
- A deep moist heat on the back or front (avoiding the precordium) is an alternative to bronchial steam.[89]
- You can adapt this entire procedure for home use, using percussion administered by a caregiver or even self-clapping administered by the client.
- Effective mechanical alternatives to postural drainage and percussion used in hospitals include intrapulmonary percussive ventilation and high-frequency chest wall compression.[253]

Elevated Resting Tension of Respiratory Muscles

Relevant Outcomes

- Decreased resting tension in respiratory muscles
- Reduced muscle tone

Clinical Relevance

What follows is a specialized version of the treatment for elevated resting tension described elsewhere in this chapter. We include it here because it is an important adjunct to treatment for respiratory conditions, such as chronic obstructive pulmonary disease, asthma, and cystic fibrosis, in which the client's inspiration is prolonged and labored. You can also use this treatment for clients on bed rest and athletes competing in aerobic or endurance events.

Treatment Considerations

The respiratory muscles that are affected include the scalenes, sternocleidomastoid, and the diaphragm. Learn to recognize the **trigger point** referral patterns for these muscles, since these trigger points are a common occurrence (see Chapter 9). Treat trigger points and other coexisting impairments, such as stress and adaptive shortening of the affected muscle(s), at the same time as your treatment for the primary impairment. Note that some of the clinical conditions associated with **hypertrophic** respiratory muscles have their own cautions and contraindications related to the client's medical and pharmaceutical management.

Guidelines for Using Massage Techniques

Use specific neuromuscular and connective tissue techniques for the scalenes, sternocleidomastoid, and diaphragm. If necessary, review the general descriptions of petrissage, stripping, specific compression, myofascial release, and direct fascial technique in Chapters 9 and 10, as well as Figures 9-10, 9-20, 9-23, 9-29, 10-2, 10-9, and 10-16 and other texts that have regional atlases of techniques.[261-264]

Complementary Modalities

- Relevant therapeutic exercise includes stretching of the scalenes and sternocleidomastoid muscles.
- Client education on diaphragmatic breathing and other breathing exercises is essential.[230]
- Educate clients on the roles of the diaphragm, scalenes, sternocleidomastoid, and abdominal muscles during normal and forced inspiration and expiration.
- Therapists may find progressive aerobic exercise useful for some conditions.

Chest Wall Tightness

Relevant Outcomes

- Increased chest wall mobility

Treatment Considerations

Chest wall tightness is associated with impairments or clinical conditions that result in restricted breathing such as stress, postural malalignment such as scoliosis and kyphosis, trigger points in certain muscles, respiratory conditions such as emphysema, and prolonged bed rest or inactivity. Because treatment involves the use of pressure on the client's chest wall, identify whether mechanical massage techniques are contraindicated for the client's condition. This would be the case for osteoporosis, osteomalacia, chest wounds, or a flail chest. Note that longstanding postural dysfunction or organ pathology, such as barrel chest in emphysema, may limit improvements in chest wall mobility.

Guidelines for Using Massage Techniques

- The first phase of treatment involves freeing restrictions in the muscles and connective tissue superficial to the ribs. Work with the client in side-lying, supine, and prone. In each position, apply general neuromuscular and connective tissue techniques, such as wringing and the myofascial release arm pull, to muscles of the trunk from the pubis/sacrum to the clavicle.[179]
- Apply specific neuromuscular techniques and connective tissue techniques to all the intercostal spaces. Systematically work your fingertips or thumbs ("stripping" or "rib-raking") *into* the intercostal spaces and

around the clavicle and costal arch. This specific work may take you 1 or 2 hours, and you may have to split it between several interventions.
- After you have freed restrictions in muscle or connective tissue, apply rhythmic mobilization ("rib springing"), rib compressions, and rocking to the rib cage.

Complementary Modalities

- Stretching and facilitated stretching to the thorax increase thoracic mobility.[230]
- For self-care, teach your client a combination of controlled deep breathing and stretching exercises of the large muscle groups of the thorax, such as the pectorals and spinal extensors.
- Systemic or regional application of heat can precede massage techniques or exercise.
- **Hatha yoga** is an appropriate home practice for people with chest wall tightness.

Abnormal or Altered Breathing Patterns

Relevant Outcomes

- Improved or normalized breathing patterns

Clinical Relevance

A less than optimal breathing pattern, with an overuse of accessory muscles of inspiration and an underuse of the diaphragm, occurs frequently in the general population. In addition, altered breathing patterns are associated with multiple impairments and clinical conditions that restrict breathing, including stress, postural malalignment, trigger points in certain muscles, respiratory conditions, the use of tobacco, and prolonged bed rest or inactivity.

Treatment Considerations

Begin your treatment by identifying the abnormalities in your client's breathing pattern. Determine whether she presents with a "paradoxical" breathing pattern, in which the abdominal diameter decreases during inspiration.[265] In addition, understand how your client's clinical condition or impairments contribute to her abnormal breathing pattern.

Guidelines for Using Massage Techniques

- Treat your client's other respiratory impairments, such as chest wall tightness and elevated resting tension of respiratory muscles, with relevant massage techniques prior to initiating education on normal respiration.

Complementary Modalities

- Education is the main approach to normalizing clients' breathing patterns. First, help your client develop an awareness of his current pattern of breathing. Have him place his hands on specified structures (scalenes, sternocleidomastoid, and the chest and abdominal walls) to monitor them for muscular contraction or shifts in position during inspiration and expiration. Looking in a mirror may also help the client to become familiar with his current habits of breathing. Once he has grasped these concepts, teach him how to perform diaphragmatic breathing and how to notice the difference between this breathing pattern and upper chest breathing and lateral costal breathing.[230]
- Diaphragm strengthening (breathing with weights, "sandbag breathing")[230,266] can be extremely important in respiratory diseases.[230]
- Improved postural awareness may facilitate a normalized breathing pattern.

INTERVENTIONS FOR IMPAIRMENTS RELATED TO MUSCLE

Unnecessary Muscle Tension

Relevant Outcomes

- Voluntary release of unnecessary muscle tension
- Improved awareness of unnecessary muscle tension

Clinical Relevance

Unnecessary muscle tension is a very common cause or result of elevated resting tension in response to situational stress (see the sections on stress in this chapter).

Treatment Considerations

There are no contraindications associated with this impairment. Two issues to explore prior to treatment are situations in the client's life that may be contributing to situational stress and the client's medications, which may affect resting muscle tension.[257]

Guidelines for Using Massage Techniques

- Begin with complementary techniques for increasing the client's awareness of unnecessary tension outlined in this section.
- Follow the general approach for a relaxing treatment outlined in the section on stress.
- Once a client has released unnecessary tension, apply the massage techniques that can reduce resting tension (see section "Elevated Resting Tension"). Whenever a palpable change in resting tension occurs, bring this change to the client's attention to familiarize her with the feeling of her muscles being relaxed and loose.
- The process of facilitating release of unnecessary tension and then decreasing resting tension to a level that makes an impression on the client is a lengthy one. It may take several 1-hour sessions for a given region and up to several months of treatment before your client can recognize and start to change the physical and mental habits that lead her to tense her muscles in stressful situations.[50,267] If your client undergoes a period of increased stress, you may have to spend one or more sessions refreshing her previously acquired awareness of decreased muscle tension.

Complementary Modalities

- At the beginning of treatment, clients may not be aware of unnecessary muscle tension. Sometimes simply lifting a limb or placing your hand on an area for up to a minute will be sufficient for a client to realize that she is unnecessarily contracting a muscle. If this does not work, then direct her attention to the area of unnecessary muscle tension with comments such as, "Are you aware that you are holding on here?" "Are you aware of tension here?" "Can you find a way to let this tension go?" Be wary of using language, such as directive commands, that suggests that effort on the client's part is required because the opposite is true.
- Passive movement techniques (see Chapter 11) often assist the client in releasing unnecessary muscle tension.

Elevated Resting Tension

Relevant Outcomes

- Reduced resting tension[268]

Clinical Relevance

Elevated resting tension of skeletal muscle is one of the most common reasons that people seek treatment with massage techniques. This impairment is associated with several clinical conditions and activities, such as stress,[267] athletic performance, overuse injuries, orthopedic injuries, postural malalignment, trigger points, **fibromyalgia**, arthritis, and connective tissue diseases.

Treatment Considerations

Prior to beginning treatment to decrease resting muscle tension, ensure that the client has released **unnecessary muscle tension**, using the approach described for that impairment. Resting tension is a complex phenomenon that has passive (material) and active (contractile) components (see section "Scientific Basis of Soft Tissue Examination" in Chapter 4). Consequently, you need to assess the degree and quality of elevated resting tension in normally innervated muscle using palpation and highly developed manual skills. In addition, identify the cautions and contraindications for the client's clinical condition.

Guidelines for Using Massage Techniques

- Use massage techniques that **engage** muscle and related fascia, especially neuromuscular techniques, connective tissue techniques, and passive movement techniques. *When applying neuromuscular techniques, such as petrissage and stripping, you must engage the layer of muscle in which you wish to change resting tension.*
- Connective tissue techniques, such as myofascial release and direct fascial release, have a local effect on resting tension. In addition, because of the interconnected nature of the fascial layers, they may also have regional effects.
- Using soothing techniques, such as rocking, to achieve a general sedative effect may produce a marginal systemic decrease in resting muscle tension.

Complementary Modalities

- Heat, either local or systemic, temporarily reduces resting tension.[89,252]
- Systematic stretching also reduces resting tension.[230]
- Aerobic and strength training exercises generally raise resting muscle tension, at least temporarily. Postexercise stretching may counteract this effect.

Trigger Points, Myofascial Pain

Relevant Outcomes

- Decreased trigger point activity[220,269-271]
- Decreased myofascial pain[265,272]
- Increased range of motion[273]

Treatment Considerations

Myofascial pain can be excruciating. Therefore, you must respect the client's pain during examination and treatment. Trigger points can mimic visceral disease, such as a heart attack,[272] and result in unusual pain referrals and symptoms that seem unrelated to activity.[274,275] In the case of trauma or repetitive strain, finding the exact mechanism of injury can help you identify the muscle(s) with trigger points.

Pain referral patterns for single trigger points are defined in several texts.[265,272] Referrals that are commonly seen in a clinical practice include trapezius, sternocleidomastoid, iliocostalis, longissimus, scalenes, pectoralis major and minor, splenius capitis and cervicis, subscapularis, infraspinatus, gluteus medius, tensor fascia lata, hamstrings, quadriceps, tibialis anterior, and tibialis posterior. Table 14-2 describes common myofascial pain syndromes. When a client has multiple trigger points, the referral patterns combine in an overlapping fashion. As a result, the client may perceive a wider distribution of pain that does not correspond to any one trigger point referral map. Identify key trigger points because their treatment may eliminate the need to treat the satellite trigger points.[272] In addition, identify perpetuating factors, as far as possible.

You may have to distinguish between the tender points of fibromyalgia and trigger points.[276] The tender points of fibromyalgia are not trigger points. In addition, the diagnosis of fibromyalgia requires the presence of at least 11 specific tender points and an associated sleep disturbance. Nevertheless, clients with fibromyalgia may also have trigger points that may respond favorably to treatment.[117]

Guidelines for Using Massage Techniques

- Treatment by any method seeks to restore full, pain-free range of motion.
- Stripping and specific compression (trigger point pressure release) are massage techniques designed to treat trigger points (see Chapter 9). You may precede and follow these techniques with regional massage techniques, which include petrissage, myofascial release, or direct fascial technique applied with a broad contact surface.
- Identify and treat primary trigger points first, if possible, since their treatment will reduce symptoms in satellites. Identify and treat all trigger points in a functional unit including agonists, antagonists, and synergists.[272]

Table 14-2   Myofascial Pain Syndromes[265,272]

Syndrome	Trigger Points Involved
Tension headache	Five common causes of tension headache are trigger points in ■ upper trapezius ■ sternocleidomastoid ■ splenius capitis and cervicis ■ suboccipitals ■ temporalis
Temporomandibular joint dysfunction	Temporomandibular joint dysfunction may involve actual joint pathology or it can be due to trigger point activity in the lateral pterygoid, with secondary involvement of the medial pterygoid, masseter, and temporalis
Frozen shoulder	Frozen shoulder is a clinical term that may involve fibrosis of the glenohumeral capsule (adhesive capsulitis); it may also be due to trigger points in subscapularis, with secondary involvement of the other rotator cuff muscles
Thoracic outlet syndrome	Thoracic outlet syndrome is often caused by entrapment of the trunks of the brachial plexus in between the anterior and medial scalenes or underneath pectoralis minor; trigger points in these muscles may also contribute to the client's pain
Trigger finger	This syndrome may involve trigger points in the long finger flexors of the forearm
Weeder's thumb	This syndrome may involve trigger points in opponens pollicis
Lumbago or back pain	"Lumbago" is an archaic term for lower back pain that has many causes and requires differential assessment; lower back pain can be caused solely by trigger points in the gluteus medius, spinal extensors (erector spinae and multifidi), or psoas, with additional involvement of quadratus lumborum
Pseudosciatica	Travell and Simons use this term to refer to an imitation of lumbar **radiculopathy** caused by trigger points in gluteus minimus
Piriformis syndrome	This complex syndrome, which may involve entrapment of the sciatic nerve in piriformis, can be caused or perpetuated by trigger points in the piriformis and the other lateral rotators
Entrapment syndromes	An entrapment syndrome involves continuous pressure on a peripheral nerve or trunk that causes a **neurapraxia**, with resulting neurological symptoms; an example of an entrapment syndrome that is caused by trigger points is thoracic outlet syndrome; there are many other less common examples detailed in longer texts[265,272]

Trigger points contribute to pain and dysfunction of virtually all soft tissue injuries such as sprains, repetitive strain injuries, and fractures. However, they can appear on their own, as trigger point syndromes or myofascial pain syndromes. Some myofascial pain syndromes are common enough to have names of their own. This table lists the conditions in which trigger points are either the sole cause of pain or a major factor in the condition.

Complementary Modalities

■ Follow massage techniques for trigger point release immediately with passive movement through the full range of motion of that muscle (do not overstretch), active movement through the full range of motion, and the application of moist heat.[265,272]

■ Moist heat before treatment or by itself is beneficial.[277]

■ Since ice packs will increase the activity of trigger points, do not use them on or around trigger points unless you are treating an acute orthopedic injury. Once the acute stage of an injury has resolved, treat the trigger points as described elsewhere in this chapter. Use ice in the context of the very specific "ice-and-stretch" protocol described in other texts.[272]

■ Use gentle stretching or the combination of stretching after proprioceptive neuromuscular facilitation techniques (agonist contract, hold-relax, and rhythmic stabilization) or postisometric relaxation.[272] When you are using stretching, ensure that you orient the stretch along the affected muscle fibers and avoid producing pain in a related joint (a "positive stretch sign").[271]

■ **Strain–counterstrain** (**positional release**) and high-velocity, low-amplitude techniques may be of value.[278]

■ For self-care, teach clients a protocol that includes local heat, self-massage, self-stripping, self-compression with a small firm ball, and stretching (or hold-relax), followed by full active range of motion.[277]

■ When teaching self-compression with a ball, limit the treatment time to a few 30-second applications, followed by the appropriate stretch and heat. Clients are prone to overdo self-compression because it feels good; this can cause **reactive cramping** or unbalance the function around a joint. If a client reports that he has to compress a muscle frequently to maintain relief, then conduct a client re-examination to identify factors that are perpetuating the trigger points.

Muscle Spasm

Relevant Outcomes

- Reduced muscle spasm[279]

Clinical Relevance

Muscle spasm is associated with spasmodic **torticollis**, traumatic orthopedic injuries, disk lesions and other conditions that compress nerves or nerve roots, athletic performance, acute visceral conditions such as appendicitis, arterial disorders including intermittent claudication, and pregnancy. It can also be the side effect of some medications, such as lithium, and the result of nutritional deficiencies. Exposure to cold, dehydration, preexisting trigger points, and postural imbalance exacerbate muscle spasm.

Treatment Considerations

If your client presents with acute muscle spasm, attempt to find the cause of the spasm since this may require a referral to a physician, as in the case of recent trauma or metabolic imbalance in a runner. Furthermore, your assessment of the acuity of the client's condition can guide your approach to treatment.

Guidelines for Using Massage Techniques and Complementary Modalities

- Do not stretch a muscle that is in extreme spasm.
- Incorporate all techniques for relaxation, such as diaphragmatic breathing and relaxing or sedative massage techniques, away from the site of spasm.
- On the site of spasm, attempt the following ordered progression of techniques, while ensuring that you *do not increase your client's pain.* Perform all techniques within the client's tolerance.
  1. Contract the antagonist. This activity moves the muscle in spasm into a lengthened position. Repeat this active lengthening between other techniques.
  2. Apply specific compression and cross-fiber petrissage on the attachments of the muscle. Combine these with active movement within the client's tolerance.[279,280]

3. Apply specific compression using your thumbs to drag the two attachments of the muscle in spasm toward the muscle belly ("muscle approximation").[260]
4. Use superficial reflex techniques such as superficial stroking (caution with fine vibration) on site.
5. Apply gentle petrissage on site.
6. Have the client perform gentle stretching.
7. Use hold-relax techniques that engage the muscle.
8. Use strain–counterstrain or positional release techniques.[281]
9. Adapt techniques 1, 5, 6, and 7 above for self-care.

- Apply heat or cold based on the stage of the client's clinical condition and his response to treatment.
- Strengthening the client's antagonist muscles may be an appropriate long-term goal.

Muscle Weakness Associated with Reduced Resting Tension or Neuromuscular Tone

Relevant Outcomes

- Increased **strength** and **power**

Clinical Relevance

Weakness can occur after trauma, orthopedic injury, surgery, illness, and bed rest. It is also a common result of inactivity in the elderly. Furthermore, muscle weakness can be associated with neurological conditions such as Parkinson's disease and hemiplegia.

Treatment Considerations

Before initiating treatment, determine the cause of the client's weakness and relevant cautions and contraindications. It is also important for you to distinguish between weakness, **fatigue**, and deconditioning. For example, some clients with neurological conditions, such as Parkinson's disease or hemiplegia, present with weakness that is secondary to other impairments that affect movement, such as **spasticity**.

Guidelines for Using Massage Techniques and Complementary Modalities

- There are no massage techniques that you can use to increase muscle strength in normally innervated tissues.
- Therapeutic exercise is the primary treatment technique that you can use to treat muscle weakness in normally innervated tissues.

- Regular application of massage techniques may indirectly improve strength in clients with neurological problems such as carpal tunnel syndrome, spinal cord injury, and multiple sclerosis.[31,70,74] Physical therapy texts describe facilitation techniques (see following Complementary Modalities section) that may produce short-term increases in an abnormally innervated muscle's ability to contract.[282] Use these techniques immediately *prior to exercise* to facilitate the contraction of a weakened muscle.
- Therapists often use regional or general massage techniques to prepare client's muscles for exercise in athletic settings.[119]

Complementary Modalities

- Use therapeutic exercise for increasing muscle performance. The full range of strengthening methods is described in numerous texts on therapeutic exercise.[230,283,284]
- Joint traction and approximation, quick stretch, fine vibration, light touch, and repetitive stroking ("brushing") can be used to increase neuromuscular tone and facilitate movement.[282]
- Short applications of cold may stimulate arousal and indirectly facilitate resistance exercise.[252]
- Conversely, prolonged heat and prolonged cold temporarily reduce strength.[252]

INTERVENTIONS FOR CONNECTIVE TISSUE IMPAIRMENTS

Decreased Connective Tissue Mobility

This category includes impairments in which poor tissue modeling compromises normal connective tissue mobility such as **adhesions**, **scarring**, decreased mobility of skin and/or fascia, **fascial restrictions**, and **contractures**. Therapists use a similar treatment approach for this group of impairments.

Relevant Outcomes

- Increased mobility of connective tissue, including decreased adhesions, improved mobility of scar tissue, increased mobility of skin and fascia, reduced fascial restriction, and reduced contracture[285]
- Increased range of motion[286,287]

Clinical Relevance

There are several possible causes of decreased connective tissue mobility. First, it often occurs during the chronic stage of inflammatory repair and is, therefore, relevant for orthopedic injuries such as fractures and sprains, various types of arthritis, inflammatory connective tissue diseases, trauma, surgery, and burns. Second, decreased connective tissue mobility can be the result of prolonged periods of reduced mobility that is associated with illness or hospitalization. Finally, it is associated with postural conditions in the form of adaptive tissue shortening. Microscarring and a reduced capacity to adjust to loads may be associated with **repetitive strain injuries** such as **tendinitis** and **tendinosis**.[229]

Treatment Considerations

Cautions and contraindications for the techniques that therapists use to treat connective tissue restriction include malignancy, cellulitis, fever, systemic or local infection, acute circulatory conditions, osteomyelitis, aneurysm, obstructive edema, acute rheumatoid arthritis, open wounds, sutures, hematomas, healing fractures, osteoporosis, anticoagulant therapy, advanced diabetes, and hypersensitivity of the skin.[288] Prior to treating decreased connective tissue mobility, *ensure that the client has no signs of local acute inflammation.* Some orthopedic conditions, such as repeated sprains or rheumatoid arthritis, may involve joint laxity or instability. Do not treat these joints with techniques that attempt to lengthen the already lengthened or weakened connective tissue. Finally, do not treat any area of connective tissue in isolation; local treatment will have a systemic effect that will facilitate postural changes.

Guidelines for Using Massage Techniques

- Skin rolling, myofascial release, direct fascial technique, and friction (see Chapter 10) are the main techniques for treating decreased connective tissue mobility.[263,264,280,289-292] When a large amount of tissue is affected, as with postural adaptive shortening or contracture of a large joint, use broad surfaces and more general techniques. These include myofascial release with widely positioned hands and direct fascial techniques delivered with the forearm. To treat smaller amounts of tissue, for example, localized fibrosis within a tendon[293] or a capsule,[286] use specific techniques such as friction applied with fingers or thumb(s). In addition, you may find petrissage and stripping beneficial if you apply them slowly and with sufficient drag; avoiding the use of too much oil will enable you to achieve this.

- When multiple layers of tissue are affected, begin at the surface and progress treatment through the restrictions in deeper layers.
- Early-stage treatment of burns, to prevent or reduce the formation of scar tissue, involves highly specialized protocols that are beyond the scope of this text.[285,294] Key Points 14-3 outlines some "scar techniques" that may be appropriate for use on *mature* scar tissue.
- **Rhythmic mobilization** applied *after* the treatment of connective tissue may enhance the client's movement patterns.
- Myofascial trigger points often coexist with many varieties of connective tissue restriction.[265,272,295-297] See guidelines for treatment of trigger points presented elsewhere in this chapter and in Chapter 9 in the sections on stripping and specific compression.
- If connective tissue restriction is associated with poor posture, refer to the section on adaptive shortening elsewhere in this chapter.

- Monitor the treatment effects, before and after treatment, using a postural scan.
- Long-lasting lengthening of connective tissue happens quickly, provided that you use the correct technique. In fact, with some conditions, you can see positive treatment effects within several minutes. Consequently, small, uncomplicated, and recently matured scars may respond in a single session. Long-standing conditions will require several local treatment sessions to achieve lasting change, as well as more general treatments to address compensations that exist throughout the client's body. Widespread fascial restriction, which is seen with postural conditions, can take more than 15 hours of treatment.

Complementary Modalities

- Use stretching exercises within the full range of motion.[230]
- Use higher grade **joint mobilization** if adhesions affect the joint capsule.[229,230]
- Use active exercises, within the full range of motion, after you have restored muscle length. Both stretching and active exercises are also effective within the client's self-care program.
- Follow changes in alignment with postural awareness exercises (see section "Decreased Postural and Kinesthetic Awareness").
- Consider therapeutic exercise for increasing muscle performance (strength, endurance, and power) once you have restored mobility.[294]
- Local heat is appropriate before massage techniques (allow several minutes to elapse before applying connective tissue techniques) or stretching. Before you apply heat, ensure that there are no signs of acute inflammation.

Restriction of Joint Capsule or Ligaments

Relevant Outcomes

- Increased mobility of joint capsule or ligaments[298]

Clinical Relevance

Restrictions of the joint capsule or ligaments accompany capsulitis, adhesive capsulitis, osteoarthritis, inflammatory arthritic conditions, and systemic connective tissue diseases, such as lupus, where there is joint involvement.

Key Points: 14-3

Scar Techniques for Mature Scars

So-called scar techniques that are used to model a *mature* scar are simply examples of all the connective tissue techniques previously described in detail in Chapter 10. Apply these in an orderly sequence that begins with light pressure to engage superficial layers and then proceeds to engage deeper layers of restriction. Remember that the area of reduced mobility often extends far to the sides of a visible scar and far below the surface.

Skin rolling. Grasp and roll the skin and subcutaneous fascia along like a wave. Vary the lifting force and direction of the stroke during repeated passes. Use this as an introductory technique and to periodically assess the mobility of the superficial tissues as treatment proceeds.[229]

Myofascial release. Using fingertip or palmar contact, take the slack out of the skin and subcutaneous tissues.[229] Then hold this position, without gliding, for 90 seconds or longer while **creep** occurs. Increase pressure with successive applications to engage the deeper tissue layers. Vary the direction of the force. Use two-handed releases with widely positioned hands if the restriction affects a large area.

Direct fascial technique. Use one or two slowly gliding digits to bow the scar tissue into a C shape or an S shape[9,229] or make the stroke follow a J pattern.[290] Use your grouped fingers or your entire palm if the restriction affects a large area.

Friction. Use friction, applied with your fingertips or thumbs on very dense hard areas, until palpable softening occurs. Orient strokes transverse or parallel to the scar or use circles.[229] Use a broad surface such as your palm for a large restriction.

Treatment Considerations

Prior to treating decreased connective tissue mobility, *ensure that the client has no signs of* **acute inflammation**. Some orthopedic conditions, such as repeated sprains or rheumatoid arthritis, may involve joint laxity or instability. Do not treat these joints with techniques that attempt to lengthen the already lengthened or weakened connective tissue.

Guidelines for Using Massage Techniques

■ This is a special case of impairment of decreased connective tissue mobility.

■ Apply general connective tissue techniques to all fascial layers that cross the client's joint. The most beneficial approach may be the application of specific techniques, such as friction, to the affected ligament(s) or capsule.[299]

Complementary Modalities

■ In addition to hydrotherapy and exercises mentioned for decreased mobility of connective tissue, use joint traction and joint mobilization techniques to mobilize the joint capsule,[229,230] as your scope of practice permits.

Hypermobility (Laxity) of Joint Capsule or Ligaments

Relevant Outcomes

■ Increased joint integrity
■ Increased joint stability

Clinical Relevance

Ligament or capsular laxity can be secondary to repeated joint dislocations and sprains, trauma, inflammatory arthritic conditions, systemic connective tissue disorders, pregnancy, and occupations that place a chronic load on particular joints such as dance or gymnastics.

Treatment Considerations

When treating ligament or capsular laxity, consider any cautions and contraindications stemming from the client's clinical condition such as pain level and medications. If a joint seems unstable or at risk for repeated dislocation or sprain, stabilize it with taping techniques, as your scope of practice permits, and refer your client to her physician if appropriate.

Guidelines for Using Massage Techniques

■ *No massage technique will tighten overstretched or weakened connective tissue.* Therapeutic exercise is the primary treatment modality.

■ During the application of massage techniques, avoid positions of instability or capsular stretch. Avoid performing connective tissue techniques or aggressive neuromuscular techniques on the site of laxity. When only one side of a joint is lax, as is the case with repeated inversion sprains of the ankle, cautious application of connective tissue techniques to the shortened side of the joint may facilitate functional activity.

■ Do not attempt to decrease the resting tension in the muscles that cross the joint, since these may be acting to stabilize the joint in the absence of other support. In cases of **functional instability**, general massage techniques may facilitate awareness of movement and posture, as described in the section on postural impairments.

Complementary Modalities

■ You can use therapeutic exercise to enhance muscle performance and control to stabilize the joint during active movement. In the early stages of treatment, select therapeutic exercises in the midrange and avoid the extreme ends of range. Numerous texts on therapeutic exercise detail appropriate stabilization protocols.[229,230]

■ Include postural awareness training for cases of functional instability.

INTERVENTIONS FOR POSTURAL IMPAIRMENTS

Postural Malalignment Due to Bony Deformity

Relevant Outcomes

■ Improved postural alignment

Clinical Relevance

Bony deformity, such as small hemipelvis or true leg-length discrepancy, may play a role in hyperkyphosis, hyperlordosis, and scoliosis.[265] Systemic conditions like Scheuermann's disease, tuberculosis of the spine, and bone cancer may also cause or contribute to postural conditions.

Treatment Considerations

Refer the client to an appropriate health care professional for correction of bony asymmetry with orthotics, prosthetics, or surgery.

Guidelines for Using Massage Techniques

- If possible, do not attempt to treat tissue contractures or adaptive shortening until the client has had his underlying bony malalignment corrected.
- Use neuromuscular or connective tissue techniques at a moderate depth, as required for symptomatic pain relief in areas of elevated resting tension and trigger points.[300]
- After correction of the bony malalignment, treat adaptive shortening, adaptive lengthening, and decreased postural awareness using massage techniques described in the relevant sections of this chapter.

Complementary Modalities

- After correction of the bony malalignment, use complementary modalities for adaptive shorting, adaptive lengthening, and decreased postural awareness as described in the relevant sections of this chapter.

Adaptive Shortening with Impaired Balance of Agonist/Antagonist Muscle Function

Relevant Outcomes

- Increased extensibility of muscle and fascia
- Improved balance of agonist/antagonist muscle function
- Improved postural alignment[301]

Clinical Relevance

Adaptive shortening of soft tissues may be associated with hyperkyphosis, hyperlordosis, scoliosis, iliotibial band contracture, valgus knee structure, patellofemoral syndrome, and pes planus.[1,2,230]

Treatment Considerations

Before you begin an intervention for adaptive shortening, ensure that it is not the result of asymmetrical bone structure, such as a true leg-length discrepancy[300] or small hemipelvis. If that is the case, consult the section on postural deformity for a modified approach. Study at length the relationships between fascial planes and layers that anatomy texts describe.[302] Be aware that releasing shortened structures can result in fairly quick changes in the client's postural alignment. Those changes may, in turn, change the mechanical load on other structures and result in a change in the client's symptoms.

Guidelines for Using Massage Techniques

- With postural conditions, the client's pain is frequently the result of a stretch on the antagonist muscles that oppose the shortened myofascial units. One standard approach to treatment is to *treat shortened structures first*.[230] If the client's pain is severe, you may choose to treat the lengthened structures first or concurrently with those that show adaptive shortening.
- Connective tissue techniques are the methods of choice for treating adaptive shortening.[262-264,290] Neuromuscular techniques are less effective but useful (see the Outcomes and Evidence section for Petrissage in Chapter 9). Neither superficial reflex nor superficial fluid techniques engage the relevant tissue layers of muscle and associated fascia. Furthermore, passive movement and percussive techniques do not subject the tissues to sufficient **drag**. Note that myofascial release and direct fascial technique require sustained horizontal traction force along layers to lengthen the fascia (see Chapter 10). Use specific compression and stripping,[301] since adaptively shortened structures often contain trigger points.[265,272,303] Finally, passive movement techniques, such as rhythmic mobilization, applied *after* connective tissue and neuromuscular techniques can help to restore more expansive movement patterns.[62]
- Assess the client's posture before and after interventions with a postural scan. Record treatment effects carefully.
- Key Points 14-4 presents a simple protocol for treating adaptive shortening.

Complementary Modalities

- Local heat is appropriate before massage techniques or stretching. Allow several minutes to elapse before applying connective tissue techniques.
- Use therapeutic exercise for stretching the shortened tissues.[230]
- Use active exercises within the full range of motion after you have restored muscle length.
- Include both stretching and active exercises in the client's self-care program.

A Simple Massage Protocol to Treat Adaptive Shortening

Following is a simple protocol that you can use to structure a single session of 30, 45, or 60 minutes to treat adaptive shortening.

1. Perform a **postural scan**.
2. Choose a target group of muscles that shows adaptive shortening.
3. Briefly apply broad, general direct fascial technique or myofascial release to the region.
4. Lengthen the target group of muscles with specific connective tissue techniques and then stretch them.
5. Treat the entire region with neuromuscular techniques, such as petrissage, and then rhythmic mobilization.
6. Address the opposite side similarly, following Steps 3 to 5.
7. Address the related axial skeleton with broad connective tissue techniques and neuromuscular techniques such as petrissage.
8. Be sure to include the paraspinal and neck musculature as in Step 7, if only briefly.
9. Monitor changes with a postural scan.
10. Guide the client through standing aligned posture, as described in Chapter 6.

Progress this intervention by choosing a different group of adaptively shortened muscles at each session.

- Therapeutic exercise to improve muscle performance is essential; consult texts on therapeutic exercise for details.[230]
- Follow changes in postural alignment with postural awareness exercises (see Chapter 6).

Adaptive Lengthening with Stretch Weakness[230] and Impaired Balance of Agonist/Antagonist Muscle Function

Relevant Outcomes

- Increased strength
- Improved balance of agonist/antagonist muscle function
- Improved postural alignment

Clinical Relevance

Whenever one group of muscles adapts by shortening, the antagonist group adapts by lengthening. Adaptive lengthening may be associated with hyperkyphosis, hyperlordosis,

scoliosis, iliotibial band contracture, valgus knee structure, patellofemoral syndrome, and pes planus.[230]

Treatment Considerations

When muscles and fascia lengthen adaptively, they must function in a lengthened position, which puts them at a mechanical disadvantage. As a result, they cannot develop maximum contractile force.[230] These muscles exhibit what is termed stretch weakness and are subject to fatigue, **spasm**, and **myofascial trigger points**. *Do not lengthen these muscles further* with vigorously applied connective tissue or neuromuscular techniques.

Guidelines for Using Massage Techniques

- First, treat adaptively shortened structures as described in the Adaptive Shortening with Impaired Balance of Agonist/Antagonist Muscle Function section.
- *None of the massage techniques affect weakness in normally innervated tissues.* Use various muscle performance exercises[230,283,284] to strengthen the lengthened muscles.
- Percussion may produce a marginal and transient increase in tone in abnormally innervated tissue. There is, however, no basis for using percussion on lengthened muscles with normal innervation (see Outcomes and Evidence sections for percussive techniques in Chapter 12).
- Adaptively lengthened muscles often contain taut bands and trigger points,[296,303] which applications of percussion may irritate. Furthermore, these trigger points may be satellites that will resolve once you have treated the adaptively shortened antagonists.[272,304,305] If they do not resolve, treat them with ischemic compression and short stripping strokes.

Complementary Modalities

- Increase muscle performance with appropriate therapeutic exercise.[230]
- Use moist heat, gentle stretch, and active range of motion after the massage techniques for treating trigger points.[272]

Decreased Postural and Kinesthetic Awareness

Relevant Outcomes

- Improved postural awareness

Clinical Relevance

Decreased postural awareness is associated with hyperkyphosis, hyperlordosis, scoliosis, and other postural conditions.[230]

Treatment Considerations

Decreased postural awareness often accompanies postural misalignment due to adaptive muscle shortening and lengthening. Occasionally, a decreased postural awareness, a "postural fault," will be the client's only presenting postural impairment.[230]

Guidelines for Using Massage Techniques

- Massage techniques help to increase body awareness in a general sense.[306-308]
- When adaptively shortened areas lengthen quickly during treatment, the client may immediately notice changes as soon as he stands. Nevertheless, no massage technique by itself can produce a lasting increase in a client's postural *awareness* without some guidance by the therapist.
- Our clinical experience suggests that applying deep massage techniques to the client's feet, immediately prior to the client standing at the end of an intervention, may help the client adapt to and integrate postural changes that have occurred as a result of connective tissue or neuromuscular techniques.

Complementary Modalities

- Postural exercises accompanied by verbal and tactile cues are the primary treatment method for increasing postural awareness.[230] During these exercises, position or guide the client's body into a better alignment and help the client to recognize this improved alignment. The client may then hold this position for a short period to develop muscular control.
- Do not instruct clients to practice postural exercises for extended periods since this may lead to an undesirable increase in muscular tension. It is better to suggest exercises that the client practices for up to 10 minutes once or twice a day. Over time, the client will gradually acquire improved postural habits during daily activities.
- Some examples of simple postural exercises are as follows:
  1. The client lies in an aligned position on the treatment table. Passively position the client in the best alignment possible and have the client maintain this position for 10 minutes or longer. This works well as a prelude to the following exercises.
  2. Use standing aligned posture and seated aligned posture as described in Chapter 6. Floor-length mirrors in your clinical setting and the client's home facilitate self-monitoring in these exercises. The client can also perform seated aligned posture while sitting on a Swiss ball.
  3. Pelvic tilt. Teach this in progressively more difficult positions: supine with the knees up (crook-lying), full supine, standing with the back and back of the pelvis against a wall for reference, and, lastly, free-standing.[264]

INTERVENTIONS FOR IMPAIRMENTS RELATED TO INFLAMMATION

Acute-Stage Inflammation

Relevant Outcomes

- Reduced signs and symptoms of inflammation, such as reduced edema
- Reduced pain
- Increased active range of motion

Clinical Relevance

Acute inflammation can be associated with a variety of orthopedic clinical conditions, including musculoskeletal trauma, repetitive strain injuries, and osteoarthritis. It also occurs after surgery. Finally, it can accompany various systemic conditions such as rheumatoid arthritis and related connective tissue diseases.

Treatment Considerations

Prior to treating traumatic orthopedic injuries, ensure that the client's anatomical structures are stable. If you are in doubt, refer the client for medical assessment and management. When inflammation is secondary to a repetitive strain injury, identify the causal activity and find out if the client can reduce or cease that activity. When inflammation is associated with osteoarthritis or any systemic disease, understand how the client's medical and pharmacological management affects his inflammatory process, pain, edema, and spasm.

Guidelines for Using Massage Techniques

Acute inflammation is not an impairment; instead, it is a physiological process that is associated with a *group* of impairments including primarily edema, acute nociceptive pain, and spasm. This section reviews the treatment approaches for the primary impairments associated with inflammation and includes an example of how to combine treatment techniques within a single intervention.

Initial Treatment

- First, treat any edema that is present because resolution of the edema will also reduce pain.
- You can use several techniques to facilitate the resolution of edema. Apply broad-contact compression or superficial lymph drainage (**terminus stroke**) to the junction of common lymphatic duct and vena cava in the thorax. Apply superficial fluid techniques proximal to the site of inflammation (working distally to the peripheral margin of swelling) repetitively for 20 minutes or more to drain edema (see Chapter 8). Apply neuromuscular techniques proximally to open the deep lymphatic drainage.
- To inhibit spasm, apply very gentle petrissage and gentle specific compression to unaffected portions of muscles that pass through the inflamed area (see the section on spasm in this chapter).
- To inhibit pain, apply superficial reflex techniques as tolerated to the site. When the client's lesion is more severe and local touch is contraindicated, you can achieve counterirritant analgesia by applying these techniques proximally in the related dermatome, to antagonist muscle groups, or even to the contralateral side.
- There may be a variety of other impairments away from the site of injury, such as reduced active range of motion, elevated resting tension, and trigger points, which respond to the appropriate massage techniques (see the sections on range of motion, elevated resting tension, and trigger points). When working away from the side of the edema, do not attempt to push fluid through a congested area and avoid placing excessive mechanical stress on the remote sections of structures that pass through the injury site.

Progression of Massage Techniques through the Subacute Stage

- Apply superficial fluid techniques closer to the center of the site of the injury as the edema lessens and local sensitivity at the site of the injury declines. In addition, once the local edema has resolved, increase the pressure of the massage technique through the superficial tissues to engage the investing layer of the deep fascia and then the superficial muscular layers. Introduce light neuromuscular and connective tissue techniques and small-amplitude passive movement techniques to apply a stress to the newly deposited connective tissue elements.
- You can treat off-site impairments somewhat more aggressively in the subacute stage than you could in the acute stage, as long as you keep the relevant cautions in mind.

Complementary Modalities

Initial Treatment

- To treat edema, elevate the body segment 30° to 45° and apply an ice pack. Ice promotes **retrostasis**, provides anesthesia, and reduces spasm.[89,252]
- Encourage *deep* diaphragmatic breathing.
- To inhibit pain in the region of a stable joint, use passive movements and gentle joint mobilization techniques, as the client's tolerance and your scope of practice permit.[230]
- To maintain muscle performance, have the client perform isometric muscle contractions of the muscles that pass through the inflamed area, within his level of tolerance.
- Educate the client about the nature of his condition, the requirement for rest, and the use of elevation, ice, compressive bandages, and assistive devices such as splints or crutches.[230]

Chronic-Stage Inflammation

Relevant Outcomes

- Reduced signs and symptoms of inflammation, such as improved connective tissue modeling, reduced pain, and full active range of motion.

Clinical Relevance

The chronic stage of inflammation can be associated with a variety of conditions, including trauma, orthopedic injuries, repetitive strain injuries, surgery, osteoarthritis, rheumatoid arthritis, and related connective tissue diseases.

Treatment Considerations

Assess how chronic or subacute injuries are progressing with treatment on the following dimensions. Determine whether the treatment was appropriate and successful.

Confirm the clinical stage of the injury based on findings from the client examination.[229,230] Ensure that reinjury has not exacerbated the acute stage of an orthopedic condition. Finally, when inflammation is associated with osteoarthritis or any systemic disease, understand how the client's medical and pharmacological management affects his inflammatory process, pain, and other symptoms.

Guidelines for Using Massage Techniques

- Chronic inflammation is not an impairment; instead, it is a physiological process with a *group* of associated impairments, which differ from those associated with acute inflammation. The main impairments that occur at the site of inflammation are the result of poor connective tissue modeling during the repair process. These impairments include adhesions, scarring, consolidated edema, fascial restriction, and abnormal density and reduced mobility of connective tissue structures. You can treat all of these impairments in a similar manner using connective tissue and neuromuscular techniques.
- If you are continuing an intervention in which you addressed the acute stage of the client's inflammatory process, gradually increase the force with which you apply neuromuscular and connective tissue techniques at the site of injury. You will not need to use more than moderate force because your use of massage techniques in the earlier stages of healing would promote adequate tissue modeling. The entire progression of massage techniques on the site of injury from the acute stage through the chronic stage might take 4 or more weeks for a second- or third-degree injury.
- The intervention will differ on sites of old injuries that were inadequately treated or not treated at all and when there is long-standing musculoskeletal pain after an injury.

Progression When the Client Presents with Long-Standing Chronic-Stage Tissue Restrictions
- In this case, you may have to use some force and persistence over several interventions to progress through the restrictions that exist in the different layers of muscle and connective tissue. Furthermore, compensatory changes and multiple sources of pain may complicate your progression of the client's intervention.

Compensatory Changes
- **Compensatory changes** in the musculoskeletal system that develop in response to local damage, such as restrictions in mobility, movement, and coordination,

complicate chronic injuries.[309] The severity and extent of these compensatory changes often reflect the severity of the original tissue damage and the amount of time that has elapsed since the injury. A client's complaints of chronic impairments that had an insidious onset may be the result of these compensatory changes. Furthermore, the client may be unaware of the causal relationship between a forgotten injury and his current complaints.
- Begin treatment by locating and addressing the layers of restriction *at the original site of injury*. You must also identify and treat shortening in soft tissue that has arisen as a mechanical consequence of the original injury in order to achieve a satisfactory resolution of the client's impairments and associated functional limitations. Unraveling the compensatory patterns[309] associated with a chronic injury may take more time than your treatment of the original injury.

Multiple Sources of Pain
- The client may present with multiple sources of local and referred pain in his muscles, fascia, and joints because long-standing chronic conditions can result in the development of widespread restrictions in multiple layers of soft tissue.[309] As a result, you may find it impossible to identify any one tissue or structure as the primary focus of your treatment.
- In this situation, consider performing several interventions of progressively deeper neuromuscular and connective tissue techniques at the outset of treatment in order to reduce the tension in the superficial layers of muscle and connective tissue throughout the body. This strategy may reduce both compensatory changes and multiple sources of pain. As you progressively reduce the tension in the superficial and deeper tissue layers, the client may experience a succession of both familiar and unfamiliar symptoms that endure for days or weeks. The end result is that you, and the client, will probably be able to identify one tissue or structure as the primary focus of treatment.

A Strategy for Achieving Adequate Depth in the Treatment of Chronic Lesions
- Inexperienced therapists often attempt to cover too wide an area with too general a focus when they are treating chronic lesions. As a result, their treatment fails because they have not worked deeply enough in any one area. The application of specific deep massage techniques is indispensable but time-consuming. A single area, such as the shoulder, can take anywhere from 30 to 90 minutes to treat. When you need to use

deep, specific massage techniques extensively, subdivide the client's body into smaller manageable areas and schedule the treatment of these areas for two or more consecutive sessions.

- Ensure that you include **general massage** techniques and address the client's antagonist and synergist muscle groups to minimize the potential for imbalances in the client's myofascial system.

Complementary Modalities

Complementary techniques for chronic inflammation include all forms of stretching, joint traction, and joint mobilization.

Poor strength and endurance associated with chronic inflammatory processes respond to progressive strengthening and aerobic exercise.

INTERVENTIONS RELATED TO IMPAIRMENTS IN RANGE OF MOTION

Reduced Active Range of Motion

Relevant Outcomes

- Increased active range of motion

Treatment Considerations

Reduced active range of motion is a common impairment *that you must treat by addressing one or more causal impairments or conditions.* It is extremely important for you to identify the underlying cause(s) of the reduction in range of motion before you begin treatment. Any of the following impairments or conditions can cause the client to exhibit reduced active range of motion:

- Adaptive shortening
- Joint or bone malformation
- Inflammation (trauma and surgery are two very common causes)
- Mechanical instability (from a fracture or ruptured structure)
- Scar tissue, connective tissue shortening, and adhesions
- Pain (pain itself is often secondary to other impairments)
- Trigger points
- Increased resting muscle tension
- Muscle spasm
- Muscle weakness
- General deconditioning (if severe)

- Edema
- Spastic paralysis
- Flaccid paralysis
- Rigidity
- Atrophy (due to disuse or abnormal innervation)

See the guidelines for treating many of these impairments in relevant sections of this chapter.

INTERVENTIONS FOR NEUROLOGICAL IMPAIRMENTS

Spasticity, Spastic Paralysis

Relevant Outcomes

- Reduction of spasticity[24,74,268,310-312]
- Improved or normalized movement patterns[313]

Clinical Relevance

Spasticity is associated with cerebrovascular accidents, cerebral palsy, multiple sclerosis, traumatic brain injuries, and other neurological conditions.

Treatment Considerations

Spasticity is the result of central nervous system (CNS) damage. Although the body does not replace destroyed upper motor neurons, the nervous system is capable of neuroplasticity, which is physical change in response to stimulus and activity. Neuroplasticity is the mechanism that supports therapists' treatments for re-educating movement patterns following CNS damage. Even with diagnostic imaging, therapists cannot be certain about the extent of a client's CNS damage and cannot predict the client's capacity for regaining function. Consequently, therapists assist clients to regain and maintain as much function as possible.

The treatment of neurological conditions is complex and beyond the scope of this text. The role of massage techniques in the treatment of spasticity focuses on the modulation of **neuromuscular tone** and the treatment of secondary impairments, such as contractures, fatigue, trigger points, and altered body image. The following are examples of the secondary impairments associated with neurological conditions. Clients with multiple sclerosis may also present with fatigue, incoordination, and trigger points; clients with severe spasticity may also have contractures. Furthermore, clients with neurological conditions may also present with deficits in communication that make education and informed consent a concern. Finally, clients may have functional limitations that require guidelines for client safety.

Guidelines for Using Massage Techniques

■ The treatment described in this section is for spasticity. Consult the suggested practices described elsewhere in this chapter for the treatment of coexisting impairments.
■ Position the client so that the muscle groups you are going to treat are not stretched.[314]
■ Limbs with spastic muscles are sensitive to sudden stretch and need slow, smooth handling.
■ Begin with muscle groups with less spasticity and contracture when you are treating your client's extremities.[314,315] Begin proximally on the limb, by treating the large joints, and proceed distally, to smaller joints, as the spasticity around the proximal joints releases. Appropriate massage techniques include slow, fairly deep,[1] continuous, and rhythmic[314] effleurage, kneading,[1] and broad-contact compression.[315] Combine these techniques with slow, smooth range of motion and stretching; specific compression and friction at the origins and insertions of spastic muscles[314]; stripping; and gentle rhythmic mobilization.[9] In addition, use superficial stroking down the related axial skeleton and down the affected limb itself.
■ Apply gentle tapping to the stretched muscle groups that oppose the spastic muscles immediately prior to exercise in order to facilitate contraction and active movement.[282]
■ One author suggests limiting the treatment time to less than 30 minutes.[314]

Complementary Modalities

■ Since stress exacerbates spasticity, use a sedative approach to treatment that incorporates diaphragmatic breathing and other relaxation techniques.
■ Use slow, controlled, and prolonged active and passive stretching.[1,9] Perform stretching with a gentle pumping action, if appropriate.[314]
■ Systemic heat, to promote relaxation, and local deep moist heat, to reduce resting tension of muscle, may be useful adjuncts to treatment, provided that the client does not have multiple sclerosis.[231]

Flaccidity, Flaccid Paralysis

Relevant Outcomes

■ Maintenance of the integrity of denervated tissue
■ Prevention or reduction of complications of flaccid paralysis[316]

Clinical Relevance

Flaccid paralysis is associated with neurological conditions such as polio, postpolio syndrome, and peripheral neuropathies that result from prolonged nerve compression or nerve injury. It also occurs in cases of compression **neurapraxia** such as lumbar radiculopathy, thoracic outlet syndrome, carpal tunnel syndrome, and trigger point compression syndromes.

Treatment Considerations

Consider the following issues when you are treating flaccid paralysis. First, the location and severity of your client's lesion will dictate his level of muscle function. If your client underwent surgical repair of a peripheral nerve, his prognosis will depend on his postsurgical course and the rate of nerve regrowth. Second, if the client's tissues have been denervated for any length of time and are fragile, you will need to use light pressure during treatment.[1] Flaccid areas may also have impaired sensation and are subject to the contraindications for that impairment. Finally, your focus of treatment may be on associated impairments, such as edema, weakness, or contracture in the unopposed antagonists.[1]

Guidelines for Using Massage Techniques

■ Use the traditional approach to using massage techniques for flaccid tissue of superficial, relatively stimulating techniques, which you apply with little force and without drag on the client's tissues.[1]
■ Treat the antagonist muscles that have normal innervation with moderate-pressure neuromuscular techniques, which you perform with minimal drag on the client's denervated tissues.
■ While you are waiting for nerve regeneration, it may be more important for you to treat associated edema and contracture.[1] The sections on edema and contracture in this chapter describe relevant treatment guidelines for those impairments.
■ It may be possible to use massage techniques to reduce pressure on a nerve or nerve root that is causing or contributing to paralysis. For example, you may be able to use massage techniques to
  1. Reduce lumbar spasm that increases compression on a lumbar nerve root in a disk herniation.
  2. Decrease resting tension of the scalenes and pectoralis minor, which causes compression on a brachial plexus root in thoracic outlet syndrome.

3. Reduce edema and fascial restrictions that contribute to the compression of the median nerve in a carpal tunnel syndrome.

4. Eliminate trigger point activity that contributes to some peripheral nerve compression neurapraxias.

Complementary Modalities

- Use passive and active assistive exercise if your client lacks the strength to perform active range of motion.
- Progress to active-assisted, active, and resisted exercise as the client's motor function returns.

IN CONCLUSION

The central premise of Outcome-Based Massage™ is that, rather than applying a standard treatment regimen for a clinical condition, therapists using Outcome-Based Massage™ design treatments for each client that vary with the client's presenting impairments in body structures and functions, the **outcomes** that reflect those impairments, and the client's stated treatment goals. In the case of wellness massage, where clients present without impairments in body structures and functions, therapists are guided by the clients' wellness goals. Furthermore, throughout the treatment process, therapists using Outcome-Based Massage™ also use information on the client's impairments in body structures and functions and wellness goals to guide their decisions on massage techniques, treatment progression, **contraindications** to treatment, and special treatment considerations. An additional advantage and characteristic of Outcome-Based Massage™ is that therapists can combine interventions that treat individual impairments and wellness within a **plan of care** in order to address each client's unique clinical presentation and goals.

Practice

Note: This section contains instructions and Clinical Cases that demonstrate how to use the principles of how to apply Outcome-Based Massage™ to clinical conditions and wellness that were introduced in this chapter.

Application of Outcome-Based Massage™ to Acquired Immune Deficiency Syndrome

Clinical Case: *Late-Stage Acquired Immune Deficiency Syndrome*

Patient Profile

A 48-year-old male with late-stage **acquired immune deficiency syndrome** who has been admitted to hospice from home for **palliative care**.

Subjective Findings:

Patient reports:
- Pain and stiffness at rest and with activity
- Anxiety and depression regarding terminal condition
- Difficulty sleeping because of pain and anxiety

Objective Findings:

Impairments in Body Structures or Function

- Muscle bulk: Marked wasting of upper and lower extremity muscles
- Range of motion: Active and passive range within normal limits in upper and lower extremities (pain throughout range)
- Muscle tightness: Mild muscle tightness in upper and lower extremities
- Strength: Grade 3/5 strength in upper and lower extremities
- Exercise tolerance: General debility, complains of fatigue and pain with less than 5 minutes of activity

Activity Limitations

- Bed mobility: Requires moderate assistance of one person
- Transfers: Requires maximal assistance of one person for lying to/from sitting and sitting to/from standing and side of bed
- Self-care: Requires moderate assistance of one person for dressing and feeding
- Mood: Appears anxious and depressed
- Social interaction: Limited social interaction

Analysis:

Treatment Rationale

The aim of treatment is to provide relief of pain, stiffness, anxiety, and depression as the patient's functional level declines.

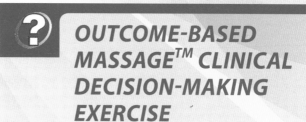

OUTCOME-BASED MASSAGE™ CLINICAL DECISION-MAKING EXERCISE

Develop a Plan of Care for the patient outlined above using the following steps in the Outcome-Based Massage™ clinical decision-making process.

1. Analyze the findings and generate the Clinical Problem List of impairments in body structure or function and activity limitations.
2. Identify the impairments in body structure or function that could respond to treatment (treatable impairments).
3. Identify which of the treatable impairments are appropriate for treatment using massage techniques.
4. Establish appropriate outcomes for each of the impairments.
5. Select one or more massage techniques to use to achieve each outcome.
6. Select other complementary techniques that you can use within treatment.

Reader: Do not turn page until you have completed the exercise!

Sample Plan of Care for Late-Stage Acquired Immune Deficiency Syndrome

Problem List:

Impairment in Body Structure or Function	Outcomes and Role of Massage
■ Pain	■ Decreased complaints of pain ■ Direct effect: pain reduction through counterirritant analgesia
■ Decreased muscle **extensibility**	■ Increased muscle extensibility ■ Direct effect: increased muscle extensibility
■ Muscle wasting	■ Decreased muscle wasting ■ Improbable effect; wasting is due to disuse
■ Muscle weakness	■ Increased muscle strength ■ Improbable effect; weakness is due primarily to disuse ■ Possible indirect effect: pain reduction may facilitate willingness to perform movement through range
■ Poor **exercise tolerance**	■ Improved exercise tolerance ■ Improbable effect; poor exercise tolerance is due primarily to disuse ■ Possible indirect effect: pain reduction may facilitate willingness to perform activities
■ Anxiety	■ Decreased anxiety ■ Direct effect: anxiety relief and systemic sedation
■ Depression	■ Improved mood ■ Indirect effect; sensory arousal may ease some symptoms of depression and lethargy
Activity Limitation	*Functional Outcomes*
■ Decreased ability to perform self-care activities	■ Able to perform feeding and dressing with assistance as required with decreased complaints of pain and stiffness ■ Indirect effect: increased function secondary to improvements in impairments
■ Decreased ability to perform transfers	■ Able to perform bed mobility and transfers with assistance as required with decreased complaints of pain and stiffness ■ Indirect effect: increased function secondary to improvements in impairments
■ Decreased social interaction	■ Increased social interaction with decreased complaints of depression ■ Indirect effect: increased function secondary to improvements in impairments
■ Impaired sleep	■ Increased duration of sleep with decreased complaints of pain and anxiety interfering with sleep ■ Indirect effect: increased function secondary to improvements in impairments

Massage Techniques:

■ Static contact, soothing superficial stroking, and manually produced fine vibration as tolerated to reduce pain and anxiety.

■ Machine-produced fine vibration, superficial effleurage, and gentle petrissage may be tolerated depending on the patient's sensitivity, level of debility, and previous familiarity with massage.

Other Complementary Techniques:

■ Passive and active assisted range of motion; assisted activities of daily living; assisted bed mobility and transfers; referral for counseling or pastoral care.

Application of Outcome-Based Massage™ to Asthma

Clinical Case: *Asthma*

Patient Profile

A 39-year-old contractor with a history of controlled asthma presents with stiffness and achiness of his neck and rib cage, especially upon waking in the morning. Though his asthma symptoms are generally minimal and under control, he recently experienced a short period of breathing difficulties, possibly due to seasonal allergies. His physician prescribed a course of steroids which he completed 10 days ago and the acute episode has resolved.

Subjective Findings:

Patient reports:
- Achiness and stiffness of the neck and rib cage
- Occasional shortness of breath with activity

Objective Findings:

Impairments in Body Structures or Function

- Range of motion: 10% decrease in lateral flexion and extension of the cervical spine with complaints of tightness at end of range
- Resting muscle tension: increased resting muscle tension in accessory muscles of respiration (sternocleidomastoid and scalenes)
- Breathing pattern: diaphragmatic breathing pattern with minimal increase in accessory muscle use
- Rib cage mobility: decreased mobility; limited movement of the rib cage and clavicles during respiration

Activity Limitations

- Self-care: occasional and minimal reduction of ability to perform self-care activities due to shortness of breath. This is relieved by a short rest.

Analysis:

Treatment Rationale

The aim of treatment is to reduce hypertonicity in muscles of respiration and to reduce adhesions and hypertonicity intended to increase rib cage mobility.

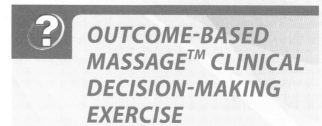

OUTCOME-BASED MASSAGE™ CLINICAL DECISION-MAKING EXERCISE

Develop a Plan of Care for the patient outlined above using the following steps in the Outcome-Based Massage™ clinical decision-making process.

1. Analyze the findings and generate the Clinical Problem List of impairments in body structures or function and activity limitations.
2. Identify the impairments in body structures or function that could respond to treatment (treatable impairments).
3. Identify which of the treatable impairments are appropriate for treatment using massage techniques.
4. Establish appropriate outcomes for each of the impairments.
5. Select one or more massage techniques to use to achieve each outcome.
6. Select other complementary techniques that you can use within treatment.

Reader: Do not turn page until you have completed the exercise!

Sample Plan of Care for Asthma

Impairment in Body Structure or Function	Outcomes and Role of Massage
■ Muscle tightness ■ Decreased cervical spine range of motion	■ Increased muscle extensibility ■ Increased cervical spine range of motion ■ Direct effect: increased muscle extensibility and increased joint mobility
■ Increased resting muscle tension	■ Decreased resting muscle tension ■ Direct effect: reduction of resting muscle tension ■ Indirect effect: general increase in relaxation and reduction of anxiety
■ Decreased rib cage mobility	■ Increased rib cage mobility ■ Direct effect: increased muscle extensibility and increased joint mobility
■ Accessory muscle use	■ Decreased accessory muscle use ■ Indirect effect: accessory muscle use reflects an increased work of breathing[3,4] that is not directly affected by the use of massage techniques. Secondary effects of increased muscle extensibility and increased relaxation
■ Dyspnea	■ Decreased dyspnea ■ Indirect effect: secondary to increased relaxation and increased airway clearance
Activity Limitation	**Functional Outcomes**
■ Shortness of breath with self-care activities	■ Able to complete activities of daily living without frequent complaints of shortness of breath ■ Indirect effect: increased function secondary to improvements in impairments

Massage Techniques:

■ Direct fascial techniques on the anterior neck/chest, inferior costal margin, along the intercostal spaces, and along the costal attachments of the diaphragm
■ Petrissage to anterior and posterior thoracic and cervical muscles
■ Stripping and lengthening of sternocleidomastoid and scalene muscles
■ Coarse vibration combined with broad-contact compression of the rib cage

■ Wringing of the rib cage

General Issues

Percussion is contraindicated for acute asthma.

Other Complementary Techniques:

■ Stretching exercises for neck muscles; diaphragmatic breathing exercises

Application of Outcome-Based Massage™ to Cystic Fibrosis

Clinical Case: *Cystic Fibrosis*

Patient Profile

A 10-year-old boy with cystic fibrosis who was admitted to an acute care setting with an acute exacerbation of cystic fibrosis. His clinical condition has responded to medical management and he is in the later stages of therapy.

Subjective Findings:

Patient reports:

- Shortness of breath at rest and during activity
- Perceived dyspnea measured using the Borg perceived exertion rating scale[56]

Objective Findings:

Impairments in Body Structures or Function

- Sputum: increased sputum production and persistent productive cough
- Airway clearance: impaired/ineffective airway clearance secondary to increased sputum production and ineffective cough and other airway clearance mechanisms
- Rib cage mobility: increased anterior–posterior diameter of the chest with decreased lateral costal and diaphragmatic expansion of the rib cage during respiration
- Respiratory pattern: sternal respiratory pattern with increased accessory muscle use and intercostal indrawing during respiration
- Breath sounds: scattered polyphonic wheezing and crackles throughout the ventilatory cycle audible during auscultation

Activity Limitations

- Ambulation tolerance 50 feet, secondary to shortness of breath
- Inability to complete activities of daily living, such as dressing tasks, without frequent rest periods secondary to shortness of breath
- Poor endurance and decreased levels of oxygen saturation during functional activity

Analysis:

Treatment Rationale

The aim of treatment is to enhance airway clearance and facilitate decreased dyspnea and increased rib cage mobility.

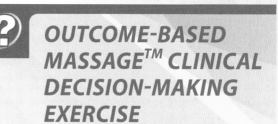

OUTCOME-BASED MASSAGE™ CLINICAL DECISION-MAKING EXERCISE

Develop a Plan of Care for the patient outlined above using the following steps in the Outcome-Based Massage™ clinical decision-making process.

1. Analyze the findings and generate the Clinical Problem List of impairments in body structures or function and activity limitations.
2. Identify the impairments in body structures or function that could respond to treatment (treatable impairments).
3. Identify which of the treatable impairments are appropriate for treatment using massage techniques.
4. Establish appropriate outcomes for each of the impairments.
5. Select one or more massage techniques to use to achieve each outcome.
6. Select other complementary techniques that you can use within treatment.

Reader: Do not turn page until you have completed the exercise!

Sample Plan of Care for Cystic Fibrosis

Problem List:

Impairment in Body Structure or Function	Outcomes and Role of Massage
■ Impaired airway clearance	■ Increased airway clearance ■ Direct effect: mobilization of sputum, especially when used with postural drainage
■ Decreased rib cage mobility	■ Increased rib cage mobility ■ Direct effect: increased muscle extensibility and increased joint mobility
■ Accessory muscle use	■ Decreased accessory muscle use ■ Indirect effect: accessory muscle use reflects an increased work of breathing[3,4] that is not directly affected by the use of massage techniques. Secondary effects of increased muscle extensibility and increased relaxation
■ Increased resting muscle tension	■ Decreased resting muscle tension ■ Direct effect: reduction of resting muscle tension ■ Indirect effect: general increase in relaxation and reduction of anxiety
■ Dyspnea	■ Decreased dyspnea ■ Indirect effect: secondary to increased relaxation and increased airway clearance
Activity Limitation	**Functional Outcomes**
■ Decreased ambulation	■ Able to ambulate 100 feet without a decrease in oxygen saturation and complaints of shortness of breath ■ Indirect effect: increased function secondary to improvements in impairments
■ Shortness of breath and decreased endurance for self-care activities	■ Able to complete self-care activities, such as dressing, without frequent complaints of shortness of breath and fatigue ■ Indirect effect: increased function secondary to improvements in impairments

Massage Techniques:

- ■ Clapping of the thorax with postural drainage (as skill level and scope of practice permit)
- ■ Rib springing
- ■ Coarse vibration combined with broad-contact compression of the rib cage
- ■ Petrissage to anterior and posterior thoracic and cervical muscles
- ■ Wringing of the rib cage
- ■ Stripping of sternocleidomastoid and scalene muscles
- ■ Direct fascial techniques on the inferior costal margin and along the intercostal spaces

Other Complementary Techniques:

- ■ Effective coughing techniques; forced expiration or audible huffing to facilitate airway clearance; diaphragmatic breathing exercises; education in energy-conservation techniques; exercise program; encourage fluid replacement; review of home postural drainage and mechanical percussion program

Application of Outcome-Based Massage™ to Lateral Epicondylitis

Clinical Case: *Lateral Epicondylitis*

Patient Profile

A 20-year-old male computer programmer with right-sided lateral epicondylitis (repetitive strain injury) secondary to keyboarding, poor posture, and poor ergonomics.

Subjective Findings:

Patient reports:

1. Pain at rest and while keyboarding
2. Inability to keyboard for greater than 10 minutes without severe pain
3. Dropping objects held in his right hand during work and self-care activities because of pain and a feeling of weakness
4. Mild swelling after work
5. Visual analog scale pain rating = 8.5
6. Lack of ergonomic modifications to work station
7. Poor knowledge of ergonomics and self-care

Objective Findings:

Impairments in Body Structures or Function

- Pain: Pain elicited on resisted right wrist and finger extension
- Grip strength: right grip weaker than left
- Palpation: Fascial shortening in area of the right common extensor origin and forearm musculature
- Posture: kyphotic, forward head posture

Activity limitations

- Work tasks: Unable to keyboard for greater than 10 minutes or perform job requirements as a computer programmer secondary to pain.
- Self-care: Compromised ability to perform self-care to pain and weakness—drops objects held in his right hand.
- Recreation: Unable to perform recreation activity of racquetball secondary to pain.

Analysis:

Treatment Rationale

The aim of treatment is to reduce the pain and inflammation associated with lateral epicondylitis and to provide education on self-care and ergonomics to prevent future exacerbations of this condition.

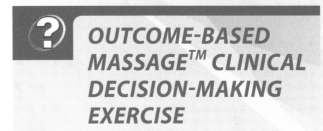

OUTCOME-BASED MASSAGE™ CLINICAL DECISION-MAKING EXERCISE

Develop a Plan of Care for the patient outlined above using the following steps in the Outcome-Based Massage™ clinical decision-making process.

1. Analyze the findings and generate the Clinical Problem List of impairments in body structure or function and activity limitations.
2. Identify the impairments in body structure or function that could respond to treatment (treatable impairments).
3. Identify which of the treatable impairments are appropriate for treatment using massage techniques.
4. Establish appropriate outcomes for each of the impairments.
5. Select one or more massage techniques to use to achieve each outcome.
6. Select other complementary techniques that you can use within treatment.

Reader: Do not turn page until you have completed the exercise!

Sample Plan of Care for Lateral Epicondylitis
Problem List:

Impairment in Body Structure or Function	Outcomes and Role of Massage
■ Pain	■ Decreased pain ■ Direct effect: pain reduction through counterirritant analgesia and decrease in inflammation
■ Inflammation	■ Decreased inflammation ■ Direct effect: reduction of inflammation
■ Fascial shortening	■ Normalized fascial extensibility ■ Direct effect: fascial lengthening
■ Postural malalignment	■ Normalized postural alignment ■ Direct effect: improved posture secondary to fascial lengthening
■ Decreased strength	■ Increased strength ■ Indirect effect: increased strength secondary to reduction in pain and inflammation
Activity Limitation	**Functional Outcomes**
■ Decreased ability to keyboard	■ Able to keyboard with the use of ergonomic modifications for 1 hour with appropriate stretching and rest periods without complaints of pain ■ Indirect effect: increased function secondary to improvements in impairments
■ Decreased ability to perform household tasks	■ Able to carry 10 lb weight in his right hand for 25 feet without complaints of pain or dropping the weight ■ Indirect effect: increased function secondary to improvements in impairments
■ Decreased ability to perform athletic tasks	■ Able to play racquetball for 20 minutes following appropriate warm up without complaints of pain ■ Indirect effect: increased function secondary to improvements in impairments

Massage Techniques:
■ Petrissage, myofascial technique, direct fascial technique applied to shortened muscles related to kyphosis and forward head posture.
■ Superficial effleurage, petrissage, myofascial release, and direct fascial technique applied to the entire forearm, especially muscles of the extensor compartment.
■ Friction to the common extensor origin.
■ Some work on the contralateral arm may be required to maintain right–left balance.
■ Some work on the flexors of the affected arm may be required to maintain antagonist balance.

Other Complementary Techniques:
■ Ice post-friction if signs of overtreatment are present; wrist and hand stretches; wrist and hand strengthening exercises; postural stretches; postural education; ergonomic examination; education in ergonomics; and self-care.

Application of Outcome-Based Massage™ to Low Back Pain

Clinical Case: *Low Back Pain*

Patient Profile

A 65-year-old male professional writer who has a long history of chronic low back pain. The more recent acute episode of low back pain has resolved but he is now experiencing tightness and discomfort in his low back muscles during long periods of sitting.

Subjective Findings:

Patient reports:

- Tight muscles and generalized achiness in his low back.
- Discomfort is a distraction and he wants to be able to sit long enough to finish his novel.
- Acute episode of low back pain has improved and referrals into buttocks and left leg have ceased.

Objective Findings:

Impairments in Body Structures or Function

- Posture: hyperlordotic
- Resting muscle tension: increased resting muscle tension in quadratus lumborum, gluteals, piriformis, lumbar erector spinae, rectus femoris, psoas, iliacus, and tensor fascia latae
- Range of motion: lumbar range of motion within normal limits. Patient reports feeling of tightness at end of range for lumbar flexion
- Trigger points: trigger points in lumbar quadratus lumborum, gluteals, and piriformis

Activity Limitations

- Unable to sit for greater than 30 minutes without discomfort. Pain is distracting and he needs to be able to focus on writing to meet a deadline.

Analysis:

Treatment Rationale

The aim of treatment is to reduce muscle tightness and discomfort in low back during sitting so that patient can work without distraction.

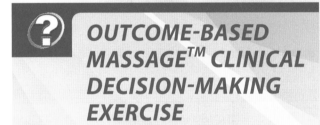

OUTCOME-BASED MASSAGE™ CLINICAL DECISION-MAKING EXERCISE

Develop a Plan of Care for the patient outlined above using the following steps in the Outcome-Based Massage™ clinical decision-making process.

1. Analyze the findings and generate the Clinical Problem List of impairments in body structures or function and activity limitations.
2. Identify the impairments in body structures or function that could respond to treatment (treatable impairments).
3. Identify which of the treatable impairments are appropriate for treatment using massage techniques.
4. Establish appropriate outcomes for each of the impairments.
5. Select one or more massage techniques to use to achieve each outcome.
6. Select other complementary techniques that you can use within treatment.

Reader: Do not turn page until you have completed the exercise!

Sample Plan of Care for Low Back Pain

Problem List:

Impairment in Body Structure or Function	Outcomes and Role of Massage
■ Hyperlordosis	■ Lengthen shortened hip flexor, lumbar erector spinae, and gluteal muscles to facilitate decreased lordosis ■ Direct effect: increased muscle extensibility
■ Increased resting muscle tension	■ Decreased resting muscle tension ■ Direct effect: decreased resting muscle tension
■ Muscle tightness	■ Increased muscle extensibility ■ Direct effect: increased muscle extensibility
■ Trigger points	■ Alleviated trigger points in lumbar erector spinae, gluteals, piriformis, rectus femoris, tensor fasciae latae, and iliopsoas ■ Direct effect: deactivate trigger points
■ Less than optimal ease of movement	■ Less than optimal ease of movement ■ Indirect effect: rhythmic mobilization facilitates neuromuscular patterning
Activity Limitation	*Functional Outcomes*
■ Unable to sit for greater than 30 minutes due to pain	■ Able to sit and write for greater than 30 minutes without discomfort ■ Indirect effect: increased function secondary to improvements in impairments

Massage Techniques:

- Superficial effleurage and petrissage to the lumbar, anterior thigh, and gluteal regions
- Lengthening strokes to tight/shortened muscles associated with hyperlordosis including rectus femoris, quadratus lumborum, tensor fasciae latae, and lumbar erector spinae
- Direct fascial technique to thoracolumbar fascia
- Trigger point pressure release to alleviate trigger points followed by cross-fiber strokes and passive stretching for muscles with trigger points
- Rhythmic mobilization within pain tolerance to reduce muscle tone and restore neuromuscular function
- Consider treatment of iliopsoas if skill level and scope of practice permit

Other Complementary Techniques:

- Low back, rectus femoris, and psoas stretching; heat; education on sitting posture; and relaxation (visualization or progressive muscle relaxation)

Application of Outcome-Based Massage™ to Lymphedema

Clinical Case: *Lymphedema*

Patient Profile

A 45-year-old female with breast cancer in remission presents 1 month after mastectomy with chronic lymphedema of the right arm and hand. She has had 50% of her axillary lymph nodes and some breast tissue removed and has had no radiation.

Subjective Findings:

Patient reports:

- Right-handed pain and swelling that interferes with function
- Feeling self-conscious about appearance of her arm

Objective Findings:

Impairments in Body Structure or Function

- Edema: gross edema, pitting from shoulder to fingers; girth recorded
- Limb volume: right greater than left; measured with volumetric analysis
- Strength: grade 3—for shoulder, elbow, and wrist movements on right
- Range of motion:
  - Right shoulder: flexion = 85°, extension = 5°, abduction = 70°, adduction = 10°, external rotation = 30°, internal rotation = 5°
  - Right elbow: flexion = 95°, extension = neutral, pronation = 45°, supination = 30°
  - Right wrist: flexion = 25°, extension = 35°, radial deviation = 5°, ulnar deviation = 10°
  - Right hand metacarpophalangeals: flexion = 45°, extension = neutral; interphalangeals: flexion = 50°, extension = neutral

Activity Limitations

- Unable to comb hair with right arm
- Difficulty dressing and performing self-care
- Unable to reach object placed above shoulder level
- Unable to carry objects in right hand

Analysis:

Treatment Rationale

The aim of treatment is to reduce the patient's edema and address the secondary weakness, pain, distorted body image, and activity limitations.

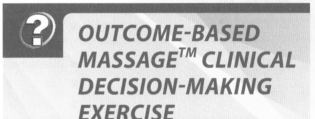

OUTCOME-BASED MASSAGE™ CLINICAL DECISION-MAKING EXERCISE

Develop a Plan of Care for the patient outlined above using the following steps in the Outcome-Based Massage™ clinical decision-making process.

1. Analyze the findings and generate the Clinical Problem List of impairments in body structure or function and activity limitations.
2. Identify the impairments in body structure or function that could respond to treatment (treatable impairments).
3. Identify which of the treatable impairments are appropriate for treatment using massage techniques.
4. Establish appropriate outcomes for each of the impairments.
5. Select one or more massage techniques to use to achieve each outcome.
6. Select other complementary techniques that you can use within treatment.

 Reader: Do not turn page until you have completed the exercise!

Sample Plan of Care for Lymphedema
Problem List:

Impairment in Body Structure or Function	Outcomes and Role of Massage
■ Edema (impaired lymph drainage)	■ Decreased edema ■ Direct effect: increased lymphatic drainage
■ Range of motion	■ Increased range of motion to within normal limits ■ Direct effect (range is limited by edema): increased lymphatic drainage, increased joint mobility
■ Strength	■ Increased strength to grade 5/5 throughout ■ Possible indirect effect; weakness is primarily due to disuse; decreased edema may facilitate strengthening and will provide increased range for strengthening
■ Altered body image	■ Improved body image ■ Possible direct effect: enhanced body image ■ Indirect effect: secondary to reduced edema since gross edema contributes to altered image
Activity Limitation	Functional Outcomes
■ Decreased ability to perform self-care activities	■ Able to carry a 10-lb object in her right hand while ambulating 100 feet ■ Able to perform self-care activities (dressing, bathing, and toileting) without adaptive equipment ■ Able to reach object placed 3 feet above head with her right hand ■ Able to lift 1-lb object from overhead shelf with her right hand ■ Indirect effect: increased function secondary to improvements in impairments
■ Decreased social interaction	■ Increased social interaction with fewer complaints of self-consciousness regarding the appearance of her arm ■ Indirect effect: increased function secondary to improvements in impairments

Massage Techniques:
■ Superficial effleurage, briefly, and then superficial lymph drainage technique. These are applied in sequence each session, thoroughly to the contralateral quadrant first (including intercostal and sternal areas) and then to proximal areas of the affected quadrant, especially to axillary, intercostal, and parasternal areas. The clinician gradually works more distally into the patient's arm and then alternates back and forth between proximal and distal segments.

■ At the outset of each intervention, repetitive broad-contact compression delivered over the junctions of the right lymphatic and thoracic ducts with the vena cava may also be useful.

Other Complementary Techniques:
■ Bandaging or pressure garments, skin hygiene, range-of-motion exercises, functional activity, strengthening exercises, and adaptive equipment for short-term use.

Application of Outcome-Based Massage™ to Pregnancy

Clinical Case: *Pregnancy*

Patient Profile

A 35-year-old woman with a high-risk pregnancy who has been hospitalized at 28 weeks of gestation for evaluation and modification of pharmacologic management of premature onset of labor. Prior to hospitalization, she was bed bound for 6 weeks. Medication: terbutaline (β-adrenergic stimulant).

Subjective Findings:

Patient reports:
1. Muscle and joint achiness
2. Generalized weakness
3. Stress related to the high-risk pregnancy, rating of perceived stress using a visual analog scale: 8/10
4. Reported stress-related symptoms: altered sleep patterns; headaches and muscle tension in shoulder, neck, and back muscles; anxiety about the pregnancy; and depression

Objective Findings:

Impairments in Body Structures or Function

- Fetal monitor in situ.
- Range of motion: Within normal limits for neck and upper and lower extremity range of motion. Complaints of achiness during range of motion.
- Strength: Unable to assess formally; resisted movement is contraindicated. Risk of ongoing decrease in strength because of restricted activity level.
- Resting muscle tension: Increased level of resting muscle tension in neck, shoulder, and erector spinae muscles.

Activity Limitations

- Bed mobility: Performed rolling side-to-side and scooting independently with use of monkey bar. Complaints of achiness and weakness
- Transfers: Performed lying-to-sit, sit-to-stand, stand-to-toilet, and toilet-to-stand with contact guard assistance secondary to complaints of weakness and achiness
- Ambulation: 10 feet with minimal assistance of one person secondary to poor balance and complaints of weakness

Analysis:

Treatment Rationale

The aim of treatment is to (a) prevent further deterioration of health status and functional level because of inactivity and (b) reduce

stress-related symptoms as a means of increasing the patient's comfort level and facilitating maternal and fetal well-being.

- Precautions: Maternal and fetal monitors.
- Activity restrictions: Valsalva maneuver, resisted movements, and abdominal exercises are contraindicated. Ensure adequate hydration during treatment and encourage frequent emptying of the bladder.
- Side effects of β-adrenergic medication: Maternal and fetal tachycardia and hypotension.

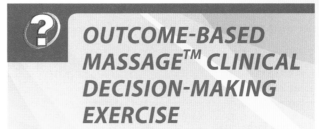

OUTCOME-BASED MASSAGE™ CLINICAL DECISION-MAKING EXERCISE

Develop a Plan of Care for the patient outlined above using the following steps in the Outcome-Based Massage™ clinical decision-making process.

1. Analyze the findings and generate the Clinical Problem List of impairments in body structure or function and activity limitations.
2. Identify the impairments in body structure or function that could respond to treatment (treatable impairments).
3. Identify which of the treatable impairments are appropriate for treatment using massage techniques.
4. Establish appropriate outcomes for each of the impairments.
5. Select one or more massage techniques to use to achieve each outcome.
6. Select other complementary techniques that you can use within treatment.

Reader: Do not turn page until you have completed the exercise!

Sample Plan of Care for Pregnancy

Problem List:

Impairment in Body Structure or Function	Outcomes and Role of Massage
■ Anxiety	■ Decreased anxiety ■ Direct effect: reduction of perceived anxiety
■ Perceived stress and stress-related symptoms	■ Decreased stress-related symptoms ■ Direct and indirect effect: increased relaxation
■ Increased resting muscle tension	■ Decreased resting muscle tension ■ Direct effect: reduction of resting muscle tension ■ Indirect effect: general increase in relaxation and reduction of anxiety
■ Muscle and joint pain ("achiness")	■ Decreased muscle and joint pain ("achiness") ■ Direct effect: pain reduction through counterirritant analgesia and sedation
■ Fatigue	■ Decreased fatigue ■ Possible indirect effect: secondary to increased sensory arousal
■ Muscle weakness	■ Increased muscle strength ■ No effect
Activity Limitation	**Functional Outcomes**
■ Decreased ability to transfers and bed mobility	■ Able to perform bed mobility independently with use of monkey bar ■ Able to perform transfers with contact guard assistance ■ Indirect effect: increased function secondary to improvements in impairments
■ Decreased ambulation	■ Maintain ability to ambulate 10 feet to bathroom with minimal assistance of one person ■ Indirect effect: increased function secondary to improvements in impairments

Massage Techniques:

■ Gentle superficial effleurage and broad-contact petrissage in a rhythmic and soothing manner to the limbs, back, and shoulders for the specific aim of producing and sustaining sedation during the course of the massage.

■ Rhythmic and gentle specific petrissage to the patient's hands, feet, and face.

■ More specific neuromuscular techniques, such as stripping and specific compression, in areas of increased resting muscle tension.

■ Precede or follow massage techniques with diaphragmatic breathing and gentle passive stretches of the muscles.

■ Instruct patient on how to apply static contact and superficial stroking to her own abdomen.

General Issues

■ Work in close consultation with the attending physician throughout treatment to understand all cautions and contraindications. Limit depth of application of techniques to the most superficial muscle layer and avoid passive movement techniques such as rocking.

Other Complementary Techniques:

■ Relaxing music, relaxation training (guided imagery and meditation); stress management instruction; stretching exercises and gentle, active range of motion exercise in lying; ankle pumping; breathing training; referral for counseling.

Application of Outcome-Based Massage™ to Shin Splints (Tibial Stress Syndrome)

Clinical Case: *Shin Splints (Tibial Stress Syndrome)*

Patient Profile

A 60-year-old woman who has had neuromuscular massage therapy sessions due to mild-to-moderate chronic pain in her back, shoulders, and neck with good success. She returned to her clinician with shin and foot pain after a 3-week vacation during which she did extensive walking.

Subjective Findings:

Patient reports:

- Dull aching pain in the front of her lower legs along her shin bones and feelings of weakness, especially when coming downstairs
- Achiness on the top of both feet

Objective Findings:

Impairments in Body Structures or Function

- Ambulation: slow, antalgic gait
- Range of motion: within normal limits for the ankle and knee, but patient complains of feeling of tightness during movement
- Resisted movement: pain on (a) resisted ankle dorsiflexion and eversion and (b) toe extension bilaterally
- Strength: grade 4 ankle dorsiflexors and toe extensors secondary to pain
- Pain: pain on palpation along the lateral border of the tibia bilaterally and the dorsum of the foot
- Resting muscle tension: increased bilaterally at the tibialis anterior and extensor digitorum muscles
- Trigger points: active trigger points in tibialis anterior muscles

Activity Limitations

- Needs to hold handrail for support when coming downstairs secondary to pain
- Needs to use arm rests of chairs to rise from a chair
- Difficulty walking for greater than 30 feet secondary to pain

Analysis:

Treatment Rationale

The aim of treatment is to reduce pain, decrease resting muscle tension, and alleviate trigger points that are contributing to shin and foot pain.

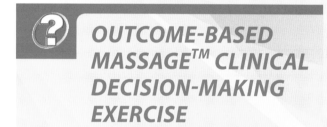

OUTCOME-BASED MASSAGE™ CLINICAL DECISION-MAKING EXERCISE

Develop a Plan of Care for the patient outlined above using the following steps in the Outcome-Based Massage™ clinical decision-making process.

1. Analyze the findings and generate the Clinical Problem List of body structures or functions related to client's wellness goals.
2. Identify the body structures or functions that could respond to treatment.
3. Identify which of the body structures and functions and wellness goals are appropriate for treatment using massage techniques.
4. Establish appropriate outcomes for each of the wellness goals.
5. Select one or more massage techniques to use to achieve each outcome.
6. Select other complementary techniques that you can use within treatment.

Reader: Do not turn page until you have completed the exercise!

Sample Plan of Care for Shin Splints (Tibial Stress Syndrome)

Problem List:

Impairment in Body Structure or Function	Outcomes and Role of Massage
■ Antalgic gait	■ Normalize gait ■ Indirect effect: improvements in gait secondary to reduction of pain and muscle tightness
■ Tight muscles	■ Increase muscle extensibility ■ Direct effect: increase extensibility of muscles
■ Decreased strength	■ Increased strength ■ Indirect effect: improvement in strength secondary to pain reduction
■ Pain	■ Decreased pain on palpation and with activity ■ Direct effect: pain reduction and deactivation of trigger points in the anterior and lateral leg compartments
■ Increased resting muscle tension	■ Normalized resting muscle tension ■ Direct effect: reduction of resting muscle tension
Activity Limitation	*Functional Outcomes*
■ Needs to hold handrail for support when coming down stairs secondary to pain	■ Ability to ascend and descend stairs without the need of additional support ■ Indirect effect: increased function secondary to improvements in impairments
■ Needs to use arm rests of chairs to rise from a chair	■ Ability to sit and rise from chair without additional support ■ Indirect effect: increased function secondary to improvements in impairments
■ Difficulty walking for greater than 30 feet secondary to pain	■ Ability to walk distances required to participate in her usual self-care and recreational activities ■ Indirect effect: increased function secondary to improvements in impairments

Massage Techniques:

- Superficial effleurage and petrissage to help sooth muscles in general at the hips, thighs, and legs, beginning in prone and proceeding in supine.
- Muscle stripping to the tibialis anterior, extensor digitorum longus, peroneus longus, and peroneus brevis beginning superficially and ending deep.
- Deep transverse friction is provided to the same areas along with the retinaculum of the ankles and the tendons of the muscles involved.

- Trigger point pressure release to alleviate trigger points followed by cross-fiber strokes and passive stretching for muscles with trigger points.
- Passive stretching for low leg and foot muscles.

Other Complementary Techniques:

- Ice, hydrotherapy, orthotics (custom or over-the-counter), range of motion and stretching exercises, tensor bandage or neoprene sleeve.

Application of Outcome-Based Massage™ to Sports

Clinical Case: *Precompetition Sports*

Patient Profile
A 25-year-old female professional pentathlete at competition, prior to the javelin throw.

Subjective Findings:
Patient reports:
- No complaints
- Wants to be physically and mentally prepared to perform optimally during the event

Objective Findings:
Impairments in Body Structures or Function
- Possibility of muscle strain of upper extremity and trunk muscles during propulsive motion
- Less than optimal tissue extensibility of upper extremity and trunk muscles
- Coordination may be less than optimal for peak performance
- Less than optimal ease of movement through range for peak performance in the javelin throw

Activity Limitations
- Not sufficiently prepared physically and mentally to give peak athletic performance during the competitive javelin event without risking an injury

Analysis:
Treatment Rationale
The aim of treatment is to assist the athlete with physical and preparation for peak performance during a competitive event.

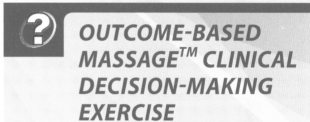

OUTCOME-BASED MASSAGE™ CLINICAL DECISION-MAKING EXERCISE

Develop a Plan of Care for the patient outlined above using the following steps in the Outcome-Based Massage™ clinical decision-making process.

1. Analyze the findings and generate the Clinical Problem List of impairments in body structures or function and activity limitations.
2. Identify the impairments in body structures or function that could respond to treatment (treatable impairments).
3. Identify which of the treatable impairments are appropriate for treatment using massage techniques.
4. Establish appropriate outcomes for each of the impairments.
5. Select one or more massage techniques to use to achieve each outcome.
6. Select other complementary techniques that you can use within treatment.

Reader: Do not turn page until you have completed the exercise!

Sample Plan of Care for Precompetition Sports Massage
Problem List:

Impairment in Body Structure or Function	Outcomes and Role of Massage
■ Risk of muscle tear	■ Decreased risk of muscle tear ■ Direct effect: decreased tissue viscosity and decreased resting muscle tension
■ Less than optimal tissue extensibility	■ Optimized tissue extensibility ■ Direct effect: increased tissue extensibility
■ Less than optimal coordination	■ Enhanced coordination ■ Indirect effect: rhythmic mobilization facilitates neuromuscular patterning
■ Less than optimal ease of movement	■ Enhanced optimal ease of movement ■ Indirect effect: increased tissue extensibility will facilitate ease of movement
■ Less than optimal mental arousal	■ Enhanced mental arousal ■ Direct effect: increased arousal second ary to the faster movement techniques
Activity Limitation	*Functional Outcomes*
■ Less than optimal athletic performance	■ Enhanced athletic performance during the javelin event with decreased risk of injury ■ Indirect effect: increased function secondary to improvements in impairments

Massage Techniques:
■ Rhythmic mobilization and fast shaking interspersed with repetitive, broad-contact compression and fast petrissage.

Other Complementary Techniques:
■ Stretching, passive range of motion, and visualization of her performance.

Application of Outcome-Based Massage™ for Wellness

Clinical Case: *Wellness*

History of Present Illness

An active 35-year-old man who is in good health. As a result of his concerns about his relatively sedentary lifestyle as a bus driver, he recently started a fitness program and improved his diet. He would like to include massage in his overall wellness regimen. His medical history is unremarkable.

Subjective Findings:

Patient reports:
- He hopes that massage will help him feel more relaxed, yet energized
- Would like muscles to feel looser and to be more aware of his posture as a way of maintaining good posture since he sits a lot at work
- Would like to learn how to massage his own neck and shoulder muscles

Objective Findings:

Status of Body Structure or Function

- Resting muscle tension: within normal limits
- Posture: no postural malalignment noted
- Range of motion: full and pain-free active range of motion in upper and lower extremity joints, neck, and back

Activity Limitations

- None reported
- Self-care and recreation: Able to participate fully in social roles and activities of daily living

Analysis:

Treatment Rationale

The aim of treatment is to increase the patient's well-being and relaxation and to optimize his postural awareness.

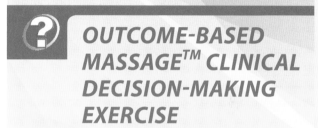

OUTCOME-BASED MASSAGE™ CLINICAL DECISION-MAKING EXERCISE

Develop a Plan of Care for the patient outlined above using the following steps in the Outcome-Based Massage™ clinical decision-making process.

1. Analyze the findings and generate the Clinical Problem List of body structures or functions related to the client's wellness goals.
2. Identify the body structures or functions that could respond to treatment.
3. Identify which of the body structures or functions are appropriate for treatment using massage techniques.
4. Establish appropriate outcomes for each of the wellness goals.
5. Select one or more massage techniques to use to achieve each outcome.
6. Select other complementary techniques that you can use within treatment.

Reader: Do not turn page until you have completed the exercise!

Sample Plan of Care for Wellness
Wellness Outcomes:

Wellness Goal	Outcomes and Role of Massage
■ Increased relaxation	■ Increased relaxation ■ Decreased levels of cortisol, epinephrine, and norepinephrine ■ Direct effect: increased relaxation ■ Potential, though not proven, effect: decreased levels of cortisol, epinephrine, and norepinephrine
■ Decreased resting muscle tension	■ Decreased resting muscle tension ■ Direct effect: reduction of level of resting muscle tension ■ Indirect effect: general increase in relaxation
■ Improved postural awareness	■ Increased postural awareness ■ Optimized tissue extensibility ■ Optimized postural alignment ■ Direct effect: fascial lengthening ■ Direct effect: increased tissue extensibility
■ Increased well-being	■ Increased well-being ■ Indirect effect: increased relaxation, decreased resting muscle tension, and increased tissue extensibility and postural awareness
Activity Limitation	*Functional Outcomes*
■ Enhanced quality of life	■ Enhanced quality of life and participation in social roles ■ Indirect effect: increased function secondary to improvements in impairments

Massage Techniques:
- Rhythmic gentle rocking to the whole body
- Gentle superficial effleurage and broad-contact petrissage to the limbs, back, and shoulders
- Rhythmic and gentle specific petrissage to the patient's hands, feet, and face
- Specific compression for the neck, shoulder, and low back muscles
- Gentle passive stretches of the muscle groups being massaged

Other Complementary Techniques:
- Relaxing music during treatment; relaxation training (progressive muscle relaxation, guided imagery, and meditation); breathing training; movement therapy; self-massage of neck and shoulder muscles; stretching exercises.

SECTION REVIEW

TAKEAWAYS

1. Outcome-Based Massage™ suggests that clinicians recognize that patients with clinical conditions present with related impairments in body structures and functions, secondary to pathophysiology, that clinicians must assess and treat.

2. Clinicians using Outcome-Based Massage™ design treatments for each patient that vary with the patient's presenting impairments in body structures and functions, the outcomes that reflect those impairments, and the patient's stated treatment goals.

3. In the case of wellness massage, where patients present without impairments in body structures and functions, clinicians are guided by the patients' wellness goals.

4. Throughout the treatment process, clinicians using Outcome-Based Massage™ also use information on the patient's impairments in body structures and functions and wellness goals to guide their decisions on massage techniques, treatment progression, contraindications to treatment, and special treatment considerations.

5. Clinicians typically have to address multiple impairments or wellness goals within a single intervention. In doing so, they must combine interventions for different impairments, wellness goals, and body structures into a single plan of care.

6. Clinicians need to consider the contraindications and cautions to treatment for each impairment, wellness goal, and massage technique. They may have to exclude some techniques from the intervention entirely or modify how you apply them locally based on these contraindications and cautions.

7. The relative priority of impairments or wellness goals will guide your choice and progression of techniques. Give priority to impairments that are more severe (greater grade) and that cause other impairments. In addition, consider the patient's priorities for care.

8. The treatment of a patient's clinical condition progresses through stages that reflect the clinical course and prognosis of that condition and patient.

9. The appropriate number of interventions using massage techniques will also vary with other factors, including the cause, severity, acuity, and complexity of the patient's clinical condition; the use of complementary modalities; and the patient's overall health status and age. For this reason, clinicians should try to avoid using a standard plan of care for all patients with a given clinical condition.

10. The development of interventions that include or focus on wellness-related outcomes follows a similar process to that for clinical conditions. Prior to embarking on a wellness intervention, it is very important that clinicians first identify any impairments in body structures and functions that are present.

Critical Thinking Questions

1. How does the process of developing interventions to address impairments in body structures and function (medical massage) differ from the process for developing interventions to address wellness goals? How are they similar?

2. Describe the guidelines that you would use when you have conflicting cautions and contraindications for your patient's presenting clinical conditions and the massage techniques that you intend you use.

3. Outline the thought process and guidelines that you would use to prioritize treatment outcomes when you and your patient have multiple outcomes for the massage intervention.

4. What strategies and information would you use to guide your progression of the intervention for a patient with a clinical condition?

5. How does treatment differ for early and later stages of the general adaptation syndrome?

6. What are the similarities and differences between your outcomes and treatment approaches for acute nociceptive pain and chronic pain syndrome?

7. You are using superficial fluid techniques to increase fluid return. In which direction would you orient your strokes: proximal to distal or distal to proximal? Would your pressure be centripetal or centrifugal? Explain your answers.

8. What are the similarities and differences between unnecessary resting tension and elevated resting tension? How would your treatment approaches for these two impairments differ?

9. In interventions that address postural conditions, why treat shortened areas earlier in the intervention?

10. What are the similarities and differences between your treatment approach for acute-stage inflammation and chronic-stage inflammation?

References for Chapter 14 begin on p. 481.

Quick Treatment Guide for Adhesive Capsulitis (Frozen Shoulder Syndrome)

Description

Progressive pain and decreased range of motion of the glenohumeral joint that is associated with inflammation, thickening, and shortening of the glenohumeral joint capsule.[318-321] The etiology of adhesive capsulitis is unclear and the condition often resolves within 2 years.

Relevant Anatomy

Glenohumeral joint, acromioclavicular joint, joint capsule, coracohumeral ligament

Relevant Examination Techniques, Impairments, and Activity Limitations

Examination Techniques	Impairments in Body Structure or Function
■ Pain visual analog scale	■ Pain
■ Palpation	■ Pain
	■ Increased resting muscle tension
	■ Adhesions
■ Postural examination	■ Postural malalignment
■ Selective tissue tension testing	■ Impaired muscle integrity
■ Shoulder muscle strength testing	■ Impaired muscle performance
■ Shoulder passive accessory motion testing	■ Impaired joint mobility and joint integrity
■ Shoulder range of motion measurements	■ Impaired joint mobility
	■ Impaired muscle extensibility

Examination Techniques	Activity Limitations
■ Functional examination	■ Limitations in overhead and behind the back work, recreational, and self-care activities

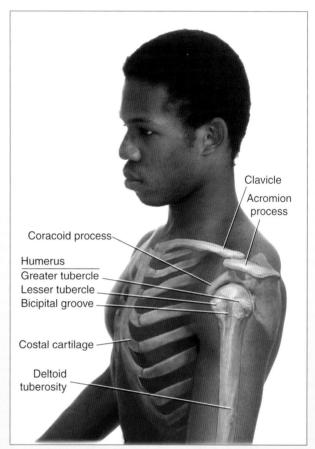

FIGURE 14-1 Anatomy of the shoulder. Reprinted from Clay JH, Pounds DM. *Basic Clinical Massage Therapy: Integrating Anatomy and Treatment.* 2nd ed. Philadelphia, PA: Lippincott Williams & Wilkins; 2008.

Labels: Coracoid process, Humerus, Greater tubercle, Lesser tubercle, Bicipital groove, Costal cartilage, Deltoid tuberosity, Clavicle, Acromion process

Relevant Outcomes and Massage Techniques

- Decreased pain: superficial effleurage, myofascial release, direct fascial technique, shaking, rhythmic mobilization
- Decreased resting muscle tension (primary and compensatory): effleurage, petrissage, stripping, specific compression, myofascial release, direct fascial technique, rhythmic mobilization, rocking, shaking
- Increased joint mobility and normalized posture: direct fascial techniques, friction, myofascial release, rhythmic mobilization, rocking
- Normalized joint and muscle integrity; decreased adhesions; increased muscle extensibility: cross fiber and longitudinal strokes, petrissage, stripping, specific compression, direct fascial techniques, friction, myofascial release
- Increased muscle performance: rhythmic mobilization, rocking, percussive techniques

Note: See Quick Treatment Guide for Rotator Cuff Strain

Relevant Complementary Techniques

Hydrotherapy, muscle energy techniques, pendular exercises

Contraindications and Precautions

Be cautious of vessels and nerves in the axilla. Do range of motion techniques only within the client's comfortable range of motion.

Helpful Hints

Trigger points in any muscle that crosses the glenohumeral joint may be a contributory factor.

Quick Treatment Guide for Ankle Sprain (Lateral)

Description

Stretching or tearing of the ligamentous structures of the lateral ankle resulting in pain, inflammation, and loss of function that is often caused by quick or extreme supination.[318-321] It has similar characteristics to a strain, but the pain and edema subside more slowly.

Relevant Anatomy

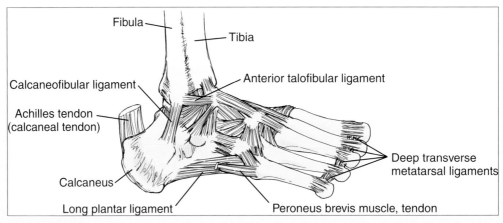

FIGURE 14-2 Anatomy of lateral ankle ligaments. Reprinted from Hendrickson T. *Massage for Orthopedic Conditions.* 2nd ed. Baltimore, MD: Lippincott Williams & Wilkins; 2009.

Relevant Examination Techniques, Impairments, and Activity Limitations

Examination Techniques	Impairments in Body Structure or Function
■ Ankle and lower leg girth measurement	■ Edema
■ Ankle ligament stability tests	■ Impaired ligament stability
	■ Impaired joint integrity
■ Ankle range of motion measurement	■ Impaired joint mobility
■ Foot and ankle muscle strength testing	■ Impaired muscle performance
■ Gait analysis	■ Gait dysfunction
■ Pain visual analog scale	■ Pain
■ Palpation	■ Pain
	■ Edema
	■ Increased resting muscle tension

Examination Techniques	Activity Limitations
■ Functional examination	■ Limitations in weight-bearing work, recreational, and self-care activities

Relevant Outcomes and Massage Techniques

■ Decreased edema: superficial effleurage, superficial lymph drainage techniques, broad-contact compression, petrissage

■ Normalized joint integrity: cross fiber friction and longitudinal strokes for ankle ligaments, petrissage, stripping, specific compression, direct fascial techniques, myofascial release

■ Increased joint mobility: direct fascial techniques, friction, myofascial release, rhythmic mobilization, rocking

■ Decreased resting muscle tension (primary and compensatory); normalized neuromuscular tone: effleurage, petrissage, stripping, specific compression, myofascial release, direct fascial technique, rhythmic mobilization, rocking, shaking

■ Increased muscle performance: rhythmic mobilization, rocking, percussive techniques

■ Decreased pain: superficial effleurage, myofascial release, direct fascial technique, shaking, rhythmic mobilization

Relevant Complementary Techniques

■ Hydrotherapy, muscle energy techniques, ankle stretching and strengthening exercises

Contraindications and Precautions

■ Be cautious when treating a third degree sprain in the acute stage

Helpful Hints

■ Tissues surrounding the injured ligament and the affected area may develop compensatory patterns including hypertonicity, trigger points, and joint dysfunction.

 Andrade, *Outcome-Based Massage*™ Quick Treatment Guides © 2014 Lippincott Williams & Wilkins

Quick Treatment Guide for Hamstring Strain

Description

Stretching or tearing of the hamstring muscles resulting in pain, inflammation, and loss of function.[318-321] Hamstring strains are a common sports injury.

Relevant Anatomy

Semimembranosus, semitendinosus, biceps femoris

Relevant Examination Techniques, Impairments, and Activity Limitations

Examination Techniques	Impairments in Body Structure or Function
■ Gait analysis	■ Gait dysfunction
■ Hip and knee joint range of motion measurement	■ Impaired joint mobility
	■ Impaired joint integrity
■ Hip and knee muscle extensibility testing	■ Impaired muscle extensibility
■ Hip and knee muscle strength testing	■ Impaired muscle performance
■ Pain visual analog scale	■ Pain
■ Palpation	■ Pain
	■ Increased resting muscle tension
■ Selective tissue tension testing	■ Impaired muscle integrity

Examination Techniques	Activity Limitations
■ Functional examination	■ Limitations in weight-bearing work, recreational, and self-care activities

FIGURE 14-3 Anatomy of the hamstrings. Reprinted from Clay JH, Pounds DM. *Basic Clinical Massage Therapy: Integrating Anatomy and Treatment.* 2nd ed. Philadelphia, PA: Lippincott Williams & Wilkins; 2008.

Relevant Outcomes and Massage Techniques

- Increased joint mobility: direct fascial techniques, friction, myofascial release, rhythmic mobilization, rocking
- Increased muscle performance: rhythmic mobilization, rocking, percussive techniques
- Decreased pain: superficial effleurage, myofascial release, direct fascial technique, shaking, rhythmic mobilization
- Decreased resting muscle tension (primary and compensatory); normalized neuromuscular tone: effleurage, petrissage, stripping, specific compression, myofascial release, direct fascial technique, rhythmic mobilization, rocking, shaking
- Normalized muscle and joint integrity; increased muscle extensibility: cross fiber and longitudinal strokes, petrissage, stripping, specific compression, direct fascial techniques, friction, myofascial release

Relevant Complementary Techniques

- Hydrotherapy, stretching and strengthening exercises

Contraindications and Precautions

- Be cautious when treating a severe strain in the acute stage
- Be cautious when treating a new injury. Do not work deeply if fresh bruises are present or if torn tissues have not yet developed scar tissue

Helpful Hints

- Quick or strong eccentric contraction of taut or weakened hamstrings may contribute to strain.
- Shortened, hypertonic hip flexors or hyperlordosis may be a contributing factor

Quick Treatment Guide for Iliotibial Band (ITB) Tightness

Description

Tightness and inflammation of the fibrous ITB that may result from biomechanical abnormalities, unbalanced repetitive exercise, or injury.[318-321] It may contribute to ITB syndrome with its associated lateral knee or hip pain.

Relevant Anatomy

ITB, tensor fasciae latae, lateral tibial condyle, rectus femoris, gluteus maximus, biceps femoris

Relevant Examination Techniques, Impairments, and Activity Limitations

Examination Techniques	Impairments in Body Structure or Function
■ Gait analysis	■ Gait dysfunction
■ Hip and knee joint range of motion measurement	■ Impaired joint mobility
■ ITB, hip and knee muscle extensibility tests	■ Impaired connective tissue integrity and mobility
■ Pain visual analog scale	■ Pain
■ Palpation (skin and fascial mobility)	■ Adhesions
	■ Decreased connective tissue mobility
■ Postural examination	■ Postural malalignment

Examination Techniques	Activity Limitations
■ Functional examination	■ Limitations in weight-bearing work, recreational, and self-care activities

Relevant Outcomes and Massage Techniques

■ Increased joint mobility: direct fascial techniques, friction, myofascial release, rhythmic mobilization, rocking
■ Increased connective tissue mobility and integrity; decreased adhesions: cross fiber and longitudinal strokes, petrissage, stripping, specific compression, direct fascial techniques, myofascial release, friction
■ Decreased pain: superficial effleurage, myofascial release, direct fascial technique, shaking, rhythmic mobilization
■ Normalized neuromuscular tone: compression, deep effleurage, petrissage

Relevant Complementary Techniques

■ Hydrotherapy, ITB stretches

Contraindications and Precautions

■ Avoid exerting pressure on the vessels and nerves in the femoral triangle.
■ In the early stages of treatment, be cautious not to reduce tension that is compensating for injured tissues or stabilizing the joint.

FIGURE 14-4 Anatomy of the iliotibial band. Reprinted from Clay JH, Pounds DM. *Basic Clinical Massage Therapy: Integrating Anatomy and Treatment*. 2nd ed. Philadelphia, PA: Lippincott Williams & Wilkins; 2008.

Helpful Hints

■ ITB contracture is often associated with postural malalignment of the hip, knee, ankle, and foot.
■ Trigger points in the anterior aspect of gluteus minimus and vastus lateralis may refer pain along the ITB.

Quick Treatment Guide for Lateral Epicondylitis

Description

Pain in the region of the common extensor origin associated with tendinitis (inflammation) or tendinosis (degeneration) of the tendons of the wrist and finger extensor muscles.[318-321] It is often the result of overuse or injury.

Relevant Anatomy

Lateral epicondyle, extensor carpi radialis longus and brevis, extensor carpi ulnaris, extensor digitorum

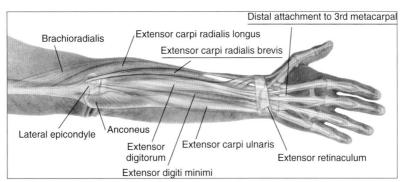

FIGURE 14-5 Anatomy of wrist and finger extensors. Reprinted from Clay JH, Pounds DM. *Basic Clinical Massage Therapy: Integrating Anatomy and Treatment.* 2nd ed. Philadelphia, PA: Lippincott Williams & Wilkins; 2008.

Relevant Examination Techniques, Impairments, and Activity Limitations

Examination Techniques	Impairments in Body Structure or Function
Elbow and wrist joint range of motion measurement	Impaired joint mobility
Grip strength testing	Impaired muscle performance
Muscle extensibility tests	Impaired muscle extensibility
Pain visual analog scale	Pain
Palpation of common extensor origin	Pain
Selective tissue tension testing	Impaired muscle integrity
Trigger point examination	Trigger points

Examination Techniques	Activity Limitations
Functional examination	Limitations in work, recreational, and self-care activities

Relevant Outcomes and Massage Techniques

- Increased joint mobility: direct fascial techniques, friction, myofascial release, rhythmic mobilization, rocking
- Increased muscle performance: rhythmic mobilization, rocking, percussive techniques
- Increased muscle extensibility; normalized muscle integrity: cross fiber strokes to the tendons, myofascial release, direct fascial technique, friction, petrissage, stripping, specific compression
- Decreased pain: superficial effleurage, myofascial release, direct fascial technique, shaking, rhythmic mobilization
- Deactivated trigger points: trigger point pressure release, cross fiber strokes, passive stretching
- Normalized neuromuscular tone: compression, deep effleurage, petrissage

Relevant Complementary Techniques

- Cyriax friction, hydrotherapy, stretching and strengthening exercises

Contraindications and Precautions

- To avoid the risk of re-injury, ensure that acute pain and inflammatory processes have resolved prior to applying deep friction to the tendon
- If repeated cross fiber strokes produce inflammation, end with cool or cold local hydrotherapy

Helpful Hints

- Muscles that oppose wrist extension may be weak when lateral epicondylitis has developed. Recommend strengthening exercises for wrist flexors to balance strength.

Quick Treatment Guide for Low Back Pain (Muscle Strain or Tension)

Description

Acute or chronic pain in the lumbar region stemming from (a) an increased resting muscle tension of the muscles of the lumbar region or (b) a strain of the muscles of the lumbar region and/or the ligaments of the lumbar spine.[318-321] It may result from injury or postural imbalance.

Relevant Anatomy

Quadratus lumborum, erector spinae, thoracolumbar fascia, latissimus dorsi

Relevant Examination Techniques, Impairments, and Activity Limitations

Examination Techniques	Impairments in Body Structure or Function
■ Abdominal, hip extensor and hip flexor muscle testing	■ Impaired muscle performance
■ Gait analysis	■ Gait dysfunction
■ Pain visual analog scale	■ Pain
■ Palpation	■ Muscle spasm
	■ Impaired connective tissue mobility
	■ Increased resting muscle tension
■ Postural examination	■ Postural malalignment
■ Thoracic and lumbar spine passive accessory joint range of motion measurement	■ Impaired joint mobility and joint integrity
■ Thoracic and lumbopelvic range of motion measurement	■ Impaired joint mobility

Examination Techniques	Activity Limitations
■ Functional examination	■ Limitations in work, recreational, and self-care activities

Relevant Outcomes and Massage Techniques

■ Increased muscle performance: rhythmic mobilization, rocking, percussive techniques
■ Decreased pain: superficial effleurage, myofascial release, direct fascial technique, shaking, rhythmic mobilization
■ Increased connective tissue mobility; normalized joint integrity and posture: cross fiber and longitudinal strokes, petrissage, stripping, specific compression, direct fascial techniques, myofascial release, friction
■ Decreased resting muscle tension (primary and compensatory) and muscle spasm; normalized neuromuscular tone: effleurage, petrissage, stripping, specific compression, myofascial release, direct fascial technique, rhythmic mobilization, rocking, shaking
■ Increased joint mobility: direct fascial techniques, friction, myofascial release, rhythmic mobilization, rocking

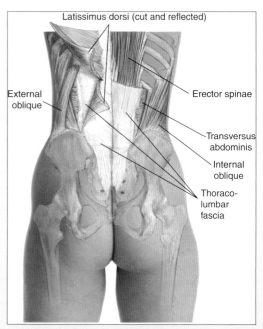

FIGURE 14-6 Anatomy of the lower back. Reprinted from Clay JH, Pounds DM. *Basic Clinical Massage Therapy: Integrating Anatomy and Treatment.* 2nd ed. Philadelphia, PA: Lippincott Williams & Wilkins; 2008.

Relevant Complementary Techniques

■ Hydrotherapy, body mechanics, and back care education

Contraindications and Precautions

■ A detailed health history may reveal herniated discs, a space-occupying lesion, or systemic conditions that require caution or may be contraindications to treatment.
■ Refer the client to his health-care provider if you suspect a non-musculoskeletal cause.
■ Be cautious not to compress nerves or cause numbness and tingling.

Helpful Hints

■ Imbalances in abdominal and lower extremity muscle length and/or strength and lower extremity postural malalignment may contribute to low back pain.
■ Wearing high heels may increase the lumbar lordotic curve and contribute to low back pain.
■ Trigger points in rectus abdominis, lumbar multifidi, lumbar erector spinae, and gluteus medius may be contributory factors.

Quick Treatment Guide for Plantar Fasciitis

Description

Acute or chronic pain (usually heel pain), thickening and/or inflammation of the plantar fascia, a band of connective tissue on the plantar surface of the foot that lies between the calcaneus and the toes.[318-321] It may be caused by overuse, a sudden increase in activity, or postural imbalance.

Relevant Anatomy

Plantar fascia, flexor digitorum brevis, abductor hallucis

Relevant Examination Techniques, Impairments, and Activity Limitations

Examination Techniques	Impairments in Body Structure or Function
▪ Ankle and foot muscle extensibility testing	▪ Impaired muscle extensibility
▪ Gait analysis	▪ Gait dysfunction
▪ Pain visual analog scale	▪ Pain
▪ Palpation	▪ Impaired connective tissue integrity
	▪ Pain
▪ Postural examination	▪ Postural malalignment

Examination Techniques	Activity Limitations
▪ Functional examination	▪ Limitations in weight-bearing work, recreational, and self-care activities

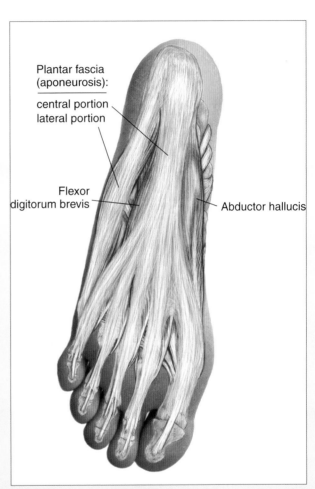

FIGURE 14-7 Anatomy of the plantar fascia. Reprinted from Clay JH, Pounds DM. *Basic Clinical Massage Therapy: Integrating Anatomy and Treatment.* 2nd ed. Philadelphia, PA: Lippincott Williams & Wilkins; 2008.

Relevant Outcomes and Massage Techniques

- Decreased pain: superficial effleurage, myofascial release, direct fascial technique, shaking, rhythmic mobilization
- Normalized connective tissue integrity; increased muscle extensibility: cross fiber and longitudinal strokes, petrissage, stripping, specific compression, direct fascial techniques, myofascial release, friction
- Decreased resting muscle tension (primary and compensatory); normalized neuromuscular tone: effleurage, petrissage, stripping, specific compression, myofascial release, direct fascial technique, rhythmic mobilization, rocking, shaking

Relevant Complementary Techniques

- Hydrotherapy, stretching and strengthening exercises for calf and intrinsic foot muscles

Contraindications and Precautions

- Be cautious when treating in the region of the vessels in the tarsal tunnel.

- Avoid deep treatment of the leg of a client who is at risk for developing blood clots.

Helpful Hints

- Trigger points in gastrocnemius, abductor hallucis, tibialis posterior, flexor digitorum longus, and soleus refer into the plantar surface of the foot.

Quick Treatment Guide for Piriformis Syndrome

Description

Pain in the gluteal region and posterior thigh resulting from compression or irritation of the sciatic nerve by a hypertonic piriformis muscle or trigger points in the piriformis muscle.[318-321] It may be caused by overuse, postural imbalance, or injury.

Relevant Anatomy

Piriformis, greater sciatic notch, gluteus medius, gluteus minimus, sciatic nerve

Relevant Examination Techniques, Impairments, and Activity Limitations

Examination Techniques	Impairments in Body Structure or Function
■ Gait analysis	■ Gait dysfunction
■ Hip range of motion measurement	■ Impaired joint mobility
■ Hip muscle extensibility testing	■ Impaired muscle extensibility
■ Hip muscle strength testing	■ Impaired muscle performance
■ Neurodynamic tension tests	■ Impaired neurodynamics
■ Pain visual analog scale	■ Pain
■ Palpation	■ Pain
	■ Increased resting muscle tension
■ Trigger point examination	■ Trigger points

Examination Techniques	Activity Limitations
■ Functional examination	■ Limitations in weight-bearing work, recreational, and self-care activities

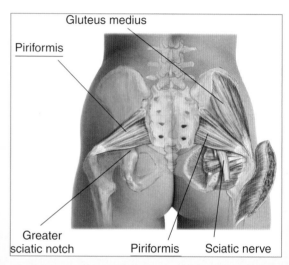

FIGURE 14-8 Anatomy of piriformis. Reprinted from Clay JH, Pounds DM. *Basic Clinical Massage Therapy: Integrating Anatomy and Treatment*. 2nd ed. Philadelphia, PA: Lippincott Williams & Wilkins; 2008.

Relevant Outcomes and Massage Techniques

■ Increased joint mobility: direct fascial techniques, friction, myofascial release, rhythmic mobilization, rocking
■ Increased muscle extensibility: cross fiber strokes, myofascial release, direct fascial technique, friction, petrissage, stripping, specific compression
■ Increased muscle performance: rhythmic mobilization, rocking, percussive techniques
■ Decreased pain: superficial effleurage, myofascial release, direct fascial technique, shaking, rhythmic mobilization
■ Decreased resting muscle tension (primary and compensatory): effleurage, petrissage, stripping, specific compression, myofascial release, direct fascial technique, rhythmic mobilization, rocking, shaking

■ Deactivated trigger points: trigger point pressure release, cross fiber strokes, passive stretching

Relevant Complementary Techniques

■ Hydrotherapy, muscle energy techniques, stretching and strengthening exercises

Contraindications and Precautions

■ Take care not to compress the sciatic nerve with enough pressure or duration to reproduce symptoms
■ Be cautious of other causes of hip and leg pain including disc herniations and space-occupying lesions

Helpful Hints

■ The smaller lateral rotators of the hips are frequently hypertonic when the piriformis is hypertonic; address these as needed.
■ Trigger points in gluteus medius, gluteus minimus, and piriformis may contribute to symptoms.

Quick Treatment Guide for Rotator Cuff Strain

Description

Pain, inflammation, and decreased range of motion of the glenohumeral joint resulting from a stretching or tearing of the muscles of the rotator cuff.[318-321] This may be the result of injury, postural imbalance, or overuse.

Relevant Anatomy

Supraspinatus, infraspinatus, teres minor, subscapularis

Relevant Examination Techniques, Impairments, and Activity Limitations

Examination Techniques	Impairments in Body Structure or Function
■ Pain visual analog scale	■ Pain
■ Palpation	■ Pain
	■ Increased resting muscle tension
■ Postural examination	■ Postural malalignment
■ Selective tissue tension testing	■ Impaired muscle integrity
■ Shoulder muscle strength testing	■ Impaired muscle performance
■ Shoulder passive accessory motion testing	■ Impaired joint mobility and joint integrity
■ Shoulder range of motion measurements	■ Impaired joint mobility

Examination Techniques	Activity Limitations
■ Functional examination	■ Limitations in overhead and behind the back work, recreational, and self-care activities

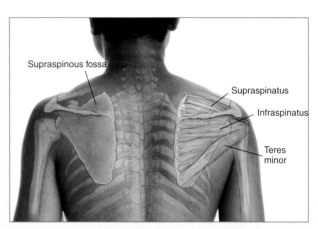

FIGURE 14-9 Anatomy of supraspinatus, infraspinatus, and teres minor. Reprinted from Clay JH, Pounds DM. *Basic Clinical Massage Therapy: Integrating Anatomy and Treatment.* 2nd ed. Philadelphia, PA: Lippincott Williams & Wilkins; 2008.

Relevant Outcomes and Massage Techniques

- Decreased pain: superficial effleurage, myofascial release, direct fascial technique, shaking, rhythmic mobilization
- Decreased resting muscle tension (primary and compensatory); normalized muscle tone: effleurage, petrissage, stripping, specific compression, myofascial release, direct fascial technique, rhythmic mobilization, rocking, shaking
- Normalized muscle and joint integrity; normalized posture: cross fiber and longitudinal strokes, petrissage, stripping, specific compression, direct fascial techniques, friction, myofascial release
- Increased muscle performance: rhythmic mobilization, rocking, percussive techniques
- Increased joint mobility: direct fascial techniques, friction, myofascial release, rhythmic mobilization, rocking

Relevant Complementary Techniques

- Hydrotherapy, therapeutic exercise, body mechanics education, muscle energy techniques

Contraindications and Precautions

- Be cautious of vessels and nerves in the axilla.
- Avoid placing the arm in painful ranges such as above 80° of shoulder flexion.

Helpful Hints

- Trigger points in any muscle that crosses the glenohumeral joint may be contributory factors.

Quick Treatment Guide for Scar Remodeling

Description

Formation of fibrous scar tissue during the wound healing process.[318-321] Abnormal tissue repair resulting from a variety of factors including impaired immune response, infection, and malnutrition may result in hypertrophic scars and keloids.

Relevant Anatomy

Epithelial cells, granulation tissue, blood vessels, fibrous scar

Relevant Examination Techniques, Impairments, and Activity Limitations

Examination Techniques	Impairments in Body Structure or Function
■ Girth measurements at, proximal to, and distal to location of scar	■ Edema
■ Measurement of dimensions of scar	■ Increased scar dimensions
■ Palpation of scar, skin and fascial mobility	■ Adhesions
	■ Decreased connective tissue mobility
	■ Pain
■ Visual inspection of scar and skin	■ Abnormal scar tissue

Examination Techniques	Activity Limitations
■ Functional examination	■ Possible limitations in work, recreational, and self-care activities

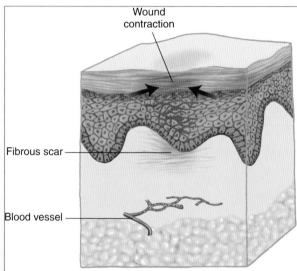

FIGURE 14-10 Anatomy of scar formation. Reprinted from Porth C, Matfin G. *Pathophysiology: Concepts of Altered Health States.* 8th ed. Baltimore, MD: Lippincott Williams & Wilkins; 2009.

Relevant Outcomes and Massage Techniques

- Decreased edema: superficial effleurage, superficial lymph drainage techniques, broad-contact compression, petrissage
- Increased connective tissue mobility; decreased adhesions; normalized scar tissue: cross fiber and longitudinal strokes, petrissage, stripping, specific compression, direct fascial techniques, myofascial release, friction
- Decreased pain: superficial effleurage, myofascial release, direct fascial technique, shaking, rhythmic mobilization
- Normalized neuromuscular tone in underlying muscles: compression, deep effleurage, and petrissage

Relevant Complementary Techniques

- Hydrotherapy. Hot wax can be effective in softening the scar tissue. Dry brushing across the scar helps in restoring sensation.

Contraindications and Precautions

- Scars and their stories need to be respected. Some scars result in feelings of pride but others may hold a complex history of trauma and emotional pain. Be aware that some clients may be reluctant, or unable, to provide a detailed history of their scars nor articulate their goals for treatment.
- Be cautious when working deeply on a new scar to avoid additional tearing of tissues.

Helpful Hints

- Scars can be superficial or deep. Evaluate the tissues carefully so that scar tissue treatment is focused on the relevant tissues.
- If edema is present, ensure that you manage the scar and edema simultaneously. For example, work fascially, then drain or vice versa until the scar is pliable and the edema is under control.

Quick Treatment Guide for Stiff Neck

Description

Sudden onset of pain, decreased range of motion, and muscle tightness of the cervical spine.[318-321] It can have multiple causes such as muscle strain, poor body mechanics or positioning, or psychosocial stress.

Relevant Anatomy

Levator scapulae, sternocleidomastoid

Relevant Examination Techniques, Impairments, and Activity Limitations

Examination Techniques	Impairments in Body Structure or Function
■ Cervical spine passive accessory motion testing	■ Impaired joint mobility and joint integrity
■ Cervical spine range of motion measurement	■ Impaired joint mobility
■ Pain visual analog scale	■ Pain
■ Palpation	■ Pain
	■ Muscle spasm
	■ Increased resting muscle tension
■ Postural examination	■ Postural malalignment

Examination Techniques	Activity Limitations
■ Functional examination	■ Limitations in work, recreational, and self-care activities

Relevant Outcomes and Massage Techniques

- Normalized joint integrity and posture: cross fiber and longitudinal strokes, petrissage, stripping, specific compression, direct fascial techniques, friction, myofascial release
- Increased joint mobility: direct fascial techniques, friction, myofascial release, rhythmic mobilization, rocking
- Decreased pain: superficial effleurage, myofascial release, direct fascial technique, shaking, rhythmic mobilization
- Decreased resting muscle tension (primary and compensatory); spasm normalized neuromuscular tone: effleurage, petrissage, stripping, specific compression, myofascial release, direct fascial technique, rhythmic mobilization, rocking, shaking

Relevant Complementary Techniques

- Hydrotherapy, body mechanics education, neck stretching and strengthening exercises

FIGURE 14-11 Anatomy of the neck muscles. Reprinted from Clay JH, Pounds DM. *Basic Clinical Massage Therapy: Integrating Anatomy and Treatment*. 2nd ed. Philadelphia, PA: Lippincott Williams & Wilkins; 2008.

Contraindications And Precautions

- Be cautious near the vessels and nerves in the anterior and posterior triangles of the neck
- Be cautious of other causes of neck pain including disc herniations and space-occupying lesions
- If the client presents with fever, vomiting, or severe headache, refer to a physician for investigation of infection such as meningitis.

Helpful Hints

- If the client presents with head forward posture, treat anterior tissues from inferior to superior, and lateral to medial.

Quick Treatment Guide for Stress, Anxiety, or Depression

Description

Chronic stress is a prolonged and heightened state of arousal that has negative physiological and psychological consequences.[318-321] Chronic stress responses occur over the cognitive, physiological, affective, or behavioral domains and may have consequences such as impaired cognitive function, depression, anxiety, muscle tension, and impaired social functioning.

Depression is a mood disorder that is characterized by feelings of sadness, worthlessness, or hopelessness; disturbances in sleep and eating; and a variety of other symptoms.[318-321] It may be classified as either a major depressive disorder or a mild depression (dysthymia).

Anxiety is an increase in fear, worrying, or nervousness in response to a situation or event.[318-321] This is different from anxiety disorders, such as panic disorders or post-traumatic stress disorder, in which individuals experience intense episodes of fearfulness and require medical management.

Relevant Examination Techniques, Impairments, and Activity Limitations

Examination Techniques

- Interview for perceived stress levels and symptoms and reports of depression or anxiety
- Pain diagram
- Palpation of area of reported symptoms
- Self-report stress measures
- Trigger point examination

Impairments in Body Structure or Function

- Reported stress, depression, or anxiety
- Pain or tenderness
- Increased resting muscle tension
- Reported increased stress
- Trigger points

Examination Techniques

- Functional examination

Activity Limitations

- Possible limitations in work, recreational, and self-care activities

FIGURE 14-12 Map of specific functional areas in the cerebral cortex. Reprinted from Porth C, Matfin G. *Pathophysiology: Concepts of Altered Health States*. 8th ed. Baltimore, MD: Lippincott Williams &Wilkins; 2009.

Relevant Outcomes and Massage Techniques

- Increased relaxation and decreased resting muscle tension: effleurage, petrissage, stripping, specific compression, myofascial release, direct fascial technique, rhythmic mobilization, rocking, shaking
- Increased arousal (for depressed mood): percussive techniques
- Decreased pain: superficial effleurage, myofascial release, direct fascial technique, shaking, rhythmic mobilization
- Deactivated trigger points: trigger point pressure release, cross fiber strokes, passive stretching

Relevant Complementary Techniques

- Relaxed breathing, relaxing music, relaxation technique (meditation and progressive relaxation), gentle exercise

Contraindications and Precautions

- Clients who present with a primary complaint of stress may have associated anxiety and depression; screen for these during the client interview.
- Refer the patient for counseling if the patient is showing signs of distress or reports that stress, anxiety, or depression is a significant concern.
- When client reports high levels of stress or anxiety, avoid techniques that stimulate the nervous system (e.g., percussive techniques, fast moving strokes, and ice).
- Avoid excess pressure or deep stroking that may cause pain or stimulate the nervous system.
- Refer the client to the physician if the patient has symptoms suggesting a chronic pain syndrome.

Helpful Hints

- Ending the session with gentle massage to the head, face, or hands can be relaxing.
- Scents, sounds, and light may stimulate the nervous system of a stressed, anxious, or depressed client.
- Assess the client for tension headaches and the presence of trigger points in the neck and shoulder muscles since these may occur in people who complain of stress, anxiety, or depression.

Quick Treatment Guide for Tension Headaches (Temporal and Suboccipital)

Description

Episodic or chronic dull, aching headache that may be caused by muscle tension and trigger points.[318-321] Temporal headaches may arise from the temporal muscles while suboccipital headaches may result from the suboccipital muscles.

Relevant Anatomy

Temporal: Frontalis, temporalis, occipitalis
Suboccipital: Suboccipital muscles, semispinalis capitis and cervicis, longissimus capitis, trapezius

Relevant Examination Techniques, Impairments, and Activity Limitations

Examination Techniques	Impairments in Body Structure or Function
■ Cervical spine range of motion (for suboccipital headaches)	■ Impaired joint mobility
■ Pain visual analog scale	■ Pain
■ Palpation	■ Muscle spasm
	■ Increased resting muscle tension
■ Passive accessory motion of cervical spine (for suboccipital headaches)	■ Impaired joint mobility and joint integrity
■ Postural examination	■ Postural malalignment
■ Trigger point examination	■ Trigger points

Examination Techniques	Activity Limitations
■ Functional examination	■ Limitations in work, recreational, and self-care activities

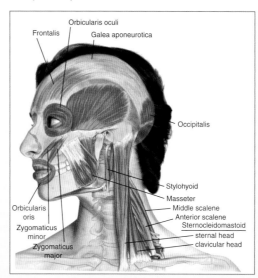

FIGURE 14-13 Anatomy of the head and neck muscles. Reprinted from Clay JH, Pounds DM. *Basic Clinical Massage Therapy: Integrating Anatomy and Treatment*. 2nd ed. Philadelphia, PA: Lippincott Williams & Wilkins; 2008.

Relevant Outcomes and Massage Techniques

- Increased joint mobility: direct fascial techniques, friction, myofascial release, rhythmic mobilization, rocking
- Decreased pain: superficial effleurage, myofascial release, direct fascial technique, shaking, rhythmic mobilization
- Decreased resting muscle tension (primary and compensatory) and muscle spasm; normalized neuromuscular tone: effleurage, petrissage, stripping, specific compression, myofascial release, direct fascial technique, rhythmic mobilization, rocking, shaking
- Increased joint mobility: direct fascial techniques, friction, myofascial release, rhythmic mobilization, rocking
- Normalized joint integrity and posture: cross fiber and longitudinal strokes, petrissage, stripping, specific compression, direct fascial techniques, friction, myofascial release
- Deactivated trigger points: trigger point pressure release, cross fiber strokes, passive stretching

Note: See Quick Treatment Guide for Stiff Neck for information pertinent to suboccipital headaches.

Relevant Complementary Techniques

- Gentle pulling of the hair may help reduce tension in relevant anatomy. Asking the client to open/close the mouth and eyes while applying techniques may enhance treatment results.
- Hydrotherapy, muscle energy techniques

Contraindications and Precautions

- For sudden, acute episodes and long-term chronic cases of headaches, be certain to understand the client's health history and any non-musculoskeletal factors that may contribute to headaches (e.g., neurological, infectious, and space-occupying lesion).
- Be cautious of vessels and nerves in the anterior and posterior triangles of the neck.
- Take care not to sustain techniques or pressure that may increase symptoms.
- Take care not to stretch tissues that are hypotonic or overstretched.
- Refer client to their health-care provider if you suspect a cause other than musculoskeletal.

Helpful Hints

- Temporomandibular joint issues may contribute to temporal headaches.
- There are a variety of trigger points that have referral patterns that mimic or contribute to headaches such as trapezius, splenii, temporalis, masseter, sternocleidomastoid, and suboccipitals.
- Scents, sounds, and light may disturb a client with an active headache.

Quick Treatment Guide for Thoracic Outlet Syndrome (TOS)

Description

Compression of the nerves and/or blood vessels that pass through the thoracic outlet resulting in gradual onset of pain, numbness and tingling, or edema in the neck, arm, and hand.[318-321] Progression of TOS may lead to decreased strength and tone of the involved muscles. The causes include anatomical abnormalities, postural imbalance, injury, or overuse.

Relevant Anatomy

Scalenes, first rib, subclavian artery, brachial plexus, clavicle

Relevant Examination Techniques, Impairments, and Activity Limitations

Examination Techniques	Impairments in Body Structure or Function
■ Pain diagram	■ Pain
	■ Paresthesia
■ Pain visual analog scale	■ Pain
■ Palpation	■ Increased resting muscle tension
■ Postural examination	■ Postural malalignment
■ Respiratory pattern examination (chest vs. diaphragmatic)	■ Abnormal respiratory pattern
■ Special tests for TOS	■ Confirmation of TOS
■ Trigger point examination	■ Trigger points
■ Upper extremity muscle strength testing	■ Impaired muscle performance
■ Upper extremity neurody-namic tension tests	■ Impaired neurodynamics

Examination Techniques	Activity Limitations
■ Functional examination	■ Limitations in work, recreational, and self-care activities

Relevant Outcomes and Massage Techniques

- Decreased pain: superficial effleurage, myofascial release, direct fascial technique, shaking, rhythmic mobilization
- Decreased resting muscle tension (primary and compensatory); normalized neuromuscular tone: effleurage, petrissage, stripping, specific compression, myofascial release, direct fascial technique, rhythmic mobilization, rocking, shaking
- Normalized posture: myofascial release, direct fascial technique
- Increased rib cage mobility: broad-contact compression, petrissage
- Deactivated trigger points: trigger point pressure release, cross fiber strokes, passive stretching
- Increased muscle performance: rhythmic mobilization, rocking, percussive techniques

Note: See Quick Treatment Guides for Tension Headache (posterior), Stiff Neck, and Upper Crossed Syndrome

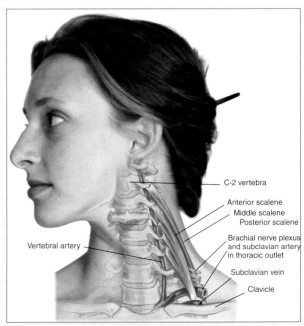

FIGURE 14-14 Anatomy of the scalenes and the thoracic outlet. Reprinted from Clay JH, Pounds DM. *Basic Clinical Massage Therapy: Integrating Anatomy and Treatment*. 2nd ed. Philadelphia, PA: Lippincott Williams & Wilkins; 2008.

Relevant Complementary Techniques

- Hydrotherapy, muscle energy techniques, relaxation techniques, diaphragmatic breathing, therapeutic exercise

Contraindications and Precautions

- Be cautious near the vessels and nerves in the anterior and posterior triangles of the neck.
- Be cautious not to stretch tissues that are already lengthened.
- Refer client to health-care provider if you suspect a cause other than musculoskeletal.

Helpful Hints

- Protraction of the shoulder girdles leading to internal rotation of glenohumeral joint often accompanies TOS. As time permits, lengthen the medial rotators of the arm.
- The head forward posture frequently accompanies TOS. In forward head posture the deep anterior muscles (e.g., longus colli) are lengthened and weak and the posterior muscles are short. As time permits, lengthen the muscles of the posterior neck.
- Trigger points in pectoralis minor, scalenes, and subclavius may contribute to or mimic symptoms of TOS.

Quick Treatment Guide for Upper Crossed Syndrome (Neck/Upper Back Pain)

Description

Dr. Janda defined upper crossed syndrome as a muscle imbalance in which there is increase tone of the upper trapezius, levator, sterno-cleidomastoid, and pectoralis muscles, accompanied by decreased tone of the deep cervical flexors, lower trapezius, and serratus anterior.[322] This muscle imbalance and associated weakness results in pain and postural imbalance.

Relevant Anatomy

Levator scapulae, trapezius, rhomboids, pectoralis major, pectoralis minor, sternocleidomastoid, serratus anterior

Relevant Examination Techniques, Impairments, and Activity Limitations

Examination Techniques	Impairments in Body Structure or Function
■ Cervical and thoracic spine passive accessory motion testing	■ Impaired joint mobility and joint integrity
■ Cervical and thoracic spine range of motion measurement	■ Impaired joint mobility
■ Pain visual analog scale	■ Pain
■ Palpation	■ Pain
	■ Increased resting muscle tension
■ Postural examination	■ Postural malalignment
■ Trigger point examination	■ Trigger points

Examination Techniques	Activity Limitations
■ Functional examination	■ Limitations in work, recreational, and self-care activities

FIGURE 14-15 Upper crossed syndrome. Reprinted from Hendrickson T. *Massage for Orthopedic Conditions*. 2nd ed. Baltimore, MD: Lippincott Williams & Wilkins; 2009.

Relevant Outcomes and Massage Techniques

- Normalized joint integrity and posture: cross fiber and longitudinal strokes, petrissage, stripping, specific compression, direct fascial techniques, friction, myofascial release
- Increased joint mobility: direct fascial techniques, friction, myofascial release, rhythmic mobilization, rocking
- Decreased pain: superficial effleurage, myofascial release, direct fascial technique, shaking, rhythmic mobilization
- Decreased resting muscle tension (primary muscles with increased tone and compensatory muscles: effleurage, petrissage, stripping, specific compression, myofascial release, direct fascial technique, rhythmic mobilization, rocking, shaking
- Deactivated trigger points: trigger point pressure release, cross fiber strokes, passive stretching
- Normalized neuromuscular tone and performance (muscles with decreased tone): compression, deep effleurage, petrissage, and percussive techniques

Note: See Quick Treatment Guide for Stiff Neck

Relevant Complementary Techniques

- Hydrotherapy, muscle energy techniques, neck and upper back stretching and strengthening exercises, body mechanics education

Contraindications and Precautions

- Be cautious near the vessels and nerves in the anterior and posterior triangles of the neck.
- Be cautious not to stretch tissues that are already lengthened.
- Be cautious of other causes of neck pain including disc herniations and space-occupying lesions.

Helpful Hints

- In forward head posture the deep anterior muscles (e.g., longus colli) are lengthened and weak and the posterior muscles are short. As time permits, lengthen the muscles of the posterior neck.

Quick Treatment Guide for Whiplash

Description

Injury of the muscles, ligaments, joints, and nerve roots of the cervical region following a rapid or extreme neck flexion and/or extension.[318-321] This can result in a variety of symptoms such as pain, decreased range of motion of the cervical spine, muscle tightness, and paresthesia.

Relevant Anatomy

Sternocleidomastoid, trapezius, splenius capitis and cervicis, suboccipital muscles, semispinalis capitis and cervicis, longissimus capitis, levator scapulae
Note: See anatomy in Quick Treatment Guides for Tension Headaches, Stiff Neck

Relevant Examination Techniques, Impairments, and Activity Limitations

Examination Techniques	Impairments in Body Structure or Function
■ Cervical spine range of motion testing	■ Impaired joint mobility
■ Pain diagram	■ Pain
	■ Paresthesia
■ Pain visual analog scale	■ Pain
■ Palpation	■ Pain
	■ Increased resting muscle tension
	■ Muscle spasm
■ Passive accessory motion of cervical spine	■ Impaired joint mobility and joint integrity
■ Postural examination	■ Postural malalignment
■ Trigger point examination	■ Trigger points

Examination Techniques	Activity Limitations
■ Functional examination	■ Limitations in work, recreational, and self-care activities

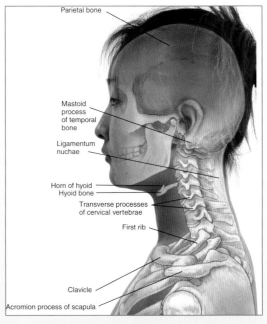

FIGURE 14-16 Anatomy of the lateral head and neck. Reprinted from Clay JH, Pounds DM. *Basic Clinical Massage Therapy: Integrating Anatomy and Treatment*. 2nd ed. Philadelphia, PA: Lippincott Williams & Wilkins; 2008.

Relevant Outcomes and Massage Techniques

- Increased joint mobility: direct fascial techniques, friction, myofascial release, rhythmic mobilization, rocking
- Decreased pain: superficial effleurage, myofascial release, direct fascial technique, shaking, rhythmic mobilization
- Decreased resting muscle tension (primary and compensatory) and muscle spasm; normalized neuromuscular tone: effleurage, petrissage, stripping, specific compression, myofascial release, direct fascial technique, rhythmic mobilization, rocking, shaking
- Increased joint mobility: direct fascial techniques, friction, myofascial release, rhythmic mobilization, rocking
- Normalized muscle integrity and posture: cross fiber and longitudinal strokes, petrissage, stripping, specific compression, direct fascial techniques, friction, myofascial release
- Deactivated trigger points: trigger point pressure release, cross fiber strokes, passive stretching

Note: See Quick Treatment Guides for Tension Headaches, Stiff Neck

Relevant Complementary Techniques

- Hydrotherapy, relaxation techniques, therapeutic exercise as tolerated, body mechanics education

Contraindications and Precautions

- When whiplash is the result of an accident or fall, fractures, dislocations, or other non-muscular injuries may be present. Take care to understand the client's circumstances and discuss with medical professionals when necessary.
- If client has developed confusion; difficulty seeing, hearing, or swallowing; or problems maintaining balance, refer to their physician for evaluation.

Helpful Hints

- If the causes of whiplash are focused primarily on one side of the neck, the opposing muscles may be weak and require strengthening.

CHAPTER 1

References

1. Sackett D, Straus S, Richardson W, Rosenberg W, Haynes R. *Evidence-Based Medicine: How to Practice and Teach EBM*, New York, NY: Churchill-Livingstone; 2000.
2. Donabedian A. Evaluating the quality of medical care. *Milbank Mem Fund Q.* 1966;44(3):166-206.
3. Dryden T, Moyer CA. *Integrating Research in Clinical Practice.* Champaign, IL: Human Kinetics; 2012.
4. IN-CAM Outcomes Database 2010. Canadian interdisciplinary network for complementary and alternative medicine research. http://www.outcomesdatabase.org/
5. Ritenbaugh C, Verhoef M, Fleishman S, Boon H, Leis A. Whole systems research: a discipline for studying complementary and alternative medicine. *Altern Ther Health Med.* 2003;9(4):32.
6. Benjamin PJ, Tappan FM. *Tappan's Handbook of Healing Massage Techniques.* 4th ed. Upper Saddle River, NJ: Pearson Prentice Hall; 2005.
7. Field TM. Massage therapy effects. *Am Psychol.* 1998;53(12):1270.
8. Oschman JL. *Energy Medicine.* Edinburgh: Churchill Livingstone; 2000.
9. Moyer CA, Rounds J, Hannum JW. A meta-analysis of massage therapy research. *Psychol Bull.* 2004;130(1):3.
10. Lewis M, Johnson MI. The clinical effectiveness of therapeutic massage for musculoskeletal pain: a systematic review. *Physiotherapy.* 2006;92(3):146-158.
11. Coelho HF, Boddy K, Ernst E. Massage therapy for the treatment of depression: a systematic review. *Int J Clin Pract.* 2008;62(2):325-333.
12. Grant KE. Steps toward massage therapy guidelines: a first report to the profession. *Int J Ther Massage Bodywork.* 2008;1(1).
13. O'Donnell MP. Definition of health promotion. Part III: expanding the definition. *Am J Health Promot.* 1989;3(3):5.
14. World Health Organization. Preamble to the constitution of the World Health Organization as adopted by the International Health Conference. *New York.* 1946;19:100.
15. World Health Organization. *Towards a Common Language for Functioning, Disability and Health: ICF—the International Classification of Functioning, Disability and Health.* Geneva, Switzerland: World Health Organization; 2002.
16. World Health Organization. *ICF Checklist.* Geneva, Switzerland: World Health Organization; 2001.
17. Goodman CC, Boissonnault WG, Fuller KS. *Pathology: Implications for the Physical Therapist.* 2nd ed. Philadelphia, PA: Saunders; 2003.
18. American Physical Therapy Association. *Interactive Guide to Physical Therapist Practice.* Alexandria, VA: American Physical Therapy Association; 2003.
19. Nemcek MA. Self nurturance: research trends and wellness model. *AAOHN J.* 2003;51(6):260-266.
20. Schuster TL, Dobson M, Jauregui M, Blanks RHI. Wellness lifestyles I: a theoretical framework linking wellness, health lifestyles, and complementary and alternative medicine. *J Altern Complement Med.* 2004;10(2):349-356.
21. Travis JW. *The Wellness Workbook: How to Achieve Enduring Health and Vitality.* 3rd ed. Berkeley, CA: Celestial Arts; 2004.
22. Soanes C, Hawker S, Elliott J. *Paperback Oxford English Dictionary.* Vol 10. New York, NY: Oxford University Press; 2006.
23. Hillman J. *A Blue Fire.* New York, NY: Harper Paperbacks; 1991.
24. Moore T. *Care of the Soul: A Guide for Cultivating Depth and Sacredness in Everyday Life.* New York, NY: Harper Paperbacks; 1994.
25. Prochaska JO, DiClemente CC. Transtheoretical therapy: toward a more integrative model of change. *Psychother Theory Res Pract.* 1982;19(3):276.
26. Mulkins AL, Verhoef M, Cormier E. The benefits of massage in Vancouver's inner city. *Massage Ther J.* 2005;44(1):102-109.
27. Bredin M. Mastectomy, body image and therapeutic massage: a qualitative study of women's experience. *J Adv Nurs.* 999;29(5):1113-1120.
28. Billhult A, Stener-Victorin E, Bergbom I. The experience of massage during chemotherapy treatment in breast cancer patients. *Clin Nurs Res.* 2007;16(2):85-99.
29. Paterson C, Allen JA, Browning M, Barlow G, Ewings P. A pilot study of therapeutic massage for people with Parkinson's disease: the added value of user involvement. *Complement Ther Clin Pract.* 2005;11(3):161-171.
30. Price C. Body-oriented therapy in recovery from child sexual abuse: an efficacy study. *Altern Ther Health Med.* 2005;11(5):46.
31. Smith JM, Sullivan SJ, Baxter GD. The culture of massage therapy: valued elements and the role of comfort, contact, connection and caring. *Complement Ther Med.* 2009;17(4):181-189.
32. Herbert CP, Bainbridge L, Bickford J, et al. Factors that influence engagement in collaborative practice. *Can Fam Physician.* 2007;53(8):1318-1325.

CHAPTER 2

References

1. Mitchell A, Cormack MA. *The Therapeutic Relationship in Complementary Health Care.* Edinburgh: Churchill Livingstone; 1998.
2. Donabedian A. Evaluating the quality of medical care. *Milbank Mem Fund Q.* 1966;44(3):166-206.
3. Bachelor A, Horvath A. The therapeutic relationship. In: Hubble M, Duncan B, Miller S, eds. *The Heart and Soul of Change.* Washington, DC: American Psychological Association; 2005;133-178.
4. Nelligan P, Grinspun D, Jonas-Simpson C, et al. Client-centered care: making the ideal real. *Hosp Q.* 2002;5(4):70-76.
5. Duncan B, Miller S, Wampold B, Hubble M. T*he Heart & Soul of Change: What Works in Therapy.* Washington, DC: American Psychological Association; 2010.
6. Canadian Physiotherapy Association. *The Code of Ethics and Rules of Conduct.* Ontario: Canadian Physiotherapy Association; 2005.
7. American Physical Therapy Association. *Code of Ethics and Guide for Professional Conduct.* Alexandria, VA: American Physical Therapy Association; 2004.
8. Quality Assurance Committee of the College of Massage Therapists of Ontario. *Code of Ethics and Standards of Practice.* Toronto, ON: College of Massage Therapists of Ontario; 2006.
9. Commission on Standards. *Occupational Therapy Code of Ethics.* Bethesda, MD: American Occupational Therapy Association; 1994.
10. International Chiropractors Association. *ICA Code of Ethics.* Arlington, VA: International Chiropractors Association; 1985.
11. American Association of Drugless Practitioners. *Code of Ethics.* Gilmern, TX: American Association of Drugless Practitioners; 2007.
12. American Massage Therapy Association. *Code of Ethics for Massage Therapists.* Evanston, IL: American Massage Therapy Association; 2005.
13. American Nurses Association. *Code of Ethics for Nurses with Interpretive Statements.* Silver Spring, MD: American Nurses Association; 2001.
14. Canadian Association of Occupational Therapists. *Canadian Framework for Ethical Occupational Therapy Practice.* Ottawa, ON: Canadian Association of Occupational Therapists; 2006.
15. Fitch P. Intimacy and attachment in massage therapy. *Massage Ther J.* 2005;43:113-121.
16. The College of Chiropractors of Ontario, College of Massage Therapists of Ontario, College of Physiotherapists of Ontario. *Where's My Line?* Toronto, ON: The College of Chiropractors of Ontario, College of Massage Therapists of Ontario, College of Physiotherapists of Ontario; 2005.

17. Benjamin BE, Sohnen-Moe C. *The Ethics of Touch: The Hands-On Practitioner's Guide to Creating a Professional, Safe and Enduring Practice.* Baltimore, MD: Lippincott, Williams & Wilkins; 2004.

18. McIntosh N. *The Educated Heart.* Memphis, TN: Dacatur Bainbridge Press; 2004.

19. Dryden T, Fitch P. Recovering body and soul from post-traumatic stress disorder. *Massage Ther J.* 2000;39:41-60.

20. Nathan B. *Touch and Emotion in Manual Therapy.* Edinburgh: Churchill Livingstone; 1999.

21. Goring S. *Relational Characterology and Embodiment: An Interpersonal Interpretation of the Characterological and Somatic Theories of Alexander Lowen and Stephen Johnson.* Unpublished master's thesis. [Master's]. Vermont College of Norwich University; 1994.

22. Rolfe I. *Rolfing: The Integration of Human Structure.* New York, NY: Harper and Row; 1977.

23. Physical therapy cures postpartum stress incontinence. *BMJ.* 2004;329(7478). doi: 10.1136/bmj.329.7478.0-f.

24. Hall ET. *The Silent Language.* Michigan: Anchor Press; 1973.

25. Van Servellen GW. *Communication Skills for the Health Care Professional: Concepts, Practice, and Evidence.* 2nd ed. Burlington, MA: Jones & Bartlett Learning; 2008.

26. Hall AM, Ferreira PH, Maher CG, Latimer J, Ferreira ML. The influence of the therapist-patient relationship on treatment outcome in physical rehabilitation: a systematic review. *Phys Ther.* 2010;90(8):1099-1110.

27. Upledger JE. *Somatoemotional Release and Beyond.* Palm Beach Gardens, FL: UI Publishing; 1990.

28. Lowen A. *Bioenergetics.* New York, NY: Penguin Books; 1975.

29. Pierrakos JC. *Core Energetics: Developing the Capacity to Love and Heal.* Mendocino, CA: LifeRhythm Publication; 1987.

30. Reich W. *The Function of the Orgasm.* New York, NY: Orgone Institute Press; 1942.

31. Nursing Practice Division. *Code of Ethics for Nurses.* Washington, DC: American Nursing Association; 2001.

32. Government of Ontario. *Regulated Health Professions Act (Ontario) Procedural Code.* 1999.

33. Fitch P. Nurturance, intimacy and attachment. *J Soft Tissue Manipulation.* 2004;12:6-9.

34. Polseno D. Enabling: the dark side of being helpful. *Massage Ther J.* 2003 (Summer);42:123-127.

35. Moyer CA, Rounds J, Hannum JW. A meta-analysis of massage therapy research. *Psychol Bull.* 2004;130(1):3.

36. Benjamin BE, Sohen-Moe C. The benefits of supervision programs: peer supervision and clinical supervision groups provide therapists with a safe harbor and forum for professional development. *Massage Ther J.* 2003;41:116-121.

37. Polseno D. Ethically speaking. Are you safe? *Massage Ther J.* 2004(43):128-130.

38. Hulka B. Patient-clinician interactions and compliance. *Compliance Health Care.* 1979:63-77.

39. Claxton AJ, Cramer J, Pierce C. A systematic review of the associations between dose regimens and medication compliance. *Clin Ther.* 2001;23(8):1296-1310.

40. Sluijs EM. A checklist to assess patient education in physical therapy practice: development and reliability. *Phys Ther.* 1991;71(8):561-569.

41. Center for Health Promotion and Education and Centers for Disease Control. *Strategies to Promote Self Management of Chronic Disease.* Atlanta, GA: Center for Health Promotion and Education and Centers for Disease Control; 1982.

42. Visser J, Keller JM. The clinical use of motivational messages: an inquiry into the validity of the ARCS model of motivational design. *Instructional Science.* 1990;19(6):467-500.

43. O'Donohue WT, Levensky ER. *Promoting Treatment Adherence: A Practical Handbook for Health Care Providers.* Thousand Oaks, CA: Sage Publications, Inc; 2006.

44. Becker MH. Theoretical models of adherence and strategies for improving adherence. In: Shumaker SA, Schron EB, Ockene JK, eds. *The Handbook of Health Behavior Change.* New York, NY: Springer; 1990:5.

45. O'Brien MK, Petrie K, Raeburn J. Adherence to medication regimens: updating a complex medical issue. *Med Care Rev.* 1992;49:435-454.

46. Haynes RB. Determinants of compliance: the disease and the mechanics of treatment. Haynes RB, Taylor DW, Sackett DL, eds. *Compliance in Health Care.* Baltimore MD: Johns Hopkins University Press; 1979;49.

47. Meichenbaum D, Turk DC. *Facilitating Treatment Adherence: A Practitioner's Guidebook.* New York, NY: Plenum Press; 1987.

48. Grueninger UJ. Arterial hypertension: lessons from patient education. *Patient Educ Couns.* 1995;26(1):37-55.

49. Sluijs EM, Kok GJ, van der Zee J. Correlates of exercise compliance in physical therapy. *Phys Ther.* 1993;73(11):771-782.

50. Donovan JL. Patient decision making. *Int J Technol Assess Health Care.* 1995;11(3):443-455.

51. Davey P, Parker S. Cost effectiveness of once-daily oral antimicrobial therapy. *J Clin Pharmacol.* 1992;32(8):706-710.

52. Dunear-Jacob J, Erlen JA, Schlenk EA, Ryan CM, Sereika SM, Doswell WM. Adherence in chronic disease. *Annu Rev Nurs Res.* 2000;18(1):48-90.

53. Popa-Lisseanu MGG, Greisinger A, Richardson M, et al. Determinants of treatment adherence in ethnically diverse, economically disadvantaged patients with rheumatic disease. *J Rheumatol.* 2005;32(5):913-919.

54. Smith BA, Shuchman M. Problem of nonadherence in chronically ill adolescents: strategies for assessment and intervention. *Curr Opin Pediatr.* 2005;17(5):613.

55. Klareskog L, Lindblad S. How is clinical progress achieved? *Best Prac Res Clin Rheumatol.* 2004;18(1):1-5.

56. Engström LO, Öberg B. Patient adherence in an individualized rehabilitation programme: a clinical follow-up. *Scand J Public Health.* 2005;33(1):11-18.

57. Reich W. *Character Analysis*, trans. VR Carfagno. New York, NY: Farrar, Straus and Giroux. 1972.

58. Scaer RC. *The Trauma Spectrum: Hidden Wounds and Human Resiliency.* New York, NY: WW Norton & Company; 2005.

59. Benoit D. *Attachment and Regulation Seminar.* Ottawa, ON: Algonquin College; November 2002.

60. American Psychiatric Association. *Diagnostic Criteria from DSM IV.* Washington, DC: American Psychiatric Association; 1994.

61. Wolf ES. *Treating the Self: Elements of Clinical Self Psychology.* New York, NY: The Guilford Press; 2002.

62. Seem M, Kaplan J. *Bodymind Energetics: Toward a Dynamic Model of Health.* Rochester, VT: Healing Arts Press; 1987.

63. Smith EWL. *The Body in Psychotherapy.* Jefferson, NC: McFarland & Co Inc Pub; 2000.

64. Mindell A, Sternback-Scott S, Goodman B. *Dreambody, the Body's Role in Revealing the Self.* Fort Collins, CO: Sigo Pr; 1982.

CHAPTER 3

References

1. Menard MB. *Making Sense of Research: A Guide to Research Literacy for Complementary Practitioners.* Toronto, ON: Curties-Overzet Publications Incorporated; 2003.

2. Eisenberg DM, Davis RB, Ettner SL, et al. Trends in alternative medicine use in the United States, 1990-1997. *JAMA.* 1998;280(18):1569-1575.

3. Ramsey SD, Spencer AC, Topolski TD, Belza B, Patrick DL. Use of alternative therapies by older adults with osteoarthritis. *Arthritis Care Res.* 2001;45(3):222-227.

4. Barnes PM, Bloom B, Nahin RL. Complementary and alternative medicine use among adults: United States, 2007. *Nat'l Health Stat Report,* 2008 Dec 10(12):1-23.

5. Esmail N. *Complementary and Alternative Medicine in Canada: Trends in Use and Public Attitudes, 1997-2006.* Vancouver: Fraser Institute; 2007.

6. Okoro CA, Zhao G, Li C, Balluz LS. Use of complementary and alternative medicine among USA adults with functional limitations: for treatment or general use? *Complement Ther Med.* 2011;19(4):208-15.

7. Ernst E. The safety of massage therapy. *Rheumatology.* 2003;42(9):1101-1106.

8. Ernst E, Pittler M, Wider B, Boddy K. Massage therapy: is its evidence-base getting stronger. *Complement Health Pract Rev.* 2007;12(3):179-183.

9. Creswell JW. *Research Design: Qualitative, Quantitative, and Mixed Methods Approaches.* Newbury Park, CA: Sage Publications, Inc; 2009.

10. Dryden T, Moyer CA. *Integrating Research in Clinical Practice.* Champaign, IL: Human Kinetics; 2012.

11. Sackett D, Straus S, Richardson W, Rosenberg W, Haynes R. *Evidence-Based Medicine: How to Practice and Teach EBM.* New York, NY: Churchill-Livingstone; 2000.

12. Straus SE, Glasziou P, Richardson SE, Haynes SE. *Evidence Based Medicine: How to Practice and Teach It.* New York, NY: Churchill Livingstone; 2010.

13. Greenhalgh T. How to read a paper. *BMJ.* 2001;322:3-5.

14. Finch PM. The evidence funnel: highlighting the importance of research literacy in the delivery of evidence informed complementary health care. *J Bodywork Movement Ther.* 2007;11(1):78-81.

15. London W. Clinical research in complementary therapies: principles, problems and solutions. *Focus Altern Complement Ther.* 2012;17(1):e3-e7.

16. Jonas WB. The evidence house: how to build an inclusive base for complementary medicine. *West J Med.* 2001;175(2):79.

17. Portney LG, Watkins MP. *Foundations of Clinical Research: Applications to Practice.* Norwalk, CT: Appleton & Lange; 1993.

18. Andrade CK, Clifford P. Qualitative research methods. In: Dryden T, Moyer CA, eds. *Massage Therapy: Integrating Research and Practice.* Champaign, IL: Human Kinetics; 2012;45-58.

19. Moyer CA, Goral K. Quantitative research methods. In: Dryden T, Moyer CA, eds. *Massage Therapy: Integrating Research and Practice.* Champaign, IL: Human Kinetics; 2012;31-44.

20. Lincoln Y, Guba E. *Naturalistic Inquiry.* Thousand Oaks, CA: Sage Publications; 1995.

21. Verhoef M. Mixed methods research. In: Dryden T, Moyer CA, eds. *Massage Therapy: Integrating Research and Practice.* Champaign, IL: Human Kinetics; 2012;59-70.

22. Guyatt G, Rennie D. *User's Guide to the Medical Literature: Essentials of Evidence-Based Clinical Practice.* Chicago, IL: American Medical Association; 2001.

23. Clifford P. Outcome based treatment planning for clients with cancer. *J Soft Tissue Manipulation.* 2003;11:3.

24. Groenewald T. A phenomenological research design illustrated. *Int J Qual Methods.* 2004;3(1):42-55.

25. Corbin JM, Strauss AL. *Basics of Qualitative Research: Techniques and Procedures for Developing Grounded Theory.* Thousand Oaks, CA: Sage Publications, Inc; 2008.

26. Preyde M. Effectiveness of massage therapy for subacute low-back pain: a randomized controlled trial. *Can Med Assoc J.* 2000;162(13):1815-1820.

27. Glaser BG, Strauss AL. *The Discovery of Grounded Theory: Strategies for Qualitative Research.* New Brunswick, NJ: Aldine; 2009.

28. Halcomb EJ, Andrew S, Brannen J. Introduction to mixed methods research. In: Andrew S, Halcomb EJ, eds. *Mixed Methods Research for Nursing and the Health Science.* Oxford: Wiley-Blackwell; 2009:13-30.

29. Boulanger KT, Moyer CA. Attitudes, beliefs, and expectations in massage therapy. In: Dryden T, Moyer CA, eds. *Massage Therapy: Integrating Research and Practice.* Champaign, IL: Human Kinetics; 2012.

30. Moyer CA, Rounds J. The attitudes toward massage (ATOM) scale: reliability, validity, and associated findings. *J Bodywork Movement Ther.* 2009;13(1):22-33.

31. Muncey T. Does mixed methods constitute a change in paradigm? In: Andrew S, Holcom E, eds. *Mixed Methods Research for Nursing and the Health Sciences.* West Sussex: Wiley-Blackwell; 2009.

32. Ritenbaugh C, Verhoef M, Fleishman S, Boon H, Leis A. Whole systems research: a discipline for studying complementary and alternative medicine. *Altern Ther Health Med.* 2003;9(4):32.

33. Glaros S. All evidence is not created equal: a discussion of levels of evidence. *PT Mag.* 2003;(11):42-52.

34. The Free Dictionary: Medical Dictionary Website. http://medical-dictionary.thefreedictionary.com/meta-analysis. Accessed November 20, 2011.

35. Gibbs LE. *Evidence-Based Practice for the Helping Professions: A Practical Guide with Integrated Multimedia,* Vol. 1. Pacific Grove, CA: Thomson Brooks/Cole; 2003:63.

36. Moyer CA, Rounds J, Hannum JW. A meta-analysis of massage therapy research. *Psychol Bull.* 2004;130(1):3.

37. Cherkin DC, Sherman KJ, Deyo RA, Shekelle PG. A review of the evidence for the effectiveness, safety, and cost of acupuncture, massage therapy, and spinal manipulation for back pain. *Ann Intern Med.* 2003;138(11):898-906.

38. Wilkinson S, Barnes K, Storey L. Massage for symptom relief in patients with cancer: systematic review. *J Adv Nurs.* 2008;63(5):430-439.

39. Haraldsson B, Gross A, Myers C, et al. Cervical overview group. Massage for mechanical neck disorders. *Cochrane Database Syst Rev.* 2006; Jul 19(3):CP004871.

40. Moraska A, Chandler C. Changes in clinical parameters in patients with tension-type headache following massage therapy: a pilot study. *J Man Manipulative Ther.* 2008;16(2):106.

41. Lawler SP, Cameron LD. A randomized, controlled trial of massage therapy as a treatment for migraine. *Ann Behav Med.* 2006;32(1):50-59.

42. Quinn C, Chandler C, Moraska A. Massage therapy and frequency of chronic tension headaches. *Am J Public Health.* 2002;92(10):1657.

43. Hernandez-Reif M, Dieter J, Field T, Swerdlow B, Diego M. Migraine headaches are reduced by massage therapy. *Int J Neurosci.* 1998;96(1-2):1-11.

44. Cherkin DC, Sherman KJ, Kahn J, et al. A comparison of the effects of 2 types of massage and usual care on chronic low back pain. *Ann Intern Med.* 2011;155(1):1.

45. Field T, Hernandez-Reif M, Diego M, Fraser M. Lower back pain and sleep disturbance are reduced following massage therapy. *J Bodywork Movement Ther.* 2007;11(2):141-145.

46. Tsao JCI. Effectiveness of massage therapy for chronic, non-malignant pain: a review. *Evid Based Complement Altern Med.* 2007;4(2):165-180.

47. Baskwill A, Kilty M, Hamilton A, Atkinson H. Massage therapy positively impacts quality of life for HIV+ individuals. *J Soft Tissue Manipulation.* 2003;11:4.

48. Furlan AD, Brosseau L, Imamura M, Irvin E. Massage for low-back pain: a systematic review within the framework of the Cochrane collaboration back review group. *Spine.* 2002;27(17):1896.

49. Bron C, De Gast A, Dommerholt J, Stegenga B, Wensing M, Oostendorp R. Treatment of myofascial trigger points in patients with chronic shoulder pain: a randomized, controlled trial. *BMC Med.* 2011;9(1):8.

50. Sherman KJ, Cherkin DC, Hawkes RJ, Miglioretti DL, Deyo RA. Randomized trial of therapeutic massage for chronic neck pain. *Clin J Pain.* 2009;25(3):233.

51. Field T, Diego M, Hernandez-Reif M, Shea J. Hand arthritis pain is reduced by massage therapy. *J Bodywork Movement Ther.* 2007;11(1):21-24.

52. Field T, Figueiredo B, Hernandez-Reif M, Diego M, Deeds O, Ascencio A. Massage therapy reduces pain in pregnant women, alleviates prenatal depression in both parents and improves their relationships. *J Bodywork Movement Ther.* 2008;12(2):146-150.

53. Post-White J, Fitzgerald M, Savik K, Hooke MC, Hannahan AB, Sencer SF. Massage therapy for children with cancer. *J Pediatr Oncol Nurs.* 2009;26(1):16-28.

54. Jane SW, Wilkie DJ, Gallucci BB, Beaton RD, Huang HY. Effects of a full-body massage on pain intensity, anxiety, and physiological relaxation in Taiwanese patients with metastatic bone pain: a pilot study. *J Pain Symptom Manage.* 2009;37(4):754-763.

55. Cunningham JE, Kelechi T, Sterba K, Barthelemy N, Falkowski P, Chin SH. Case report of a patient with chemotherapy-induced peripheral neuropathy treated with manual therapy (massage). *Support Care Cancer.* 2011:19(9):1473-6.

56. Lee A, Holdsworth M, Holland A, Button B. The immediate effect of musculoskeletal physiotherapy techniques and massage on pain and ease of breathing in adults with cystic fibrosis. *J Cyst Fibros.* 2009;8(1):79-81.

57. Furlan AD, Imamura M, Dryden T, Irvin E. Massage for low back pain: an updated systematic review within the framework of the Cochrane back review group. *Spine.* 2009;34(16):1669.

58. Little P, Lewith G, Webley F, et al. Randomised controlled trial of Alexander technique lessons, exercise, and massage (ATEAM) for chronic and recurrent back pain. *Br J Sports Med.* 2008;42(12):965-968.

59. Franke A, Gebauer S, Franke K, Brockow T. Acupuncture massage vs Swedish massage and individual exercise vs group exercise in low back pain sufferers—a randomized controlled clinical trial in a 2 × 2 factorial design. *Forsch Komplementarmed Klass Naturheilkd.* 2000;7(6):286-293.

60. Geisser ME, Wiggert EA, Haig AJ, Colwell MO. A randomized, controlled trial of manual therapy and specific adjuvant exercise for chronic low back pain. *Clin J Pain.* 2005;21(6):463.

61. Hanley J, Stirling P, Brown C. Randomised controlled trial of therapeutic massage in the management of stress. *Br J Gen Pract.* 2003;53(486):20.

62. Field T, Pickens J, Prodromidis M, et al. Targeting adolescent mothers with depressive symptoms for early intervention. *Adolescence.* 2000;35(138):381-414.

63. Field T, Diego M, Hernandez-Reif M, Schanberg S, Kuhn C. Massage therapy effects on depressed pregnant women. *J Psychosom Obstet Gynecol.* 2004;25(2):115-122.

64. Bost N, Wallis M. The effectiveness of a 15 minute weekly massage in reducing physical and psychological stress in nurses. *Aust J Adv Nurs.* 2006;23(4):28-33.

65. Moyer CA. Anxiety and depression. In: Dryden T, Moyer CA, eds. *Massage Therapy: Integrating Research and Practice.* Champaign, IL: Human Kinetics; 2012;151-165.

66. Wilkie DJ, Kampbell J, Cutshall S, et al. Effects of massage on pain intensity, analgesics and quality of life in patients with cancer pain: a pilot study of a randomized clinical trial conducted within hospice care delivery. *Hosp J.* 2000;15(3):31-53.

67. Weinrich SP, Weinrich MC. The effect of massage on pain in cancer patients. *Appl Nurs Res.* 1990;3(4):140-145.

68. Cassileth BR, Vickers AJ. Massage therapy for symptom control: outcome study at a major cancer center. *J Pain Symptom Manage.* 2004;28(3):244-249.

69. Grealish L, Lomasney A, Whiteman B. Foot massage: a nursing intervention to modify the distressing symptoms of pain and nausea in patients hospitalized with cancer. *Cancer Nurs.* 2000;23(3):237.

70. Kutner JS, Smith MC, Corbin L, et al. Massage therapy versus simple touch to improve pain and mood in patients with advanced cancer. *Ann Intern Med.* 2008;149(6):369-379.

71. Myers CD, Walton T, Small BJ. The value of massage therapy in cancer care. *Hematol Oncol Clin North Am.* 2008;22(4):649-660.

72. Billhult A, Bergbom I, Stener-Victorin E. Massage relieves nausea in women with breast cancer who are undergoing chemotherapy. *J Altern Complement Med.* 2007;13(1):53-58.

73. Billhult A, Stener-Victorin E, Bergbom I. The experience of massage during chemotherapy treatment in breast cancer patients. *Clin Nurs Res.* 2007;16(2):85-99.

74. Kohara H, Miyauchi T, Suehiro Y, Ueoka H, Takeyama H, Morita T. Combined modality treatment of aromatherapy, footsoak, and reflexology relieves fatigue in patients with cancer. *J Palliat Med.* 2004;7(6):791-796.

75. Post-White J, Kinney ME, Savik K, Gau JB, Wilcox C, Lerner I. Therapeutic massage and healing touch improve symptoms in cancer. *Integr Cancer Ther.* 2003;2(4):332.

76. Rexilius SJ, Mundt C, Erickson Megel M, Agrawal S. Therapeutic effects of massage therapy and handling touch on caregivers of patients undergoing autologous hematopoietic stem cell transplant. *Oncol Nurs Forum.* 2002;29(E35):E35.

77. Stucki MOG. Physical therapy in the treatment of fibromyalgia. *Scand J Rheumatol.* 2000;29(113):78-85.

78. Field T, Quintino O, Henteleff T, Wells-Keife L, Delvecchio-Feinberg G. Job stress reduction therapies. *Altern Ther Health Med.* 1997;3(4):54.

79. McNeely ML, Magee DJ, Lees AW, Bagnall KM, Haykowsky M, Hanson J. The addition of manual lymph drainage to compression therapy for breast cancer related lymphedema: a randomized controlled trial. *Breast Cancer Res Treat.* 2004;86(2):95-106.

80. Harris S, Hugi M, Olivotto I, Levine M. Steering committee for clinical practice guidelines for the care and treatment of breast cancer. Clinical practice guidelines for the care and treatment of breast cancer: 11. Lymphedema. *CMAJ.* 2001;164(2):191-199.

81. Andersen L, Højris I, Erlandsen M, Andersen J. Treatment of breast-cancer-related lymphedema with or without manual lymphatic drainage: a randomized study. *Acta Oncol.* 2000;39(3):399-405.

82. Preston N, Seers K, Mortimer P. Physical therapies for reducing and controlling lymphoedema of the limbs. *Cochrane Database Syst Rev.* 2004;Oct 18;(4) CD003141.

83. Johansson K, Albertsson M, Ingvar C, Ekdahl C. Effects of compression bandaging with or without manual lymph drainage treatment in patients with postoperative arm lymphedema. *Lymphology.* 1999;32(3):103-110.

84. Hernandez-Reif M, Field T, Krasnegor J, Theakston H. Lower back pain is reduced and range of motion increased after massage therapy. *Int J Neurosci.* 2001;106(3-4):131-145.

85. Field T, Diego M, Cullen C, Hernandez-Reif M, Sunshine W, Douglas S. Fibromyalgia pain and substance P decrease and sleep improves after massage therapy. *JCR: J Clin Rheumatol.* 2002;8(2):72.

86. Smith MC, Kemp J, Hemphill L, Vojir CP. Outcomes of therapeutic massage for hospitalized cancer patients. *J Nurs Sch.* 2002;34(3):257-262.

87. Escalona A, Field T, Singer-Strunck R, Cullen C, Hartshorn K. Brief report: improvements in the behavior of children with autism following massage therapy. *J Autism Dev Disord.* 2001;31(5):513-516.

88. Tsay SL, Rong JR, Lin PF. Acupoints massage in improving the quality of sleep and quality of life in patients with end-stage renal disease. *J Adv Nurs.* 2003;42(2):134-142.

89. Field T, Hernandez-Reif M, Diego M, Feijo L, Vera Y, Gil K. Massage therapy by parents improves early growth and development. *Infant Behav Dev.* 2004;27(4):435-442.

90. Williams A, Vadgama A, Franks P, Mortimer PS. A randomized controlled crossover study of manual lymphatic drainage therapy in women with breast cancer-related lymphoedema. *Eur J Cancer Care.* 2002;11(4):254-261.

91. Cullen LA, Barlow JH. A training and support programme for caregivers of children with disabilities: an exploratory study. *Patient Educ Couns.* 2004;55(2):203-209.

92. Field T. Massage and aroma therapy. *Int J Cosmetic Sci.* 2004;26(3):169-170.

93. Shen P. Two hundred cases of insomnia treated by otopoint pressure plus acupuncture. *J Tradit Chin Med.* 2004;24(3):168-169.

94. Soden K, Vincent K, Craske S, Lucas C, Ashley S. A randomized controlled trial of aromatherapy massage in a hospice setting. *Palliat Med.* 2004;18(2):87-92.

95. Weze C, Leathard HL, Stevens G. Evaluation of healing by gentle touch for the treatment of musculoskeletal disorders. *Am J Public Health.* 2004;94(1):50.

96. Dieter JNI, Field T, Hernandez-Reif M, Emory EK, Redzepi M. Stable preterm infants gain more weight and sleep less after five days of massage therapy. *J Pediatr Psychol.* 2003;28(6):403.

97. Wang XH, Yuan YD, Wang BF. Clinical observation on effect of auricular acupoint pressing in treating sleep apnea syndrome. *Zhongguo Zhong Xi Yi Jie He Za Zhi.* 2003;23(10):747-749.

98. Barlow J, Cullen L. Increasing touch between parents and children with disabilities: Preliminary results from a new programme. *J Fam Health Care.* 2002;12(1):7-9.

99. Ferber SG, Laudon M, Kuint J, Weller A, Zisapel N. Massage therapy by mothers enhances the adjustment of circadian rhythms to the nocturnal period in full-term infants. *J Dev Behav Pediatr.* 2002;23(6):410.

100. Field T. Massage therapy. *Med Clin North Am.* 2002;86(1):163-171.

101. Hernandez-Reif M, Field T, Largie S, et al. Parkinson's disease symptoms are differentially affected by massage therapy vs. progressive muscle relaxation: a pilot study. *J Bodywork Movement Ther.* 2002;6(3):177-182.

102. Tsay SL, Chen ML. Acupressure and quality of sleep in patients with end-stage renal disease—a randomized controlled trial. *Int J Nurs Stud.* 2003;40(1):1-7.

103. Agarwal KN, Gupta A, Pushkarna R, Bhargava SK, Faridi MM, Prabhu MK. Effects of massage and use of oil on growth, blood flow and sleep pattern in infants. *Indian J Med Res.* 2000;112:212-217.

104. Deng G, Cassileth BR, Yeung KS. Complementary therapies for cancer-related symptoms. *J Support Oncol.* 2004;2(5):419.

105. Ironson G, Field T, Scafidi F, et al. Massage therapy is associated with enhancement of the immune system's cytotoxic capacity. *Int J Neurosci.* 1996;84(1-4):205-217.

106. Cassar M. The application of massage in psychogenic disorders. *Positive Health.* 2004:45. www.positivehealth.com/article/massage/the.application.of.massage.in.psychogenic.diorders. Accessed August, 2012.

107. Richards K, Nagel C, Markie M, Elwell J, Barone C. Use of complementary and alternative therapies to promote sleep in critically ill patients. *Crit Care Nurs Clin North Am.* 2003;15(3):329-340.

108. Cho YC, Tsay SL. The effect of acupressure with massage on fatigue and depression in patients with end-stage renal disease. *J Nurs Res: JNR.* 2004;12(1):51.

109. Yang JH. The effects of foot reflexology on nausea, vomiting and fatigue of breast cancer patients undergoing chemotherapy. *Taehan Kanho Hakhoe Chi.* 2005;35(1):177-185.

110. Sefton JEM, Yarar C, Berry JW, Pascoe DD. Therapeutic massage of the neck and shoulders produces changes in peripheral blood flow when assessed with dynamic infrared thermography. *J Altern Complement Med.* 2010;16(7):723-732.

111. Shoemaker JK, Tiidus PM, Mader R. Failure of manual massage to alter limb blood flow: measures by Doppler ultrasound. *Med Sci Sports Exerc.* 1997;29(5):610.

112. Tiidus P, Shoemaker J. Effleurage massage, muscle blood flow and long-term post-exercise strength recovery. *Int J Sports Med.* 1995;16(7):478-483.

113. Sabir'ianov AR, Sabir'ianova ES, Epishev VV. Trends in variability of the central blood circulation in healthy individuals in response to massage of the collar cervical region. *Vopr Kurortol Fizioter Lech Fiz Kult.* 2004;(6):13-15.

114. Liu Y, Xu S, Yan J, et al. Capillary blood flow with dynamical change of tissue pressure caused by exterior force. *Sheng Wu Yi Xue Gong Cheng Xue Za Zhi.* 2004;21(5):699-703.

115. Tsarev AI, Ezhova VA, Kunitsyna LA, Slovesnov SV, Chukreeva LN, Kolesnikova EI. Aromamassage of the cervical collar region in the combined treatment of patients with atherosclerotic dyscirculatory encephalopathy. *Vopr Kurortol Fizioter Lech Fiz Kult.* 2004 Sep-Oct (5): 6-7.

116. Drust B, Atkinson G, Gregson W, French D, Binningsley D. The effects of massage on intra muscular temperature in the vastus lateralis in humans. *Int J Sports Med.* 2003;24(6): 395-399.

117. Sabir'ianov AR, Shevtsov AV, Sabir'ianova ES, et al. Effect of reflex-segmental massage on central hemodynamics in healthy people. *Vopr Kurortol Fizioter Lech Fiz Kult.* 2004 Mar-Apr (2): 5-7.

118. Prilutsky B. Medical massage and control of arterial hypertension: a pilot study. *Massage Bodywork.* 2003. www.massage and bodywork.com/articles/AugSep2003/medicalmassage.html. Accessed August, 2012.

119. Varekojis SM, Herbert Douce F, Flucke RL, et al. A comparison of the therapeutic effectiveness of and preference for postural drainage and percussion, intrapulmonary percussive ventilation, and high-frequency chest wall compression in hospitalized cystic fibrosis patients. *Respir Care.* 2003;48(1):24-28.

120. Oermann CM, Sockrider MM, Giles D, Sontag MK, Accurso FJ, Castile RG. Comparison of high-frequency chest wall oscillation and oscillating positive expiratory pressure in the home management of cystic fibrosis: a pilot study*. *Pediatr Pulmonol.* 2001;32(5):372-377.

121. Fink JB. Positioning versus postural drainage. *Respir Care.* 2002;47(7):769-777.

122. Maa SH, Sun MF, Hsu KH, et al. Effect of acupuncture or acupressure on quality of life of patients with chronic obstructive asthma: a pilot study. *J Altern Complement Med.* 2003;9(5):659-670.

123. Hess DR. The evidence for secretion clearance techniques. *Respir Care.* 2001;46(11):1276-1293.

124. Abdel Fattah M, Hamdy B. Pulmonary functions of children with asthma improve following massage therapy. *J Altern Complement Med.* 2011;17(11): 1065-1068.

125. Kosfeld M, Heinrichs M, Zak PJ, Fischbacher U, Fehr E. Oxytocin increases trust in humans. *Nature.* 2005;435(7042): 673-676.

126. Morhenn VB, Park JW, Piper E, Zak PJ. Monetary sacrifice among strangers is mediated by endogenous oxytocin release after physical contact. *Evol Hum Behav.* 2008;29(6): 375-383.

127. Shor-Posner G, Hernandez-Reif M, Miguez MJ, et al. Impact of a massage therapy clinical trial on immune status in young Dominican children infected with HIV-1. *J Altern Complement Med.* 2006;12(6):511-516.

128. Boylan M. Massage boosts immunity in breast cancer patients. *J Aust Tradit Med Soc.* 2005;11(2):59.

129. Hernandez-Reif M, Ironson G, Field T, et al. Breast cancer patients have improved immune and neuroendocrine functions following massage therapy. *J Psychosom Res.* 2004;57(1):45-52.

130. Shor-Posner G, Miguez MJ, Hernandez-Reif M, Perez-Then E, Fletcher M. Massage treatment in HIV-1 infected Dominican children: a preliminary report on the efficacy of massage therapy to preserve the immune system in children without antiretroviral medication. *J Altern Complement Med.* 2004;10(6):1093-1095.

131. Goodfellow LM. The effects of therapeutic back massage on psychophysiologic variables and immune function in spouses of patients with cancer. *Nurs Res.* 2003;52(5):318.

132. Lovas JM, Craig AR, Segal YD, Raison RL, Weston KM, Markus MR. The effects of massage therapy on the human immune response in healthy adults. *J Bodywork Movement Ther.* 2002;6(3):143-150.

133. Diego MA, Field T, Hernandez-Reif M, Shaw K, Friedman L, Ironson G. HIV adolescents show improved immune function following massage therapy. *Int J Neurosci.* 2001;106(1-2):35-45.

134. Field T, Cullen C, Diego M, et al. Leukemia immune changes following massage therapy. *J Bodywork Movement Ther.* 2001;5(4):271-274.

135. Birk TJ, McGrady A, MacArthur RD, Khuder S. The effects of massage therapy alone and in combination with other complementary therapies on immune system measures and quality of life in human immunodeficiency virus. *J Altern Complement Med.* 2000;6(5):405-414.

136. Field T, Hernandez-Reif M, Diego M, Schanberg S, Kuhn C. Cortisol decreases and serotonin and dopamine increase following massage therapy. *Int J Neurosci.* 2005;115(10):1397-1413.

137. Hernandez-Reif M, Field T, Krasnegor J, Hossain Z, Theakston H, Burman I. High blood pressure and associated symptoms were reduced by massage therapy. *J Bodywork Movement Ther.* 2000;4(1):31-38.

138. Hart S, Field T, Hernandez-Reif M, et al. Anorexia nervosa symptoms are reduced by massage therapy. *Eat Disord.* 2001;9(4):289-299.

139. McRee LD, Noble S, Pasvogel A. Using massage and music therapy to improve postoperative outcomes. *AORN.* 2003;78(3):433-447.

140. Taylor AG, Galper DI, Taylor P, et al. Effects of adjunctive Swedish massage and vibration therapy on short-term postoperative outcomes: a randomized, controlled trial. *J Altern Complement Med.* 2003;9(1):77-89.

141. Okvat HA, Oz MC, Ting W, Namerow PB. Massage therapy for patients undergoing cardiac catheterization. *Altern Ther Health Med.* 2002;8(3):68-70, 72, 74-75.

142. Simons D, Mense S. Understanding and measurement of muscle tone as related to clinical muscle pain. *Pain.* 1998;75(1):1-17.

143. Hernandez-Reif M, Field T, Largie S, et al. Cerebral palsy symptoms in children decreased following massage therapy. *Early Child Dev Care.* 2005;175(5):445-456.

144. Duval C, Lafontaine D, Hébert J, Leroux A, Panisset M, Boucher JP. The effect of Trager therapy on the level of evoked stretch responses in patients with Parkinson's disease and rigidity. *JMPT-J Manipulative Physiol Ther.* 2002;25(7): 455-464.

145. Siev-Ner I, Gamus D, Lerner-Geva L, Zaidel S, Achiron A. Reflexology treatment relieves symptoms of multiple sclerosis: a randomized controlled study. *Mult Scler.* 2003(9):356-361.

146. CONSORT. CONSORT statement. Consolidated Standards of Reporting Trials Web Site. http://www.consort-statement.org/. Accessed 2012.

147. Benjamin BE, Piltch C. Ben Benjamin's corner. Massage therapists need to embrace research. *Massage Ther J.* 2005(44):32-35.

148. Cassidy C. Methodological issues in investigations of massage/bodywork therapy. Part IV: experimental research designs. *J Bodywork Movement Ther.* 2003;7(4):240-250.

149. Cassidy C. Methodological issues in investigations of massage/bodywork therapy. Part II: making research designs and data credible: model fit validity, combining scientific soundness with the explanatory model of massage and bodywork therapies. *J Bodywork Movement Ther.* 2003;7(2):71-79.

150. Cassidy C. Methodological issues in investigations of massage/bodywork therapy. Part I. *J Bodywork Movement Ther.* 2003;7(1):2-10.

151. Cassidy CM, Hart JA. Methodological issues in investigations of massage/bodywork therapy: part III: qualitative and quantitative designs for MBT and the bias of interpretation. *J Bodywork Movement Ther.* 2003;7(3):136-141.

152. Hymel GM. Integrating research competencies in massage therapy education. *J Bodywork Movement Ther.* 2005;9(1): 43-51.

153. Hymel GM. Advancing massage therapy research competencies: dimensions for thought and action. *J Bodywork Movement Ther.* 2003;7(3):194-199.

154. Richardson J. Developing and evaluating complementary therapy services: part 1. Establishing service provision through the use of evidence and consensus development. *J Altern Complement Med.* 2001;7(3):253-260.

155. Stuttard P. Working in partnership to develop evidence-based practice within the massage profession. *Complement Ther Nurs Midwifery.* 2002;8(4):185-190.

156. American Physical Therapy Association. *Guide to Physical Therapist Practice.* 2nd ed. Alexandria, VA: American Physical Therapy Association; 1999.

157. Fellowes D, Barnes K, Wilkinson S. Aromatherapy and massage for symptom relief in patients with cancer. *Cochrane Database Syst Rev.* 2004;(2): CD002287.

158. Domholdt EA, Malone TR. Evaluating research literature: the educated clinician. *Phys Ther.* 1985;65(4):487-491.

CHAPTER 4

References

1. World Health Organization. *Towards a Common Language for Functioning, Disability and Health: ICF—The International Classification of Functioning, Disability and Health.* Geneva: World Health Organization; 2002.

2. World Health Organization. *ICF Checklist.* Geneva: World Health Organization; 2001.

3. Childs JD, Whitman JM, Sizer PS, Pugia ML, Flynn TW, Delitto A. A description of physical therapists' knowledge in managing musculoskeletal conditions. *BMC Musculoskelet Disord.* 2005;6(1):32.

4. Chaitow L. *Palpation and Assessment Skills: Assessment and Diagnosis Through Touch.* Edinburgh: Churchill-Livingston; 2003.

5. Casterline MR. Trail guide to the body: how to locate muscles, bones and more. *J Athl Train.* 1998;33(3):284.

6. Protopapas M, Cymet T. Musculoskeletal examination: a complete review. *Compr Ther.* 2005;31(1):12-20.

7. Field D. Field's anatomy, palpation and surface markings. *Recherche.* 2006;67:02.

8. Lewit K. Soft tissue and relaxation techniques in myofascial pain. In: Hamer WI, ed. *Functional Soft Tissue Examination and Treatment by Manual Methods: New Perspectives.* 2nd ed. Gaithersburg, MD: Aspen; 1999:479-532.

9. Greenman PE, Greenman PE. *Principles of Manual Medicine.* Vol. 572. Baltimore, MD: Williams & Wilkins; 1996.

10. Starkey C, Ryan JL, Ryan JL. *Evaluation of Orthopedic and Athletic Injuries.* Philadelphia, PA: FA Davis Company; 1996.

11. McKenzie AM, Taylor NF. Can physiotherapists locate lumbar spinal levels by palpation? *Physiotherapy.* 1997;83(5):235-239.

12. Najm W, Seffinger M, Mishra S, et al. Content validity of manual spinal palpatory exams—a systematic review. *BMC Complement Altern Med.* 2003;3(1):1.

13. Humphreys BK, Delahaye M, Peterson CK. An investigation into the validity of cervical spine motion palpation using subjects with congenital block vertebrae as a "gold standard". *BMC Musculoskelet Disord.* 2004;5(1):19.

14. Abbott JH, McCane B, Herbison P, Moginie G, Chapple C, Hogarty T. Lumbar segmental instability: a criterion-related validity study of manual therapy assessment. *BMC Musculoskelet Disord.* 2005;6(1):56.

15. Keating J, Matyas TA, Bach TM. The effect of training on physical therapists' ability to apply specified forces of palpation. *Phys Ther.* 1993;73(1):38-46.

16. Fritz S, ed. *Fundamentals of Therapeutic Massage.* St Louis, MO: Mosby-Lifeline; 1995.

17. Downey B, Taylor N, Niere K. Manipulative physiotherapists can reliably palpate nominated lumbar spinal levels. *Man Ther.* 1999;4(3):151-156.

18. Latimer J, Adams R, Lee M. Training with feedback improves judgements of non-biological linear elastic stiffness. *Man Ther.* 1998;3(2):85-89.

19. American Physical Therapy Association. *Guide to Physical Therapist Practice.* 2nd ed. Alexandria, VA: American Physical Therapy Association; 1999.

20. Nicholson L, Adams R, Maher C. Reliability of a discrimination measure for judgements of non-biological stiffness. *Man Ther.* 1997;2(3):150-156.

21. Simons DG, Travell JG, Simons LS. *Myofascial Pain and Dysfunction: The Trigger Point Manual: Lower Half of Body.* Vol. 2. Baltimore, MD: Williams & Wilkins; 1999.

22. DiGiovanna EL, Schiowitz S, Dowling DJ. *An Osteopathic Approach to Diagnosis and Treatment.* Philadelphia, PA: Lippincott Williams & Wilkins; 2004.

23. Cantu RI, Grodin AJ. *Myofascial Manipulation: Theory and Clinical Application.* 2nd ed. Gaithersburg, MD: Aspen Pub; 2001.

24. Thompson JS, Akesson EJ, Loeb JA, Wilson-Pauwels L. *Thompson's Core Textbook of Anatomy.* Philadelphia, PA: Lippincott Williams & Wilkins; 1990.

25. Magee DJ. *Orthopedic Physical Assessment.* 5th ed. Philadelphia, PA: WB Saunders; 2005.

26. Hoppenfeld S, Hutton R, Thomas H. *Physical Examination of the Spine and Extremities.* New York, NY: Appleton-Century-Crofts; 1976.

27. Hertling D, Kessler RM. *Management of Common Musculoskeletal Disorders: Physical Therapy Principles and Methods.* 4th ed. Philadelphia, PA: Lippincott Williams & Wilkins; 2006.

28. Faber W. Assessment of skin temperature by palpation in leprosy patients: interobserver reliability and correlation with infrared thermometry. *Int J Lepr.* 2000;68(1):65-67.

29. Oerlemans HM, Perez RSGM, Oostendorp RAB, Goris RJA. Objective and subjective assessments of temperature differences between the hands in reflex sympathetic dystrophy. *Clin Rehabil.* 1999;13(5):430-438.

30. Murff RT, Armstrong DG, Lanctot D, Lavery LA, Athanasiou KA. How effective is manual palpation in detecting subtle temperature differences? *Clin Podiatr Med Surg.* 1998;15(1):151-154.

31. Lederman E. *The Science and Practice of Manual Therapy.* 2nd ed. Edinburgh: Elsevier/Churchill Livingstone; 2005.

32. Colby LA, Kisner C. *Therapeutic Exercise: Foundations and Techniques.* 5th ed. Philadelphia, PA: FA Davis; 2007.

33. de Domenico G, Wood EC. *Beard's Massage.* 4th ed. Philadelphia, PA: WB Saunders; 1997.

34. Simons DG, Travell J, Simons LS. *Myofascial Pain and Dysfunction: The Trigger Point Manual: Upper Half of Body.* Vol. 1. Baltimore, MD: Williams & Wilkins; 1999.

35. Cox NH. Palpation of the skin—an important issue. *JRSM.* 2006;99(12):598-600.

36. Lynette Inscoe E, Witt PL, Gross MT, Mitchell RU. Reliability in evaluating passive intervertebral motion of the lumbar spine. *J Man Manipulative Ther.* 1995;3(4):135-143.

37. Scott RW. *Legal, Ethical, and Practical Aspects of Patient Care Documentation: A Guide for Rehabilitation Professionals.* 4th ed. Burlington, MA: Jones & Bartlett Learning; 2011.

38. Stedman TL. *Stedman's Medical Dictionary.* 28th ed. Baltimore, MD: Lippincott Williams & Wilkins; 2005.

39. Grindel S. Evidence based medicine in the musculoskeletal examination. *Br J Sports Med.* 1998;32(4):278-279.

40. Riegger-Krugh C, Keysor JJ. Skeletal malalignments of the lower quarter: correlated and compensatory motions and postures. *J Orthop Sports Phys Ther.* 1996;23(2):164-170.

41. Dunk NM, Lalonde J, Callaghan JP. Implications for the use of postural analysis as a clinical diagnostic tool: reliability of quantifying upright standing spinal postures from photographic images. *J Manipulative Physiol Ther.* 2005;28(6):386-392.

42. Champain N, Dupuis R, Pomero V, Mouilleseaux B, Dubousset J, Skalli W. Geometric and postural analysis of mild idiopathic scoliotic patients. *Stud Health Technol Inform.* 2002;91:267-271.

43. Dunk NM, Chung YY, Sullivan Compton D, Callaghan JP. The reliability of quantifying upright standing postures as a baseline diagnostic clinical tool. *J Manipulative Physiol Ther.* 2004;27(2):91-96.

44. Seegert E, Shapiro R. From the field-effects of alternative exercise on posture. *Clin Kinesiol.* 1999;53:41-47.

45. Grimmer K. An investigation of poor cervical resting posture. *Aust J Physiother.* 1997;43(1):7-16.

46. Villanueva MBG, Jonai H, Sotoyama M, Takeuchi Y, Saito S. Sitting posture and neck and shoulder muscle activities at different screen height settings of the visual display terminal. *Ind Health.* 1997;35:330-336.

47. Harrison AL, Barry-Greb T, Wojtowicz G. Clinical measurement of head and shoulder posture variables. *J Orthop Sports Phys Ther.* 1996;23(6):353-361.

48. Franklin ME, Chenier TC, Brauninger L, Cook H, Harris S. Effect of positive heel inclination on posture. *J Orthop Sports Phys Ther.* 1995;21(2):94-99.

49. Harrison DE, Harrison DD, Troyanovich SJ. Reliability of spinal displacement analysis of plain X-rays: a review of commonly accepted facts and fallacies with implications for chiropractic education and technique. *J Manipulative Physiol Ther.* 1998;21(4):252.

50. Tuck A, Peterson C. Accuracy and reliability of chiropractors and Anglo-European College of Chiropractic students at visually estimating the lumbar lordosis from radiographs. *Chiropr Tech.* 1998;10:19-26.

51. Capodaglio EM, Capodaglio P, Panigazzi M, Bazzini G. An ergonomic study of postures of toll collectors. *G Ital Med Lav Ergon.* 1998;20(1):24-30.

52. Novak CB, Mackinnon SE. Repetitive use and static postures: a source of nerve compression and pain. *J Hand Ther.* 1997;10(2):151-159.

53. Christensen HW. Precision and accuracy of an electrogoniometer. *J Manipulative Physiol Ther.* 1999;22(1):10-14.

54. Tsunoda K. Height loss caused by bent posture: A risk factor for stroke from ENT clinic-is it time to reconsider the physical examination? *Acta Otolaryngol.* 2011;131(10):1079-1085.

55. Conti PBM, Sakano E, Ribeiro MÂGO, Schivinski CIS, Ribeiro JD. Assessment of the body posture of mouth-breathing children and adolescents. *J Pediatr.* 2011;87(4):357-363.

56. Silva AG, Punt TD, Johnson MI. Reliability and validity of head posture assessment by observation and a four-category scale. *Man Ther.* 2010;15(5):490-495.

57. Sweeting K, Mock M. Gait and posture: assessment in general practice. *Aust Fam Physician.* 2007;36(6):398-405.

58. Sutherland C, Albert W, Wrigley A, Callaghan J. The effect of camera viewing angle on posture assessment repeatability and cumulative spinal loading. *Ergonomics.* 2007;50(6):877-889.

59. Albuquerque Baltar J, Brasileiro Santos Mdo S, Justino da Silva H. Does asthma promote changes in static posture? Systematic review. *Rev Port Pneumol.* 2010;16(3):471-476.

60. Fortin C, Ehrmann Feldman D, Cheriet F, Labelle H. Clinical methods for quantifying body segment posture: a literature review. *Disabil Rehabil.* 2011;33(5):367-383.

61. Hammer W. The use of transverse friction massage in the management of chronic bursitis of the hip or shoulder. *J Manipulative Physiol Ther.* 1993;16(2):107.

62. Antonaci F, Sand T, Lucas G. Pressure algometry in healthy subjects: interexaminer variability. *Scand J Rehabil Med.* 1998;30(1):3-8.

63. Tillman LJ, Hanks JE. Wound healing: injury and repair of dense connective tissues. In: Hertling D, Kessler RM, eds. *Management of Common Musculoskeletal Conditions.* 4th ed. Philadelphia, PA: Lippincott Williams & Wilkins; 2006:15-26.

64. Junger M, Steins A, Zuder D, Klyscz T. Physical therapy of venous diseases. *Vasa.* 1998;27(2):73-79.

65. Ogilvie-Harris D, Myerthall S. The diabetic frozen shoulder: arthroscopic release. *Arthroscopy.* 1997;13(1):1-8.

66. Capsulitis A. Adhesive capsulitis: a sticky issue. *Am Fam Physician.* 1999;59(7):1843-1850.

67. Gam A, Schydlowsky P, Rossel I, Remvig L, Jensen E. Treatment of "frozen shoulder" with distension and glucorticoid compared with glucorticoid alone: a randomised controlled trial. *Scand J Rheumatol.* 1998;27(6):425-430.

68. Schenk TJ, Brems JJ. Multidirectional instability of the shoulder: pathophysiology, diagnosis, and management. *J Am Acad Orthop Surg.* 1998;6(1):65-72.

69. Baker CL Jr, Merkley MS. Clinical evaluation of the athlete's shoulder. *J Athl Train.* 2000;35(3):256.

70. Cornelissen BP, Rijkenhuizen AB, van den Hoogen BM, Rutten VP, Barneveld A. Experimental model of synovitis/capsulitis in the equine metacarpophalangeal joint. *Am J Vet Res.* 1998;59(8):978-985.

71. Sevier TL, Wilson JK. Treating lateral epicondylitis. *Sports Med.* 1999;28(5):375-380.

72. Barozzi L, Olivieri I, De Matteis M, Padula A, Pavlica P. Seronegative spondyloarthropathies: imaging of spondylitis, enthesitis and dactylitis. *Eur J Radiol.* 1998;27:S12-S17.

73. Coari G, Paoletti F, Iagnocco A. Shoulder involvement in rheumatic diseases. Sonographic findings. *J Rheumatol.* 1999;26(3):668-673.

74. Hjelm R, Draper C, Spencer S. Anterior-inferior capsular length insufficiency in the painful shoulder. *J Orthop Sports Phys Ther.* 1996;23(3):216-222.

75. Rozzi SL, Lephart SM, Gear WS, Fu FH. Knee joint laxity and neuromuscular characteristics of male and female soccer and basketball players. *Am J Sports Med.* 1999;27(3):312-319.

76. Messina DF, Farney WC, DeLee JC. The incidence of injury in Texas high school basketball. *Am J Sports Med.* 1999;27(3):294-299.

77. Lindsay Harris N. Physical diagnosis of collateral ligament and combined ligament injuries. *Oper Tech Sports Med.* 1996;4(3):148-157.

78. Cyriax J, Coldham M. *Textbook of Orthopedic Medicine Volume 2. Treatment by Manipulation, Massage and Injection.* 11th ed. London: Bailliere Tindall; 1984.

79. Fritz JM, Delitto A, Erhard RE, Roman M. An examination of the selective tissue tension scheme, with evidence for the concept of a capsular pattern of the knee. *Phys Ther.* 1998;78(10):1046-1056.

80. Pellecchia G, Paolino J, Connell J. Intertester reliability of the Cyriax evaluation in assessing patients with shoulder pain. *J Orthop Sports Phys Ther.* 1996;23(1):34.

81. Wilk K, Andrews J, Arrigo C. The physical examination of the glenohumeral joint: emphasis on the stabilizing structures. *J Orthop Sports Phys Ther.* 1997;25(6):380.

82. Blevins FT. Rotator cuff pathology in athletes. *Sports Med.* 1997;24(3): 205-220.

83. van Dijk CN, Mol BWJ, Lim LSL, Marti RK, Bossuyt PMM. Diagnosis of ligament rupture of the ankle joint: physical examination, arthrography, stress radiography and sonography compared in 160 patients after inversion trauma. *Acta Orthop.* 1996;67(6):566-570.

84. Dias R, Cutts S, Massoud S. Frozen shoulder. *BMJ.* 2005;331(7530): 1453-1456.

85. Blakey CM, Field MH, Singh PJ, Tayar R, Field RE. Secondary capsular laxity of the hip. *Hip Int.* 2010;20(4):497-504.

86. Ng AWH, Chu C, Lo W, Lai Y, Kam C. Assessment of capsular laxity in patients with recurrent anterior shoulder dislocation using MRI. *Am J Roentgenol.* 2009;192(6):1690-1695.

87. Ivancic PC, Ito S, Tominaga Y, et al. Whiplash causes increased laxity of cervical capsular ligament. *Clin Biomech.* 2008;23(2):159-165.

88. Dewing CB, McCormick F, Bell SJ, et al. An analysis of capsular area in patients with anterior, posterior, and multidirectional shoulder instability. *Am J Sports Med.* 2008;36(3):515-522.

89. Mense S, Simons DG, Russell IJ. *Muscle Pain: Understanding Its Nature, Diagnosis, and Treatment.* Baltimore, MD: Lippincott Williams & Wilkins; 2001.

90. White DJ. Musculoskeletal assessment. In: O'Sullivan SB, Schmitz TJ, eds. *Physical Rehabilitation.* 6th ed. Philadelphia, PA: FA Davis Company; 2006:101-133.

91. Norkin W. *Measurement of Joint Motion: A Guide to Goniometry.* 3rd ed. Philadelphia, PA: FA Davis Company; 2009.

92. Gilliam J, Barstow IK. Joint range of motion. In: Van Deusen J, Brunt D, eds. *Assessment in Occupational Therapy and Physical Therapy.* Philadelphia, PA: WB Saunders; 1997.

93. MacDermid JC, Chesworth BM, Patterson S, Roth JH. Intratester and intertester reliability of goniometric measurement of passive lateral shoulder rotation. *J Hand Ther.* 1999;12(3):187-192.

94. Thoms V, Rome K. Effect of subject position on the reliability of measurement of active ankle joint dorsiflexion. *The Foot.* 1997;7(3):153-158.

95. Bruton A, Ellis B, Goddard J. Comparison of visual estimation and goniometry for assessment of metacarpophalangeal joint angle. *Physiotherapy.* 1999;85(4):201-208.

96. Somers DL, Hanson JA, Kedzierski CM, Nestor KL, Quinlivan KY. The influence of experience on the reliability of goniometric and visual measurement of forefoot position. *J Orthop Sports Phys Ther.* 1997;25(3):192-202.

97. Meyer DC, Werner CML, Wyss T, Vienne P. A mechanical equinometer to measure the range of motion of the ankle joint: interobserver and intraobserver reliability. *Foot Ankle Int.* 2006;27(3):202-205.

98. Ellis B, Bruton A, Goddard JR. Joint angle measurement: a comparative study of the reliability of goniometry and wire tracing for the hand. *Clin Rehabil.* 1997;11(4):314-320.

99. Neumann DA, Rowan EE. *Kinesiology of the Musculoskeletal System: Foundations for Physical Rehabilitation.* Philadelphia, PA: Mosby; 2002.

100. O'Sullivan SB, Schmitz TJ. *Physical Rehabilitation: Assessment and Treatment.* 6th ed. Philadelphia, PA: FA Davis; 2006.

101. Gajdosik RL. Comparison and reliability of three goniometric methods for measuring forearm supination and pronation. *Percept Mot Skills.* 2001;93(2): 353-355.

102. Flowers KR, Stephens-Chisar J, LaStayo P, Galante BL. Intrarater reliability of a new method and instrumentation for measuring passive supination and pronation: a preliminary study. *J Hand Ther.* 2001;14(1):30-35.

103. Brosseau L, Balmer S, Tousignant M, et al. Intra- and intertester reliability and criterion validity of the parallelogram and universal goniometers for measuring maximum active knee flexion and extension of patients with knee restrictions. *Arch Phys Med Rehabil.* 2001;82(3):396-402.

104. Ellis B, Bruton A. A study to compare the reliability of composite finger flexion with goniometry for measurement of range of motion in the hand. *Clin Rehabil.* 2002;16(5):562-570.

105. Menadue C, Raymond J, Kilbreath S, Refshauge K, Adams R. Reliability of two goniometric methods of measuring active inversion and eversion range of motion at the ankle. *BMC Musculoskelet Disord.* 2006;7(1):60.

106. Stam HJ, Ardon MS, den Ouden AC, Schreuders TA, Roebroeck ME. The compangle: a new goniometer for joint angle measurements of the hand. A technical note. *Eura Medicophys.* 2006;42(1):37-40.

107. Holm I, Bolstad B, Lütken T, Ervik A, Røkkum M, Steen H. Reliability of goniometric measurements and visual estimates of hip ROM in patients with osteoarthrosis. *Physiother Res Int.* 2000;5(4):241-248.

108. Chiu H, Su F. The motion analysis system and the maximal area of fingertip motion: a preliminary report. *J Hand Surg [Br].* 1996;21(5):604-608.

109. Friedrichsen K. The validity and reliability of a two-dimensional computer-assisted video gait analysis system. *Diss Abstr Int.* 1995;33(6):1863.

110. Mueller MJ, Norton BJ. Reliability of kinematic measurements of rear-foot motion. *Phys Ther.* 1992;72(10):731.

111. Maulucci R, Eckhouse R. A technique for measuring clothed range of joint motion. *J Appl Biomech.* 1997;13:316-333.

112. Williams GN, Gangel TJ, Arciero RA, Uhorchak JM, Taylor DC. Comparison of the single assessment numeric evaluation method and two shoulder rating scales. *Am J Sports Med.* 1999;27(2):214-221.

113. Love S, Gringmuth R, Kazemi M, Cornacchia P, Schmolke M. Interexaminer and intraexaminer reliability of cervical passive range of motion using the CROM and Cybex 320 EDI. *J Can Chiropractic Assoc.* 1998;42(4):222.

114. Barrett C, Singer K, Day R. Assessment of combined movements of the lumbar spine in asymptomatic and low back pain subjects using a three-dimensional electromagnetic tracking system. *Man Ther.* 1999;4(2):94-99.

115. Nitschke JE, Nattrass CL, Disler PB, Chou MJ, Ooi KT. Reliability of the American Medical Association guides' model for measuring spinal range of motion: its implication for whole-person impairment rating. *Spine.* 1999;24(3):262.

116. Evans K, Refshauge KM, Adams R. Measurement of active rotation in standing: reliability of a simple test protocol. *Percept Mot Skills.* 2006;103(2): 619-628.

117. Ng JKF, Kippers V, Richardson CA, Parnianpour M. Range of motion and lordosis of the lumbar spine: reliability of measurement and normative values. *Spine.* 2001;26(1):53.

118. Troke M, Moore A, Cheek E. Reliability of the OSI CA 6000 spine motion analyzer with a new skin fixation system when used on the thoracic spine. *Man Ther.* 1998;3(1):27-33.

119. Harrison DE, Haas JW, Cailliet R, Harrison DD, Holland B, Janik TJ. Concurrent validity of flexicurve instrument measurements: sagittal skin contour of the cervical spine compared with lateral cervical radiographic measurements. *J Manipulative Physiol Ther.* 2005;28(8):597-603.

120. Piva SR, Erhard RE, Childs JD, Hicks G, Al-Abdulmohsin H. Reliability of measuring iliac crest level in the standing and sitting position using a new measurement device. *J Manipulative Physiol Ther.* 2003;26(7):437-441.

121. Viitanen J, Kokko ML, Heikkilä S, Kautiainen H. Assessment of thoracolumbar rotation in ankylosing spondylitis: a simple tape method. *Clin Rheumatol.* 1999;18(2):152-157.

122. Hresko MT, Mesiha M, Richards K, Zurakowski D. A comparison of methods for measuring spinal motion in female patients with adolescent idiopathic scoliosis. *J Pediatr Orthop.* 2006;26(6):758.

123. Morphett AL, Crawford CM, Lee D. The use of electromagnetic tracking technology for measurement of passive cervical range of motion: a pilot study. *J Manipulative Physiol Ther.* 2003;26(3):152-159.

124. Hagins M, Brown M, Cook C, et al. Intratester and intertester reliability of the palpation meter (PALM) in measuring pelvic position. *J Man Manipulative Ther.* 1998;6(3):130-136.

125. Kaltenborn F. *Manual Mobilization of the Joints: The Extremities.* Minneapolis, MN: Orthopedic Physical Therapy Products; 2002.

126. Fjellner A, Bexander C, Faleij R, Strender LE. Interexaminer reliability in physical examination of the cervical spine. *J Manipulative Physiol Ther.* 1999;22(8):511-516.

127. Ellem D. Assessment of the wrist, hand and finger complex. *J Man Manipulative Ther.* 1995;3(1):9-14.

128. Olson KA, Paris SV, Spohr C, Gorniak G. Radiographic assessment and reliability study of the craniovertebral sidebending test. *J Man Manipulative Ther.* 1998;6(2):87-96.

129. Huber FE, Irrgang JJ, Harner C, Lephart S. Intratester and intertester reliability of the KT-1000 arthrometer in the assessment of posterior laxity of the knee. *Am J Sports Med.* 1997;25(4):479-485.

130. Malanga GA, Andrus S, Nadler SF, McLean J. Physical examination of the knee: a review of the original test description and scientific validity of common orthopedic tests. *Arch Phys Med Rehabil.* 2003;84(4):592-603.

131. Bauer BA, Cutshall SM, Wentworth LJ, et al. Effect of massage therapy on pain, anxiety, and tension after cardiac surgery: a randomized study. *Complement Ther Clin Pract.* 2010;16(2):70-75.

132. Lakhani E, Nook B, Haas M, Docrat A. Motion palpation used as a postmanipulation assessment tool for monitoring end-feel improvement: a randomized controlled trial of test responsiveness. *J Manipulative Physiol Ther.* 2009;32(7):549-555.

133. Haneline MT, Cooperstein R, Young M, Birkeland K. Spinal motion palpation: a comparison of studies that assessed intersegmental end feel vs excursion. *J Manipulative Physiol Ther.* 2008;31(8):616-626.

134. Haneline M, Cooperstein R, Young M, Birkeland K. An annotated bibliography of spinal motion palpation reliability studies. *J Can Chiropractic Assoc.* 2009;53(1):40.

135. van de Pol RJ, van Trijffel E, Lucas C. Inter-rater reliability for measurement of passive physiological range of motion of upper extremity joints is better if instruments are used: a systematic review. *J Physiother.* 2010;56(1):7-17.

136. Gatt A, Chockalingam N. Clinical assessment of ankle joint dorsiflexion. *J Am Podiatr Med Assoc.* 2011;101(1):59-69.

137. van Trijffel E, van de Pol RJ, Oostendorp R, Lucas C. Interrater reliability for measurement of passive physiological movements in lower extremity joints is generally low: a systematic review. *J Physiother.* 2010;56(4):223-235.

138. Bozic PR, Pazin NR, Berjan BB, Planic NM, Cuk ID. Evaluation of the field tests of flexibility of the lower extremity: reliability and the concurrent and factorial validity. *J Strength Cond Res.* 2010;24(9):2523.

139. Araújo CGS. Flexibility assessment: normative values for flexitest from 5 to 91 years of age. *Arq Bras Cardiol.* 2008;90(4):280-287.

140. Zchezewski JE. Improving flexibility. In: Scully RM, Barnes MR, eds. *Physical Therapy.* Philadelphia, PA: Lippincott Company; 1989.

141. Simons D, Mense S. Understanding and measurement of muscle tone as related to clinical muscle pain. *Pain.* 1998;75(1):1-17.

142. Santi MD, Botte MJ. Volkmann's ischemic contracture of the foot and ankle: evaluation and treatment of established deformity. *Foot Ankle Int.* 1995;16(6):368-377.

143. O'Dwyer N, Ada L, Neilson P. Spasticity and muscle contracture following stroke. *Brain.* 1996;119(5):1737-1749.

144. Niamane R, Birouk N, Benomar A, et al. Rigid spine syndrome. Two case-reports. *Rev Rhum Engl Ed.* 1999;66(6):347-350.

145. Noonan TJ, Garrett WE Jr. Muscle strain injury: diagnosis and treatment. *J Am Acad Orthop Surg.* 1999;7(4):262-269.

146. Almekinders LC. Tendinitis and other chronic tendinopathies. *J Am Acad Orthop Surg.* 1998;6(3):157-164.

147. Khan KM, Cook JL, Bonar F, Harcourt P, Astrom M. Histopathology of common tendinopathies: update and implications for clinical management. *Sports Med.* 1999;27(6):393-408.

148. Fredriksen H, Dagfinrud H, Jacobsen V, Maehlum S. Passive knee extension test to measure hamstring muscle tightness. *Scand J Med Sci Sports.* 1997;7(5):279-282.

149. Jones CJ, Rikli RE, Max J, Noffal G. The reliability and validity of a chair sit-and-reach test as a measure of hamstring flexibility in older adults. *Res Q Exerc Sport.* 1998;69:338-343.

150. Tyler TF, Roy T, Nicholas SJ, Gleim GW. Reliability and validity of a new method of measuring posterior shoulder tightness. *J Orthop Sports Phys Ther.* 1999;29(5):262.

151. Scully RM, Barnes MR. *Physical Therapy.* Philadelphia, PA: J. B. Lippincott Company; 1989.

152. Reese N. Use of an inclinometer to measure flexibility of the iliotibial band using the Ober test and the modified Ober test: differences in magnitude and reliability of measurements. *J Orthop Sports Phys Ther.* 2003;33:326-330.

153. Reid DA, McNair PJ. Passive force, angle, and stiffness changes after stretching of hamstring muscles. *Med Sci Sports Exerc.* 2004;36(11):1944.

154. Cornbleet SL, Woolsey NB. Assessment of hamstring muscle length in school-aged children using the sit-and-reach test and the inclinometer measure of hip joint angle. *Phys Ther.* 1996;76(8):850-855.

155. Allison GT, Weston R, Shaw R, et al. The reliability of quadriceps muscle stiffness in individuals with Osgood-Schlatter disease. *J Sport Rehab.* 1998;7:258-266.

156. Siems JJ, Breur GJ, Blevins WE, Cornell KK. Use of two-dimensional real-time ultrasonography for diagnosing contracture and strain of the infraspinatus muscle in a dog. *J Am Vet Med Assoc.* 1998;212(1):77-80.

157. Rothenberger A, Huther G. The role of psychosocial stress in childhood for structural and functional brain development: neurobiological basis of developmental psychopathology. *Prax Kinderpsychol Kinderpsychiatr.* 1997;46(9):623-644.

158. Diniz DHMP, Schor N, Blay SL. Stressful life events and painful recurrent colic of renal lithiasis. *J Urol.* 2006;176(6):2483-2487.

159. Savoia MG, Bernik M. Adverse life events and coping skills in panic disorder. *Revista do Hospital das Clínicas.* 2004;59(6):337-340.

160. Clarke D, Singh R. Life events, stress appraisals, and hospital doctors' mental health. *N Z Med J.* 2004;117(1204):U1121.

161. Holmes TH, Rahe RH. The social readjustment rating scale. *J Psychosom Res.* 1967;11:213-218.

162. Lazarus RS, Folkman S. *Manual for the Hassles and Uplifts Scales.* Palo Alto, CA: Consulting Psychologists Press; 1989.

163. Folkman S, Lazarus RS. *Ways of Coping Questionnaire Research Edition.* Palo Alto, CA: Consulting Psychologists Press; 1988.

164. Spies RA, Plake BS. *The Sixteenth Mental Measurements Yearbook.* Lincoln, NE: Buros Institute of Mental Measurements; 2005.

165. Ermis MN, Yıldırım D, Durakbasa MO, Tamam C, Ermis OE. Medial superior cluneal nerve entrapment neuropathy in military personnel; diagnosis and etiologic factors. *J Back Musculoskelet Rehabil.* 2011;24(3):137-144.

166. Rha D, Shin JC, Kim YK, Jung JH, Kim YU, Lee SC. Detecting local twitch responses of myofascial trigger points in the lower-back muscles using ultrasonography. *Arch Phys Med Rehabil.* 2011;92(10):1576-1580.

167. Grogono B. Textbook of orthopedic medicine. Vol. 1. Diagnosis of soft tissue lesions. *Can Med Assoc J.* 1976;115(1):26.

168. Ferber R, Kendall KD, Farr L. Changes in knee biomechanics after a hip-abductor strengthening protocol for runners with patellofemoral pain syndrome. *Journal of Athletic Training.* 2011;46(2):142-149.

169. Knepler C, Richard WB. Subjectivity of forces associated with manual-muscle test grades of 3, 4-and 4. *Percept Mot Skills.* 1998;87(3f):1123-1128.

170. Jain M, Smith M, Cintas H, et al. Intra-rater and inter-rater reliability of the 10-point manual muscle test (MMT) of strength in children with juvenile idiopathic inflammatory myopathies (JIIM). *Phys Occup Ther Pediatr.* 2006;26(3):5-17.

171. Fournier K, Bourbonnais D, Bravo G, Arsenault J, Harris P, Gravel D. Reliability and validity of pinch and thumb strength measurements in de Quervain's disease. *J Hand Ther.* 2006;19(1):2-11.

172. Li RC, Jasiewicz JM, Middleton J, et al. The development, validity, and reliability of a manual muscle testing device with integrated limb position sensors. *Arch Phys Med Rehabil.* 2006;87(3):411-417.

173. Hogrel JY, Ollivier G, Desnuelle C. Manual and quantitative muscle testing in neuromuscular disorders. How to assess the consistency of strength measurements in clinical trials? *Rev Neurol (Paris).* 2006;162(4):427-436.

174. Krause DA, Schlagel SJ, Stember BM, Zoetewey JE, Hollman JH. Influence of lever arm and stabilization on measures of hip abduction and adduction torque obtained by hand-held dynamometry. *Arch Phys Med Rehabil.* 2007;88(1):37-42.

175. Ladeira CE, Hess LW, Galin BM, Fradera S, Harkness MA. Validation of an abdominal muscle strength test with dynamometry. *J Strength Cond Res.* 2005;19(4):925.

176. Burns SP, Spanier DE. Break-technique handheld dynamometry: relation between angular velocity and strength measurements. *Arch Phys Med Rehabil.* 2005;86(7):1420-1426.

177. Bohannon WB. Internal consistency of manual muscle testing scores. *Percept Mot Skills.* 1997;85(2):736-738.

178. Bohannon RW. Manual muscle testing: does it meet the standards of an adequate screening test? *Clin Rehabil.* 2005;19(6):662-667.

179. Bohannon WB. Research incorporating hand-held dynamometry: publication trends since 1948. *Percept Mot Skills.* 1998;86(3c):1177-1178.

180. Reinking MF, Bockrath-Pugliese K, Worrell T, Kegerreis RL, Miller-Sayers K, Farr J. Assessment of quadriceps muscle performance by hand-held, isometric, and isokinetic dynamometry in patients with knee dysfunction. *J Orthop Sports Phys Ther.* 1996;24(3):154-159.

181. Risberg M, Holm I, Tjomsland O, Ljunggren E, Ekeland A. Prospective study of changes in impairments and disabilities after anterior cruciate ligament reconstruction. *J Orthop Sports Phys Ther.* 1999;29(7):400.

182. Binder-Macleod SA, Lee SCK, Fritz AD, Kucharski LJ. New look at force-frequency relationship of human skeletal muscle: effects of fatigue. *J Neurophysiol.* 1998;79(4):1858-1868.

183. Wilkerson G, Pinerola J, Caturano R. Invertor vs. evertor peak torque and power deficiencies associated with lateral ankle ligament injury. *J Orthop Sports Phys Ther.* 1997;26(2):78.

184. Whitcomb LJ, Kelley MJ, Leiper CI. A comparison of torque production during dynamic strength testing of shoulder abduction in the coronal plane and the plane of the scapula. *J Orthop Sports Phys Ther.* 1995;21(4):227-232.

185. Bridgewater KJ, Sharpe MH. Trunk muscle performance in early Parkinson's disease. *Phys Ther.* 1998;78(6):566-576.

186. Shirley LF, Caroline WJ, Scott MH. Effect of work glove and type of muscle action on grip fatigue. *Ergonomics.* 1997;40(6):601-612.

187. Möller M, Lind K, Styf J, Karlsson J. The reliability of isokinetic testing of the ankle joint and a heel-raise test for endurance. *Knee Surg Sports Traumatol Arthrosc.* 2005;13(1):60-71.

188. Wang SS, Normile SO, Lawshe BT. Reliability and smallest detectable change determination for serratus anterior muscle strength and endurance tests. *Physiother Theory Pract.* 2006;22(1):33-42.

189. Kaegi C, Thibault MC, Giroux F, Bourbonnais D. The interrater reliability of force measurements using a modified sphygmomanometer in elderly subjects. *Phys Ther.* 1998;78(10):1095-1103.

190. Sherrington C, Lord SR. Reliability of simple portable tests of physical performance in older people after hip fracture. *Clin Rehabil.* 2005;19(5):496-504.

191. Perell K, Gregor R, Scremin A. Lower limb cycling mechanics in subjects with unilateral cerebrovascular accidents. *J Appl Biomech.* 1998;14:158-179.

192. Bohannon RW. Alternatives for measuring knee extension strength of the elderly at home. *Clin Rehabil.* 1998;12(5):434-440.

193. Roberts HC, Denison HJ, Martin HJ, et al. A review of the measurement of grip strength in clinical and epidemiological studies: towards a standardised approach. *Age Ageing.* 2011;40(4):423-429.

194. Thorborg K, Petersen J, Magnusson S, Hölmich P. Clinical assessment of hip strength using a hand-held dynamometer is reliable. *Scand J Med Sci Sports.* 2010;20(3):493-501.

195. Rashid T, Ostermann RF. Strength-based assessment in clinical practice. *J Clin Psychol.* 2009;65(5):488-498.

196. Shalev AY, Bloch M, Peri T, Bonne O. Alprazolam reduces response to loud tones in panic disorder but not in posttraumatic stress disorder. *Biol Psychiatry.* 1998;44(1):64-68.

197. Smith LK, Weiss EL, Lehmkuhl LD. *Brunnstrom's Clin Kinesiol.* 5th ed. Philadelphia, PA: FA Davis Company; 1996.

198. Maruyama K. Connectin, an elastic protein of striated muscle. *Biophys Chem.* 1994;50(1-2):73-85.

199. Prado LG, Makarenko I, Andresen C, Krüger M, Opitz CA, Linke WA. Isoform diversity of giant proteins in relation to passive and active contractile properties of rabbit skeletal muscles. *J Gen Physiol.* 2005;126(5):461-480.

200. Campbell K, Lakie M. A cross-bridge mechanism can explain the thixotropic short-range elastic component of relaxed frog skeletal muscle. *J Physiol (Lond).* 1998;510(3):941-962.

201. O'Sullivan SB. Strategies to improve motor learning and motor control. In: O'Sullivan SB, Schmitz TJ, eds. *Physical Rehabilitation.* 6th ed. Philadelphia, PA: FA Davis Company; 2006:363-411.

202. Katavich L. Neural mechanisms underlying manual cervical traction. *J Man Manipulative Ther.* 1999;7(1):20-25.

203. Katavich L. Differential effects of spinal manipulative therapy on acute and chronic muscle spasm: a proposal for mechanisms and efficacy. *Man Ther.* 1998;3(3):132-139.

204. Kovac C, Krapf M, Ettlin T, Mennet P, Stratz T, Muller W. Methods for detection of changes in muscle tonus. *Z Rheumatol.* 1994;53(1):26-36.

205. Dvořák J. Epidemiology, physical examination, and neurodiagnostics. *Spine.* 1998;23(24):2663.

206. Walsh EG. *Muscles, Masses and Motion: The Physiology of Normality, Hypertonicity, Spasticity and Rigidity.* Vol. 125. London: Mac Kieth Press; 1992.

207. Hill D. Tension due to interaction between the sliding filaments in resting striated muscle. The effect of stimulation. *J Physiol (Lond).* 1968;199(3):637-684.

208. Masi AT, Hannon JC. Human resting muscle tone (HRMT): narrative introduction and modern concepts. *J Bodywork Movement Ther.* 2008;12(4):320-332.

209. Masi AT, Nair K, Evans T, Ghandour Y. Clinical, biomechanical, and physiological translational interpretations of human resting myofascial tone or tension. *Int J Ther Massage Bodywork.* 2010;3(4):16.

210. Reynolds R, Lakie M. Postmovement changes in the frequency and amplitude of physiological tremor despite unchanged neural output. *J Neurophysiol.* 2010;104(4):2020-2023.

211. Svensson P. Muscle pain in the head: overlap between temporomandibular disorders and tension-type headaches. *Curr Opin Neurol.* 2007;20(3):320.

212. Pluess M, Conrad A, Wilhelm FH. Muscle tension in generalized anxiety disorder: a critical review of the literature. *J Anxiety Disord.* 2009;23(1):1-11.

213. Snider KT, Snider EJ, Degenhardt BF, Johnson JC, Kribs JW. Palpatory accuracy of lumbar spinous processes using multiple bony landmarks. *J Manipulative Physiol Ther.* 2011;34(5):306-313.

214. Petrone MR, Guinn J, Reddin A, Sutlive TG, Flynn TW, Garber MP. The accuracy of the palpation meter (PALM) for measuring pelvic crest height difference and leg length discrepancy. *J Orthop Sports Phys Ther.* 2003;33(6):319-325.

215. Rolfe I. *Rolfing: The Integration of Human Structure.* New York, NY: Harper & Row; 1977.

216. Chaitow L, DeLany J. *Modern Neuromuscular Techniques.* 2nd ed. New York, NY: Churchill Livingstone; 2003.

217. Mannheim CJ. *The Myofascial Release Manual.* 3rd ed. Thorofare, NJ: Slack Inc; 2001.

218. Sucher BM. Thoracic outlet syndrome—a myofascial variant: part 1. Pathology and diagnosis. *J Am Osteopath Assoc.* 1990;90(8):686-686.

219. Sucher B, Heath D. Thoracic outlet syndrome—a myofascial variant: part 3. Structural and postural considerations. *J Am Osteopath Assoc.* 1993;93(3):334-334.

220. Boyling JD, Jull G. *Grieve's Modern Manual Therapy: The Vertebral Column.* 3rd ed. New York, NY: Churchill Livingstone; 2005.

221. Cisler T. Whiplash as a total-body injury. *J Am Osteopath Assoc.* 1994;94(2):145-145.

222. Hanten WP, Chandler SD. Effects of myofascial release leg pull and sagittal plane isometric contract-relax techniques on passive straight-leg raise angle. *J Orthop Sports Phys Ther.* 1994;20(3):138-144.

223. Drape JL, Silbermann-Hoffman O, Houvet P, et al. Complications of flexor tendon repair in the hand: MR imaging assessment. *Radiology.* 1996;198(1):219-224.

224. Tillman LJ, Chasan N, eds. Properties of dense connective tissue. In: Hertling D, Kessler RM, eds. *Management of Common Musculoskeletal Conditions.* 4th ed. Philadelphia, PA: Lippincott Williams & Wilkins; 2006.

225. Tillman LJ, Cummings GS. Biologic mechanisms of connective tissue mutability. In: Currier DP, Nelson M, ed. *Dynamics of Human Biologic Tissues.* Philadelphia, PA: FA Davis; 1992:44.

226. Hertling D. Friction massage. In: Kessler RM, Hertling D, eds. *Management of common musculoskeletal conditions. 4th ed.* Philadelphia, PA: Lippincott Williams & Wilkins; 2006.

227. Hammer WI. Friction massage. In: Hammer WI, ed. *Functional Soft Tissue Examination and Treatment by Manual Methods.* 2nd ed. Gaithersburg, MD: Aspen; 1999:463-478.

228. Palastanga N. The use of transverse frictions for soft tissue lesions. In: Grieve GP, ed. *Grieve's Modern Manual Therapy for the Vertebral Column.* New York, NY: Churchill-Livingston; 1986:819-825.

229. Brosseau L, Casimiro L, Milne S, et al. Deep transverse friction massage for treating tendinitis. *Cochrane Database Syst Rev.* 2002;4:CD003528.

230. Cyriax JH, Cyriax P. *Cyriax's Illustrated Manual of Orthopaedic Medicine.* 2nd ed. Stoneham, MA: Butterworth-Heineman; 1993.

231. Cyriax J. Deep massage. *Physiotherapy.* 1977;63(2):60-61.

232. Fernández-de-las-Peñas C, Alonso-Blanco C, Fernández-Carnero J, Carlos Miangolarra-Page J. The immediate effect of ischemic compression technique and transverse friction massage on tenderness of active and latent myofascial trigger points: a pilot study. *J Bodywork Movement Ther.* 2006;10(1):3-9.

233. Lazarus RS. Toward better research on stress and coping. *Am Psychol.* 2000;55:665-673.

234. Lutgendorf SK, Costanzo ES. Psychoneuroimmunology and health psychology: an integrative model. *Brain Behav Immun.* 2003;17(4):225-232.

235. Berczi I. The stress concept and neuroimmunoregulation in modern biology. *Ann N Y Acad Sci.* 1998;851(1):3-12.

236. Szabo S. Hans Selye and the development of the stress concept: special reference to gastroduodenal ulcerogenesis. *Ann N Y Acad Sci.* 1998;851(1):19-27.

237. Sarafino EP. *Health Psychology: Biopsychosocial Interactions .* New York, NY: Wiley; 1990.

238. Rozanski A, Blumenthal JA, Kaplan J. Impact of psychological factors on the pathogenesis of cardiovascular disease and implications for therapy. *Circulation.* 1999;99(16):2192-2217.

239. Fuchs E, Flügge G. Stress, glucocorticoids and structural plasticity of the hippocampus. *Neurosci Biobehav Rev.* 1998;23(2):295-300.

240. Wilbert-Lampen U, Trapp A, Modrzik M, Fiedler B, Straube F, Plasse A. Effects of corticotropin-releasing hormone (CRH) on endothelin-1 and NO release, mediated by CRH receptor subtype R2: a potential link between stress and endothelial dysfunction? *J Psychosom Res.* 2006;61(4):453-460.

241. Oei N, Everaerd W, Elzinga B, Van Well S, Bermond B. Psychosocial stress impairs working memory at high loads: an association with cortisol levels and memory retrieval. *Stress.* 2006;9(3):133-141.

242. Steptoe A, Donald AE, O'Donnell K, Marmot M, Deanfield JE. Delayed blood pressure recovery after psychological stress is associated with carotid intima-media thickness. *Arterioscler Thromb Vasc Biol.* 2006;26(11):2547-2551.

243. Jansen LMC, Gispen-de Wied CC, Wiegant VM, Westenberg HGM, Lahuis BE, van Engeland H. Autonomic and neuroendocrine responses to a psychosocial stressor in adults with autistic spectrum disorder. *J Autism Dev Disord.* 2006;36(7):891-899.

244. Elsenbruch S, Lucas A, Holtmann G, et al. Public speaking stress-induced neuroendocrine responses and circulating immune cell redistribution in irritable bowel syndrome. *Am J Gastroenterol.* 2006;101(10):2300-2307.

245. Duncko R, Makatsori A, Fickova E, Selko D, Jezova D. Altered coordination of the neuroendocrine response during psychosocial stress in subjects with high trait anxiety. *Prog Neuro-Psychopharmacol Biol Psychiatry.* 2006;30(6):1058-1066.

246. Keltikangas-Järvinen L, Ravaja N, Räikkönen K, Hautanen A, Adlercreutz H. Relationships between the pituitary-adrenal hormones, insulin, and glucose in middle-aged men: moderating influence of psychosocial stress. *Metab Clin Exp.* 1998;47(12):1440-1449.

247. Sanders K, Bruce N. A prospective study of psychosocial stress and fertility in women. *Hum Reprod.* 1997;12(10):2324-2329.

248. Axtelius B, Söderfeldt B, Edwardsson S, Attström R. Therapy-resistant periodontitis (I). clinical and treatment characteristics. *J Clin Periodontol.* 1997;24(9):640-645.

249. Ohl F, Fuchs E. Differential effects of chronic stress on memory processes in the tree shrew. *Cogn Brain Res.* 1999;7(3):379-387.

250. Bennett SJ, Puntenney PJ, Walker NL, Ashley ND. Development of an instrument to measure threat related to cardiac events. *Nurs Res.* 1996;45(5):266.

251. Rief W, Shaw R, Fichter MM. Elevated levels of psychophysiological arousal and cortisol in patients with somatization syndrome. *Psychosom Med.* 1998;60(2):198-203.

252. Stones A, Groome D, Perry D, Hucklebridge F, Evans P. The effect of stress on salivary cortisol in panic disorder patients. *J Affect Disord.* 1999;52(1-3): 197-201.

253. Eller NH, Netterstrøm B, Hansen ÅM. Psychosocial factors at home and at work and levels of salivary cortisol. *Biol Psychol.* 2006;73(3):280-287.

254. Rohleder N, Wolf JM, Herpfer I, Fiebich BL, Kirschbaum C, Lieb K. No response of plasma substance P, but delayed increase of interleukin-1 receptor antagonist to acute psychosocial stress. *Life Sci.* 2006;78(26):3082-3089.

255. Koo-Loeb JH, Pedersen C, Girdler SS. Blunted cardiovascular and catecholamine stress reactivity in women with bulimia nervosa. *Psychiatry Res.* 1998;80(1):13-27.

256. Demaree HA, Harrison DW. Physiological and neuropsychological correlates of hostility. *Neuropsychologia.* 1997;35(10):1405-1411.

257. Dahlgren A, Kecklund G, Akerstedt T. Overtime work and its effects on sleep, sleepiness, cortisol and blood pressure in an experimental field study. *Scand J Work Environ Health.* 2006;32(4):318-327.

258. Davis PA, Holm JE, Myers TC, Suda KT. Stress, headache, and physiological dysregulation: a time-series analysis of stress in the laboratory. *Headache.* 1998;38(2):116-121.

259. Artinian NT, Washington OGM, Flack JM, Hockman EM, Jen KLC. Depression, stress, and blood pressure in urban African-American women. *Prog Cardiovasc Nurs.* 2006;21(2):68-75.

260. Podbevsek D. Hyperlipidemia with disseminated eruptive xanthomas and hyperglycemia caused by mental stress—a case report. *Lijec Vjesn.* 2005;127(9-10):220-223.

261. Wilhelm FH, Roth WT. Acute and delayed effects of alprazolam on flight phobics during exposure. *Behav Res Ther.* 1997;35(9):831-841.

262. Schneider RH, Nidich SI, Salerno JW, et al. Lower lipid peroxide levels in practitioners of the transcendental meditation program. *Psychosom Med.* 1998;60(1):38-41.

263. Anderzén I, Arnetz BB. Psychophysiological reactions to international adjustment. *Psychother Psychosom.* 1999;68(2):67-75.

264. Schuck P. Glycated hemoglobin as a physiological measure of stress and its relations to some psychological stress indicators. *Behav Med.* 1998;24(2):89-94.

265. Spies RA, Carlson JF, Geisinger KF, eds. *The Eighteenth Mental Measurements Yearbook.* Lincoln, NE: Buros Institute of Mental Measurements; 2010.

266. Merskey H, Bogduk N. ISAP subcommittee on taxonomy, classification of chronic pain. *Pain.* 1994:S1-S226.

267. Ballantyne JC, Fishman SM, Abdi S. Massachusetts general hospital: handbook of pain management. *Recherche.* 2005;67:02.

268. Woolf CJ, Salter MW. Neuronal plasticity: increasing the gain in pain. *Science.* 2000;288(5472):1765-1768.

269. Johannes CB, Le TK, Zhou X, Johnston JA, Dworkin RH. The prevalence of chronic pain in United States adults: results of an internet-based survey. *J Pain.* 2010;11(11):1230-1239.

270. Backonja MM. Defining neuropathic pain. *Anesth Analg.* 2003;97(3): 785-790.

271. Kidd B, Urban L. Mechanisms of inflammatory pain. *Br J Anaesth.* 2001;87(1): 3-11.

272. Heitz NA, Eisenman PA, Beck CL, Walker JA. Hormonal changes throughout the menstrual cycle and increased anterior cruciate ligament laxity in females. *J Athl Train.* 1999;34(2):144.

273. Von Baeyer CL. Children's self-reports of pain intensity: scale selection, limitations and interpretation. *Pain Res Manage.* 2006;11(3):157.

274. Heck JF, Sparano JM. A classification system for the assessment of lumbar pain in athletes. *J Athl Train.* 2000;35(2):204.

275. Main CJ, de C Williams AC. Musculoskeletal pain. *BMJ.* 2002;325(7363): 534-537.

276. Goddard G, Karibe H, McNeill C. Reproducibility of visual analog scale (VAS) pain scores to mechanical pressure. *J Craniomandibular Pract.* 2004;22(3): 250-266.

277. Main C, Watson P. Psychological aspects of pain. *Man Ther.* 1999;4(4): 203-215.

278. Puttick MPE. Rheumatology: 11. Evaluation of the patient with pain all over. *Can Med Assoc J.* 2001;164(2):223-227.

279. Laslett M, McDonald B, Tropp H, Aprill C, Öberg B. Agreement between diagnoses reached by clinical examination and available reference standards: a prospective study of 216 patients with lumbopelvic pain. *BMC Musculoskelet Disord.* 2005;6(1):28.

280. Koes B, Van Tulder M, Thomas S. Diagnosis and treatment of low back pain. *BMJ.* 2006;332(7555):1430-1434.

281. Chaplin ER. Chronic pain and the injured worker: A sociobiological problem. In: Kasdan ML, ed. *Occupational hand and upper extremity injuries and diseases;* 1991:13-45.

282. Simon JM. Chronic pain syndrome: nursing assessment and intervention. *Rehabil Nurs.* 1996;21(1):13-19.

283. Van Herk R, Van Dijk M, Baar FPM, Tibboel D, De Wit R. Observation scales for pain assessment in older adults with cognitive impairments or communication difficulties. *Nurs Res.* 2007;56(1):34.

284. Carr J, Moffett J, Sharp D, Haines D. Is the pain stages of change questionnaire (PSOCQ) a useful tool for predicting participation in a self-management programme? Further evidence of validity, on a sample of UK pain clinic patients. *BMC Musculoskelet Disord.* 2006;7(1):101.

285. Fink R. Pain assessment: the cornerstone to optimal pain management. *Proc (Bayl Univ Med Cent).* 2000;13(3):236.

286. Corran TM, Farrell M, Helme RD, Gibson S. The classification of patients with chronic pain: age as a contributing factor. *Clin J Pain.* 1997;13(3):207.

287. Sluka KA. Pain mechanisms involved in musculoskeletal disorders. *J Orthop Sports Phys Ther.* 1996;24:240-254.

288. Katavich L. Pain mechanisms underlying peripheral nerve injury: implications for mobilisation of the nervous system. *NZ J Physiother.* 1999;27:24-27.

289. Khalsa PS. Muscle pain due to mechanical stimuli. *J Neuromusculoskeletal Syst.* 1999(7):1-8.

290. Seaman DR, Cleveland C III. Spinal pain syndromes: nociceptive, neuropathic, and psychologic mechanisms. *J Manipulative Physiol Ther.* 1999;22(7):458-472.

291. Hall T, Elvey R. Nerve trunk pain: physical diagnosis and treatment. *Man Ther.* 1999;4(2):63-73.

292. Ross R, LaStayo P. Clinical assessment of pain. In: Van Deusen J, Brunt D, eds. *Assessment in occupational therapy and physical therapy;* 1997:123-133.

293. Downie W, Leatham P, Rhind V, Wright V, Branco J, Anderson J. Studies with pain rating scales. *Ann Rheum Dis.* 1978;37(4):378-381.

294. McDougall JJ. Arthritis and pain neurogenic origin of joint pain. *Arthritis Res Ther.* 2006;8(6):220.

295. Weinstein SM. Cancer pain. *Phys Med Rehabil State Art Rev.* 1994;8(2): 279-296.

296. Elvey RL. Physical evaluation of the peripheral nervous system in disorders of pain and dysfunction. *J Hand Ther.* 1997;10(2):122-129.

297. Lewis J, Ramot R, Green A. Changes in mechanical tension in the median nerve: possible implications for the upper limb tension test. *Physiotherapy.* 1998;84(6):254-261.

298. Song KM, Morton AA, Koch KD, Herring JA, Browne RH, Hanway JP. Chronic musculoskeletal pain in childhood. *J Pediatr Orthop.* 1998;18(5):576.

299. Marovino T, Blackmon CB, Sherman M, Carzon M, Tworek R. Pain assessment. The accuracy and test-retest reliability of dolorimetry measurements in a healthy and chronic pain population. *Am J Pain Manage.* 995;5:94-97.

300. Hong CZ. Algometry in evaluation of trigger points and referred pain. *J Musculoskelet Pain.* 1998;6(1):47-59.

301. Scott J, Huskisson E. Vertical or horizontal visual analogue scales. *Ann Rheum Dis.* 1979;38(6):560.

302. Nussbaum EL, Downes L. Reliability of clinical pressure-pain algometric measurements obtained on consecutive days. *Phys Ther.* 1998;78(2):160-169.

303. Swift T, Brescia N. *Intra and Inter-Rater Reliability of Pressure Algometer Measurements Taken By Student Physical Therapists.* [Masters]. Oakland, CA: Samuel Merritt College; 1997.

304. Brown FF, Robinson ME, Riley JL 3rd, Gremillion HA, McSolay J, Meyers G. Better palpation of pain: reliability and validity of a new pressure pain protocol in TMD. *Cranio.* 2000;18(1):58-65.

305. Lew P, Lewis J, Story I. Inter-therapist reliability in locating latent myofascial trigger points using palpation. *Man Ther.* 1997;2(2):87-90.

306. Hsieh CYJ, Hong CZ, Adams AH, et al. Interexaminer reliability of the palpation of trigger points in the trunk and lower limb muscles. *Arch Phys Med Rehabil.* 2000;81(3):258-264.

307. Cohen H, Pertes R. Diagnosis and management of fascial pain. In: Rachin ES, ed. *Myofascial Pain and Fibromyalgia: Trigger Point Management.* St Louis, MO: Mosby Yearbook Inc; 1994:361-382.

308. Delaney GA, McKee AC. Inter- and intra-rater reliability of the pressure threshold meter in measurement of myofascial trigger point sensitivity. *Am J Phys Med Rehabil.* 1993;72(3):136-139.

309. Alvarez DJ, Rockwell PG. Trigger points: diagnosis and management. *Am Fam Physician.* 2002;65(4):653-662.

310. Rivner MH. The neurophysiology of myofascial pain syndrome. *Curr Pain Headache Rep.* 2001;5(5):432-440.

311. Ingber R. Myofascial pain in lumbar dysfunction. *Phys Med Rehabil.* 1999;13:473-498.

312. Hammond E. Electrodiagnosis of the neuromuscular system. In: Van Deusen J, Brunt D, eds. *Assessment in Occupational Therapy and Physical Therapy.* Philadelphia, PA: WB Saunders; 1997.

313. Abram SE, Miller RD. *Atlas of Anesthesia Volume 6: Pain Management.* Vol. 6. 1st ed. Philadelphia, PA: Churchill Livingstone; 1998.

314. American Psychiatric Association, American Psychiatric Association. Task Force on DSM-IV. *Diagnostic and Statistical Manual of Mental Disorders: DSM-IV-TR.* Arlington, VA: American Psychiatric Publishing; 2000.

315. Turk DC, Melzack R. *Handbook of Pain Assessment.* New York, NY: The Guilford Press; 2010.

316. Maigne JY, Doursounian L. Entrapment neuropathy of the medial superior cluneal nerve: nineteen cases surgically treated, with a minimum of 2 years' follow-up. *Spine.* 1997;22(10):1156.

317. Van Deursen RWM, Sanchez M, Derr J, Becker M, Ulbrecht J, Cavanagh P. Vibration perception threshold testing in patients with diabetic neuropathy: ceiling effects and reliability. *Diabetic Med.* 2001;18(6):469-475.

318. Billi A, Catalucci A, Barile A, Masciocchi C. Joint impingement syndrome: clinical features. *Eur J Radiol.* 1998;27:S39-S41.

319. Idler RS. General principles of patient evaluation and nonoperative management of cubital syndrome. *Hand Clin.* 1996;12(2):397-403.

320. Nakano KK. Nerve entrapment syndromes. *Curr Opin Rheumatol.* 1997;9(2):165.

321. Huang KC, Chen YJ, Hsu RW. Anterior tarsal tunnel syndrome: case report. *Changgeng Yi Xue Za Zhi.* 1999;22(3):503-507.

322. Preston DC. Distal median neuropathies. *Neurol Clin.* 1999;17(3): 407-424.

323. Lee CY. Lower limb entrapment neuropathies. *Phys Med Rehabil State Art Rev.* 1999;13:231-249.

324. Cherniack MG, Moalli D, Viscolli C. A comparison of traditional electrodiagnostic studies, electroneurometry, and vibrometry in the diagnosis of carpal tunnel syndrome. *J Hand Surg.* 1996;21(1):122-131.

325. Kleindienst A, Hamm B, Hildebrandt G, Klug N. Diagnosis and staging of carpal tunnel syndrome: comparison of magnetic resonance imaging and intraoperative findings. *Acta Neurochir.* 1996;138(2):228-233.

326. Knight CA. Peripheral vascular disease. In: O'Sullivan SB, Schmitz TJ, eds. *Physical rehabilitation: Assessment and treatment.* Philadelphia, PA: FA Davis Company; 2006:583-619.

327. Johansson K, Albertsson M, Ingvar C, Ekdahl C. Effects of compression bandaging with or without manual lymph drainage treatment in patients with postoperative arm lymphedema. *Lymphology.* 1999;32(3):103-110.

328. Moholkar K, Fenelon G. Diurnal variations in volume of the foot and ankle. *J Foot Ankle Surg.* 2001;40(5):302-304.

329. Todd J. Lymphoedema—a challenge for all healthcare professionals. *Int J Palliat Nurs.* 1998;4:230-239.

330. Ramadan A. Hand analysis. In: Van Deusen J, Brunt D, eds. *Assessment in Occupational Therapy and Physical Therapy.* Philadelphia, PA: WB Saunders; 1997.

331. Palmada M, Shah S, O'Hare K. Issues in the measurement of hand oedema. *Physiotherapy Theory Pract.* 1998;14(3):139-148.

332. Acebes O, Renau E, Sansegundo R, Santos FJ, Aguilar JJ. Evaluation of postmastectomy lymphedema. Comparative study of two measurement methods (abstract). *Rehabilitacion.* 1999;33:190-194.

333. Klauser A, Frauscher F, Halpern EJ, et al. Remitting seronegative symmetrical synovitis with pitting edema of the hands: ultrasound, color Doppler ultrasound, and magnetic resonance imaging findings. *Arthritis Care Res.* 2005;53(2):226-233.

334. del Olmo J, Espana A, Richter J. The usefulness of isotopic lymphoscintigraphy in the study of lymphedemas. *Actas Dermosifiliogr.* 2005;96(7): 419-423.

335. Khan O, Maharaj P, Rampaul R, Archibald A, Naipaul R, Loutan N. Lymphoscintigraphic evaluation of chronic lower limb edema. *West Indian Med J.* 2003;52:136-139.

336. Cornish B, Bunce I, Ward L, Jones L, Thomas B. Bioelectrical impedance for monitoring the efficacy of lymphoedema treatment programmes. *Breast Cancer Res Treat.* 1996;38(2):169-176.

337. Gorassini MA, Bennett DJ, Yang JF. Self-sustained firing of human motor units. *Neurosci Lett.* 1998;247(1):13-16.

338. O'Dwyer NJ, Ada L. Reflex hyperexcitability and muscle contracture in relation to spastic hypertonia. *Curr Opin Neurol.* 1996;9(6):451.

339. Jepsen J, Laursen L, Hagert CG, Kreiner S, Larsen A. Diagnostic accuracy of the neurological upper limb examination II: relation to symptoms of patterns of findings. *BMC Neurol.* 2006;6(1):10.

340. Agostinucci J. Upper motor neuron syndrome. In: Deusen J, Brunt D, eds. *Assessment in occupational therapy and physical therapy.* 1st ed. Philadelphia, PA: WB Saunders Company; 1997:271-293.

341. Clarkson HM, Gilewich BG. *Musculoskeletal Assessment: Joint Range of Motion and Manual Muscle Strength.* Baltimore, MD: Lippincott Williams & Wilkins; 1989.

342. Shaw J, Bially J, Deurvorst N, Macfie C, Brouwer B. Clinical and physiological measures of tone in chronic stroke. *J Neurol Phys Ther.* 1999;23(1):19.

343. Yam WKL, Leung MSM. Interrater reliability of modified Ashworth scale and modified Tardieu scale in children with spastic cerebral palsy. *J Child Neurol.* 2006;21(12):1031-1035.

344. Mehrholz J, Wagner K, Meißner D, et al. Reliability of the modified Tardieu scale and the modified Ashworth scale in adult patients with severe brain injury: a comparison study. *Clin Rehabil.* 2005;19(7):751-759.

345. Smith AW, Jamshidi M, Lo SK. Clinical measurement of muscle tone using a velocity-corrected modified Ashworth scale. *Am J Phys Med Rehabil.* 2002;81(3):202.

346. Singer B, Dunne J, Singer K, Allison G. Velocity dependent passive plantar flexor resistive torque in patients with acquired brain injury. *Clin Biomech.* 2003;18(2):157-165.

347. Smith AW, Kirtley C, Jamshidi M. Intrarater reliability of manual passive movement velocity in the clinical evaluation of knee extensor muscle tone. *Arch Phys Med Rehabil.* 2000;81(10):1428-1431.

348. Fleuren JF, Nederhand MJ, Hermens HJ. Influence of posture and muscle length on stretch reflex activity in poststroke patients with spasticity. *Arch Phys Med Rehabil.* 2006;87(7):981-988.

349. Kakebeeke T, Lechner H, Baumberger M, Denoth J, Michel D, Knecht H. The importance of posture on the isokinetic assessment of spasticity. *Spinal Cord.* 2002;40(5):236-243.

350. Lin CCK, Ju MS, Huang HW. Muscle tone in diabetic polyneuropathy evaluated by the quantitative pendulum test. *Arch Phys Med Rehabil.* 2007;88(3):368-373.

351. Lechner HE, Frotzler A, Eser P. Relationship between self-and clinically rated spasticity in spinal cord injury. *Arch Phys Med Rehabil.* 2006;87(1):15-19.

352. McDonald MF, Kevin Garrison M, Schmit BD. Length–tension properties of ankle muscles in chronic human spinal cord injury. *J Biomech.* 2005;38(12): 2344-2353.

353. Rabita G, Dupont L, Thevenon A, Lensel-Corbeil G, Pérot C, Vanvelcenaher J. Quantitative assessment of the velocity-dependent increase in resistance to passive stretch in spastic plantarflexors. *Clin Biomech.* 2005;20(7):745-753.

354. Peng Q, Shah P, Selles RW, Gaebler-Spira DJ, Zhang LQ. Measurement of ankle spasticity in children with cerebral palsy using a manual spasticity evaluator. *Conf Proc IEEE Eng Med Biol Soc.* 2004;7:4896-4899.

355. Sabari J. Motor control. In: Van Eusen J, Brunt D, eds. *Assessment in Occupational Therapy and Physical Therapy.* Philadelphia, PA: WB Saunders; 1997.

356. Vattanasilp W, Ada L. The relationship between clinical and laboratory measures of spasticity. *Aust J Physiother.* 1999;45(2):135-139.

357. Rabadi MH, Rabadi FM. Comparison of the action research arm test and the Fugl-Meyer assessment as measures of upper-extremity motor weakness after stroke. *Arch Phys Med Rehabil.* 2006;87(7):962-966.

358. Hsueh IP, Hsieh CL. Responsiveness of two upper extremity function instruments for stroke in patients receiving rehabilitation. *Clin Rehabil.* 2002;16(6):617-624.

359. de Nap Shelton F, Volpe BT, Reding M. Motor impairment as a predictor of functional recovery and guide to rehabilitation treatment after stroke. *Neurorehabil Neural Repair.* 2001;15(3):229-237.

360. Chae J, Labatia I, Yang G. Upper limb motor function in hemiparesis: concurrent validity of the arm motor ability test. *Am J Phys Med Rehabil.* 2003;82(1):1.

361. Kelly PJ, Furie KL, Shafqat S, Rallis N, Chang Y, Stein J. Functional recovery following rehabilitation after hemorrhagic and ischemic stroke. *Arch Phys Med Rehabil.* 2003;84(7):968-972.

362. Frownfelter D, Dean E. *Cardiovascular and Pulmonary Physical Therapy.* 4th ed. St. Louis, MO: Mosby; 2006.

363. Kupferberg DH, Kaplan RM, Slymen DJ, Ries AL. Minimal clinically important validity of the UCSD shortness of breath questionnaire. *J Cardiopulm Rehabil Prev.* 2005;25(6):370.

364. Gunen H, Hacievliyagil SS, Kosar F, Gulbas G, Kizkin O, Sahin I. The role of arterial blood gases, exercise testing, and cardiac examination in asthma. *Allergy Asthma Proc.* 2006;27(1):45-52.

365. Hutter BO, Wurtemberger G. Functional capacity (dyspnea) and quality of life in patients with chronic obstructive lung disease (COPD): instruments of assessment and methodological aspects (abstract). *Pneumologie.* 1999;53:133-142.

366. Geiger R, Strasak A, Treml B, et al. Six-minute walk test in children and adolescents. *J Pediatr.* 2007;150(4):395-399, e2.

367. Carlson-Catalano J, Lunney M, Paradiso C, et al. Clinical validation of ineffective breathing pattern, ineffective airway clearance, and impaired gas exchange. *J Nurs Sch.* 1998;30(3):243-248.

368. Dallimore K, Jenkins S, Tucker B. Respiratory and cardiovascular responses to manual chest percussion in normal subjects. *Aust J Physiother.* 1998;44(4):267-274.

369. McChesney JA, McChesney JW. Auscultation of the chest and abdomen by athletic trainers. *J Athl Train.* 2001;36(2):190.

370. Protas E. Cardiovascular and pulmonary function. In: Van Deusen J, Brunt D, eds. *Assessment in Occupational Therapy and Physical Therapy.* Philadelphia, PA: WB Saunders.

371. Basoglu OK, Atasever A, Bacakoglu F. The efficacy of incentive spirometry in patients with COPD. *Respirology.* 2005;10(3):349-353.

372. Thomas JR, von Gunten CF. Management of dyspnea. *J Support Oncol.* 2003;1:23-32.

373. De Torres JP, Pinto-Plata V, Ingenito E, et al. Power of outcome measurements to detect clinically significant changes in pulmonary rehabilitation of patients with COPD*. *Chest.* 2002;121(4):1092-1098.

374. Aaron SD, Vandemheen KL, Clinch JJ, et al. Measurement of short-term changes in dyspnea and disease-specific quality of life following an acute COPD exacerbation*. *Chest.* 2002;121(3):688-696.

375. Fujimoto K, Kubo K, Miyahara T, et al. Effects of muscle relaxation therapy using specially designed plates in patients with pulmonary emphysema. *Intern Med.* 1996;35(10):756-763.

376. Oberdörster G, Cox C, Gelein R. Intratracheal instillation versus intratracheal inhalation of tracer particles for measuring lung clearance function. *Exp Lung Res.* 1997;23(1):17-34.

377. Fuchs-Climent D, Le Gallais D, Varray A, Desplan J, Cadopi M, Préfaut C. Quality of life and exercise tolerance in chronic obstructive pulmonary disease: effects of a short and intensive inpatient rehabilitation program. *Am J Phys Med Rehabil.* 1999;78(4):330.

378. Resnick B. Reliability and validity testing of the self-efficacy for functional activities scale. *J Nurs Meas.* 1999;7(1):5-20.

379. Springhouse. *Professional Guide to Diseases.* 8th ed. Springhouse, PA: Springhouse Corporation; 2009.

380. Mancini I, Body J. Assessment of dyspnea in advanced cancer patients. *Support Care Cancer.* 1999;7(4):229-232.

381. Harris J, Johansen J, Pedersen S, LaPier T. Site of measurement and subject position affect chest excursion measurements. *Cardiopulm Physical Ther.* 1997;8:12-17.

382. Fruth SJ. Differential diagnosis and treatment in a patient with posterior upper thoracic pain. *Phys Ther.* 2006;86(2):254-268.

383. Barnett M. An overview of assessment and management in COPD. *Br J Community Nurs.* 2009;14(5):195-201.

384. Lansing RW, Gracely RH, Banzett RB. The multiple dimensions of dyspnea: review and hypotheses. *Respir Physiol Neurobiol.* 2009;167(1):53-60.

385. Van Deusen J, Brunt D. *Assessment in Occupational Therapy and Physical Therapy.* Philadelphia, PA: WB Saunders; 1997.

386. King PM, Tuckwell N, Barrett TE. A critical review of functional capacity evaluations. *Phys Ther.* 1998;78(8):852-866.

387. Law M. Self care. In: Van Deusen J, Brunt D, eds. *Assessment in Occupational Therapy and Physical Therapy.* Philadelphia, PA: WB Saunders; 1997.

388. Finch E, Brooks D, Stratford P, Mayo N. *Physical Rehabilitation Outcome Measures.* Philadelphia, PA: Lippincott Williams & Wilkins; 2002.

389. Mahoney FI. The Barthel Index. *Maryland State Med J.* 1965;14: 61-65.

390. De Groot IJM, Post MWM, Van Heuveln T, Van Den Berg LH, Lindeman E. Measurement of decline of functioning in persons with amyotrophic lateral sclerosis: responsiveness and possible applications of the functional independence measure, Barthel Index, rehabilitation activities profile and Frenchay Activities Index. *Amyotrophic Lat Scler.* 2006;7(3):167-172.

391. Langhammer B, Stanghelle JK. Co-variation of tests commonly used in stroke rehabilitation. *Physiother Res Int.* 2006;11(4):228-234.

392. Bennett M, Ryall N. Using the modified Barthel index to estimate survival in cancer patients in hospice: observational study. *BMJ.* 2000;321(7273): 1381-1382.

393. Ceran F, ÖZCAN A. The relationship of the functional rating index with disability, pain, and quality of life in patients with low back pain. *Medical science monitor.* 2006;12(10):CR35-CR39.

394. Engberg A, Bentzen L, Garde B. Rehabilitation after stroke: predictive power of Barthel index versus a cognitive and a motor index. *Acta Neurol Scand.* 1995;91(1):28-36.

395. Levi SJ. Posthospital setting, resource utilization, and self-care outcome in older women with hip fracture. *Arch Phys Med Rehabil.* 1997;78(9): 973-979.

396. Kakurai S, Akai M. Clinical experiences with a convertible thermoplastic knee-ankle-foot orthosis for post-stroke hemiplegic patients. *Prosthet Orthot Int.* 1996;20(3):191-194.

397. Hui E, Lum C, Woo J, Or K, Kay RLC. Outcomes of elderly stroke patients: day hospital versus conventional medical management. *Stroke.* 1995;26(9):1616-1619.

398. Jonsson B, Overend T, Kramer J. Functional measures following liver transplantation. *Physiotherapy Can.* 1998;50(2):141-146.

399. Patti F, Reggio A, Nicoletti F, Sellaroli T, Deinite G, Nicoletti F. Effects of rehabilitation therapy on parkinsonians' disability and functional independence. *Neurorehabil Neural Repair.* 1996;10(4):223-231.

400. Condie E, Jones D, Treweek S, Scott H. A one-year national survey of patients having a lower limb amputation. *Physiotherapy.* 1996;82(1):14-20.

401. Jette AM. Using health-related quality of life measures in physical therapy outcomes research. *Phys Ther.* 1993;73(8):528-537.

402. Mielenz T, Jackson E, Currey S, DeVellis R, Callahan LF. Psychometric properties of the centers for disease control and prevention health-related quality of life (CDC HRQOL) items in adults with arthritis. *Health Qual Life Outcomes.* 2006;4(1):66.

403. Whitfield K, Buchbinder R, Segal L, Osborne RH. Parsimonious and efficient assessment of health-related quality of life in osteoarthritis research: validation of the assessment of quality of life (AQoL) instrument. *Health Qual Life Outcomes.* 2006;4(1):19.

404. Ware JE Jr, Sherbourne CD. The MOS 36-item short-form health survey (SF-36): I. Conceptual framework and item selection. *Med Care.* 1992:473-483.

405. McHorney CA, Haley SM, Ware JE. Evaluation of the MOS SF-36 physical functioning scale (PF-40): II. Comparison of relative precision using Likert and Rasch scoring methods. *J Clin Epidemiol.* 1997;50(4):451-461.

406. Thumboo J, Fong KY, Ng TP, et al. Validation of the MOS SF-36 for quality of life assessment of patients with systemic lupus erythematosus in Singapore. *J Rheumatol.* 1999;26(1):97-102.

407. Daeppen JB, Krieg MA, Burnand B, Yersin B. MOS-SF-36 in evaluating health-related quality of life in alcohol-dependent patients. *Am J Drug Alcohol Abuse.* 1998;24(4):685.

408. Lam CLK, Gandek B, Ren XS, Chan M. Tests of scaling assumptions and construct validity of the Chinese (HK) version of the SF-36 health survey. *J Clin Epidemiol.* 1998;51(11):1139-1147.

409. Duncan PW, Samsa GP, Weinberger M, et al. Health status of individuals with mild stroke. *Stroke.* 1997;28(4):740-745.

410. Russo J, Trujillo CA, Wingerson D, et al. The MOS 36-item short form health survey: reliability, validity, and preliminary findings in schizophrenic outpatients. *Med Care.* 1998;36(5):752.

411. Schlenk EA, Erlen JA, Dunbar-Jacob J, et al. Health-related quality of life in chronic disorders: a comparison across studies using the MOS SF-36. *Qual Life Res.* 1997;7(1):57-65.

412. Wu AW, Hays RD, Kelly S, Malitz F, Bozzette SA. Applications of the medical outcomes study health-related quality of life measures in HIV/AIDS. *Qual Life Res.* 1997;6(6):531-554.

413. De Jong Z, van der Heijde D, McKenna S, Whalley D. The reliability and construct validity of the RAQoL: a rheumatoid arthritis-specific quality of life instrument. *Rheumatology.* 1997;36(8):878-883.

414. Vo TXH, Guillemin F, Deschamps JP. Psychometric properties of the DUKE health profile-adolescent version (DHP-A): a generic instrument for adolescents. *Qual Life Res.* 2005;14(10):2229-2234.

415. Guillemin F, Paul-Dauphin A, Virion JM, Bouchet C, Briancon S. The DUKE health profile: a generic instrument to measure the quality of life tied to health. *Sante Publique.* 1997;9(1):35-44.

416. Nanda U, McLendon PM, Andresen EM, Armbrecht E. The SIP68: an abbreviated sickness impact profile for disability outcomes research. *Qual Life Res.* 2003;12(5):583-595.

417. Lipsett PA, Swoboda SM, Campbell KA, Cornwell E III, Dorman T. Sickness impact profile score versus a modified short-form survey for functional outcome assessment: acceptability, reliability, and validity in critically ill patients with prolonged intensive care unit stays. *J Trauma.* 2000;49(4): 737.

418. Kim KU, Yoon SJ, Lee JL, et al. Validation of the Korean version of the McMaster quality of life scale in terminal cancer patients. *J Palliat Care.* 2006;22(1):40-45.

419. Reardon JZ, Lareau SC, ZuWallack R. Functional status and quality of life in chronic obstructive pulmonary disease. *Am J Med.* 2006;119(10):32-37.

420. Rubenstein L, Voelker M, Chrischilles E, Glenn D, Wallace R, Rodnitzky R. The usefulness of the functional status questionnaire and medical outcomes study short form in Parkinson's disease research. *Qual Life Res.* 1998;7(4): 279-290.

421. Fritz S. *Fundamentals of Therapeutic Massage.* 3rd ed. St. Louis, MO: Mosby-Yearbook; 2004.

422. Gajdosik RL. Passive extensibility of skeletal muscle: review of the literature with clinical implications. *Clin Biomech.* 2001;16(2):87-101.

423. McPartland JM. Travell trigger points—molecular and osteopathic perspectives. *J Am Osteopath Assoc.* 2004;104(6):244-249.

Further Reading

American Psychiatric Association, American Psychiatric Association. Task Force on DSM-IV. *Diagnostic and Statistical Manual of Mental Disorders: DSM-IV-TR.* Arlington, VA: American Psychiatric Publishing; 2000.

Backonja MM. Defining neuropathic pain. *Anesth Analg.* 2003;97(3):785-790.

Ballantyne JC, Fishman SM, Abdi S. Massachusetts General Hospital: handbook of pain management. *Recherche.* 2005;67:02.

Johannes CB, Le TK, Zhou X, Johnston JA, Dworkin RH. The prevalence of chronic pain in United States adults: results of an internet-based survey. *J Pain.* 2010;11(11):1230-1239.

Kado DM, Huang MH, Karlamangla AS, Barrett-Connor E, Greendale GA. Hyperkyphotic posture predicts mortality in older Community-Dwelling men and women: a prospective study. *J Am Geriatr Soc.* 2004;52(10):1662-1667.

Kidd B, Urban L. Mechanisms of inflammatory pain. *Br J Anaesth.* 2001;87(1):3-11.

Krause SJ, Backonja MM. Development of a neuropathic pain questionnaire. *Clin J Pain.* 2003;19(5):306.

Merskey H, Bogduk N. ISAP subcommittee on taxonomy, classification of chronic pain. *Pain.* 1994:S1-S226.

Turk DC, Melzack R. *Handbook of Pain Assessment.* New York, NY: The Guilford Press; 2010.

Woolf CJ, Salter MW. Neuronal plasticity: increasing the gain in pain. *Science.* 2000;288(5472):1765-1768.

CHAPTER 5

References

1. World Health Organization. *Towards a Common Language for Functioning, Disability and Health: ICF—The International Classification of Functioning, Disability and Health.* Geneva: World Health Organization; 2002.

2. Jensen GM, Shepard KF, Gwyer J, Hack LM. Attribute dimensions that distinguish master and novice physical therapy clinicians in orthopedic settings. *Phys Ther.* 1992;72(10):711-722.

3. May BJ, Dennis JK. Expert decision making in physical therapy—a survey of practitioners. *Phys Ther.* 1991;71(3): 190-202.

4. Payton OD. Clinical reasoning process in physical therapy. *Phys Ther.* 1985;65(6):924-928.

5. Rothstein JM, Echternach JL, Riddle DL. The hypothesis-oriented algorithm for clinicians II (HOAC II): a guide for patient management. *Phys Ther.* 2003;83(5):455-470.

6. Leach M. *Clinical Decision Making in Complementary & Alternative Medicine.* Chatswood, NSW: Elsevier Australia; 2010.

7. Dryden T, Moyer CA. *Massage Therapy: Integrating Research in Clinical Practice.* Champaign, IL: Human Kinetics; 2012.

8. Sullivan P, Markos PD. *Clinical Decision-Making in Therapeutic Exercise.* East Norwalk, CT: Appleton & Lange; 1999.

9. American Physical Therapy Association. *Guide to Physical Therapist Practice.* Alexandria, VA: American Physical Therapy Association; 2005.

10. Magee DJ. *Orthopedic Physical Assessment.* 5th ed. Philadelphia, PA: WB Saunders; 2005.

11. World Health Organization. *Towards a Common Language for Functioning, Disability and Health: ICF: The International Classification of Functioning, Disability and Health.* Geneva: World Health Organization; 2002.

12. Fritz S. *Fundamentals of Therapeutic Massage.* 3rd ed. St. Louis, MO: Mosby-Yearbook; 2004.

13. Tappan F, Benjamin P. *Tappan's Handbook of Healing Massage Techniques: Holistic, Classic, and Emerging Methods.* Upper Saddle River, NJ: Prentice Hall; 2004.

14. Werner RA, Benjamin BE. *A Massage Therapist's Guide to Pathology.* Baltimore, MD: Lippincott Williams & Wilkins; 2002.

15. de Domenico G, Wood EC. *Beard's Massage.* 4th ed. Philadelphia, PA: WB Saunders; 1997.

16. Batavia M. Contraindications for therapeutic massage: do sources agree? *J Bodywork Movement Ther.* 2004;8(1): 48-57.

17. Cohen MH, Kemper KJ. Complementary therapies in pediatrics: a legal perspective. *Pediatrics.* 2005;115(3):774-780.

18. Grant AC, Wang N. Carotid dissection associated with a handheld electric massager. *South Med J.* 2004;97(12):1262.

19. Grant KE. Massage safety: injuries reported in Medline relating to the practice of therapeutic massage—1965–2003. *J Bodywork Movement Ther.* 2003;7(4):207-212.

20. Miesler D. Geriatric massage: assessment and contraindications for the geriatric client. *Massage Bodywork.* 1996;11(66).

21. Ugboma HA, Akani CI. Abdominal massage: another cause of maternal mortality. *Niger J Med.* 2004;13(3):259.

22. Wada Y, Yanagihara C, Nishimura Y. Internal jugular vein thrombosis associated with shiatsu massage of the neck. *J Neurol Neurosurg Psychiatry.* 2005;76(1):142-143.

23. Walton T. Exploring contraindications to massage therapy. *J Soft Tissue Manipulation (JSTM).* 1999;6:5-13.

24. Whitehill W, Gustman B. Massage and skin conditions: indications and contraindications. *Athletic Therapy Today.* 2002;7(3):24-28.

25. Yokoyama T, Shimizu Y. A case of bilateral chylothorax following neck massage. *Nihon Kokyuki Gakkai Zasshi.* 2004;42(12):1034-1036.

26. National Center for Medical Rehabilitation Research (US). National Advisory Board on Medical Rehabilitation Research, National Institute of Child Health and Human Development (US). *Research plan for the national center for medical rehabilitation research.* Bethesda, Maryland: US Department of Health and Human Services, Public Health Service, National Institutes of Health, National Institute of Child Health and Human Development; 1993.

27. Herskovitz S, Strauch B, Gordon MJ. Shiatsu massage-induced injury of the median recurrent motor branch. *Muscle Nerve.* 1992;15(10):1215.

28. Salvo SG. *Massage Therapy: Principles and Practice.* 2nd ed. Philadelphia, PA: WB Saunders; 2003.

29. Sackett D, Straus S, Richardson W, Rosenberg W, Haynes R. *Evidence-Based Medicine: How to Practice and Teach EBM.* New York, NY: Churchill Livingstone; 2000.

30. Fitch P. Intimacy and attachment in massage therapy. *Massage Ther J.* 2005;43:113-121.

CHAPTER 6

References

1. Sharkey BJ, Gaskill SE. *Fitness and Health.* 4th ed. Champaign, IL: Human Kinetics Publishers; 2007.

2. Anderson B, Pearl B, Burke E. *Getting in Shape: 32 Workout Programs for Lifelong Fitness.* Bolinas, CA: Shelter Publications; 2002.

3. Moffat M, Vickery S. *The American Physical Therapy Association Book of Body Maintenance and Repair.* New York, NY: Henry Holt and Co.; 1999.

4. Alter MJ. *Science of Stretching.* Champaign, IL: Human Kinetics Books; 1988.

5. Oswald CA, Bacso SN. *Stretching for Fitness, Health & Performance: The Complete Handbook for All Ages & Fitness Levels.* New York, NY: Sterling Publications; 1998.

6. Anderson B, Anderson J. *Stretching.* Bolinas, CA: Shelter Publications; 2000.

7. Loving J. *Massage Therapy.* Stamford, CT: Appleton & Lange; 1999.

8. Fritz S. *Fundamentals of Therapeutic Massage.* 3rd ed. St. Louis, MO: Mosby-Yearbook; 2004.

9. Salvo SG. *Massage Therapy: Principles and Practice.* 2nd ed. Philadelphia, PA: WB Saunders; 2003.

10. Quality Assurance Committee of the College of Massage Therapists of Ontario. *Code of Ethics and Standards of Practice.* Toronto, ON: College of Massage Therapists of Ontario; 2006.

11. Curties D. *Breast Massage.* 3rd ed. New Brunswick: Curties-Overzet Publications; 1999.

12. Beck M. *Milady's Theory and Practice of Therapeutic Massage.* 3rd ed. Albany, NY: Milady; 1999.

13. Hollis M. *Massage for Therapists.* 2nd ed. Oxford: Blackwell Science; 1998.

CHAPTER 7

References

*Randomized Controlled Trial
†Systematic Review

1. Fritz S. *Fundamentals of Therapeutic Massage.* 3rd ed. St. Louis, MO: Mosby-Yearbook; 2004.

2. American Physical Therapy Association. *Guide to Physical Therapist Practice.* Alexandria, VA: American Physical Therapy Association; 2005.

3. Benjamin PJ, Tappan FM. *Tappan's Handbook of Healing Massage Techniques.* 4th ed. Upper Saddle River, NJ: Pearson Prentice Hall; 2005.

4. Loving J. *Massage Therapy.* Stamford, CT: Appleton & Lange; 1999.

5. de Domenico G, Wood EC. *Beard's Massage.* 4th ed. Philadelphia, PA: WB Saunders; 1997.

6. Salvo SG. *Massage Therapy: Principles and Practice.* 2nd ed. Philadelphia, PA: WB Saunders; 2003.

7. Holey E, Cook E. *Evidence-Based Therapeutic Massage.* 2nd ed. Edinburgh, Scotland: Churchill Livingstone; 2003.

8. Monroe CM. The effects of therapeutic touch on pain. *J Holist Nurs.* 2009;27(2):85-92.

9. Hawranik P, Johnston P, Deatrich J. Therapeutic touch and agitation in individuals with Alzheimer's disease. *West J Nurs Res.* 2008;30(4):417.

10. Maville JA, Bowen JE, Benham G. Effect of healing touch on stress perception and biological correlates. *Holist Nurs Pract.* 2008;22(2):103.

11. Jackson E, Kelley M, McNeil P, Meyer E, Schlegel L, Eaton M. Does therapeutic touch help reduce pain and anxiety in patients with cancer? *Clin J Oncol Nurs.* 2008;12(1):113-120.

†12. Ernst E. Massage therapy for cancer palliation and supportive care: a systematic review of randomised clinical trials. *Support Care Cancer.* 2009;17(4):333-337.

†13. Lee M, Pittler M, Ernst E. Effects of reiki in clinical practice: a systematic review of randomised clinical trials. *Int J Clin Pract.* 2008;62(6):947-954.

*14. Henricson M, Ersson A, Maatta S, Segesten K, Berglund AL. The outcome of tactile touch on stress parameters in intensive care: a randomized controlled trial. *Complement Ther Clin Pract.* 2008;14(4):244-254.

15. Dunbar R. The social role of touch in humans and primates: behavioural function and neurobiological mechanisms. *Neurosci Biobehav Rev.* 2010;34(2):260-268.

16. McGlone F, Vallbo AB, Olausson H, Loken L, Wessberg J. Discriminative touch and emotional touch. *Can J Exp Psychol.* 2007;61(3):173.

17. Ashfeld M. *Effect of Therapeutic Touch in Treating Agitation of Persons with Alzheimer's Disease* [Masters]. St. Paul, MN: St. Catherine University; 2011.

*18. Gomes VM, Silva MJP, Araújo EAC. Gradual effects of therapeutic touch in reducing anxiety in university students. *Rev Bras Enferm.* 2008;61(6):841-846.

*19. Lindgren L, Rundgren S, Winsö O, et al. Physiological responses to touch massage in healthy volunteers. *Auton Neurosci.* 2010;158(1-2):105-110.

20. Moraska A, Pollini RA, Boulanger K, Brooks MZ, Teitlebaum L. Physiological adjustments to stress measures following massage therapy: a review of the literature. *Evid Based Complement Alternat Med.* 2008;7(4):409-418.

*21. Sefton JEM, Yarar C, Carpenter DM, Berry JW. Physiological and clinical changes after therapeutic massage of the neck and shoulders. *Man Ther.* 2011;16(5):487-494.

22. Kerr CE, Wasserman RH, Moore CI. Cortical dynamics as a therapeutic mechanism for touch healing. *J Altern Complement Med.* 2007;13(1):59-66.

*23. Rapaport MH, Schettler P, Bresee C. A preliminary study of the effects of a single session of Swedish massage on hypothalamic–pituitary–adrenal and immune function in normal individuals. *J Altern Complement Med.* 2010;16(10):1079-1088.

*24. Marta IER, Baldan SS, Berton AF, Pavam M, Silva MJP. The effectiveness of therapeutic touch on pain, depression and sleep in patients with chronic pain: clinical trial. *Rev Escola Enfermagem USP.* 2010;44(4):1100-1106.

*25. Assefi N, Bogart A, Goldberg J, Buchwald D. Reiki for the treatment of fibromyalgia: a randomized controlled trial. *J Altern Complement Med.* 2008;14(9):1115-1122.

*26. Woods DL, Beck C, Sinha K. The effect of therapeutic touch on behavioral symptoms and cortisol in persons with dementia. *Forschende Komplementärmedizin/Res Complement Med.* 2009;16(3):181-189.

27. Domínguez Rosales R, Albar Marín M, Tena Gazcía B. Effectiveness of the application of therapeutic touch on weight, complications, and length of hospital stay in preterm newborns attended in a neonatal unit. *Enferm Clin.* 2009;1:11-15.

28. Rosa L, Rosa E, Sarner L, Barrett S. A close look at therapeutic touch. *JAMA.* 1998;279(13):1005.

29. Wesa K, Cassileth B, Jain S. The effectiveness of biofield therapies for decreasing symptoms of pain and anxiety, and improving QoL. *Focus Altern Complement Ther.* 2011;16(1):62-65.

30. Movaffaghi Z, Farsi M. Biofield therapies: Biophysical basis and biological regulation? *Complement Ther Clin Pract.* 2009;15(1):35-37.

31. Harris M, Richards KC. The physiological and psychological effects of slow-stroke back massage and hand massage on relaxation in older people. *J Clin Nurs.* 2010;19(7-8):917-926.

32. Field T, Diego M, Hernandez-Reif M. Preterm infant massage therapy research: a review. *Infant Behav Dev.* 2010;33(2):115-124.

*33. Beider S, Moyer CA. Randomized controlled trials of pediatric massage: a review. *Evid Based Complement Alternat Med.* 2007;4(1):23-34.

*34. Gill H, Hoffmann A. The timing of onset of mechanical systole and diastole in reference to the QRS-T complex: A study to determine performance criteria for a non-invasive diastolic timed vibration massage system in treatment of potentially unstable cardiac disorders. *Cardiovascular Engineering.* 2010;10(4):235-245.

35. McCorkle R. Effects of touch on seriously ill patients. *Nurs Res.* 1974;23(2):125-132.

36. Knable J. Handholding: one means of transcending barriers of communication. *Heart Lung.* 1981;10(6):1106.

37. Linn LS, Kahn KL. Physician attitudes toward the "laying on of hands" during the AIDS epidemic. *Acad Med.* 1989;64(7):408.

38. Anonymous. Research: reiki induces relaxation, liminal state of awareness. *Massage Mag.* 2002;129.

39. Oh HJ, Park JS. Effects of hand massage and hand holding on the anxiety in patients with local infiltration anesthesia. *Taehan Kanho Hakhoe Chi.* 2004;34(6):924-933.

40. Post-White J, Kinney ME, Savik K, Gau JB, Wilcox C, Lerner I. Therapeutic massage and healing touch improve symptoms in cancer. *Integr Cancer Ther.* 2003;2(4):332.

41. Engebretson J, Wardell DW. Research: Reiki induces relaxation, liminal state of awareness. *Alternative Therapies in Health and Medicine.* 2002;8(2):48-53.

42. Lynch JJ. The effects of human contact on cardiac arrhythmia in coronary care patients. *J Nerv Ment Dis.* 1974;158(2):88-99.

43. Lynch JJ, Flaherty L, Emrich C, Mills ME, Katcher A. Effects of human contact on the heart activity of curarized patients in a shock-trauma unit. *Am Heart J.* 1974;88(2):160-169.

44. McCaffery M, Wolff M. Pain relief using cutaneous modalities, positioning, and movement. *Hosp J.* 1992;8:121-153.

45. Werner RA, Benjamin BE. *A Massage Therapist's Guide to Pathology.* Baltimore, MD: Lippincott Williams & Wilkins; 2002.

46. Apostle-Mitchell M, MacDonald G. An innovative approach to pain management in critical care: therapeutic touch. *Off J Can Assoc Crit Care Nurs.* 1997;8(3):19-22.

47. Bracciante LE. Scientific validation for healing touch. *Massage Bodywork.* 2004;19:12.

*48. Cook C, Guerrerio J, Slater V. Healing touch and quality of life in women receiving radiation treatment for cancer: a randomized controlled trial. *Altern Ther Health Med.* 2004;10(3):34.

49. Weze C, Leathard HL, Grange J, Tiplady P, Stevens G. Evaluation of healing by gentle touch in 35 clients with cancer. *Eur J Oncol Nurs.* 2004;8(1):40-49.

50. Colby LA, Kisner C. *Therapeutic Exercise: Foundations and Techniques.* 5th ed. Philadelphia, PA: FA Davis; 2007.

51. Krieger D. The response of in-vivo human hemoglobin to an active healing therapy by direct laying on of hands. *Hum Dimens.* 1972;1:12-15.

52. Krieger D. Healing by the laying on of hands as a facilitator of bio-energetic change: the response of in vivo human hemoglobin. *Psychoenergetic Syst.* 1976;1(2):121-129.

53. Krieger D. Therapeutic touch: the imprimatur of nursing. *Am J Nurs.* 1975;75(5):784-787.

54. Krieger D, Peper E, Ancoli S. Physiologic indices of therapeutic touch. *Am J Nurs.* 1979;4:660-662.

55. Krieger D. *The Therapeutic Touch: How to Use Your Hands to Help or to Heal.* New York, NY: Prentice-Hall; 1979.

56. Seidman M. *Like a Hollow Flute: A Guide to Polarity Therapy.* Santa Cruz, CA: Elan Press; 1982.

57. Gordon R. *Your Healing Hands: The Polarity Experience.* Santa Cruz, CA: Unity Press; 1979.

58. Stein D. *Essential Reiki: A Complete Guide to an Ancient Healing Art.* Freedom, CA: Crossing Press; 1995.

59. Richards K, Nagel C, Markie M, Elwell J, Barone C. Use of complementary and alternative therapies to promote sleep in critically ill patients. *Crit Care Nurs Clin North Am.* 2003;15(3):329-340.

60. Moyer CA, Rounds J, Hannum JW. A meta-analysis of massage therapy research. *Psychol Bull.* 2004;130(1):3.

61. Oschman JL. *Energy Medicine.* Edinburgh: Churchill Livingstone; 2000.

62. Oschman JL. Energy and the healing response. *J Bodywork Mov Ther.* 2005;9(1):3-15.

63. Oschman JL. Clinical aspects of biological fields: an introduction for health care professionals. *J Bodywork Mov Ther.* 2002;6(2):117-125.

64. Oschman J. The electromagnetic environment: implications for bodywork. *J Bodywork Mov Ther.* 2000;4:56-67.

65. Oschman JL. Energy circles: energy review part 6B. *J Bodywork Mov Ther.* 1998;2:59-61.

66. Oschman JL. What is healing energy? Part 4: vibrational medicines. *J Bodywork Mov Ther*. 1997;1(4):239-247.

67. Oschman JL. What is healing energy? Part 6: conclusions: is energy medicine the medicine of the future? *J Bodywork Mov Ther*. 1998;2(1):46-59.

68. Oschman JL. What is healing energy? Part 2: measuring the fields of life energy review part 2A. *J Bodywork Mov Ther*. 1997;1:117-121.

69. Oschman JL. Polarity, therapeutic touch, magnet therapy and related methods. *J Bodywork Mov Ther*. 1996;1:123-128.

70. Chaitow L. *Palpation and Assessment Skills: Assessment and Diagnosis through Touch*. Edinburgh, Scotland: Churchill-Livingston; 2003.

71. Weiss S. Psychophysiologic effects of caregiver touch on incidence of cardiac dysrhythmia. *Heart Lung*. 1986;15(5):495.

72. Nathan B. *Touch and Emotion in Manual Therapy*. Edinburgh, Scotland: Churchill Livingstone; 1999.

73. Fowlie L. *Heat and Cold as Therapy*. Toronto, ON: Curties-Overzet Publications; 2006.

74. Upledger JE, Vredevoogd JD. *Craniosacral Therapy*. Seattle, WA: Eastland Press; 1983.

75. Hollis M. *Massage for Therapists*. 2nd ed. Oxford, England: Blackwell Science; 1998.

76. Mennell JB. Physical treatment by movement, manipulation and massage. *Am J Med Sci*. 1947;213(1):125.

77. Björnsdotter M, Löken L, Olausson H, Vallbo Å, Wessberg J. Somatotopic organization of gentle touch processing in the posterior insular cortex. *J Neurosci*. 2009;29(29):9314.

78. Selden ST. Tickle. *J Am Acad Dermatol*. 2004;50(1):93-97.

79. Ruggieri V, Sabatini N, Milizia M. Muscular tone at rest: relationship with cutaneous pleasurable experience, an interpretation according to the dimensional approach to cerebral dominance. *Percept Mot Skills*. 1983;57(1):187-198.

80. Longworth J. Psychophysiological effects of slow stroke back massage in normotensive females. *ANS Adv Nurs Sci*. 1982;4(4):44.

81. Sims S. Slow stroke back massage for cancer patients. *Nurs Times*. 1986;82(47):47-50.

82. Fakouri C, Jones P. Relaxation treatment: slow stroke back rub. *J Gerontol Nurs*. 1987;13:32-35.

83. Meek SS. Effects of slow stroke back massage on relaxation in hospice clients. *J Nurs Sch*. 1993;25(1):17-22.

84. Lewis P, Nichols E, Mackey G, et al. The effect of turning and backrub on mixed venous oxygen saturation in critically ill patients. *Am J Crit Care*. 1997;6(2):132-140.

85. Mok E, Pang Woo C. The effects of slow-stroke back massage on anxiety and shoulder pain in elderly stroke patients. *Complement Ther Nurs Midwifery*. 2004;10(4):209-216.

86. Muller-Oerlinghausen B, Berg C, Scherer P, Mackert A, Moestl HP, Wolf J. Effects of slow-stroke massage as complementary treatment of depressed hospitalized patients. *Dtsch Med Wochenschr*. 2004;129(24):1363-1368.

87. Rowe M, Alfred D. The effectiveness of slow-stroke massage in diffusing agitated behaviors in individuals with Alzheimer's disease. *J Gerontol Nurs*. 1999;25(6):22.

88. Holland B, Pokorny ME. Slow stroke back massage: its effect on patients in a rehabilitation setting. *Rehabil Nurs*. 2001;26(5):182-186.

89. Lund I, Lundeberg T, Kurosawa M, Uvnäs-Moberg K. Sensory stimulation (massage) reduces blood pressure in unanaesthetized rats. *J Auton Nerv Syst*. 1999;78(1):30-37.

90. Lund I, Yu LC, Uvnas-Moberg K, et al. Repeated massage-like stimulation induces long-term effects on nociception: contribution of oxytocinergic mechanisms. *Eur J Neurosci*. 2002;16(2):330-338.

91. Kurosawa M, Lundeberg T, Agren G, Lund I, Uvnas-Moberg K. Massage-like stroking of the abdomen lowers blood pressure in anesthetized rats: influence of oxytocin. *J Auton Nerv Syst*. 1995;56:26-30.

92. Agren G, Lundeberg T, Uvnäs-Moberg K, Sato A. The oxytocin antagonist 1-deamino-2--tyr-(oet)-4-thr-8-orn-oxytocin reverses the increase in the withdrawal response latency to thermal, but not mechanical nociceptive stimuli following oxytocin administration or massage-like stroking in rats. *Neurosci Lett*. 1995;187(1):49-52.

93. Brouwer B, de Andrade VS. The effects of slow stroking on spasticity in patients with multiple sclerosis: a pilot study. *Physiother Theory Pract*. 1995;11(1):13-21.

*94. Aly H, Moustafa MF, Hassanein SM, Massaro AN, Amer HA, Patel K. Physical activity combined with massage improves bone mineralization in premature infants: a randomized trial. *J Perinatol*. 2004;24(5):305-309.

95. Dieter JNI, Field T, Hernandez-Reif M, Emory EK, Redzepi M. Stable preterm infants gain more weight and sleep less after five days of massage therapy. *J Pediatr Psychol*. 2003;28(6):403.

96. Ferber SG, Kuint J, Weller A, et al. Massage therapy by mothers and trained professionals enhances weight gain in preterm infants. *Early Hum Dev*. 2002;67(1):37-45.

97. Field T. Preterm infant massage therapy studies: an American approach. *Semin Neonatol*. 2002;7(6):487-494.

98. Field T. Massage therapy facilitates weight gain in preterm infants. *Curr Dir Psychol Sci*. 2001;10(2):51.

99. Field T. *Massage Therapy Research*. 1st ed. Edinburgh: Churchill Livingstone Elsevier; 2006.

100. Hayes JA, Adamson-Macedo EN, Perera S. The mediating role of cutaneous sensitivity within neonatal psychoneuroimmunology. *Neuro Endocrinol Lett*. 2000;21(3):187-193.

101. Hayes JA. TAC-TIC therapy: a non-pharmacological stroking intervention for premature infants. *Complement Ther Nurs Midwifery*. 1998;4(1):25-27.

102. Mathai S, Fernandez A, Mondkar J, Kanbur W. Effects of tactile-kinesthetic stimulation in preterms—a controlled trial. *Indian Pediatr*. 2001;38(10):1091-1098.

103. Vickers A, Ohlsson A, Lacy J, Horsley A. Massage for promoting growth and development of preterm and/or low birth-weight infants. *Cochrane Database Syst Rev*. 2004;2:CD000390.

104. Field TM, Schanberg SM, Scafidi F, et al. Tactile/kinesthetic stimulation effects on preterm neonates. *Pediatrics*. 1986;77(5):654.

105. Schanberg SM, Evoniuk G, Kuhn CM. Tactile and nutritional aspects of maternal care: specific regulators of neuroendocrine function and cellular development. *Exp Biol Med*. 1984;175(2):135.

106. Jay SS. The effects of gentle human touch on mechanically ventilated very-short-gestation infants. *Matern Child Nurs*. 1982;11(4):199-259.

107. White JL, Labarba RC. The effects of tactile and kinesthetic stimulation on neonatal development in the premature infant. *Dev Psychobiol*. 1976;9(6):569-577.

108. Kramer M, Chamorro I, Green D, Knudtson F. Extra tactile stimulation of the premature infant. *Nurs Res*. 1975;24(5):324.

109. Kattwinkel J, Nearman HS, Fanaroff AA, Katona PG, Klaus MH. Apnea of prematurity: comparative therapeutic effects of cutaneous stimulation and nasal continuous positive airway pressure. *J Pediatr*. 1975;86(4):588-592.

110. Solkoff N, Matuszak D. Tactile stimulation and behavioral development among low-birthweight infants. *Child Psychiatry Hum Dev*. 1975;6(1):33-37.

111. Lewis S. Utilising paediatric massage in an intensive care unit (PICU) in Saudi Arabia. *Aust J Holist Nurs*. 2000;7(2):29-33.

112. Onozawa K, Glover V, Adams D, Modi N, Kumar RC. Infant massage improves mother-infant interaction for mothers with postnatal depression. *J Affect Disord*. 2001;63(1-3):201-207.

113. Kim TI, Shin YH, White-Traut RC. Multisensory intervention improves physical growth and illness rates in Korean orphaned newborn infants. *Res Nurs Health*. 2003;26(6):424-433.

114. Agarwal KN, Gupta A, Pushkarna R, Bhargava SK, Faridi MM, Prabhu MK. Effects of massage & use of oil on growth, blood flow & sleep pattern in infants. *Indian J Med Res*. 2000;112:212-217.

115. Kuhn CM, Schanberg SM. Responses to maternal separation: mechanisms and mediators. *Int J Dev Neurosci*. 1998;16(3-4):261-270.

*116. Bellieni CV, Bagnoli F, Perrone S, Nenci A, Cordelli D, Fusi M. Effect of multisensory stimulation on analgesia in term neonates: a randomized controlled trial. *Pediatr Res*. 2002;51(4):460.

117. Davanzo R. Newborns in adverse conditions: issues, challenges, and interventions. *J Midwifery Womens Health*. 2004;49(S1):29-35.

118. Field T, Hernandez-Reif M, Diego M, Feijo L, Vera Y, Gil K. Massage therapy by parents improves early growth and development. *Infant Behav Dev*. 2004;27(4):435-442.

119. Darmstadt G, Mao-Qiang M, Chi E, et al. Impact of topical oils on the skin barrier: Possible implications for neonatal health in developing countries. *Acta Paediatr*. 2002;91(5):546-554.

120. Ferber SG, Laudon M, Kuint J, Weller A, Zisapel N. Massage therapy by mothers enhances the adjustment of circadian rhythms to the nocturnal period in full-term infants. *J Dev Behav Pediatr*. 2002;23(6):410.

121. Dennis C. Treatment of postpartum depression, part 2: a critical review of nonbiological interventions. *J Clin Psychiatry*. 2004;65(9):1252.

122. Field T. Early interventions for infants of depressed mothers. *Pediatrics*. 1998;102(suppl E1):1305.

123. Field T. Maternal depression effects on infants and early interventions. *Prev Med*. 1998;27(2):200-203.

124. Glover V, Onozawa K, Hodgkinson A. Benefits of infant massage for mothers with postnatal depression. *Semin Neonatol*. 2002;7(6):495-500.

125. Porter LS, Porter BO. A blended infant massage-parenting enhancement program for recovering substance-abusing mothers. *Pediatr Nurs*. 2004;30(5):363-372.

126. Brooks WW, Conrad CH, Nedder AP, Bing OHL, Slawsky MT. Thoracic massage permits use of echocardiography in unanesthetized rats. *Comp Med.* 2003;53(3):288-292.

127. Oschman JL. Therapeutic entrainment. *J Bodywork Mov Ther.* 1997;1: 189-194.

128. Oschman JL. What is healing energy? Part 3: silent pulses. *J Bodywork Mov Ther.* 1997;1(3):179-189.

129. Rider MS, Floyd JW, Kirkpatrick J. The effect of music, imagery, and relaxation on adrenal corticosteroids and the re-entrainment of circadian rhythms. *J Music Ther.* 1985;22(1):46-58.

130. McCaffrey R, Locsin RC. Music listening as a nursing intervention: a symphony of practice. *Holist Nurs Pract.* 2002;16(3):70.

131. Labyak SE, Metzger BL. The effects of effleurage backrub on the physiological components of relaxation: a meta-analysis. *Nurs Res.* 1997;46(1):59.

132. Hansson P, Ekblom A. Acute pain relieved by vibratory stimulation. *Br Dent J.* 1981;151(7):213.

133. Lundeberg T, Ottoson D, Hakansson S, et al. Vibratory stimulation for the control of intractable chronic orofacial pain. *Adv Pain Res Ther.* 1983;5: 555-561.

134. Ottoson D, Ekblom A, Hansson P. Vibratory stimulation for the relief of pain of dental origin. *Pain.* 1981;10(1):37-45.

135. Lundeberg T. Vibratory stimulation for the alleviation of pain. *Am J Chin Med.* 1984;12(1-4):60-70.

136. Bini G, Cruccu G, Hagbarth KE, Schady W, Torebjörk E. Analgesic effect of vibration and cooling on pain induced by intraneural electrical stimulation. *Pain.* 1984;18(3):239-248.

137. Lundeberg T. The pain suppressive effect of vibratory stimulation and transcutaneous electrical nerve stimulation (TENS) as compared to aspirin. *Brain Res.* 1984;294(2):201-209.

138. Lundeberg T. A comparative study of the pain alleviating effect of vibratory stimulation, transcutaneous electrical nerve stimulation, electroacupuncture and placebo. *Am J Chin Med.* 1984;12(1-4):72-79.

139. Lundeberg T. Long-term results of vibratory stimulation as a pain relieving measure for chronic pain. *Pain.* 1984;20(1):13-23.

140. Lundeberg T, Nordemar R, Ottoson D. Pain alleviation by vibratory stimulation. *Pain.* 1984;20(1):25-44.

141. Ekblom A, Hansson P. Extrasegmental transcutaneous electrical nerve stimulation and mechanical vibratory stimulation as compared to placebo for the relief of acute oro-facial pain. *Pain.* 1985;23(3):223-229.

142. Lundeberg T. Naloxone does not reverse the pain-reducing effect of vibratory stimulation. *Acta Anaesthesiol Scand.* 1985;29(2):212-216.

143. Lundeberg T. Relief of pain from a phantom limb by peripheral stimulation. *J Neurol.* 1985;232(2):79-82.

144. Sherer CL, Clelland JA, O'Sullivan P, Doleys DM, Canan B. The effect of two sites of high frequency vibration on cutaneous pain threshold. *Pain.* 1986;25(1):133-138.

145. Lundeberg T, Abrahamsson P, Bondesson L, Haker E. Effect of vibratory stimulation on experimental and clinical pain. *Scand J Rehabil Med.* 1988;20(4):149-159.

146. Palmesano TJ, Clelland JA, Sherer C, Stullenbarger E, Canan B. Effect of high-frequency vibration on experimental pain threshold in young women when applied to areas of different size. *Clin J Pain.* 1989;5(4):337.

147. Guieu R, Tardy-Gervet M, Blin O, Pouget J. Pain relief achieved by transcutaneous electrical nerve stimulation and/or vibratory stimulation in a case of painful legs and moving toes. *Pain.* 1990;42(1):43-48.

148. Guieu R, Tardy-Gervet MF, Roll JP. Analgesic effects of vibration and transcutaneous electrical nerve stimulation applied separately and simultaneously to patients with chronic pain. *Can J Neurol Sci.* 1991;18(2):113.

149. Guieu R, Tardy-Gervet MF, Giraud P. Met-enkephalin and beta-endorphin are not involved in the analgesic action of transcutaneous vibratory stimulation. *Pain.* 1992;48(1):83-88.

150. Tardy-Gervet M, Guieu R, Ribot-Ciscar E, Roll J. Transcutaneous mechanical vibrations: analgesic effect and antinociceptive mechanisms. *Rev Neurol.* 1993;149(3):177.

151. Yarnitsky D, Kunin M, Brik R, Sprecher E. Vibration reduces thermal pain in adjacent dermatomes. *Pain.* 1997;69(1-2):75-77.

152. Cody F, Richardson HC, MacDermott N, Ferguson I. Stretch and vibration reflexes of wrist flexor muscles in spasticity. *Brain.* 1987;110(2):433.

153. O'sullivan SB, Schmitz TJ. *Physical Rehabilitation: Assessment and Treatment.* 6th ed. Philadelphia, PA: FA Davis; 2006.

154. Hagbarth KE, Eklund G. The muscle vibrator—a useful tool in neurological therapeutic work. *Scand J Rehabil Med.* 1969;1(1):26-34.

155. Matheson D, Edelson R, Hiatrides D, Newkirk J, Twinem K, Thurston S. Relaxation measured by EMG as a function of vibrotactile stimulation. *Appl Psychophysiol Biofeedback.* 1976;1(1):285-292.

156. Spicher C, Kohut G. A significant increase in superficial sensation, a number of years after a peripheral neurologic lesion, using transcutaneous vibratory stimulation. *Ann Chir Main Memb Super.* 1997;16(2):124-129.

157. Roy EA, Hollins M, Maixner W. Reduction of TMD pain by high-frequency vibration: a spatial and temporal analysis. *Pain.* 2003;101(3):267-274.

158. Strelis AA, Strelis AK, Roskoshnykh VK. Vibration massage in the prevention of postresection complications and in the clinical rehabilitation of patients with pulmonary tuberculosis after surgical interventions. *Probl Tuberk Bolezn Legk.* 2004;11:29-34.

159. Murillo N, Kumru H, Vidal-Samso J, et al. Decrease of spasticity with muscle vibration in patients with spinal cord injury. *Clin Neurophysiol.* 2010;122(6): 1183-1189.

160. Hertling D, Kessler RM. *Management of Common Musculoskeletal Disorders: Physical Therapy Principles and Methods.* 4th ed. Philadelphia, PA: Lippincott Williams & Wilkins; 2006.

161. Michlovitz S. *Thermal Agents in Rehabilitation.* 3rd ed. Philadelphia, PA: FA Davis; 1996.

Further Reading

Anonymous. Research: reiki induces relaxation, liminal state of awareness. *Massage Mag.* 2002;129.

Benjamin PJ. A look back: massage in the nursery 100 years ago. *Massage Ther J.* 2004;43:144-148.

Bond C. Positive touch and massage in the neonatal unit: a British approach. *Semin Neonatol.* 2002;7(6):477-486.

Bracciante LE. Scientific validation for healing touch. *Massage Bodywork.* 2004;19:12.

Bruce DN, Tachiki KH. Autonomic and skeletal muscle responses to nonelectrical cutaneous stimulation. *Percept Mot Skills.* 1991;72(2):575-584.

Burke D, Hagbarth KE, Löfstedt L, Wallin BG. The responses of human muscle spindle endings to vibration of non-contracting muscles. *J Physiol (Lond).* 1976;261(3):673.

Carter A, Sanderson H. Complementary therapy. The use of touch in nursing practice. *Nurs Stand.* 1995;9(16):31-35.

Cashar L, Dixson B. The therapeutic use of touch. *J Psychiatr Nurs.* 1967;5(5):442-451.

Ching M. The use of touch in nursing practice. *Aust J Adv Nurs.* 1993;10(4):4-9.

Cody F, Plant T. Vibration-evoked reciprocal inhibition between human wrist muscles. *Exp Brain Res.* 1989;78(3):613-623.

Darmstadt GL, Saha SK. Traditional practice of oil massage of neonates in Bangladesh. *J Health Popul Nutr.* 2011;20(2):184-188.

Darmstadt GL, Saha SK. Neonatal oil massage. *Indian Pediatr.* 2003;40(11):1098-1099.

Doering TJ, Fieguth HG, Steuernagel B, et al. External stimuli in the form of vibratory massage after heart or lung transplantation. *Am J Phys Med Rehabil.* 1999;78(2):108.

Doraisamy P. The management of spasticity—a review of options available in rehabilitation. *Ann Acad Med Singapore.* 1992;21(6):807-812.

Engle VF, Graney MJ. Biobehavioral effects of therapeutic touch. *J Nurs Sch.* 2000;32(3):287-293.

Fakouri C, Jones P. Relaxation treatment: slow stroke back rub. *J Gerontol Nurs.* 1987;13:32-35.

Feldman R, Eidelman A. Intervention programs for premature infants: How and do they affect development? *Clin Perinatol.* 1998;25(3):613-626.

Fowlie L. *Heat and Cold as Therapy.* Toronto, ON: Curties-Overzet Publications; 2006.

Geis F, Viksne V. Touching: physical contact and level of arousal. *Proc Ann Convent Am Psychol Assoc.* 1972;7:179-180.

Gharavi B, Schott C, Linderkamp O. Value of kangaroo care, basal stimulation, kinesthesis awareness and baby massage in development promoting nursing of premature infants. *Kinderkrankenschwester.* 2004;23(9):368-372.

Helmig O. Vibrator therapy. History repeats itself. *Ugeskr Laeger.* 2001;163(51):7286-7288.

Hertling D, Kessler RM. *Management of Common Musculoskeletal Disorders: Physical Therapy Principles and Methods.* 4th ed. Philadelphia, PA: Lippincott Williams & Wilkins; 2006.

Huhtala V, Lehtonen L, Heinonen R, Korvenranta H. Infant massage compared with crib vibrator in the treatment of colicky infants. *Pediatrics.* 2000;105(6):e84.

Issurin V, Tenenbaum G. Acute and residual effects of vibratory stimulation on explosive strength in elite and amateur athletes. *J Sports Sci.* 1999;17(3): 177-182.

Jones JE, Kassity N. Varieties of alternative experience: complementary care in the neonatal intensive care unit. *Clin Obstet Gynecol.* 2001;44(4):750.

Kubsch SM, Neveau T, Vandertie K. Effect of cutaneous stimulation on pain reduction in emergency department patients. *Accid Emerg Nurs*. 2001;9(3): 143-151.

Kubsch SM, Neveau T, Vandertie K. Effect of cutaneous stimulation on pain reduction in emergency department patients. *Complement Ther Nurs Midwifery*. 2000;6(1):25-32.

Kuntz A. Anatomic and physiologic properties of cutaneo-visceral vasomotor reflex arcs. *J Neurophysiol*. 1945;8(6):421-429.

Malaquin-Pavan E. Therapeutic benefit of touch-massage in the overall management of demented elderly. *Rech Soins Infirm*. 1997;(49):11-66.

Mansour AA, Beuche M, Laing G, Leis A, Nurse J. A study to test the effectiveness of placebo reiki standardization procedures developed for a planned reiki efficacy study. *J Altern Complement Med*. 1998;5(2):153-164.

Matthews P. The reflex excitation of the soleus muscle of the decerebrate cat caused by vibration applied to its tendon. *J Physiol (Lond)*. 1966;184(2): 450.

Megharfi W, Bughin V. Physical therapy-massage of children in a sterile isolator. *Rev Infirm*. 2002;(86):33.

Miriutova NF, Levitskii EF, Abdulkina NG. Electromagnetic and mechanical vibrations in the therapy of myofascial pains. *Vopr Kurortol Fizioter Lech Fiz Kult*. 2000;(1):14-16.

Modrcin-Talbott MA, Harrison LL, Groer MW, Younger MS. The biobehavioral effects of gentle human touch on preterm infants. *Nurs Sci Q*. 2003;16(1):60-67.

Mullany LC, Darmstadt GL, Khatry SK, Tielsch JM. Traditional massage of newborns in Nepal: implications for trials of improved practice. *J Trop Pediatr*. 2005;51(2): 82-86.

Oschman JL. Energy circles: energy review part 6B. *J Bodywork Mov Ther*. 1998;2:59-61.

Oschman JL. What is healing energy? Part 2: measuring the fields of life energy review part 2A. *J Bodywork Mov Ther*. 1997;1:117-121.

Oschman JL. Healing energy part 1: historical background. *J Bodywork Mov Ther*. 1996;1(1):34-39.

Sansone P, Schmitt L. Providing tender touch massage to elderly nursing home residents: a demonstration project. *Geriatr Nurs*. 2000;21(6):303-308.

Seraia EV, Lapshin VP, Loginov LP, Artemova VV. Comparative efficacy of various massage techniques in the rehabilitation treatment of patients with inhalation trauma early after admission to the hospital. *Vopr Kurortol Fizioter Lech Fiz Kult*. 2002;(5):32-33.

Spencer KM. The primal touch of birth: midwives, mothers and massage. *Midwifery Today Int Midwife*. 2004;(70):11-13, 67.

Stiles KG. A new look at energy work. *Massage Ther J*. 2005;44:88-99.

Tovar MK, Cassmeyer VL. Touch. The beneficial effects for the surgical patient. *AORN J*. 1989;49(5):1356-1361.

Tyler DO, Winslow EH, Clark AP, White KM. Effects of a 1-minute back rub on mixed venous oxygen saturation and heart rate in critically ill patients. *Heart Lung*. 1990;19(5 pt 2): 562-565.

Ulm G. The current significance of physiotherapeutic measures in the treatment of Parkinson's disease. *J Neural Transm Suppl*. 1995;46:455-460.

Wang R. Treatment of 40 cases of hydroceles with massage at qichong (st 30). *J Tradit Chin Med*. 1998;18(3):218-219.

White-Traut R. Providing a nurturing environment for infants in adverse situations: multisensory strategies for newborn care. *J Midwifery Womens Health*. 2004;49(4):36-41.

CHAPTER 8

References

*Randomized Controlled Trial

†Systematic Review

1. Fritz S. *Fundamentals of Therapeutic Massage*. 3rd ed. St. Louis, MO: Mosby-Yearbook; 2004.
2. American Physical Therapy Association. *Guide to Physical Therapist Practice*. 2nd ed. Alexandria, VA: American Physical Therapy Association; 1999.
3. Benjamin PJ, Tappan FM. *Tappan's Handbook of Healing Massage Techniques*. 4th ed. Upper Saddle River, NJ: Pearson Prentice Hall; 2005.
4. Loving J. *Massage Therapy*. Stamford, CT: Appleton & Lange; 1999.
5. Salvo SG. *Massage Therapy: Principles and Practice*. 2nd ed. Philadelphia, PA: WB Saunders; 2003.
6. de Domenico G, Wood EC. *Beard's Massage*. 4th ed. Philadelphia, PA: WB Saunders; 1997.
7. Holey E, Cook E. *Evidence-Based Therapeutic Massage*. 2nd ed. Edinburgh, Scotland: Churchill Livingstone; 2003.

8. Hollis M. *Massage for Therapists*. 2nd ed. Oxford, England: Blackwell Science; 1998.
*9. Kimber L, McNabb M, Haines A, Brocklehurst P. Massage or music for pain relief in labour: a pilot randomised placebo controlled trial. *Eur J Pain*. 2008;12(8):961-969.
†10. Beider S, Moyer CA. Randomized controlled trials of pediatric massage: a review. *Evid Based Complement Alternat Med*. 2007;4(1):23-34.
11. Harris M, Richards KC. The physiological and psychological effects of slow-stroke back massage and hand massage on relaxation in older people. *J Clin Nurs*. 2010;19(7-8): 917-926.
*12. Seers K, Crichton N, Martin J, Coulson K, Carroll D. A randomised controlled trial to assess the effectiveness of a single session of nurse administered massage for short term relief of chronic non-malignant pain. *BMC Nurs*. 2008;7(1):10.
*13. Cherkin DC, Sherman KJ, Kahn J, et al. Effectiveness of focused structural massage and relaxation massage for chronic low back pain: protocol for a randomized controlled trial. *Trials*. 2009;10(1):96.
14. Bazzichi L, Dini M, Rossi A, et al. A combination therapy of massage and stretching increases parasympathetic nervous activity and improves joint mobility in patients affected by fibromyalgia. *Health*. 2010;2(8): 919-926.
15. Lindgren L, Rundgren S, Winsö O, et al. Physiological responses to touch massage in healthy volunteers. *Auton Neurosci*. 2010;158(1-2):105-110.
†16. Schiff A. Literature review of back massage and similar techniques to promote sleep in elderly people. *Pflege*. 2006;19(3):163-173.
17. Tiidus P, Shoemaker J. Effleurage massage, muscle blood flow and long-term post-exercise strength recovery. *Int J Sports Med*. 1995;16(7):478-483.
18. Shoemaker JK, Tiidus PM, Mader R. Failure of manual massage to alter limb blood flow: measures by Doppler ultrasound. *Med Sci Sports Exerc*. 1997;29(5):610.
19. Schmid-Schonbein G. Microlymphatics and lymph flow. *Physiol Rev*. 1990;70(4):987.
20. Grieve GP. Episacroiliac lipoma. *Physiotherapy*. 1990;76(6):308-310.
21. Mason M. The treatment of lymphoedema by complex physical therapy. *Aust J Physiother*. 1993;39:41-45.
22. Groer M, Mozingo J, Droppleman P, Davis M, Jolly ML. Measures of salivary secretory immunoglobulin A and state anxiety after a nursing back rub. *Appl Nurs Res*. 1994;7(1):2-6.
23. Labyak SE, Metzger BL. The effects of effleurage backrub on the physiological components of relaxation: a meta-analysis. *Nurs Res*. 1997;46(1):59.
*24. Fischer RL, Bianculli KW, Sehdev H, Hediger ML. Does light pressure effleurage reduce pain and anxiety associated with genetic amniocentesis? A randomized clinical trial. *J Matern Fetal Neonatal Med*. 2000;9(5):294-297.
25. Goldberg J, Sullivan SJ, Seaborne DE. The effect of two intensities of massage on H-reflex amplitude. *Phys Ther*. 1992;72(6):449.
26. Sullivan SJ, Seguin S, Seaborne D, Goldberg J. Reduction of H-reflex amplitude during the application of effleurage to the triceps surae in neurologically healthy subjects. *Physiother Theory Pract*. 1993;9(1):25-31.
27. Larsen JH. Infants' colic and belly massage. *Practitioner*. 1990;234(1487): 396-397.
28. Emly M. Abdominal massage. *Nurs Times*. 1993;89(3):34-36.
29. Yates J. *A Physician's Guide to Therapeutic Massage*. 3rd ed. Toronto, ON: Curties Overset; 2004.
30. Dunbar S, Redick E. Should patients with acute myocardial infarctions receive back massage? *Focus Crit Care*. 1986;13(3):42-46.
31. Tyler DO, Winslow EH, Clark AP, White KM. Effects of a 1-minute back rub on mixed venous oxygen saturation and heart rate in critically ill patients. *Heart Lung*. 1990;19(5 pt 2):562-565.
32. Leduc A, Lievens P, Dewald J. The influence of multidirectional vibrations on wound healing and on regeneration of blood- and lymph vessels. *Lymphology*. 1981;14(4):179-185.
33. Ueda W, Katataka Y, Sagara Y. Effect of gentle massage on regression of sensory analgesia during epidural block. *Anesth Analg*. 1993;76(4):783.
34. American Physical Therapy Association. *Guide to Physical Therapist Practice*. Alexandria, VA: American Physical Therapy Association; 2005.
35. Ciocon JO, Galindo-Ciocon D, Galindo DJ. Raised leg exercises for leg edema in the elderly. *Angiology*. 1995;46(1):19.
36. Wittlinger H, Wittlinger G. *Textbook of Dr. Vodder's Manual Lymphatic Drainage, Volume 1: Basic Course*. 3rd ed. Heidelberg: Karl F Haug Verlag; 1982.
37. Kurz I. *Textbook of Dr. Vodder's Manual Lymph Drainage*. Vol 2. 4th ed. Heidelberg: Karl F Haug Verlag; 1997.
38. Kurz I. *Textbook of Dr. Vodder's Manual Lymph Drainage*. Vol 3. 2nd ed. Heidelberg: Karl F Haug Verlag; 1990.
39. Kasseroller RG. The Vodder school: the Vodder method. *Cancer*. 1998;83(S12B):2840-2842.

40. Harris R. An introduction to manual lymph drainage: the Vodder method *Massage Ther J.* 1992;Winter:55-66.
41. Fritsch C, Tomson D. The usefulness of lymphatic drainage. *Schweiz Rundsch Med Prax.* 1991;80(15):383-386.
42. Casley-Smith JR, Boris M, Weindorf S, Lasinski B. Treatment for lymphedema of the arm—the Casley-Smith method. *Cancer.* 1998;83(S12B):2843-2860.
43. Leduc O, Leduc A, Bourgeois P, Belgrado JP. The physical treatment of upper limb edema. *Cancer.* 1998;83(S12B):2835-2839.
44. Lerner R. Complete decongestive physiotherapy and the Lerner lymphedema services academy of lymphatic studies (the Lerner school). *Cancer.* 1998;83(S12B):2861-2863.
45. Kurz W, Kurz R, Litmanovitch Y, Romanoff H, Pfeifer Y, Sulman F. Effect of manual lymphdrainage massage on blood components and urinary neurohormones in chronic lymphedema. *Angiology.* 1981;32(2):119.
46. Foeldi M, Strössenreuther RHK. *Foundations of Manual Lymph Drainage.* St. Louis, MO: Elsevier Mosby; 2005.
47. Reul-Hirche H. Manual lymph drainage when added to advice and exercise may not be effective in preventing lymphoedema after surgery for breast cancer. *J Physiother.* 2011;57(4):258.
*48. Devoogdt N, Christiaens MR, Geraerts I, et al. Effect of manual lymph drainage in addition to guidelines and exercise therapy on arm lymphoedema related to breast cancer: randomised controlled trial. *BMJ.* 2011;343: d5326.
49. Bongi SM, Del Rosso A, Passalacqua M, Miccio S, Cerinic MM. Manual lymph drainage improving upper extremity edema and hand function in patients with systemic sclerosis in edematous phase. *Arthritis Care Res.* 2011;63(8):1134-1141.
50. Ochałek K, Grądalski T. Manual lymph drainage may not be a necessary component in lymphedema treatment. *J Pain Symptom Manage.* 2010;39(5):e1-e2.
51. Kim SJ, Kwon OY, Yi CH. Effects of manual lymph drainage on cardiac autonomic tone in healthy subjects. *Int J Neurosci.* 2009;119(8):1105-1117.
52. Francois A, Richaud C, Bouchet J, Franco A, Comet M. Does medical treatment of lymphedema act by increasing lymph flow. *Vasa.* 1989;18(4):281-286.
53. Hutzschenreuter P, Brummer H, Ebberfeld K. Experimental and clinical studies of the mechanism of effect of manual lymph drainage therapy. *Z Lymphol.* 1989;13(1):62-64.
54. Hutzschenreuter P, Ehlers R. Effect of manual lymph drainage on the autonomic nervous system. *Z Lymphol.* 1986;10(2):58-60.
55. Liao SF, Huang MS, Chou YH, Wei TS. Successful complex decongestive physiotherapy for lymphedema and lymphocutaneous reflux of the female external genitalia after radiation therapy. *J Formosan Med Assoc.* 2003;102(6):404-406.
56. Cheville AL, McGarvey CL, Petrek JA, Russo SA, Taylor ME, Thiadens SRJ. Lymphedema management. *Semin Radiat Oncol.* 2003;13(3):290-301.
*57. Williams A, Vadgama A, Franks P, Mortimer PS. A randomized controlled crossover study of manual lymphatic drainage therapy in women with breast cancer-related lymphedema. *Eur J Cancer Care.* 2002;11(4):254-261.
58. Kriederman B, Myloyde T, Bernas M, et al. Limb volume reduction after physical treatment by compression and/or massage in a rodent model of peripheral lymphedema. *Lymphology.* 2002;35(1):23-27.
†59. Kasseroller RG, Schrauzer GN. Treatment of secondary lymphedema of the arm with physical decongestive therapy and sodium selenite: a review. *Am J Ther.* 2000;7(4):273.
60. Ko DSC, Lerner R, Klose G, Cosimi AB. Effective treatment of lymphedema of the extremities. *Archiv Surg.* 1998;133(4):452.
61. Franzeck U, Spiegel I, Fischer M, Börtzler C, Stahel HU, Bollinger A. Combined physical therapy for lymphedema evaluated by fluorescence microlymphography and lymph capillary pressure measurements. *J Vasc Res.* 1997;34(4):306-311.
62. Herpertz U. Outcome of various inpatient lymph drainage procedures. *Z Lymphol.* 1996;20(1):27-30.
63. Boris M, Weindorf S, Lasinski B, Boris G. Lymphedema reduction by noninvasive complex lymphedema therapy. *Oncology (Williston Park).* 1994;8(9):95-106; discussion 109-110.
64. Földi E. The treatment of lymphedema. *Cancer.* 1998;83 (S12B):2833-2834.
65. Gillham L. Lymphoedema and physiotherapists: control not cure. *Physiotherapy.* 1994;80(12):835-843.
66. Ruger K. Lymphedema of the head in clinical practice. *Z Lymphol.* 1993;17(1):6-11.
67. Barrellier MT. Lymphedema: is there a treatment? *Rev Med Interne.* 1992;13(1):49-57.
68. Lerner R. The ideal treatment for lymphedema. *Massage Ther J.* 1992; Winter: 37-39.
69. Clodius L, Foldi E, Foldi M. On nonoperative management of chronic lymphedema. *Lymphology.* 1990;23(1):2-3.
70. Cluzan R, Miserey G, Barrey P, Alliot F. Principles and results of physiotherapeutic therapy in mechanical lymphatic insufficiency of secondary or primary nature. *Phlebologie.* 1988;41(2):401-408.
71. Einfeld TH, Henkel M, Schmidt-Aufurth T, et al. Therapeutic and palliative lymph drainage in the treatment of face and neck edema. *HNO (German).* 1986;(34):365-367.
72. Földi E, Földi M, Weissleder H. Conservative treatment of lymphoedema of the limbs. *Angiology.* 1985;36(3):171.
73. Kurz W, Wittlinger G, Litmanovitch YI, et al. Effect of manual lymph drainage massage on urinary excretion of neurohormones and minerals in chronic lymphedema. *Angiology.* 1978;29(10):764-772.
74. Howell D, Watson M. Evaluation of a pilot nurse-led, community-based treatment programme for lymphoedema. *Int J Palliat Nurs.* 2005;11(2):62-69.
75. Campisi C, Boccardo F, Zilli A, et al. Lymphedema secondary to breast cancer treatment: possibility of diagnostic and therapeutic prevention. *Ann Ital Chir.* 2002;73(5):493.
76. Enig B, Mogensen M, Jorgensen RJ. Lymphedema in patients treated for breast cancer. A cross-sectional study in the county of Ribe. The need of manual lymph drainage; risk factors. *Ugeskr Laeger.* 1999;161(22):3293-3298.
77. Johansson K, Albertsson M, Ingvar C, Ekdahl C. Effects of compression bandaging with or without manual lymph drainage treatment in patients with postoperative arm lymphedema. *Lymphology.* 1999;32(3):103-110.
78. Fiaschi E, Francesconi G, Fiumicelli S, Nicolini A, Camici M. Manual lymphatic drainage for chronic post-mastectomy lymphoedema treatment. *Panminerva Med.* 1998;40(1):48-50.
*79. Johansson K, Lie E, Ekdahl C, Lindfeldt J. A randomized study comparing manual lymph drainage with sequential pneumatic compression for treatment of postoperative arm lymphedema. *Lymphology.* 1998;31(2):56-64.
80. Ferrandez JC, Laroche JP, Serin D, Felix-Faure C, Vinot JM. Lymphoscintigraphic aspects of the effects of manual lymphatic drainage. *J Mal Vasc.* 1996;21(5):283-289.
81. Cluzan RV, Alliot F, Ghabboun S, Pascot M. Treatment of secondary lymphedema of the upper limb with CYCLO 3 FORT. *Lymphology.* 1996;29(1):29-35.
82. Mirolo BR, Bunce IH, Chapman M, et al. Psychosocial benefits of postmastectomy lymphedema therapy. *Cancer Nurs.* 1995;18(3):197.
83. Gruffaz J. Management by the angiologist of sequellae of radiosurgical treatment of breast cancer. *J Mal Vasc.* 1995;20(2):150-152.
84. Bunce IH, Mirolo BR, Hennessy JM, Ward LC, Jones LC. Post-mastectomy lymphoedema treatment and measurement. *Med J Aust.* 1994;161(2):125-128.
85. Bertelli G, Venturini M, Forno G, Macchiavello F, Dini D. An analysis of prognostic factors in response to conservative treatment of postmastectomy lymphedema. *Surg Gynecol Obstet.* 1992;175(5):455-460.
86. Casley-Smith JR, Casley-Smith JR. Modern treatment of lymphoedema I. Complex physical therapy: the first 200 Australian limbs. *Australas J Dermatol.* 1992;33(2):61-68.
87. Zanolla R, Monzeglio C, Balzarini A, Martino G. Evaluation of the results of three different methods of postmastectomy lymphedema treatment. *J Surg Oncol.* 1984;26(3):210-213.
†88. Preston N, Seers K, Mortimer P. Physical therapies for reducing and controlling lymphoedema of the limbs. *Cochrane Database Syst Rev.* 2004(4): CD003141.
*89. McNeely ML, Magee DJ, Lees AW, Bagnall KM, Haykowsky M, Hanson J. The addition of manual lymph drainage to compression therapy for breast cancer related lymphedema: a randomized controlled trial. *Breast Cancer Res Treat.* 2004;86(2):95-106.
90. Harris R, Piller N. Three case studies indicating the effectiveness of manual lymph drainage on patients with primary and secondary lymphedema using objective measuring tools. *J Bodywork Mov Ther.* 2003;7(4):213-221.
91. Harris S, Hugi M, Olivotto I, Levine M. Steering committee for clinical practice guidelines for the care and treatment of breast cancer. Clinical practice guidelines for the care and treatment of breast cancer: 11. Lymphedema. *CMAJ.* 2001;164(2):191-199.
*92. Andersen L, Højris I, Erlandsen M, Andersen J. Treatment of breast-cancer-related lymphedema with or without manual lymphatic drainage: a randomized study. *Acta Oncol.* 2000;39(3):399-405.
93. Kessler T, de Bruin E, Brunner F, Vienne P, Kissling R. Effect of manual lymph drainage after hindfoot operations. *Physiother Res Int.* 2003;8(2):101-110.
94. Härén K, Backman C, Wiberg M. Effect of manual lymph drainage as described by Vodder on oedema of the hand after fracture of the distal radius: a prospective clinical study. *Scand J Plast Reconstr Surg Hand Surg.* 2000;34(4):367-372.

95. Weiss JM. Treatment of leg edema and wounds in a patient with severe musculoskeletal injuries. *Phys Ther.* 1998;78(10): 1104.

96. Trettin H. Craniocerebral trauma caused by sports. Pathogenic mechanism, clinical aspects and physical therapy with special reference to manual lymph drainage. *Z Lymphol.* 1993;17(2):36-40.

97. Valentin J, Leonhardt D, Perrin M. Prevention of venous thromboses and cutaneous necroses using physical methods and pressure therapy in the surgery of chronic venous insufficiency of the lower limbs. *Phlebologie.* 1988;41(3): 690-696.

98. Asdonk J. Physical lymph drainage and therapy of edema in chronic venous insufficiency. *Z Lymphol.* 1981;5(2):107-111.

99. Chomard D, Habault P, Ledemeney M, Haon C. Prognostic aspects of TcPO2 in iloprost treatment as an alternative to amputation. *Angiology.* 1999;50(4):283.

100. Husmann MJ, Roedel C, Leu AJ, et al. Lymphoedema, lymphatic microangiopathy and increased lymphatic and interstitial pressure in a patient with Parkinson's disease (abstract only). *Schweiz Med Wochenschr (German).* 1999;129:410-412.

101. Klyscz T, Bogenschutz O, Junger M, Rassner G. Microangiopathic changes and functional disorders of nail fold capillaries in dermatomyositis. *Hautarzt.* 1996;47(4):289-293.

102. Zahumensky E, Rybka J, Adamikova A. New aspects of pharmacologic and general prophylactic care of the diabetic foot. *Vnitr Lek.* 1995;41(8): 531-534.

103. Bringezu G. Combating fatigue in sports physical therapy with reference to manual lymph drainage (abstract only). *Z Lymphol (German).* 1994;18: 12-15.

104. Joos E, Bourgeois P, Famaey J. Lymphatic disorders in rheumatoid arthritis. *Semin Arthritis Rheum.* 1993;22(6):392-398.

105. Trettin H. Neurologic principles of edema in inactivity. *Z Lymphol.* 1992;16(1):14-16.

106. Kaaja R, Tiula E. Manual lymph drainage in nephrotic syndrome during pregnancy. *Lancet.* 1989;2(8669):990.

*107. Uher EM, Vacariu G, Schneider B, Fialka V. Comparison of manual lymph drainage with physical therapy in complex regional pain syndrome, type I. A comparative randomized controlled therapy study. *Wien Klin Wochenschr.* 2000;112(3):133-137.

†108. Preston N, Seers K, Mortimer P. Physical therapies for reducing and controlling lymphoedema of the limbs. *Cochrane Database Syst Rev.* 2004(4): CD003141. Reassessed 2008

109. Preisler VK, Hagen R, Hoppe F. Indications and risks of manual lymph drainage in head-neck tumors. *Laryngorhinootologie.* 1998;77(4):207-212.

110. Herpertz U. Malignant lymphedema (abstract only). *Z Lymphol (German).* 1990;14:17-23.

111. Wittlinger G, Wittlinger H. *Textbook of Dr. Vodder's Manual Lymph Drainage.* Vol 1. Heidelberg: Thieme; 2004.

Further Reading

Adcock J. Rehabilitation of the breast cancer patient. In: McGarvey CL, ed. *Physical therapy for the cancer patient.* New York, NY: Churchill Livingstone; 1990:67-87.

Asdonk J. Effectiveness, indications and contraindications of manual lymph drainage therapy in painful edema. *Z Lymphol.* 1995;19(1):16-22.

†Bakker EWP, Verhagen AP, van Trijffel E, Lucas C, Koes BW. Spinal mechanical load as a risk factor for low back pain: a systematic review of prospective cohort studies. *Spine.* 2009;34(8):E281.

Bauer WC, Dracup KA. Physiologic effects of back massage in patients with acute myocardial infarction. *Focus Crit Care.* 1987;14(6):42-46.

Bernas M, White M, Kriederman B, Summers P, Witte C. Massage therapy in the treatment of lymphedema. *Eng Med Biol Magazine, IEEE.* 2005;24(2): 58-68.

*Bertelli G, Venturini M, Forno G, Macchiavello F, Dini D. Original article: conservative treatment of postmastectomy lymphedema: a controlled, randomized trial. *Ann Oncol.* 1991;2(8):575.

Bringezu G. Combating fatigue in sports physical therapy with reference to manual lymph drainage (abstract only). *Z Lymphol (German).* 1994;18: 12-15.

Calnan J, Pflug J, Reis N, Taylor L. Lymphatic pressures and the flow of lymph1. *Br J Plast Surg.* 1970;23:305-317.

Campisi C, Boccardo F, Casaccia M. Post-mastectomy lymphedema: surgical therapy. *Ann Ital Chir.* 2002;73(5):473.

Carriere B. Edema: its development and treatment using lymph drainage massage. *Clin Manage Phys Ther.* 1988;8(5):19-21.

Casley-Smith J. Estimation of optimal massage pressure: is this possible. *Folia Angiol.* 1981;29:154-156.

Casley-Smith JR. Changes in the microcirculation at the superficial and deeper levels in lymphoedema: the effects and results of massage, compression, exercise and benzopyrones on these levels during treatment. *Clin Hemorheol Microcirc.* 2000;23(2-4):335-343.

Casley-Smith JR. Measuring and representing peripheral oedema and its alterations. *Lymphology.* 1994;27(2):56-70.

Chikly B. Post-mastectomy care and lymph drainage therapy. *J Bodywork Mov Ther.* 1999;3(1):11-16.

Downie PA, Innocenti D, Jackson S. *Cash's Textbook of Chest, Heart and Vascular Disorders for Physiotherapists.* London: Royal Marsden Hospital; 1987.

Drinker CK, Yoffey JM. *Lymphatics, Lymph, and Lymphoid Tissue. Their Physiological and Clinical Significance.* Cambridge, MA: Harvard University Press; 1941.

Einfeld TH, Henkel M, Schmidt-Aufurth T, et al. Therapeutic and palliative lymph drainage in the treatment of face and neck edema. *HNO (German).* 1986;34:365-367.

Evrard-Bras M, Coupe M, Laroche JP, Janbon C. Manual lymphatic drainage. *Rev Prat.* 2000;50(11):1199-1203.

Flowers KR. String wrapping versus massage for reducing digital volume. *Phys Ther.* 1988;68(1):57.

Földi E. Massage and damage to lymphatics. *Lymphology.* 1995;28(1):1-3.

Földi E, Sauerwald A, Hennig B. Effect of complex decongestive physiotherapy on gene expression for the inflammatory response in peripheral lymphedema. *Lymphology.* 2000;33(1):19.

Foldi M. Anatomical and physiological basis for physical therapy of lymphedema. *Experientia Suppl.* 1978;33:15-18.

Gironet N, Baulieu F, Giraudeau B, et al. Lymphedema of the limb: predictors of efficacy of combined physical therapy. *Ann Dermatol Venereol.* 2004;131(8-9):775-779.

Herpertz U. Malignant lymphedema (abstract only). *Z Lymphol (German).* 1990;14:17-23.

Herpertz U. Significance of radiogenic damage for lymphology. *Z Lymphol.* 1990;14(2):62-67.

Husmann MJ, Roedel C, Leu AJ, et al. Lymphoedema, lymphatic microangiopathy and increased lymphatic and interstitial pressure in a patient with Parkinson's disease (abstract only). *Schweiz Med Wochenschr (German).* 1999;129:410-412.

Kaya TI, Kokturk A, Polat A, Tursen U, Ikizoglu G. A case of cutaneous lymphangiectasis secondary to breast cancer treatment. *Int J Dermatol.* 2001;40(12):760-761.

Kirshbaum M. Using massage in the relief of lymphoedema. *Prof Nurse.* 1996;11(4):230-232.

Kurz I. *Textbook of Dr. Vodder's Manual Lymph Drainage, Volume 2: Therapy.* 4th ed. Heidelberg: Karl F Haug Verlag; 1997.

Kurz I. *Textbook of Dr. Vodder's Manual Lymph Drainage.* Vol 3. 2nd ed. Heidelberg: Karl F Haug Verlag; 1990.

Leduc A, Caplan I, Lievens P. *Traitement physique de l'œdème du bras.* Paris: Masson; 1981.

Lindemayr H, Santler R, Jurecka W. Compression therapy of lymphedema (author's transl). *MMW Munch Med Wochenschr.* 1980;122(22):825-828.

Little L, Porche DJ. Manual lymph drainage (MLD). *J Assoc Nurs AIDS Care.* 1998;9(1):78-81.

Morgan R, Casley-Smith JR, Mason M, Casley-Smith J. Complex physical therapy for the lymphoedematous arm. *J Hand Surg J Br Soc Surg Hand.* 1992;17(4):437-441.

Mortimer PS, Simmonds R, Rezvani M, Robbins M, Hopewell JW, Ryan TJ. The measurement of skin lymph flow by isotope clearance—reliability, reproducibility, injection dynamics, and the effect of massage. *J Invest Dermatol.* 1990;95(6):677-682.

Mortimer P. Therapy approaches for lymphedema. *Angiology.* 1997;48(1):87.

Pastura G, Mesiti M, Saitta M, et al. Lymphedema of the upper extremity in patients operated for carcinoma of the breast: clinical experience with coumarinic extract from melilotus officinalis. *Clin Ter.* 1999;150(6): 403-408.

Reiss M, Reiss G. Manual lymph drainage as therapy of edema in the head and neck area. *Praxis (Bern 1994).* 2003;92(7):271-274.

Rinehart-Ayres ME. Conservative approaches to lymphedema treatment. *Cancer.* 1998;83(S12B):2828-2832.

Rubin A, Hoefflin SM, Rubin M. Treatment of postoperative bruising and edema with external ultrasound and manual lymphatic drainage. *Plast Reconstr Surg.* 2002;109(4):1469.

Ruger K. Diagnosis and therapy of malignant lymphedema. *Fortschr Med.* 1998;116(12):28-30, 32, 34.

Stahel HU. Manual lymph drainage. *Curr Probl Dermatol.* 1999;27: 148-152.

Strossenreuther RH, Dax I, Emde C. Lymphedema—treatment. *MMW Fortschr Med*. 2004;146(3-4):28-30, 32-33.

Swedborg I. Effectiveness of combined methods of physiotherapy for post-mastectomy lymphoedema. *Scand J Rehabil Med*. 1980;12(2):77-85.

Thiadens SRJ. Current status of education and treatment resources for lymphedema. *Cancer*. 1998;83(S12B):2864-2868.

*Uher EM, Vacariu G, Schneider B, Fialka V. Comparison of manual lymph drainage with physical therapy in complex regional pain syndrome, type I. A comparative randomized controlled therapy study. *Wien Klin Wochenschr*. 2000;112(3):133-137.

Vasudevan SV, Melvin JL. Upper extremity edema control: rationale of the techniques. *Am J Occup Ther*. 1979;33(8):520-523.

Vignes S, Champagne A, Poisson O. Management of lymphedema: experience of the Cognacq-Jay Hospital. *Rev Med Interne*. 2002;23(suppl 3): 414s-420s.

Vodder E. Lymphdrainage ad modem Vodder. *Aesthetic Med*. 1965;14:190.

Williams C. Compression therapy for lymphoedema from vernon-carus. *Br J Nurs*. 1998;7(6):339-343.

Woods M. The experience of manual lymph drainage as an aspect of treatment for lymphoedema. *Int J Palliat Nurs*. 2003;9(8):336-342; discussion 342.

Worthington EL, Martin GA, Shumate M. Which prepared-childbirth coping strategies are effective? *JOGN Nurs*. 1982;11(1):45-51.

CHAPTER 9

References

1. Fritz S. *Fundamentals of Therapeutic Massage*. 3rd ed. St. Louis, MO: Mosby-Yearbook; 2004.
2. Benjamin PJ, Tappan FM. *Tappan's Handbook of Healing Massage Techniques*. 4th ed. Upper Saddle River, NJ: Pearson Prentice Hall; 2005.
3. Salvo SG. *Massage Therapy: Principles and Practice*. 2nd ed. Philadelphia, PA: WB Saunders; 2003.
4. Yates J. *A Physician's Guide to Therapeutic Massage*. 3rd ed. Toronto, ON: Curties Overzet; 2004.
5. Loving J. *Massage Therapy*. Stamford, CT: Appleton & Lange; 1999.
6. Holey E, Cook E. *Evidence-Based Therapeutic Massage*. 2nd ed. Edinburgh, Scotland: Churchill Livingstone; 2003.
7. Lowe W. *Orthopedic Massage: Theory and Technique*. Edinburgh, Scotland: Mosby; 2003.
8. Benjamin PJ, Lamp SP. *Understanding Sports Massage*. Champaign, IL: Human Kinetics; 1996.
9. Murrell W. *Massotherapeutics or Massage as a Mode of Treatment*. Philadelphia, PA: Blakiston; 1890.
10. Palmer MD. *Lessons on Massage (Illustrated Edition)*. 4th ed. London: Balliere Tindall and Cox; 1912.
11. Kellogg JH. *The Art of Massage*. Battle Creek, MI: Modern Medicine Publishing; 1923.
12. de Domenico G, Wood EC. *Beard's Massage*. 4th ed. Philadelphia, PA: WB Saunders; 1997.
13. Dery M, Yonuschot G, Winterson B. The effects of manually applied intermittent pulsation pressure to rat ventral thorax on lymph transport. *Lymphology*. 2000;33(2):58.
14. DiGiovanna EL, Schiowitz S, Dowling DJ. *An Osteopathic Approach to Diagnosis and Treatment*. Philadelphia, PA: Lippincott Williams & Wilkins; 2004.
15. Greenman PE, Greenman PE. *Principles of Manual Medicine*. Vol. 572. Baltimore, MD: Williams & Wilkins; 1996.
16. Field TM. Massage therapy effects. *Am Psychol*. 1998;53(12):1270.
17. Mair P, Kornberger E, Schwarz B, Baubin M, Hoermann C. Forward blood flow during cardiopulmonary resuscitation in patients with severe accidental hypothermia: an echocardiographic study. *Acta Anaesthesiol Scand*. 1998;42(10):1139-1144.
18. Boczar ME, Howard MA, Rivers EP, et al. A technique revisited: hemodynamic comparison of closed-and open-chest cardiac massage during human cardiopulmonary resuscitation. *Crit Care Med*. 1995;23(3):498.
19. Redberg RF, Tucker KJ, Cohen TJ, Dutton JP, Callaham ML, Schiller NB. Physiology of blood flow during cardiopulmonary resuscitation. A transesophageal echocardiographic study. *Circulation*. 1993;88(2):534-542.
20. Horiuchi K, Johnson R, Weissman C. Influence of lower limb pneumatic compression on pulmonary artery temperature: effect on cardiac output measurements. *Crit Care Med*. 1999;27(6):1096.
21. Malone MD, Cisek PL, Comerota AJ, Holland B, Eid IG. High-pressure, rapid-inflation pneumatic compression improves venous hemodynamics in healthy volunteers and patients who are post-thrombotic. *J Vasc Surg*. 1999;29(4): 593-599.

22. Liu K, Chen LE, Seaber AV, Johnson GW, Urbaniak JR. Intermittent pneumatic compression of legs increases microcirculation in distant skeletal muscle. *J Orthop Res*. 1999;17(1):88-95.
23. Vanek VW. Meta-analysis of effectiveness of intermittent pneumatic compression devices with a comparison of thigh-high to knee-high sleeves. *Am Surg*. 1998;64(11):1050.
24. Ricci MA, Fisk P, Knight S, Case T. Hemodynamic evaluation of foot venous compression devices. *J Vasc Surg*. 1997;26(5):803-808.
25. Allegra C, Bartolo M Jr, Martocchia R. Therapeutic effects of Vascupump treatment patients with Fontaine Stage II B arteriopathy. *Minerva Cardioangiol*. 2001;49(3):189-195.
26. Valtonen EJ, Lilius HG. The effect of syncardial massage produced without synchronization and with different pressure impulse frequencies. *Ann Chir Gynaecol Fenn*. 1973;62(2):69-72.
27. McGeown J, McHale N, Thornbury K. The role of external compression and movement in lymph propulsion in the sheep hind limb. *J Physiol (Lond)*. 1987;387(1):83.
28. Colby LA, Kisner C. *Therapeutic Exercise: Foundations and Techniques*. 5th ed. Philadelphia, PA: FA Davis; 2007.
29. Frownfelter DL, Dean E. *Principles and Practice of Cardiopulmonary Physical Therapy*. 3rd ed. St Louis, MO: Mosby; 1996.
30. Frownfelter DL. *Chest Physical Therapy and Pulmonary Rehabilitation: An Interdisciplinary Approach*. Chicago, IL: Year Book Medical; 1987.
31. McGeown J, McHale N, Thornbury K. Effects of varying patterns of external compression on lymph flow in the hindlimb of the anaesthetized sheep. *J Physiol (Lond)*. 1988;397(1):449.
32. Madenci E, Altindag O, Koca I, Yilmaz M, Gur A. Reliability and efficacy of the new massage technique on the treatment in the patients with carpal tunnel syndrome. *Rheumatol Int*. 2011; published online September 28: 1-9.
33. Hayes J, Cox C. Immediate effects of a five-minute foot massage on patients in critical care. *Intensive Crit Care Nurs*. 1999;15(2):77-82.
34. Ahles TA, Tope DM, Pinkson B, et al. Massage therapy for patients undergoing autologous bone marrow transplantation. *J Pain Symptom Manage*. 1999;18(3):157-163.
35. Field T, Hemandez-Reif M, Hart S, Theakston H, Schanberg S, Kuhn C. Pregnant women benefit from massage therapy. *J Psychosom Obstet Gynecol*. 1999;20(1):31-38.
36. Richards K. Effect of a back massage and relaxation intervention on sleep in critically ill patients. *Am J Crit Care*. 1998;7(4):288-299.
37. MacDonald G. Massage as a respite intervention for primary caregivers. *Am J Hosp Palliat Med*. 1998;15(1):43-47.
38. Field T, Schanberg S, Kuhn C, et al. Bulimic adolescents benefit from massage therapy. *Adolescence*. 1998;33:555-564.
39. Field T, Peck M, Krugman S, et al. Burn injuries benefit from massage therapy. *J Burn Care Res*. 1998;19(3):241.
40. Field T, Hernandez-Reif M, Seligmen S, et al. Juvenile rheumatoid arthritis: benefits from massage therapy. *J Pediatr Psychol*. 1997;22(5):607-617.
41. Ironson G, Field T, Scafidi F, et al. Massage therapy is associated with enhancement of the immune system's cytotoxic capacity. *Int J Neurosci*. 1996;84(1-4):205-217.
42. Fraser J, Kerr JR. Psychophysiological effects of back massage on elderly institutionalized patients. *J Adv Nurs*. 1993;18(2):238-245.
43. Field T, Morrow C, Valdeon C, Larson S, Kuhn C, Schanberg S. Massage reduces anxiety in child and adolescent psychiatric patients. *J Am Acad Child Adolesc Psychiatry*. 1992;31(1):125-131.
44. Field T, Ironson G, Scafidi F, et al. Massage therapy reduces anxiety and enhances EEG pattern of alertness and math computations. *Int J Neurosci*. 1996;86(3-4):197-205.
45. Field T. Maternal depression effects on infants and early interventions. *Prev Med*. 1998;27(2):200-203.
46. Field T, Grizzle N, Scafidi F, Schanberg S. Massage and relaxation therapies' effects on depressed adolescent mothers. *Adolescence*. 1996;31:903-912.
47. Field TM, Quintino O, Hernandez-Reif M, Koslovsky G. Adolescents with attention deficit hyperactivity disorder benefit from massage therapy. *Adolescence*. 1998;33:103-108.
48. Field T, Lasko D, Mundy P, et al. Brief report: autistic children's attentiveness and responsivity improve after touch therapy. *J Autism Dev Disord*. 1997;27(3):333-338.
49. Leivadi S, Hernandez-Reif M, Field T, et al. Massage therapy and relaxation effects on university dance students. *J Dance Med Sci*. 1999;3(3): 108-112.
50. Blackman P, Simmons LR, Crossley KM. Treatment of chronic exertional anterior compartment syndrome with massage: a pilot study. *Clin J Sport Med*. 1998;8(1):14.

51. Field DA, Miller S. Cosmetic breast surgery. *Am Fam Physician*. 1992;45(2):711-719.

52. Gam AN, Warming S, Larsen LH, et al. Treatment of myofascial trigger-points with ultrasound combined with massage and exercise-a randomised controlled trial. *Pain*. 1998;77(1):73-79.

53. Gluck NI. Passive care and active rehabilitation in a patient with failed back surgery syndrome. *J Manipulative Physiol Ther*. 1996;19(1):41-47.

54. Hammill JM, Cook TM, Rosecrance JC. Effectiveness of a physical therapy regimen in the treatment of tension-type headache. *Headache*. 1996;36(3):149-153.

55. Inoue M, Ohtsu I, Tomioka S, et al. Effects of pulmonary rehabilitation on vital capacity in patients with chronic pulmonary emphysema. *Nihon Kyobu Shikkan Gakkai Zasshi*. 1996;34(11):1182-1188.

56. Pope MH, Phillips RB, Haugh LD, Hsieh C, MacDonald L, Haldeman S. A prospective randomized three-week trial of spinal manipulation, transcutaneous muscle stimulation, massage and corset in the treatment of subacute low back pain. *Spine*. 1994;19(22):2571.

57. Waylonis GW, Perkins RH. Post-traumatic fibromyalgia. A long-term follow-up. *Am J Phys Med Rehabil*. 1994;73(6):403-412.

58. Levoska S, Keinänen-Kiukaanniemi S. Active or passive physiotherapy for occupational cervicobrachial disorders? A comparison of two treatment methods with a 1-year follow-up. *Arch Phys Med Rehabil*. 1993;74(4):425.

59. Zhao A. Study of effects of traditional Chinese massage. *Chin J Sports Med*. 1982;(1):46-48.

60. Schachner L, Field T, Hernandez-Reif M, Duarte AM, Krasnegor J. Atopic dermatitis symptoms decreased in children following massage therapy. *Pediatr Dermatol*. 1998;15(5):390-395.

61. Hoehn-Saric R. Psychic and somatic anxiety: worries, somatic symptoms and physiological changes. *Acta Psychiatr Scand*. 1998;98:32-38.

62. Millenson JR. *Mind Matters: Psychological Medicine in Holistic Practice*. Seattle, WA: Eastland Press; 1995.

63. Lundberg U. Muscle tension. *J Soft Tissue Manipulation*. 2006;13:3.

64. Crosman LJ, Chateauvert SR, Weisberg J. The effects of massage to the hamstring muscle group on range of motion. *J Orthop Sports Phys Ther*. 1984;6(3):168-172.

65. Van Den Dolder PA, Roberts DL. A trial into the effectiveness of soft tissue massage in the treatment of shoulder pain. *Aust J Physiother*. 2003;49(3):183-194.

66. Barlow A, Clarke R, Johnson N, Seabourne B, Thomas D, Gal J. Effect of massage of the hamstring muscle group on performance of the sit and reach test. *Br J Sports Med*. 2004;38(3):349-351.

67. Henriksen M, Højrup A, Lund H, Christensen L, Danneskiold-Samsøe B, Bliddal H. The effect of stimulating massage of thigh muscles on knee joint position sense. *Adv Physiother*. 2004;6(1):29-36.

68. Shipman M, Boniface D, Tefft M, McCloghry F. Antenatal perineal massage and subsequent perineal outcomes: a randomised controlled trial. *BJOG*. 1997;104(7):787-791.

69. Vendittelli F, Tabaste JL, Janky E. Antepartum perineal massage: review of randomized trials. *J Gynecol Obstet Biol Reprod (Paris)*. 2001;30(6):565-571.

70. Stamp G, Kruzins G, Crowther C. Perineal massage in labour and prevention of perineal trauma: randomised controlled trial. *BMJ*. 2001;322(7297):1277-1280.

71. Eason E, Labrecque M, Wells G, Feldman P. Preventing perineal trauma during childbirth: a systematic review. *Obstet Gynecol*. 2000;95(3):464.

72. Labrecque M, Eason E, Marcoux S. Randomized trial of perineal massage during pregnancy: perineal symptoms three months after delivery. *Obstet Gynecol*. 2000;182(1):76-80.

73. Morelli M, Chapman C, Sullivan S. Do cutaneous receptors contribute to the changes in the amplitude of the H-reflex during massage? *Electromyogr Clin Neurophysiol*. 1999;39(7):441.

74. Morelli M, Sullivan SJ, Chapman CE. Inhibitory influence of soleus massage onto the medial gastrocnemius H-reflex. *Electromyogr Clin Neurophysiol*. 1998;38(2):87-93.

75. Goldberg J, Seaborne DE, Sullivan SJ, Leduc BE. The effect of therapeutic massage on H-reflex amplitude in persons with a spinal cord injury. *Phys Ther*. 1994;74(8):728-737.

76. Goldberg J, Sullivan SJ, Seaborne DE. The effect of two intensities of massage on H-reflex amplitude. *Phys Ther*. 1992;72(6):449.

77. Sullivan SJ, Williams LRT, Seaborne DE, Morelli M. Effects of massage on alpha motoneuron excitability. *Phys Ther*. 1991;71(8):555-560.

78. Morelli M, Seaborne D, Sullivan S. H-reflex modulation during manual muscle massage of human triceps surae. *Arch Phys Med Rehabil*. 1991;72(11):915.

79. Morelli M, Seaborne D, Sullivan S. Changes in H-reflex amplitude during massage of triceps surae in healthy subjects. *J Orthop Sports Phys Ther*. 1990;12(2):55.

80. Dishman J, Bulbulian R. Comparison of effects of spinal manipulation and massage on motoneuron excitability. *Electromyogr Clin Neurophysiol*. 2001;41(2):97-106.

81. Newham DJ, Lederman E. Effect of manual therapy techniques on the stretch reflex in normal human quadriceps. *Disabil Rehabil*. 1997;19(8):326-331.

82. Lederman E. *The Science and Practice of Manual Therapy*. Edinburgh, Scotland: Elsevier/Churchill Livingstone; 2005.

83. Hernandez-Reif M, Field T, Krasnegor J, Martinez E, Schwartzman M, Mavunda K. Children with cystic fibrosis benefit from massage therapy. *J Pediatr Psychol*. 1999;24(2):175.

84. Beeken JE, Parks D, Cory JA, Montopoli G. The effectiveness of neuromuscular release massage therapy in five individuals with chronic obstructive lung disease. *Clin Nurs Res*. 1998;7(3):309.

85. Field T, Henteleff T, Hernandez-Reif M, et al. Children with asthma have improved pulmonary functions after massage therapy. *J Pediatr*. 1998;132(5):854-858.

86. Ernst E, Matrai A, Magyarosy I, Liebermeister R, Eck M, Breu M. Massages cause changes in blood fluidity. *Physiotherapy*. 1987;73(1):43-47.

87. Arkko P, Pakarinen A, Kari-Koskinen O. Effects of whole body massage on serum protein, electrolyte and hormone concentrations, enzyme activities and hematological parameters. *Int J Sports Med*. 1983;4(4):265-267.

88. Liu Y, Xu S, Yan J, et al. Capillary blood flow with dynamical change of tissue pressure caused by exterior force. *Sheng Wu Yi Xue Gong Cheng Xue Za Zhi*. 2004;21(5):699-703.

89. Shoemaker JK, Tiidus PM, Mader R. Failure of manual massage to alter limb blood flow: measures by Doppler ultrasound. *Med Sci Sports Exerc*. 1997;29(5):610.

90. Wyper D, McNiven D. Effects of some physiotherapeutic agents on skeletal muscle blood flow. *Physiotherapy*. 1976;62(3):83.

91. Hovind H, Nielsen SL. Effect of massage on blood flow in skeletal muscle. *Scand J Rehabil Med*. 1974;6(2):74-77.

92. Hansen TI, Kristensen JH. Effect of massage, shortwave diathermy and ultrasound upon 133Xe disappearance rate from muscle and subcutaneous tissue in the human calf. *Scand J Rehabil Med*. 1973;5(4):179-182.

93. Hinds T, McEwan I, Perkes J, Dawson E, Ball D, George K. Effects of massage on limb and skin blood flow after quadriceps exercise. *Med Sci Sports Exerc*. 2004;36(8):1308.

94. Linde B. Dissociation of insulin absorption and blood flow during massage of a subcutaneous injection site. *Diabetes Care*. 1986;9(6):570-574.

95. Martin NA, Zoeller RF, Robertson RJ, Lephart SM. The comparative effects of sports massage, active recovery, and rest in promoting blood lactate clearance after supramaximal leg exercise. *J Athl Train*. 1998;33(1):30.

96. Gupta S, Goswami A, Sadhukhan A, Mathur D. Comparative study of lactate removal in short term massage of extremities, active recovery and a passive recovery period after supramaximal exercise sessions. *Int J Sports Med*. 1996;17(2):106-110.

97. Dolgener FA, Morien A. The effect of massage on lactate disappearance. *J Strength Cond Res*. 1993;7(3):159.

98. Bale P, James H. Massage, warm-down and rest as recuperative measures after short term intense exercise. *Physiother Sport*. 1991;13(2):4-7.

99. Hemmings B, Smith M, Graydon J, Dyson R. Effects of massage on physiological restoration, perceived recovery, and repeated sports performance. *Br J Sports Med*. 2000;34(2):109-114.

100. Monedero J, Donne B. Effect of recovery interventions on lactate removal and subsequent performance. *Int J Sports Med*. 2000;21(8):593-597.

101. Boone T, Tanner M, Radosevich A. Effects of a 10-minute back rub on cardiovascular responses in healthy subjects. *Am J Chin Med*. 2001;29(1):47-52.

102. Anonymous. Trends in slow wave variability of the central circulation in healthy individuals in response to massage of the collar cervical region. *Vopr Kurortol Fizioter*. 2004;6:13-15.

103. Mortimer PS, Simmonds R, Rezvani M, Robbins M, Hopewell JW, Ryan TJ. The measurement of skin lymph flow by isotope clearance—reliability, reproducibility, injection dynamics, and the effect of massage. *J Invest Dermatol*. 1990;95(6):677-682.

104. Yamazaki Z, Idezuki Y, Nemoto T, Togawa T. Clinical experiences using pneumatic massage therapy for edematous limbs over the last 10 years. *Angiology*. 1988;39(2):154.

105. Yamazaki Z, Fujimori Y, Wada T, Togawa T, Yamakoshi K, Shimazu H. Admittance plethysmographic evaluation of undulatory massage for the edematous limb. *Lymphology*. 1979;12(1):40-42.

106. De Godoy J, Batigalia F. Preliminary evaluation of a new, more simplified physiotherapy technique for lymphatic drainage. *Lymphology*. 2002;35(2):91.

107. Aksenova AM, Teslenko OI, Boganskaia OA. Changes in the immune status of peptic ulcer patients after combined treatment including deep massage. *Vopr Kurortol Fizioter Lech Fiz Kult*. 1999;(2):19-20.

108. Makarova MR, Kuznetsov OF, Markina LP, Gusarova SA, Stiazhkina EM. The effect of massage on the neuromuscular apparatus and blood coagulating system of patients with chronic salpingo-oophoritis. *Vopr Kurortol Fizioter Lech Fiz Kult*. 1998;(6):45-48.

109. Aksenova AM, Romanova MM. The effect of reflex muscle massage on the body regulator processes of peptic ulcer patients with concomitant diseases. *Vopr Kurortol Fizioter Lech Fiz Kult (Russian)*. 1998;6:24-26.

110. Gusarova SA, Kuznetsov OF, Gorbunov FE, Maslovskaia SG. The characteristics of the effect of point and classical massage on the hemodynamics of patients with a history of transient ischemic attacks in the vertebrobasilar system. *Vopr Kurortol Fizioter Lech Fiz Kult*. 1998;(5):7-9.

111. Kuznetsov OF, Makarova MR, Markina LP. The comparative effect of classic massage of different intensities on patients with chronic salpingo-oophoritis. *Vopr Kurortol Fizioter Lech Fiz Kult*. 1998;(2):20-23.

112. Aksenova AM. A new method for deep reflex muscular massage. *Vopr Kurortol Fizioter Lech Fiz Kult*. 1997;(4):30-32.

113. Aksenova AM, Reznikov KM, Andreeva VV. The effect of deep massage and physical exercises on the cerebral circulation in osteochondrosis of the cervicothoracic spine. *Vopr Kurortol Fizioter Lech Fiz Kult*. 1997;(3):19-21.

114. Gusarova SA, Kuznetsov OF, Maslovskaia SG. The effect of the massage of different areas of the body on the cerebral hemodynamics in patients with a history of acute disorders of the cerebral circulation. *Vopr Kurortol Fizioter Lech Fiz Kult*. 1996;(1):14-16.

115. Richaud C, Bouchet JY, Bosson JL, Pichot O, Carpentier PH, Franco A. Manual fragmentation of deep vein thrombosis. *J Mal Vasc*. 1995;20(3):166-171.

116. Labrecque M, Nouwen A, Bergeron M, Rancourt JF. A randomized controlled trial of nonpharmacologic approaches for relief of low back pain during labor. *J Fam Pract*. 1999;48(4):259-263.

117. Field T, Hemandez-Reif M, Taylor S, Quintino O, Burman I. Labor pain is reduced by massage therapy. *J Psychosom Obstet Gynecol*. 1997;18(4):286-291.

118. Yildirim G, Sahin NH. The effect of breathing and skin stimulation techniques on labour pain perception of Turkish women. *Pain Res Manage*. 2004;9(4):183-187.

119. Nixon M, Teschendorff J, Finney J, Karnilowicz W. Expanding the nursing repertoire: the effect of massage on post-operative pain. *Aust J Adv Nurs*. 1997;14(3):21-26.

120. Ferrell-Torry AT, Glick OJ. The use of therapeutic massage as a nursing intervention to modify anxiety and the perception of cancer pain. *Cancer Nurs*. 1993;16(2):93.

121. Weinrich SP, Weinrich MC. The effect of massage on pain in cancer patients. *Appl Nurs Res*. 1990;3(4):140-145.

122. Akbayrak T, Citak I, Demirturk F, Akarcali I. Manual therapy and pain changes in patients with migraine? An open pilot study. *Adv Physiother*. 2001;3(2):49-54.

123. Puustjärvi K, Airaksinen O, Pöntinen P. The effects of massage in patients with chronic tension headache. *Acupunct Electrother Res*. 1990;15(2):159.

124. Danneskiold-Samsøe B, Christiansen E, Andersen RB. Myofascial pain and the role of myoglobin. *Scand J Rheumatol*. 1986;15(2):174-178.

125. Field T, Diego M, Cullen C, Hernandez-Reif M, Sunshine W, Douglas S. Fibromyalgia pain and substance P decrease and sleep improves after massage therapy. *J Clin Rheumatol*. 2002;8(2):72.

126. Ernst E. Massage therapy for low back pain: a systematic review. *J Pain Symptom Manage*. 1999;17(1):65-69.

127. Preyde M. Effectiveness of massage therapy for subacute low-back pain: a randomized controlled trial. *Can Med Assoc J*. 2000;162(13):1815-1820.

128. Carreck A. The effect of massage on pain perception threshold. *Manipulation Ther*. 1994;26:10-16.

129. Day JA, Mason RR, Chesrown SE. Effect of massage on serum level of β-endorphin and β-lipotropin in healthy adults. *Phys Ther*. 1987;67(6):926-930.

130. Tiidus PM. Manual massage and recovery of muscle function following exercise: a literature review. *J Orthop Sports Phys Ther*. 1997;25(2):107-112.

131. Callaghan MJ. The role of massage in the management of the athlete: a review. *Br J Sports Med*. 1993;27(1):28-33.

132. Cafarelli E, Flint F. The role of massage in preparation for and recovery from exercise. An overview. *Sports Med (Auckland, NZ)*. 1992;14(1):1.

133. Harmer PA. The effect of pre-performance massage on stride frequency in sprinters. *J Athl Train*. 1991;26(1):55-59.

134. Boone T, Cooper R, Thompson W. A physiologic evaluation of the sports massage. *J Athl Train*. 1991;26:51-54.

135. Wiktorsson-Moller M, Öberg B, Ekstrand J, Gillquist J. Effects of warming up, massage, and stretching on range of motion and muscle strength in the lower extremity. *Am J Sports Med*. 1983;11(4):249.

136. Ernst E. Does post-exercise massage treatment reduce delayed onset muscle soreness? A systematic review. *Br J Sports Med*. 1998;32(3):212.

137. Weber M, Servedio F, Woodall W. The effects of three modalities on delayed onset muscle soreness. *J Orthop Sports Phys Ther*. 1994;20(5):236.

138. Smith LL, Keating MN, Holbert D, et al. The effects of athletic massage on delayed onset muscle soreness, creatine kinase, and neutrophil count: a preliminary report. *J Orthop Sports Phys Ther*. 1994;19(2):93.

139. Cheung K, Hume PA, Maxwell L. Delayed onset muscle soreness: treatment strategies and performance factors. *Sports Med*. 2003;33(2):145-164.

140. Farr T, Nottle C, Nosaka K, Sacco P. The effects of therapeutic massage on delayed onset muscle soreness and muscle function following downhill walking. *J Sci Med Sport*. 2002;5(4):297-306.

141. Hilbert JE, Sforzo G, Swensen T. The effects of massage on delayed onset muscle soreness. *Br J Sports Med*. 2003;37(1):72.

142. Rinder A, Sutherland C. An investigation of the effects of massage on quadriceps performance after exercise fatigue. *Complement Ther Nurs Midwifery*. 1995;1(4):99-102.

143. Tiidus PM. Massage and ultrasound as therapeutic modalities in exercise-induced muscle damage. *Can J Appl Physiol*. 1999;24(3):267-278.

144. Rodenburg J, Steenbeek D, Schiereck P, Bar P. Warm-up, stretching and massage diminish harmful effects of eccentric exercise. *Int J Sports Med*. 1994;15(7):414-419.

145. Drews T, Kreider RB, Drinkard B, Jackson CW. Effects of post-event massage therapy on psychological profiles of exertion, feeling and mood during a 4-day ultra endurance cycling. *Med Sci Sports Exerc*. 1991;23:91.

146. Drews T, Kreider R, Drinkard B, et al. Effects of post-event massage therapy on repeated ultra-endurance cycling. *Int J Sports Med*. 1990;11:407.

147. Weinberg RS, Jackson AJ, Kolodny K. The relationship of massage and exercise to mood enhancement. *The Sport Psychologist*. 1988;2:202-211.

148. Robertson A, Watt J, Galloway S. Effects of leg massage on recovery from high intensity cycling exercise. *Br J Sports Med*. 2004;38(2):173-176.

149. Jönhagen S, Ackermann P, Eriksson T, Saartok T, Renström PAFH. Sports massage after eccentric exercise. *Am J Sports Med*. 2004;32(6):1499.

150. Lane KN, Wenger H. Effect of selected recovery conditions on performance of repeated bouts of intermittent cycling separated by 24 hours. *J Strength Cond Res*. 2004;18(4):855.

151. Tanaka T, Leisman G, Mori H, Nishijo K. The effect of massage on localized lumbar muscle fatigue. *BMC Complement Altern Med*. 2002;2(1):9.

152. Eliska O, Eliskova M. Are peripheral lymphatics damaged by high pressure manual massage? *Lymphology*. 1995;28(1):21-30.

153. Lindsay W, Pitcaithly D, Geelen N, Buntin L, Broxholme S, Ashby M. A comparison of the effects of four therapy procedures on concentration and responsiveness in people with profound learning disabilities. *J Intellect Disabil Res*. 1997;41(3):201-207.

154. Brooker DJR, Snape M, Johnson E, Ward D, Payne M. Single case evaluation of the effects of aromatherapy and massage on disturbed behaviour in severe dementia. *Br J Clin Psychol*. 1997;36(2):287-296.

155. Simons DG, Travell J, Simons LS. *Myofascial Pain and Dysfunction: The Trigger Point Manual: Upper Half of Body*. Vol. 1. Baltimore, MD: Williams & Wilkins; 1999.

156. Travell JG, Simons DG. *Myofascial Pain and Dysfunction: The Trigger Point Manual*. Vol. 1. Baltimore, MD: Lippincott Williams & Wilkins; 1983.

157. Chaitow L, DeLany J. *Modern Neuromuscular Techniques*. 2nd ed. New York, NY: Churchill Livingstone; 2003.

158. Mannheim CJ. *The Myofascial Release Manual*. 3rd ed. Thorofare, NJ: Slack; 2001.

159. Leikind ER, Harlin HC. Relief of back and sciatic pain by prostato-vesicular massage-stripping. *Clin Med*. 1962;69:1073-1082.

160. Travell JG, Simons DG. *Myofascial Pain and Dysfunction: The Trigger Point Manual*. Vol. 2. Baltimore, MD: Lippincott Williams & Wilkins; 1992.

161. Murphy GJ. Physical medicine modalities and trigger point injections in the management of temporomandibular disorders and assessing treatment outcome. *Oral Surg Oral Med Oral Pathol Oral Radiol Endod*. 1997;83(1):118-122.

162. Fricton JR. Management of masticatory myofascial pain. *Semin Orthod*. 1995;1(4):229-243.

163. Clark GT, Seligman DA, Solberg WK, Pullinger AG. Guidelines for the treatment of temporomandibular disorders. *J Craniomandib Disord*. 1990;4(2):80-88.

164. Seaman DR, Cleveland C III. Spinal pain syndromes: nociceptive, neuropathic, and psychologic mechanisms. *J Manipulative Physiol Ther*. 1999;22(7):458-472.

165. Kovacs FM, Abraira V, Pozo F, et al. Local and remote sustained trigger point therapy for exacerbations of chronic low back pain: a randomized, double-blind, controlled, multicenter trial. *Spine*. 1997;22(7):786.

166. Ingber RS. Iliopsoas myofascial dysfunction: a treatable cause of "failed" low back syndrome. *Arch Phys Med Rehabil*. 1989;70(5):382-386.

167. Morris CE. Chiropractic rehabilitation of a patient with S1 radiculopathy associated with a large lumbar disk herniation. *J Manipulative Physiol Ther.* 1999;22(1):38-44.

168. Hawk C, Long C, Azad A. Chiropractic care for women with chronic pelvic pain: a prospective single-group intervention study. *J Manipulative Physiol Ther.* 1997;20(2):73.

169. Hughes KH. Painful rib syndrome. A variant of myofascial pain syndrome. *AAOHN J.* 1998;46(3):115-120.

170. Antonelli MA, Vawter RL. Nonarticular pain syndromes. Differentiating generalized, regional, and localized disorders. *Postgrad Med.* 1992;91(2):95-98, 103-104.

171. Gerwin RD. Myofascial pain syndromes in the upper extremity. *J Hand Ther.* 1997;10(2):130-136.

172. Simons DG, Travell JG, Simons LS. *Myofascial Pain and Dysfunction: The Trigger Point Manual: Lower Half of Body.* Vol. 2. Baltimore, MD: Williams & Wilkins; 1999.

173. Simons DG, Mense S. Diagnosis and therapy of myofascial trigger points. *Schmerz.* 2003;17(6):419-424.

174. Granger J. *Neuromuscular Therapy Manual.* Baltimore, MD: Lippincott Williams & Wilkins; 2010.

175. Davies C, Davies A, Simons DG. *The Trigger Point Therapy Workbook: Your Self Treatment Guide for Pain Relief.* 2nd ed. Oakland, CA: New Harbinger; 2004.

176. Danneskiold-Samsoe B, Christiansen E, Lund B, Andersen RB. Regional muscle tension and pain ("fibrositis"). Effect of massage on myoglobin in plasma. *Scand J Rehabil Med.* 1983;15(1):17-20.

177. Buchberger D. Use of Active Release techniques in the postoperative shoulder: a case report. *J Sports Chiropract Rehabil.* 1999;13:60-66.

178. Hannon J. The man who mistook his patient for a chair: a speculation regarding sitting mechanical treatment of lower back pain. *J Bodywork Mov Ther.* 1998;2(2):88-100.

179. Morhenn VB. Firm stroking of human skin leads to vasodilatation possibly due to the release of substance P. *J Dermatol Sci.* 2000;22(2):138-144.

180. Lew P, Lewis J, Story I. Inter-therapist reliability in locating latent myofascial trigger points using palpation. *Man Ther.* 1997;2(2):87-90.

181. Han SC, Harrison P. Myofascial pain syndrome and trigger-point management. *Reg Anesth Pain Med.* 1997;22(1):89-101.

182. Chaitow L. *Positional Release Techniques.* New York, NY: Elsevier Health Sciences; 2002.

183. Prudden B. *Pain Erasure: The Bonnie Prudden Way.* New York, NY: Evans; 1980.

184. Prudden B. *Myotherapy: Bonnie Prudden's Complete Guide to Pain Free Living.* New York, NY: Dial Press; 1988.

185. Masunaga S, Ohashi W. *Zen Shiatsu: How to Harmonize Yin and Yang for Better Health.* Tokyo: Japan Publications; 1977.

186. Yamamoto S, McCarty P. *The Shiatsu Handbook: A Guide to the Traditional Art of Shiatsu Acupressure.* New York, NY: Avery; 1996.

187. Tappan FM. Finger pressure to acupuncture points. In: Tappan FM, Benjamin PJ, eds. *Tappan's Handbook of Healing Massage Techniques.* 3rd ed. Stamford, CT: Appleton & Lange; 1998:243-268.

188. Wolf JE, Teegarden IM. Jin shin do. In: Benjamin PJ, Tappan FM, eds. *Handbook of Healing Massage Techniques.* 4th ed. Upper Saddle River, NJ: Pearson Prentice Hall; 2005:363-376.

189. Dougans I. *The Complete Illustrated Guide to Reflexology: Therapeutic Foot Massage for Health and Well-Being.* Boston, MA: Element Books; 1996.

190. Byers DC. *Better Health with Foot Reflexology: The Original Ingham Method.* St Petersburg, FL: Ingham; 1996.

191. Hjelmstedt A, Shenoy ST, Stener-Victorin E, et al. Acupressure to reduce labor pain: a randomized controlled trial. *Acta Obstet Gynecol Scand.* 2010;89(11):1453-1459.

192. Kimber L, McNabb M, Haines A, Brocklehurst P. Massage or music for pain relief in labour: a pilot randomised placebo controlled trial. *Eur J Pain.* 2008;12(8):961-969.

193. Hou CR, Tsai LC, Cheng KF, Chung KC, Hong CZ. Immediate effects of various physical therapeutic modalities on cervical myofascial pain and trigger-point sensitivity. *Arch Phys Med Rehabil.* 2002;83(10):1406-1414.

194. McPartland JM. Travell trigger points—molecular and osteopathic perspectives. *J Am Osteopath Assoc.* 2004;104(6):244-249.

195. O'Sullivan SB. Strategies to improve motor control. In: O'Sullivan SB, Schmitz J, eds. *Physical Rehabilitation, Assessment and Treatment.* Philadelphia, PA: FA Davis; 1988.

196. Leone JA, Kukulka CG. Effects of tendon pressure on alpha motoneuron excitability in patients with stroke. *Phys Ther.* 1988;68(4):475-480.

197. Kukulka CG, Haberichter PA, Mueksch AE, Rohrberg MG. Muscle pressure effects on motoneuron excitability. *Phys Ther.* 1987;67(11):1720-1722.

198. Kukulka CG, Beckman SM, Holte JB, Hoppenworth PK. Effects of intermittent tendon pressure on alpha motoneuron excitability. *Phys Ther.* 1986;66(7):1091-1094.

199. Kukulka CG, Fellows WA, Oehlertz JE, VanderWilt SG. Effect of tendon pressure on alpha motoneuron excitability. *Phys Ther.* 1985;65(5):595-600.

200. Siev-Ner I, Gamus D, Lerner-Geva L, Zaidel S, Achiron A. Reflexology treatment relieves symptoms of multiple sclerosis: a randomized controlled study. *Mult Scler.* 2003;9:356-361.

201. Stephenson NN, Weinrich SP, Tavakoli AS. The effects of foot reflexology on anxiety and pain in patients with breast and lung cancer. *Oncol Nurs Forum.* 2000;27:67-72.

202. Kesselring A. Foot reflexology massage: a clinical study. *Forsch Komplementarmed.* 1999;6(suppl 1):38-40.

203. Sudmeier I, Bodner G, Egger I, Mur E, Ulmer H, Herold M. Changes of renal blood flow during organ-associated foot reflexology measured by color Doppler sonography. *Forsch Komplementarmed.* 1999;6(3):129-134.

204. Baerheim A, Algroy R, Skogedal KR, Stephansen R, Sandvik H. Feet—a diagnostic tool? *Tidsskr Nor Laegeforen.* 1998;118(5):753-755.

205. Kesselring A, Spichiger E, Muller M. Foot reflexology: an intervention study. *Pflege.* 1998;11(4):213-218.

206. Kristof O, Schlumpf M, Saller R. Foot reflex zone massage—a review. *Wien Med Wochenschr.* 1997;147(18):418-422.

207. Omura Y. Accurate localization of organ representation areas on the feet & hands using the bi-digital O-ring test resonance phenomenon: its clinical implication in diagnosis & treatment—part I. *Acupunct Electrother Res.* 1994;19(2-3):153-190.

208. Kesselring A. Foot reflex zone massage. *Schweiz Med Wochenschr Suppl.* 1994;62:88-93.

209. Oleson T, Flocco W. Randomized controlled study of premenstrual symptoms treated with ear, hand, and foot reflexology. *Obstet Gynecol.* 1993;82:906-911.

210. Petersen LN, Faurschou P, Olsen OT, Svendsen UG. Foot zone therapy and bronchial asthma—a controlled clinical trial. *Ugeskr Laeger.* 1992;154(30):2065-2068.

211. Brygge T, Heinig J, Collins P, et al. Reflexology and bronchial asthma. *Respir Med.* 2001;95(3):173-179.

212. Mollart L. Single-blind trial addressing the differential effects of two reflexology techniques versus rest, on ankle and foot oedema in late pregnancy. *Complement Ther Nurs Midwifery.* 2003;9(4):203-208.

213. Ross C, Hamilton J, Macrae G, Docherty C, Gould A, Cornbleet M. A pilot study to evaluate the effect of reflexology on mood and symptom rating of advanced cancer patients. *Palliat Med.* 2002;16(6):544.

214. Stephenson N, Dalton JA, Carlson J. The effect of foot reflexology on pain in patients with metastatic cancer. *Appl Nurs Res.* 2003;16(4):284-286.

215. Tovey P. A single-blind trial of reflexology for irritable bowel syndrome. *Br J Gen Pract.* 2002;52(474):19.

216. White A, Williamson J, Hart A, Ernst E. A blinded investigation into the accuracy of reflexology charts. *Complement Ther Med.* 2000;8(3):166-172.

217. Williamson J, White A, Hart A, Ernst E. Randomised controlled trial of reflexology for menopausal symptoms. *BJOG.* 2002;109(9):1050-1055.

218. Kannathal N, Paul JK, Lim C, Chua K, Sadasivan P. Effect of reflexology on EEG—a nonlinear approach. *Am J Chin Med.* 2004;32(4):641-650.

219. Mur E, Schmidseder J, Egger I, et al. Influence of reflex zone therapy of the feet on intestinal blood flow measured by color Doppler sonography. *Forsch Komplementarmed Klass Naturheilkd.* 2001;8(2):86-89.

220. Bennedbaek O, Viktor J, Carlsen KS, Roed H, Vinding H, Lundbye-Christensen S. Infants with colic. A heterogenous group possible to cure? Treatment by pediatric consultation followed by a study of the effect of zone therapy on incurable colic. *Ugeskr Laeger.* 2001;163(27):3773-3778.

221. Yang JH. The effects of foot reflexology on nausea, vomiting and fatigue of breast cancer patients undergoing chemotherapy. *Taehan Kanho Hakhoe Chi.* 2005;35(1):177-185.

222. Hodgson H. Does reflexology impact on cancer patients' quality of life? *Nurs Stand.* 2000;14(31):33.

223. Kohara H, Miyauchi T, Suehiro Y, Ueoka H, Takeyama H, Morita T. Combined modality treatment of aromatherapy, footsoak, and reflexology relieves fatigue in patients with cancer. *J Palliat Med.* 2004;7(6):791-796.

224. Wright S, Courtney U, Donnelly C, Kenny T, Lavin C. Clients' perceptions of the benefits of reflexology on their quality of life. *Complement Ther Nurs Midwifery.* 2002;8(2):69-76.

225. Porkert M, Hempen CH, Pao C. *Classical Acupuncture: The Standard Textbook.* Dinkelscherben: Phainon Editions & Media GmbH; 1995.

226. Helms JM. *Acupuncture Energetics. A Clinical Approach for Physicians.* Berkeley, CA: Medical Acupuncture Publishers; 1995.

227. Kielkowska A. *Your Health in Your Hands.* Gdansk: Kolmio; 1995.

228. Melzack R. Myofascial trigger points: relation to acupuncture and mechanisms of pain. *Arch Phys Med Rehabil.* 1981;62(3):114.

229. Melzack R, Stillwell DM, Fox EJ. Trigger points and acupuncture points for pain: correlations and implications. *Pain.* 1977;3(1):3-23.

230. Shenkman Z, Holzman RS, Kim C, et al. Acupressure-acupuncture antiemetic prophylaxis in children undergoing tonsillectomy. *Anesthesiology.* 1999;90(5):1311.

231. Harmon D, Ryan M, Kelly A, Bowen M. Acupressure and prevention of nausea and vomiting during and after spinal anaesthesia for caesarean section. *Br J Anaesth.* 2000;84(4):463.

232. Murphy PA. Alternative therapies for nausea and vomiting of pregnancy. *Obstet Gynecol.* 1998;91(1):78-81.

233. Stein DJ, Birnbach DJ, Danzer BI, Kuroda MM, Grunebaum A, Thys DM. Acupressure versus intravenous metoclopramide to prevent nausea and vomiting during spinal anesthesia for cesarean section. *Anesth Analg.* 1997;84(2): 342.

234. Ho CM, Hseu SS, Tsai SK, Lee TY. Effect of P-6 acupressure on prevention of nausea and vomiting after epidural morphine for post-cesarean section pain relief. *Acta Anaesthesiol Scand.* 1996;40(3):372-375.

235. Agarwal A, Pathak A, Gaur A. Acupressure wristbands do not prevent postoperative nausea and vomiting after urological endoscopic surgery. *Can J Anaesth.* 2000;47(4):319-324.

236. Collins KB, Thomas DJ. Acupuncture and acupressure for the management of chemotherapy-induced nausea and vomiting. *J Am Acad Nurse Pract.* 2004;16(2):80-84.

237. Cummings M. Hand acupressure reduces postoperative vomiting after strabismus surgery (*n* = 50). *Acupunct Med.* 2001;19(1):53-54.

238. Dibble SL, Chapman J, Mack KA, Shih AS. Acupressure for nausea: results of a pilot study. *Oncol Nurs Forum.* 2000;27(1):41-47.

239. Eizember FL, Tomaszewski CA, Kerns WP. Acupressure for prevention of emesis in patients receiving activated charcoal. *Clin Toxicol.* 2002;40(6):775-780.

240. Vellacott I, Cooke E, James C. Nausea and vomiting in early pregnancy. *Int J Gynecol Obstet.* 1988;27(1):57-62.

241. Klein J, Griffiths P. Acupressure for nausea and vomiting in cancer patients receiving chemotherapy. *Br J Community Nurs.* 2004;9(9):383-388.

242. Lu DP, Lu GP, Reed JF 3rd. Acupuncture/acupressure to treat gagging dental patients: a clinical study of anti-gagging effects. *Gen Dent.* 2000;48(4): 446-452.

243. Norheim AJ, Pedersen EJ, Fønnebø V, Berge L. Acupressure treatment of morning sickness in pregnancy. A randomised, double-blind, placebo-controlled study. *Scand J Prim Health Care.* 2001;19(1):43-47.

244. Roscoe JA, Morrow GR, Hickok JT, et al. The efficacy of acupressure and acustimulation wrist bands for the relief of chemotherapy-induced nausea and vomiting: a University of Rochester Cancer Center Community Clinical Oncology Program multicenter study. *J Pain Symptom Manage.* 2003;26(2): 731-742.

245. Schlager A, Boehler M, Pühringer F. Korean hand acupressure reduces postoperative vomiting in children after strabismus surgery. *Br J Anaesth.* 2000;85(2):267.

246. Shin YH, Kim TI, Shin MS, Juon HS. Effect of acupressure on nausea and vomiting during chemotherapy cycle for Korean postoperative stomach cancer patients. *Cancer Nurs.* 2004;27(4):267.

247. Slotnick RN. Safe, successful nausea suppression in early pregnancy with P-6 acustimulation. *J Reprod Med.* 2001;46(9):811-814.

248. Steele NM, French J, Gatherer-Boyles J, Newman S, Leclaire S. Effect of acupressure by Sea-Bands on nausea and vomiting of pregnancy. *J Obstet Gynecol Neonatal Nurs.* 2001;30(1):61-70.

249. Stern RM, Jokerst MD, Muth ER, Hollis C. Acupressure relieves the symptoms of motion sickness and reduces abnormal gastric activity. *Altern Ther Health Med.* 2001;7(4):91-94.

250. Tiran D. Nausea and vomiting in pregnancy: safety and efficacy of self-administered complementary therapies. *Complement Ther Nurs Midwifery.* 2002;8(4):191-196.

251. Vachiramon A, Wang WC. Acupressure technique to control gag reflex during maxillary impression procedures. *J Prosthet Dent.* 2002;88(2):236.

252. Wright LD. The use of motion sickness bands to control nausea and vomiting in a group of hospice patients. *Am J Hosp Palliat Med.* 2005;22(1):49-53.

253. Sakurai M, Suleman MI, Morioka N, Akça O, Sessler DI. Minute sphere acupressure does not reduce postoperative pain or morphine consumption. *Anesth Analg.* 2003;96(2):493.

254. Samad K, Afshan G, Kamal R. Effect of acupressure on postoperative nausea and vomiting in laparoscopic cholecystectomy. *J Pak Med Assoc.* 2003;53(2):68-72.

255. Schultz AA, Andrews AL, Goran SF, Mathew T, Sturdevant N. Comparison of acupressure bands and droperidol for reducing post-operative nausea and vomiting in gynecologic surgery patients. *Appl Nurs Res.* 2003;16(4):256-265.

256. Windle PE, Borromeo A, Robles H, Ilacio-Uy V. The effects of acupressure on the incidence of postoperative nausea and vomiting in postsurgical patients. *J Perianesth Nurs.* 2001;16(3):158-162.

257. Kober A, Scheck T, Schubert B, et al. Auricular acupressure as a treatment for anxiety in prehospital transport settings. *Anesthesiology.* 2003;98(6):1328.

258. Brady LH, Henry K, Luth JF, Casper-Bruett KK. The effects of shiatsu on lower back pain. *J Holist Nurs.* 2001;19(1):57.

259. Chung UL, Hung LC, Kuo SC, Huang CL. Effects of LI4 and BL 67 acupressure on labor pain and uterine contractions in the first stage of labor. *J Nurs Res.* 2003;11(4):251-260.

260. Hsieh LLC, Kuo CH, Yen MF, Chen THH. A randomized controlled clinical trial for low back pain treated by acupressure and physical therapy. *Prev Med.* 2004;39(1):168-176.

261. Kober A, Scheck T, Greher M, et al. Prehospital analgesia with acupressure in victims of minor trauma: a prospective, randomized, double-blinded trial. *Anesth Analg.* 2002;95(3):723.

262. Lee TA. Chinese way of easing pain-acupressure. *Int J Altern Med.* 2001;1(1): 1-12.

263. Yip Y, Tse S. The effectiveness of relaxation acupoint stimulation and acupressure with aromatic lavender essential oil for non-specific low back pain in Hong Kong: a randomised controlled trial. *Complement Ther Med.* 2004;12(1):28-37.

264. Chen ML, Lin LC, Wu SC, Lin JG. The effectiveness of acupressure in improving the quality of sleep of institutionalized residents. *J Gerontol A Biol Sci Med Sci.* 1999;54(8):M389.

265. Shen P. Two hundred cases of insomnia treated by otopoint pressure plus acupuncture. *J Tradit Chin Med.* 2004;24(3):168-169.

266. Tsay SL, Rong JR, Lin PF. Acupoints massage in improving the quality of sleep and quality of life in patients with end-stage renal disease. *J Adv Nurs.* 2003;42(2):134-142.

267. Wang XH, Yuan YD, Wang BF. Clinical observation on effect of auricular acupoint pressing in treating sleep apnea syndrome. *Zhongguo Zhong Xi Yi Jie He Za Zhi.* 2003;23(10):747-749.

268. Chen LL, Hsu SF, Wang MH, Chen CL, Lin YD, Lai JS. Use of acupressure to improve gastrointestinal motility in women after trans-abdominal hysterectomy. *Am J Chin Med.* 2003;31(5):781-790.

269. Jeon SY, Jung HM. The effects of abdominal meridian massage on constipation among CVA patients. *Taehan Kanho Hakhoe Chi.* 2005;35(1):135.

270. Maa SH, Sun MF, Hsu KH, et al. Effect of acupuncture or acupressure on quality of life of patients with chronic obstructive asthma: a pilot study. *J Altern Complement Med.* 2003;9(5):659-670.

271. Maa S, Gauthier D, Turner M. Acupressure as an adjunct to a pulmonary rehabilitation program. *J Cardiopulm Rehabil Prev.* 1997;17(4):268.

272. Beal MW. Acupuncture and acupressure. *J Midwifery Womens Health.* 1999;44(3):217-230.

273. Chen HM, Chen CH. Effects of acupressure at the Sanyinjiao point on primary dysmenorrhoea. *J Adv Nurs.* 2004;48(4):380-387.

274. Taylor D, Miaskowski C, Kohn J. A randomized clinical trial of the effectiveness of an acupressure device (relief brief) for managing symptoms of dysmenorrhea. *J Altern Complement Med.* 2002;8(3):357-370.

275. Cho Y, Tsay S. The effect of acupressure with massage on fatigue and depression in patients with end-stage renal disease. *J Nurs Res.* 2004;12(1):51.

276. Herskovitz S, Strauch B, Gordon MJ. Shiatsu massage-induced injury of the median recurrent motor branch. *Muscle Nerve.* 1992;15(10):1215.

277. Andrade C, Randall T, Swift T, Brescia N, eds. *The Effect of a Self-Managed Manual Trigger Point Pressure Program with a Hand-Held Massage Device on Trigger Point Sensitivity, Perceived Pain Levels, and Frequency of Self-Care in Adults with Chronic Myofascial Neck Pain.* Oakland, CA: Samuel Merritt College; 1997.

Further Reading

Physical therapy cures postpartum stress incontinence. *BMJ.* 2004;329(7478). doi:10.1136/bmj.329.7478.0-f.

Airaksinen O, Partanen K, Kolari PJ, Soimakallio S. Intermittent pneumatic compression therapy in posttraumatic lower limb edema: computed tomography and clinical measurements. *Arch Phys Med Rehabil.* 1991;72(9): 667-670.

Airaksinen O. Changes in posttraumatic ankle joint mobility, pain, and edema following intermittent pneumatic compression therapy. *Arch Phys Med Rehabil.* 1989;70(4):341-344.

Aldridge S. Brain-injured turn to CAM therapies. *Massage Magazine.* 2003; Nov/Dec(106):28.

Alexander R, Bennet-Clark H. Storage of elastic strain energy in muscle and other tissues. *Nature.* 1977;265(5590):114.

Allardice P. The no-surgery face lift. *Nat Way for Better Health.* 1997;3(22).

Angus S. Massage therapy for sprinters and runners. *Clin Podiatr Med Surg.* 2001;18(2):329-336.

Ause-Ellias KL, Richard R, Miller SF, Finley RK Jr. The effect of mechanical compression on chronic hand edema after burn injury: a preliminary report. *J Burn Care Res.* 1994;15(1):29.

Balke B, Anthony J, Wyatt F. The effects of massage treatment on exercise fatigue. *Clin Sports Med.* 1989;1:189-196.

Balla JI. The late whiplash syndrome. *Aust N Z J Surg.* 1980;50(6):610-614.

Barr J, Taslitz N. The influence of back massage on autonomic functions. *Phys Ther.* 1970;50(12):1679.

Bell GW. Aquatic sports massage therapy. *Clin Sports Med.* 1999;18(2): 427-435, ix.

Benjamin PJ. A look back: mechanical massage at the battle creek sanitarium. *Massage Ther J.* 2004;43(138):140.

Bodian M. Use of massage following lid surgery. *Eye Ear Nose Throat Mon.* 1969;48(9):542-547.

Bonica JJ. Management of myofascial pain syndromes in general practice. *J Am Med Assoc.* 1957;164(7):732.

Bork K, Korting GW, Faust G. Serum enzyme levels after a whole body massage. *Arch Dermatol Forsch.* 1971;240:342.

Braverman D, Schulman R. Massage techniques in rehabilitation medicine. *Phys Med Rehabil Clin N Am.* 1999;10(3):631.

Burovych AA, Samtsova IA, Manilov IA. An investigation of the effects of individual variants of sports massage on muscle blood circulation. *Sov Sports Sci Rev.* 1989;24:197.

Buskila D. Fibromyalgia, chronic fatigue syndrome, and myofascial pain syndrome. *Curr Opin Rheumatol.* 2001;13(2):117.

Cailliet R. *Soft tissue pain and disability 3/E.* 3rd ed. Philadelphia, PA: F. A. Davis Company; 1996.

Carrier E. Studies on the physiology of capillaries: V. The reaction of the human skin capillaries to drugs and other stimuli. *Am J Physiol.* 1922;61(3):528-547.

Cawley N. A critique of the methodology of research studies evaluating massage. *Eur J Cancer Care (Engl).* 1997;6(1):23-31.

Chaitow L. What is NMT? *J Bodywork Mov Ther.* 1999;3:1.

Chor H, Cleveland D, Davenport H, Dolkart RE, Beard G. Atrophy and regeneration of the gastrocnemius-soleus muscles. *J Am Med Assoc.* 1939;113(11):1029.

Chor H, Dolkart RE. A study of "simple disuse atrophy" in the monkey. *Am J Physiol.* 1936;117(4):626-630.

Curties D. Could massage therapy promote cancer metastasis? *Massage Ther J.* 2000;39(3):83-88.

Danneskiold-Samsoe B, Christiansen E. The effect of massage on muscle infiltrations as assessed by myoglobin in the blood. *Ugeskr Laeger.* 1985;147(4): 269-271.

Datta S. Handbook of chronic pain management. *JAMA.* 1989;262(17):2453.

Davidson K, Jacoby S, Brown MS. Prenatal perineal massage: preventing lacerations during delivery. *J Obstet Gynecol Neonatal Nurs.* 2000;29(5):474-479.

de las Peñas CF, Sohrbeck Campo M, Fernández Carnero J, Miangolarra Page JC. Manual therapies in myofascial trigger point treatment: a systematic review. *J Bodywork Mov Ther.* 2005;9(1):27-34.

Dejung B. Manual trigger point treatment in chronic lumbosacral pain. *Schweiz Med Wochenschr Suppl.* 1994;62:82-87.

Delaney GA, McKee AC. Inter-and intra-rater reliability of the pressure threshold meter in measurement of myofascial trigger point sensitivity. *Am J Phys Med Rehabil.* 1993;72(3):136-139.

Delaney J, Leong KS, Watkins A, Brodie D. The short-term effects of myofascial trigger point massage therapy on cardiac autonomic tone in healthy subjects. *J Adv Nurs.* 2002;37(4):364-371.

Donatelli R. *Physical Therapy of the Shoulder.* New York, NY: Churchill Livingstone; 1991.

Drust B, Atkinson G, Gregson W, French D, Binningsley D. The effects of massage on intra muscular temperature in the vastus lateralis in humans. *Int J Sports Med.* 2003;24(6):395-399.

Dubrovsky V. Changes in muscle and venous blood flow after massage. *Sov Sports Rev.* 1983;18(3):134-135.

Dunn C, Sleep J, Collett D. Sensing an improvement: an experimental study to evaluate the use of aromatherapy, massage and periods of rest in an intensive care unit. *J Adv Nurs.* 1995;21(1):34-40.

E Stamp G, Kruzins GS. A survey of midwives who participated in a randomised trial of perineal massage in labour. *Aust J Midwifery.* 2001;14(1):15-21.

Edgecombe W, Bain W. The effect of baths, massage and exercise on the blood-pressure. *Lancet.* 1899;153(3954):1552-1557.

Eichelberger G. Study on foot reflex zone massage. Alternative to tablets. *Krankenpfl Soins Infirm.* 1993;86(5):61-63.

Elkins EC, Herrick JF, Grindlay JH, Mann FC, De Forest RE. Effect of various procedures on the flow of lymph. *Arch Phys Med Rehabil.* 1953;34(1):31-39.

Elliott M. What future, medical massage? *Massage Bodywork.* 1999;14:128.

Evans RW. Some observations on whiplash injuries. *Neurol Clin.* 1992;10(4):975-997.

Felhendler D, Lisander B. Effects of non-invasive stimulation of acupoints on the cardiovascular system. *Complement Ther Med.* 1999;7(4):231-234.

Field T, Hernandez-Reif M, Shaw K, LaGreca A, Schanberg S, Kuhn C. Glucose levels decreased after giving massage therapy to children with diabetes mellitus. *Diabetes Spectr.* 1997;10:23-25.

Field T, Quintino O, Henteleff T, Wells-Keife L, Delvecchio-Feinberg G. Job stress reduction therapies. *Altern Ther Health Med.* 1997;3(4):54.

Field T, Seligman S, Scafidi F, Schanberg S. Alleviating posttraumatic stress in children following hurricane Andrew. *J Appl Dev Psychol.* 1996;17(1):37-50.

Field TM, Sunshine W, Hernandez-Reif M, et al. Massage therapy effects on depression and somatic symptoms in chronic fatigue syndrome. *J Chronic Fatigue Syndrome.* 1997;3(3):43-51.

Fire M. Providing massage therapy in a psychiatric hospital. *Int J Altern Complement Med.* 1984.

Fischer AA. Documentation of myofascial trigger points. *Arch Phys Med Rehabil.* 1988;69(4):286-291.

Fishbain D, Goldberg M, Steele R, Rosomoff H. DSM-III diagnoses of patients with myofascial pain syndrome (fibrositis). *Arch Phys Med Rehabil.* 1989;70(6):433.

Foda MI, Kawashima T, Nakamura S, Kobayashi M, Oku T. Composition of milk obtained from unmassaged versus massaged breasts of lactating mothers. *J Pediatr Gastroenterol Nutr.* 2004;38(5):484.

Fricton JR, Kroening R, Haley D, Siegert R. Myofascial pain syndrome of the head and neck: a review of clinical characteristics of 164 patients. *Oral Surg Oral Med Oral Pathol Oral Radiol Endod.* 1985;60(6):615-623.

Fricton JR. Clinical care for myofascial pain. *Dent Clin North Am.* 1991;35(1):1-28.

Gardner A, Fox R, Lawrence C, Bunker T, Ling R, MacEachern A. Reduction of post-traumatic swelling and compartment pressure by impulse compression of the foot. *J Bone Joint Surg Br.* 1990;72(5):810.

Goats G. Massage—the scientific basis of an ancient art: part 1. The techniques. *Br J Sports Med.* 1994;28(3):149.

Goats G. Massage—the scientific basis of an ancient art: part 2. Physiological and therapeutic effects. *Br J Sports Med.* 1994;28(3):153-156.

Goldman LB, Rosenberg NL. Myofascial pain syndrome and fibromyalgia. *Semin Neurol.* 1991;11(3):274-280.

Graff-Radford SB, Reeves JL, Baker RL, Chiu D. Effects of transcutaneous electrical nerve stimulation on myofascial pain and trigger point sensitivity. *Pain.* 1989;37(1):1-5.

Grimsby D, Grimsby K. Electromyographic and range of motion evaluation to compare the results of two treatment approaches: soft tissue massage versus a segmental manipulation off the cervical spine. *Ned Tijdschr Manuele Ther.* 1993;12:2.

Guan Z, Zheng G. The effects of massage on the left heart functions in patients of coronary heart disease. *J Tradit Chin Med.* 1995;15:59.

Gulla J, Singer AJ. Use of alternative therapies among emergency department patients. *Ann Emerg Med.* 2000;35(3):226-228.

Gunn C. *Treating Myofascial Pain: Intramuscular Stimulation (IMS) for Myofascial Pain Syndromes of Neuropathic Origin.* Seattle, WA: Multidisciplinary Pain Center, University of Washington Medical School; 1989.

Gusarova SA, Kuznetsov OF, Gorbunov FE, Maslovskaia SG. The use of point massage in patients with circulatory encephalopathy. *Vopr Kurortol Fizioter Lech Fiz Kult.* 1997;(6):11-13.

Hack GD, Robinson WL, Koritzer RT. Previously undescribed relation between muscle and dura. *Proceedings of the Congress of Neurological Surgeons San Francisco, CA.* 1995.

Hargens AR. *Tissue Nutrition and Viability.* New York, NY: Springer; 1986.

Hawk C, Long CR, Reiter R, Davis CS, Cambron JA, Evans R. Issues in planning a placebo-controlled trial of manual methods: results of a pilot study. *J Altern Complement Med.* 2002;8(1):21-32.

Hernandez-Reif M, Martinez A, Field T, Quintero O, Hart S, Burman I. Premenstrual symptoms are relieved by massage therapy. *J Psychosom Obstet Gynecol.* 2000;21(1):9-15.

Hey LR, Helewa A. Myofascial pain syndrome: a critical review of the literature. *Physiol Can.* 1994;46:28.

Hinz B. Perineal massage in pregnancy. *J Midwifery Womens Health.* 2005;50(1):63-64.

Hobbs S, Davies PD. Critical review of how nurses research massage therapy: are they using the best methods? *Complement Ther Nurs Midwifery.* 1998;4(2):35-40.

Hondras M, Linde K, Jones A. Manual therapy for asthma. *Cochrane Database Syst Rev.* 2005;2(April 18):CD001002.

Hong CZ, Simons DG. Pathophysiologic and electrophysiologic mechanisms of myofascial trigger points. *Arch Phys Med Rehabil.* 1998;79(7):863-872.

Huang FY, Huang LM. Effect of local massage on vaccination: DTP and DTPa. *Acta Paediatr Taiwan.* 1999;40(3):166-170.

Hulme J, Waterman H, Hillier V. The effect of foot massage on patients' perception of care following laparoscopic sterilization as day case patients. *J Adv Nurs.* 1999;30:460-468.

Issel C. The roots of reflexology. *Massage Bodywork.* 2003;18:52.

Jacobs M. Massage for the relief of pain: anatomical and physiological considerations. *Phys Ther Rev.* 1960;40:93-98.

Jami L. Golgi tendon organs in mammalian skeletal muscle: functional properties and central actions. *Physiol Rev.* 1992;72(3):623.

Janda V, Lewit K. On the concept of postural muscles and posture in man. *Aust J Physiother.* 1983;29:83-84.

Jimenez A, Lane M. Serial determinations of pressure threshold tolerance in chronic pain patients. *Arch Phys Med Rehabil.* 1985;66:545-546.

Jones DA, Round JM. *Skeletal Muscle in Health and Disease.* Vol. 3. Manchester: Manchester University Press; 1990:5.

Jones NA, Field T. Massage and music therapies attenuate frontal EEG asymmetry in depressed adolescents. *Adolescence.* 1999;34:529-534.

Jordan KD, Jessup D. The recuperative effects of sports massage as compared to rest. *Massage Ther J.* 1990;57.

Katz J, Wowk A, Culp D, Wakeling BA. A randomized, controlled study of the pain- and tension-reducing effects of 15 minute workplace massage treatments versus seated rest for nurses in a large teaching hospital. *Pain Res Manage.* 1999;4:81.

Katz J, Wowk A, Culp D, Wakeling H. Pain and tension are reduced among hospital nurses after on-site massage treatments: a pilot study. *J Perianesth Nurs.* 1999;14(3):128-133.

Kinney BM. External fatty tissue massage (the "endermologie" and "silhouette" procedures). *Plast Reconstr Surg.* 1997;100(7):1903.

Kraus H. *Diagnosis and Treatment of Muscle Pain.* Chicago, IL: Quintessence Publishing; 1988.

Krilov V. The use of restorative massage in the training of high level basketball players. *Soviet Sports Review.* 1985;20(1):7-9.

Kristof O, Schlumpf M, Saller R. Foot reflex zone massage—general practice and evaluation. *Fortschr Med.* 1998;116(29):50-54.

Labrecque M, Eason E, Marcoux S. Perineal massage in pregnancy: such massage significantly decreases perineal trauma at birth. *BMJ.* 2001;323(7315):753.

Labrecque M, Eason E, Marcoux S. Women's views on the practice of prenatal perineal massage. *BJOG.* 2001;108(5):499-504.

Ladd MP, Kottke FJ, Blanchard RS. Studies of the effect of massage on the flow of lymph from the foreleg of the dog. *Arch Phys Med Rehabil.* 1952;33(10):604-612.

Le Vu B, Dumortier A, Guillaume MV, Mouriesse H, Barreau-Pouhaer L. Efficacy of massage and mobilization of the upper limb after surgical treatment of breast cancer. *Bull Cancer.* 1997;84(10):957-961.

Lee YH. The effects of a foot-reflexo-massage education program on foot care in diabetic patients. *Taehan Kanho Hakhoe Chi.* 2003;33(5):633-642.

Lett A. The scope and limitations of treatment. An interview with Ann Lett, Principle, British School—Reflex Zone Therapy of the Feet. *Complement Ther Nurs Midwifery.* 2001;7(3):146-149.

Li Z, Liu J, Wu Y, et al. Effect of massotherapy on the in vivo free radical metabolism in patients with prolapse of lumbar intervertebral disc and cervical spondylopathy. *J Tradit Chin Med.* 1995;15(1):53-58.

Linde K, Vickers A, Hondras M, et al. Systematic reviews of complementary therapies—an annotated bibliography. Part 1: acupuncture. *BMC Complement Altern Med.* 2001;1(1):3.

Linde B, Philip A. Massage-enhanced insulin absorption—increased distribution or dissociation of insulin? *Diabetes Res.* 1989;11(4):191-194.

Lipton SA. Prevention of classic migraine headache by digital massage of the superficial temporal arteries during visual aura. *Ann Neurol.* 1986;19(5):515-516.

Losito JM, O'Neil J. Rehabilitation of foot and ankle injuries. *Clin Podiatr Med Surg.* 1997;14(3):533-557.

Lowe JC, Homeyman-Lowe G. Facilitating the decrease in fibromyalgic pain during metabolic rehabilitation: an essential role for soft tissue therapies. *J Bodywork Mov Ther.* 1998;2(4):208-217.

Lucas KR, Polus BI, Rich PA. Latent myofascial trigger points: their effects on muscle activation and movement efficiency. *J Bodywork Mov Ther.* 2004;8(3):160-166.

Lund I, Lundeberg T, Kurosawa M, Uvnäs-Moberg K. Sensory stimulation (massage) reduces blood pressure in unanaesthetized rats. *J Auton Nerv Syst.* 1999;78(1):30-37.

Lynn J. Using complementary therapies: reflexology. *Prof Nurse.* 1996;11(5):321-322.

Manyam BV, Sanchez-Ramos JR. Traditional and complementary therapies in Parkinson's disease. *Adv Neurol.* 1999;80:565-574.

McCaffrey R, Taylor N. Effective anxiety treatment prior to diagnostic cardiac catheterization. *Holist Nurs Pract.* 2005;19(2):70.

McCain GA, Scudds RA. The concept of primary fibromyalgia (fibrositis): clinical value, relation and significance to other chronic musculoskeletal pain syndromes. *Pain.* 1988;33(3):273-287.

McCandlish R. Perineal trauma: prevention and treatment. *J Midwifery Womens Health.* 2001;46(6):396-401.

McGain CA. Treatment of fibromyalgia and myofascial pain syndromes. In: Rachlin ES, ed. *Myofascial Pain and Fibromyalgia.* St Louis, MO: Mosby Year Book; 1994.

Miller L, Smith A, Mehler B. *The Stress Audit Manual.* Brookline, MA: Biobehavioral Associates; 1988.

Molea D, Murcek B, Blanken C, Burns R, Chila A, Howell J. Evaluation of two manipulative techniques in the treatment of postexercise muscle soreness. *J Am Osteopath Assoc.* 1987;87(7):477-483.

Nguyen HP, Le DL, Tran QM, Nguyen VT, Nguyen NO. Chromassi: a therapy advice system based on chrono-massage and acupression using the method of ZiWuLiuZhu. *Medinfo.* 1995;8(pt 2):998.

Nordschow M, Bierman W. The influence of manual massage on muscle relaxation: effect on trunk flexion. *J Am Phys Ther Assoc.* 1962;42:653.

Nussbaum EL, Downes L. Reliability of clinical pressure-pain algometric measurements obtained on consecutive days. *Phys Ther.* 1998;78(2):160-169.

Omura Y. Simple and quick non-invasive evaluation of circulatory condition of cerebral arteries by clinical application of the "bi-digital O-ring test." *Acupunct Electrother Res.* 1985;10(3):139-161.

Ortego NE. Acupressure: an alternative approach to mental health counseling through body-mind awareness. *Nurs Pract Forum.* 1994;5:72.

Oschman JL. Acupuncture and related methods: energy review part 1B. *J Bodywork Mov Ther.* 1996;1:40.

Paikov V. Means of restoration in the training of speed skaters. *Sov Sports Rev.* 1985;20:9-12.

Partsch H, Mostbeck A, Leitner G. Experimental studies on the efficacy of pressure wave massage (lymphapress) in lymphedema. *Z Lymphol.* 1981;5(1):35-39.

Pfaffenrath V, Rehm M. Migraine in pregnancy: what are the safest treatment options? *Drug Saf.* 1998;19(5):383-388.

Polisena CG. Case problem: presenting conventional and complementary approaches for relieving nausea in a breast cancer patient undergoing chemotherapy. *J Am Diet Assoc.* 2000;100(2):257-258.

Potapov IA, Abisheva TM. The action of massage on lymph formation and transport. *Vopr Kurortol Fizioter Lech Fiz Kult.* 1989;(5):44-47.

Poznick-Patewitz E. Cephalic spasm of head and neck muscles. *Headache.* 1976;15:261.

Rachlin ES. Musculofascial pain syndromes. *Med Times.* 1984:34.

Rachlin ES. *Myofascial Pain and Fibromyalgia: Trigger Point Management.* St Louis, MO: Mosby Year Book; 1994.

Rachlin I. Therapeutic massage in the treatment of myofascial pain syndromes and fibromyalgia. In: Rachlin ES, ed. *Myofascial Pain and Fibromyalgia.* St Louis, MO: Mosby Year Book; 1994:173-195.

Ragan C. Connective tissues. Transactions of the second conference. *South Med J.* 1953;46(8):830.

Reeves JL, Jaeger B, Graff-Radford SB. Reliability of the pressure algometer as a measure of myofascial trigger point sensitivity. *Pain.* 1986;24(3):313-321.

Roberts JR, Hedges JR. *Clinical Procedures in Emergency Medicine.* Philadelphia, PA: Saunders/Elsevier; 2010.

Rubin D. Myofascial trigger point syndromes: an approach to management. *Arch Phys Med Rehabil.* 1981;62(3):107.

Sa'adah S. Perineal massage to prevent perineal trauma during pregnancy. *J Fam Pract.* 1999;48(7):494-495.

Sander M, Siegert R, Gundlach KK. Results of physiotherapy for patients with myofacial dysfunction. *Dtsch Zahnarztl Z.* 1989;44(11 Spec No):S12-S14.

Sandler S. The physiology of soft tissue massage. *J Bodywork Mov Ther.* 1999;3(2):118-122.

Schneider W, Dvorak J. Functional treatment of diseases and injuries of the cervical spine. *Orthopade.* 1996;25(6):519-523.

Schuler L. A new fix for old injuries. *Men's Health.* 1999;14(9):80-81.

Scifres C. Neuromuscular therapy for groin strain. *J Bodywork Mov Ther.* 1998;2:148.

Scifres C. Neuromuscular therapy management of tenosynovitis. *J Bodywork Mov Ther.* 1997;1(3):150-154.

Scudds RA, Trachsel LC, Luckhurst BJ, Percy JS. A comparative study of pain, sleep quality and pain responsiveness in fibrositis and myofascial pain syndrome. *J Rheumatol Suppl.* 1989;19:120-126.

Severini V, Venerando A. The physiological effects of massage on the cardio-vascular system. *Eura Medicophys.* 1967;3:165.

Simons DG. Muscular pain syndromes. In: Fricton JR, Awad EA, eds. *Advances in Pain Research and Therapy.* Vol. 17. New York, NY: Raven Press; 1990.

Simons DG, Mense S. Diagnosis and therapy of myofascial trigger points. *Schmerz.* 2003;17(6):419-424.

Sinyakov A, Belov E. Restoration of work capacity of gymnasts. *Gymnastika.* 1982;1:48-51.

Snyder-Mackler L, Bork C, Bourbon B, Trumbore D. Effect of helium-neon laser on musculoskeletal trigger points. *Phys Ther.* 1986;66(7):1087-1090.

Sola A, Rodenberger M, Gettys B. Incidence of hypersensitive areas in posterior shoulder muscles; a survey of two hundred young adults. *Am J Phys Med.* 1955;34(6):585.

Stephenson NLN, Dalton JA. Using reflexology for pain management. *J Holist Nurs.* 2003;21(2):179-191.

Steven H, Jones GE. Massage therapy as a workplace intervention for reduction of stress. *Percept Mot Skills.* 1997;84(1):157-158.

Strong TH. Alternative therapies of morning sickness. *Clin Obstet Gynecol.* 2001;44(4):653.

Sullivan SJ, Blumberger J, Lachowicz C, Raymond D. Does massage decrease laryngeal tension in a subject with complete tetraplegia? *Percept Mot Skills.* 1997;84(1):169-170.

Sunshine W, Field T, Schanberg S. Massage therapy and transcutaneous electrical stimulation effects on fibromyalgia. *J Clin Rheumatol.* 1997;2:18.

Suskind MI, Hajek NM, Hines HM. Effects of massage on denervated skeletal muscle. *Arch Phys Med Rehabil.* 1946;27:133-135.

Takeuchi H, Jawad MSM, Eccles R. The effects of nasal massage of the "yingxiang" acupuncture point on nasal airway resistance and sensation of nasal airflow in patients with nasal congestion associated with acute upper respiratory tract infection. *Am J Rhinol.* 1999;13(2):77-79.

Travell J, Rinzler SH. The myofascial genesis of pain. *Postgrad Med.* 1952;11(5):425-434.

Tunnell PW. Protocol for visual assessment: postural evaluation of the muscular system through visual inspection. *J Bodywork Mov Ther.* 1996;1(1):21-27.

Urba SG. Nonpharmacologic pain management in terminal care. *Clin Geriatr Med.* 1996;12(2):301.

Valtonen EJ. Syncardial massage for treating extremities swollen by traumata, vein diseases or idiopathic lymphoedema. *Acta Chir Scand.* 1967;133(5):363-367.

Wakim KG, Martin GM, Krusen FH. Influence of centripetal rhythmic compression on localized edema of an extremity. *Arch Phys Med Rehabil.* 1955;36:98.

Wakim KG, Martin GM. The effects of massage on the circulation in normal and paralyzed extremities. *Arch Phys Med Rehabil.* 1949;30(3):135-144.

Walker DeLany J. Neuromuscular therapy management. *J Bodywork Mov Ther.* 1996;1(1):16-18.

Walling AD. From other journals perineal massage during labor offers limited benefit. *Am Fam Physician.* 2001;64(11):1888-1889.

Warfield CA, Bajwa ZH. *Principles and Practice of Pain Management.* New York, NY: McGraw-Hill; 1993.

Watson S, Watson S. The effects of massage: an holistic approach to care. *Nurs Stand.* 1997;11(47):45-47.

Weerapong P, Hume PA, Kolt GS. The mechanisms of massage and effects on performance, muscle recovery and injury prevention. *Sports Med.* 2005;35(3):235-256.

Weinrich SP, Weinrich MC. The effect of massage on pain in cancer patients. *Appl Nurs Res.* 1990;3(4):140-145.

Wilkinson S, Aldridge J, Salmon I, Cain E, Wilson B. An evaluation of aromatherapy massage in palliative care. *Palliat Med.* 1999;13(5):409-417.

Williams P, Goldspink G. Changes in sarcomere length and physiological properties in immobilized muscle. *J Anat.* 1978;127(pt 3):459.

Yessis M, Birukov AA, Pogosyan NM. Special means of restoration of work capacity of wrestlers in the periods between bouts. *Sov Sports Rev.* 1983;21(29):191.

Yunus MB. Fibromyalgia syndrome and myofascial pain syndrome: clinical features, laboratory tests, diagnosis, and pathophysiologic mechanisms. In: *Myofascial Pain and Fibromyalgia: Trigger Point Management.* St Louis, MO: Mosby; 1994:3-29.

Yunus M, Kalyan-Raman U, Kalyan-Raman K. Primary fibromyalgia syndrome and myofascial pain syndrome: clinical features and muscle pathology. *Arch Phys Med Rehabil.* 1988;69(6):451.

Yunus MB, Masi AT, Aldag JC. A controlled study of primary fibromyalgia syndrome: clinical features and association with other functional syndromes. *J Rheumatol Suppl.* 1989;19:62-71.

Zalessky M. Restoration for middle, long-distance, steeplechase and marathon runners and speed walkers. *Legkaya Atletika.* 1980;3:10.

Zalessky M. Coaching, medico-biological and psychological means of restoration. *Legkaya Atletika.* 1979;2:20.

Zeitlin D, Keller SE, Shiflett SC, Schleifer SJ, Bartlett JA. Immunological effects of massage therapy during academic stress. *Psychosom Med.* 2000;62(1):83-84.

CHAPTER 10

References

*Randomized controlled trial

1. Holey E, Cook E. *Evidence-Based Therapeutic Massage.* 2nd ed. Edinburgh, Scotland: Churchill Livingstone; 2003.

2. Yates J. *A Physician's Guide to Therapeutic Massage.* 3rd ed. Toronto, ON: Curties Overset; 2004.

3. Cantu RI, Grodin AJ. *Myofascial Manipulation: Theory and Clinical Application.* 2nd ed. Gaithersburg, MD: Aspen; 2001.

4. Chaitow L. *Palpation and Assessment Skills: Assessment and Diagnosis through Touch.* Edinburgh, Scotland: Churchill-Livingston; 2003.

5. Fritz S. *Fundamentals of Therapeutic Massage.* 3rd ed. St. Louis, MO: Mosby-Yearbook; 2004.

6. Maigne R. Low back pain of thoracolumbar origin. *Arch Phys Med Rehabil.* 1980;61(9):389-395.

7. Greenman PE, Greenman PE. *Principles of Manual Medicine.* Vol. 572. Baltimore, MD: Williams & Wilkins; 1996.

8. Benjamin PJ, Tappan FM. *Tappan's Handbook of Healing Massage Techniques.* 4th ed. Upper Saddle River, NJ: Pearson Prentice Hall; 2005.

9. Salvo SG. *Massage Therapy: Principles and Practice.* 2nd ed. Philadelphia, PA: WB Saunders; 2003.

10. de Domenico G, Wood EC. *Beard's Massage.* 4th ed. Philadelphia, PA: WB Saunders; 1997.

11. American Physical Therapy Association. *Guide to Physical Therapist Practice.* Alexandria, VA: American Physical Therapy Association; 2005.

12. American Physical Therapy Association. *Guide to Physical Therapist Practice.* 2nd ed. Alexandria, VA: American Physical Therapy Association; 1999.

13. Tillman LJ, Cummings GS. Biologic mechanisms of connective tissue mutability. In: Currier DP, Nelson M, eds. *Dynamics of Human Biologic Tissues.* Philadelphia, PA: FA Davis; 1992:44.

14. Taylor DC, Dalton JD, Seaber AV, Garrett WE. Viscoelastic properties of muscle-tendon units. *Am J Sports Med.* 1990;18(3):300-309.

15. Frank C, Amiel D, Woo S, Akeson W. Normal ligament properties and ligament healing. *Clin Orthop.* 1985;196:15.

16. Dunn MG, Silver FH. Viscoelastic behavior of human connective tissues: relative contribution of viscous and elastic components. *Connect Tissue Res.* 1983;12(1):59-70.

17. Sapega A, Quedenfeld T, Moyer R, Butler R. Biophysical factors in range-of-motion exercise. *Physician Sportsmed.* 1981;9(12):57-65.

18. Light KE, Nuzik S, Personius W, Barstrom A. Low-load prolonged stretch vs. high-load brief stretch in treating knee contractures. *Phys Ther.* 1984;64(3):330-333.

19. Hooley C, McCrum N, Cohen R. The viscoelastic deformation of tendon. *J Biomech.* 1980;13(6):521-528.

20. Warren CG, Lehmann JF. Heat and stretch procedures: an evaluation using rat tail tendon. *Arch Phys Med Rehabil.* 1976;57:122-126.

21. Chaitow L, DeLany J. *Modern Neuromuscular Techniques.* 2nd ed. New York, NY: Churchill Livingstone; 2003.

22. Lagrana NA, Alexander H, Stauchler I, Mehta A, Ricci J. Effect of mechanical load in wound healing. *Ann Plastic Surg.* 1983;10:200-208.

23. Magonne T, DeWitt MT, Handeley CJ. In vitro responses of chondrocytes to mechanical loading: the effect of short term mechanical tension. *Connect Tissue Res.* 1984;12:97-109.

24. Arem AJ, Madden JW. Effects of stress on healing wounds: I. Intermittent noncyclical tension. *J Surg Res.* 1976;20(2):93.

25. Woo S, Matthews JV. Connective tissue response to immobility. *Arthritis Rheum.* 1975;18:257-264.

26. Akeson WH, Amiel D. Connective tissue response to immobility: an accelerated aging process. *Arthritis Rheum.* 1968;18(3):257-301.

27. Hilton J. *The Influence of Mechanical and Physiological Rest in the Treatment of Accidents and Surgical Diseases, and the Diagnostic Value of Pain.* London, England: Bell and Daldy; 1863.

28. Editors of the American Heritage Dictionaries. *The American Heritage Medical Dictionary.* Boston, MA: Houghton Mifflin Company; 2007.

29. Kellogg JH. *The Art of Massage in Early American Manual Therapy Volume.* Vol. 6. Virginia Beach, VA: McMillin Media; 2011.

30. Taylor P, Tole G, Vernon H. Skin rolling technique as an indicator of spinal joint dysfunction. *J Can Chiropr Assoc.* 1990;34(2):82.

31. Tillman LJ, Chasan NP. Wound healing: injury and repair of dense connective tissues. In: Hertling D, Kessler RM, eds. *Management of Common Musculoskeletal Conditions.* Philadelphia, PA: Lippincott Williams and Wilkins; 2006:15-26.

32. Colby LA, Kisner C. *Therapeutic Exercise: Foundations and Techniques.* 5th ed. Philadelphia, PA: FA Davis; 2007.

33. Lederman E. *The Science and Practice of Manual Therapy.* Edinburgh, Scotland: Elsevier/Churchill Livingstone; 2005.

34. Mannheim CJ. *The Myofascial Release Manual.* 3rd ed. Thorofare, NJ: Slack Inc.; 2001.

35. Barnes JF. Myofascial release. In: Hammer WI, ed. *Functional Soft Tissue Examination and Treatment by Manual Methods.* 2nd ed. Gaithersburg, MD: Aspen; 1999:533-548.

36. DiGiovanna EL, Schiowitz S, Dowling DJ. *An Osteopathic Approach to Diagnosis and Treatment.* Philadelphia, PA: Lippincott Williams & Wilkins; 2004.

37. Sucher B, Heath D. Thoracic outlet syndrome—a myofascial variant: part 3. Structural and postural considerations. *JAOA: J Am Osteopath Assoc.* 1993;93(3):334.

38. Sucher BM. Thoracic outlet syndrome—a myofascial variant: part 1. Pathology and diagnosis. *JAOA: J Am Osteopath Assoc.* 1990;90(8):686.

39. Sucher BM. Thoracic outlet syndrome—a myofascial variant: part 2. Treatment. *JAOA: J Am Osteopath Assoc.* 1990;90(9):810.

40. Sucher B. Myofascial manipulative release of carpal tunnel syndrome: documentation with magnetic resonance imaging. *JAOA: J Am Osteopath Assoc.* 1993;93(12):1273.

41. Sucher BM. Myofascial release of carpal tunnel syndrome. *JAOA: J Am Osteopath Assoc.* 1993;93(1):92.

42. Cisler T. Whiplash as a total-body injury. *JAOA: J Am Osteopath Assoc.* 1994;94(2):145.

43. Hanten WP, Chandler SD. Effects of myofascial release leg pull and sagittal plane isometric contract-relax techniques on passive straight-leg raise angle. *J Orthop Sports Phys Ther.* 1994;20(3):138-144.

*44. Radjieski J, Lumley M, Cantieri M. Effect of osteopathic manipulative treatment of length of stay for pancreatitis: a randomized pilot study. *JAOA: J Am Osteopath Assoc.* 1998;98(5):264.

45. Barnes MF. Efficacy study of the effect of a myofascial release treatment technique on obtaining pelvic symmetry. *J Bodywork Movement Ther.* 1997;1(5):289-296.

46. Konczak CR, Ames R. Relief of internal snapping hip syndrome in a marathon runner after chiropractic treatment. *J Manipulative Physiol Ther.* 2005;28(1):e1-e7.

47. Anonymous. Massage reduces headache frequency. *Massage Magazine.* 2003(109).

48. Crawford JS, Simpson J, Crawford P. Myofascial release provides symptomatic relief from chest wall tenderness occasionally seen following lumpectomy and radiation in breast cancer patients. *Int J Radiat Oncol Biol Phys.* 1996;34(5):1188-1189.

49. Moore MK. Upper crossed syndrome and its relationship to cervicogenic headache. *J Manipulative Physiol Ther.* 2004;27(6):414-420.

50. Hou CR, Tsai LC, Cheng KF, Chung KC, Hong CZ. Immediate effects of various physical therapeutic modalities on cervical myofascial pain and trigger-point sensitivity. *Arch Phys Med Rehabil.* 2002;83(10):1406-1414.

51. MacDonald G. Massage offers respite for primary caregivers. *The American Journal of Hospice & Palliative Care.* 1998;15(1):43-47.

52. Upledger JE, Vredevoogd JD. *Craniosacral Therapy.* Seattle, WA: Eastland Press; 1983.

53. Anonymous. Tips for bodyworkers working with cancer patients. *Massage Bodywork.* 1999;14:19.

54. Schultz RL, Feitis R, Sallas D. *The Endless Web: Fascial Anatomy and Physical Reality.* Berkeley, CA: North Atlantic Books; 1996.

55. Rolfe I. *Rolfing: The Integration of Human Structure.* New York, NY: Harper & Row; 1977.

56. Myers TW. *Anatomy Trains.* Edinburgh, Scotland: Churchill Livingstone; 2001.

57. Stanborough M. *Direct Release Myofascial Technique.* Vol. 4. Edinburgh, Scotland: Churchill Livingstone; 2004.

58. Smith J. *Structural Bodywork.* Edinburgh, Scotland: Elsevier Churchill Livingstone; 2005.

59. McCutcheon B. Fascial integration: a global approach for specific results. *J Soft Tissue Manipulation.* 2007;7:4-7.

60. McCutcheon B. Fascial gait analysis. *J Soft Tissue Manipulation.* 2000;7:3-7.

61. Myers TW. The "anatomy trains:" part 2. *J Bodywork Movement Ther.* 1997;1:134-145.

62. Erickson S. How to understand tissue memory and its implications. *Massage Ther J.* 2003;42:70-77.

63. Cummings GS, Tillman LJ. Remodeling of dense connective tissue in normal adult tissues. In: Currier DP, Nelson RM, eds. *Dynamics of Human Biologic Tissues.* Philadelphia, PA: FA Davis; 1992:45-73.

64. Barlow W. *The Alexander Technique.* New York, NY: Alfred A. Knopf; 1973.

65. Quality Assurance Committee of the College of Massage Therapists of Ontario. *Code of Ethics and Standards of Practice.* Toronto, ON: College of Massage Therapists of Ontario; 2006.

66. Ebner M. *Connective Tissue Manipulations: Theory and Therapeutic Application.* 3rd ed. Malabar, FL: RE Krieger Publishing Company; 1985.

67. Rolf I, Feitis R. *Rolfing and Physical Reality.* Rochester, VT: Healing Arts Press; 1990.

68. Jones TA. Rolfing. *Phys Med Rehabil Clin N Am.* 2004;15(4):799-809, vi.

69. Myers TW. Structural integration—developments in Ida Rolf's "recipe"—I. *J Bodywork Movement Ther.* 2004;8(2):131-142.

70. Myers TW. Structural integration—developments in Ida Rolf's "recipe"—part 3. An alternative form. *J Bodywork Movement Ther.* 2004;8(4):249-264.

71. Myers TW. Structural integration: developments in Ida Rolf's "recipe"—part 2. *J Bodywork Movement Ther.* 2004;8(3):189-198.

72. Stillerman E. *The Encyclopedia of Bodywork.* New York, NY: Facts on File; 1996.

73. Holey EA. Connective tissue massage: a bridge between complementary and orthodox approaches. *J Bodywork Movement Ther.* 2000;4(1):72-80.

74. Cottingham JT, Porges SW, Richmond K. Shifts in pelvic inclination angle and parasympathetic tone produced by Rolfing soft tissue manipulation. *Phys Ther.* 1988;68(9):1364-1370.

75. Cottingham JT, Maitland J. A three-paradigm treatment model using soft tissue mobilization and guided movement-awareness techniques for a patient with chronic low back pain: a case study. *J Orthop Sports Phys Ther.* 1997;26(3):155-167.

76. Perry J, Jones MH, Thomas L. Functional evaluation of Rolfing in cerebral palsy. *Dev Med Child Neurol.* 1981;23:717-729.

77. Anonymous. World-class pianist recovers with Rolfing. *Massage Magazine.* 1996;148.

78. Hunt VV, Massey W. Electromyographic evaluation of structural integration techniques. *Psychoenerg Syst.* 1977;2:199-210.

79. Cottingham JT, Porges SW, Lyon T. Effects of soft tissue mobilization (Rolfing pelvic lift) on parasympathetic tone in two age groups. *Phys Ther.* 1988;68(3):352-356.

80. McKechnie AA, Wilson F, Watson N, Scott D. Anxiety states: a preliminary report on the value of connective tissue massage. *J Psychosom Res.* 1983;27(2):125-129.

81. Weinberg RS, Hunt VV. Effects of structural integration on state-trait anxiety. *J Clin Psychol.* 1979;35(2):319-322.

82. Silverman J, Rappaport M, Hopkins HK, et al. Stress, stimulus intensity control, and the structural integration technique. *Confin Psychiatr.* 1973;16(3):201-219.

83. Reed BV, Held JM. Effects of sequential connective tissue massage on autonomic nervous system of middle-aged and elderly adults. *Phys Ther.* 1988;68(8):1231-1234.

84. Kisner CD, Taslitz N. Connective tissue massage: influence of the introductory treatment on autonomic functions. *Phys Ther.* 1968;48(2):107-119.

85. Kaada B, Torsteinb O. Increase of plasma [beta]-endorphins in connective tissue massage. *Gen Pharmacol.* 1989;20(4):487-489.

86. Kaada B, Torsteinbų O. Vasoactive intestinal polypeptides in connective tissue massage. With a note on VIP in heat pack treatment. *Gen Pharmacol.* 1987;18(4):379-384.

87. Gross D. Physical therapy and rheumatism of soft tissues. *Schweiz Med Wochenschr.* 1982;112(35):1214-1218.

88. Frazer FW. Persistent post-sympathetic pain treated by connective tissue massage. *Physiotherapy.* 1978;64(7):211-212.

89. Akbayrak T, Citak I, Demirturk F, Akarcali I. Manual therapy and pain changes in patients with migraine? An open pilot study. *Adv Physiother.* 2001;3(2):49-54.

90. Brattberg G. Connective tissue massage in the treatment of fibromyalgia. *Eur J Pain.* 1999;3(3):235-244.

91. Enebo B. Conservative management of chronic low back pain using mobilization: a single-subject descriptive case study. *Chiropr Tech.* 1998;10:58-74.

92. Schleip R. Fascial plasticity—a new neurobiological explanation: part 1. *J Bodywork Movement Ther.* 2003;7(1):11-19.

93. Gifford J, Gifford L. Connective tissue massage. In: Wells PE, Frampton V, Bowsher D, eds. *Pain Management by Physiotherapy.* 2nd ed. London, UK: Butterworth-Heinemann; 1994:213-227.

94. Holey LA. Connective tissue zones: an introduction. *Physiotherapy.* 1995;81(7):366-368.

95. Holey LA, Watson MJ. Inter-rater reliability of connective tissue zones recognition. *Physiotherapy.* 1995;81(7):369-372.

96. Holey LA. Connective tissue manipulation: towards a scientific rationale. *Physiotherapy.* 1995;81:730-739.

97. Michalsen A, Buhring M. Connective tissue massage. *Wien Klin Wochenschr.* 1993;105(8):220-227.

98. Goats G, Keir K. Connective tissue massage. *Br J Sports Med.* 1991;25(3):131-133.

99. Palastanga N. Connective tissue massage. In: Grieve GP, ed. *Modern Manual Therapy for the Vertebral Column.* New York, NY: Churchill-Livingston; 1986:827-833.

100. Ebner M. Connective tissue massage. *Physiotherapy.* 1978;64(7):208-210.

101. Gonin M, Gerster JC. Pigmentation disorders in systemic scleroderma. *Schweiz Rundsch Med Prax.* 1994;83(2):42-45.

102. Predel K. Physical therapy in gastroenterology. *Z Gesamte Inn Med.* 1987;42(4):112-114.

103. Sabir'ianov AR, Shevtsov AV, Sabir'ianova ES, et al. Effect of reflex-segmental massage on central hemodynamics in healthy people. *Vopr Kurortol Fizioter Lech Fiz Kult.* 2004;(2)(2):5-7.

104. Nekorkina OA. Segmental-reflex massage in rehabilitation of patients with ischemic heart disease. *Vopr Kurortol Fizioter Lech Fiz Kult.* 2005;1(1):45-49.

105. Nansel D, Szlazak M. Somatic dysfunction and the phenomenon of visceral disease simulation: a probable explanation for the apparent effectiveness of somatic therapy in patients presumed to be suffering from true visceral disease. *J Manipulative Physiol Ther.* 1995;18(6):379-397.

106. Hertling D. Friction massage. In: Kessler RM, Hertling D, eds. *Management of common musculoskeletal conditions.* 4th ed. Philadelphia, PA: Lippincott Williams & Wilkins; 2006.

107. Madenci E, Altindag O, Koca I, Yilmaz M, Gur A. Reliability and efficacy of the new massage technique on the treatment in the patients with carpal tunnel syndrome. *Rheumatol Int.* 2011; published online September 28:1-9.

108. Hammer WI. Friction massage. In: Hammer WI, ed. *Functional Soft Tissue Examination and Treatment by Manual Methods.* 2nd ed. Gaithersburg, MD: Aspen; 1999:463-478.

109. Palastanga N. The use of transverse frictions for soft tissue lesions. In: Grieve GP, ed. *Greive's Modern Manual Therapy for the Vertebral Column.* New York, NY: Churchill-Livingston; 1986:819-825.

110. Cyriax J, Coldham M. *Textbook of Orthopedic Medicine Volume 2. Treatment by Manipulation, Massage and Injection.* 11th ed. London, UK: Bailliere Tindall; 1984.

111. Cyriax J. Deep massage. *Physiotherapy.* 1977;63(2):60-61.

112. Lowe W. *Orthopedic Massage: Theory and Technique.* Edinburgh, Scotland: Mosby; 2003.

113. Walker JM. Deep transverse frictions in ligament healing*. *J Orthop Sports Phys Ther.* 1984;6(2):89-94.

114. De Bruijn R. Deep transverse friction: its analgesic effect. *Int J Sports Med.* 1984;5:35-36.

115. Bajuk S, Jelnikar T, Ortar M. Rehabilitation of patient with brachial plexus lesion and break in axillary artery: case study. *J Hand Ther.* 1996;9(4): 399-403.

116. Guler-Uysal F, Kozanoglu E. Comparison of the early response to two methods of rehabilitation in adhesive capsulitis. *Swiss Med Wkly.* 2004;134(23-24): 353-358.

*117. Nilsson N, Christensen HW, Hartvigsen J. Lasting changes in passive range motion after spinal manipulation: a randomized, blind, controlled trial. *J Manipulative Physiol Ther.* 1996;19(3):165.

*118. Nilsson N. A randomized controlled trial of the effect of spinal manipulation in the treatment of cervicogenic headache. *J Manipulative Physiol Ther.* 1995;18(7):435.

119. O'sullivan SB, Schmitz TJ. *Physical Rehabilitation: Assessment and Treatment.* 6th ed. Philadelphia, PA: FA Davis; 2006.

120. Patino O, Novick C, Merlo A, Benaim F. Massage in hypertrophic scars. *J Burn Care Rehabil.* 1999;20(3):268-271.

121. Sevier TL, Wilson JK. Treating lateral epicondylitis. *Sports Med.* 1999;28(5):375-380.

122. Hammer W. The use of transverse friction massage in the management of chronic bursitis of the hip or shoulder. *J Manipulative Physiol Ther.* 1993;16(2):107.

123. Fritschy D, de Gautard R. Jumper's knee and ultrasonography. *Am J Sports Med.* 1988;16(6):637-640.

124. Hunter SC, Poole RM. The chronically inflamed tendon. *Clin Sports Med.* 1987;6(2):371-388.

125. Woodman RM, Pare L. Evaluation and treatment of soft tissue lesions of the ankle and forefoot using the Cyriax approach. *Phys Ther.* 1982;62(8): 1144-1147.

126. Brosseau L, Casimiro L, Milne S, et al. Deep transverse friction massage for treating tendinitis. *Cochrane Database Syst Rev.* 2002;4:CD003528.

127. Boisaubert B, Brousse C, Zaoui A, Montigny JP. Nonsurgical treatment of tennis elbow. *Ann Readapt Med Phys.* 2004;47(6):346-355.

Further Reading

Adcock D, Paulsen S, Jabour K, Davis S, Nanney LB, Bruce Shack R. Analysis of the effects of deep mechanical massage in the porcine model. *Plast Reconstr Surg.* 2001;108(1):233.

Akeson WH, Amiel D. Connective tissue response to immobility: an accelerated aging process. *Arthritis Rheum.* 1968;18(3):257-301.

Anonymous. Clinical perspectives. Connective tissue perspectives: part 2. *J Bodywork Movement Ther.* 2002;(6):220-227.

Barnes J. Myofascial release in treatment of thoracic outlet syndrome. *J Bodywork Movement Ther.* 1996;1(1):53-57.

Barnes JF. The myofascial release approach. Part III: the fascial cranium and intuitive therapy. *Massage Magazine.* 1994;84.

Barnes JF. The myofascial release approach: the missing link. *Massage Magazine.* 1994;36.

Barnes J. The myofascial release approach, part II the mind/body connection. *Massage Magazine.* 1994;58.

Barnes M. The basic science of myofascial release. *J Bodywork Movement Ther.* 1997;1(4):231-238.

Barnes JF. Myofascial release for craniomandibular pain and dysfunction. *Int J Orofacial Myology.* 1996;22:20-22.

Bernau-Eigen M. Rolfing: a somatic approach to the integration of human structures. *Nurse Pract Forum.* 1998;9(4):235-242.

Cook J, Khan K. What is the most appropriate treatment for patellar tendinopathy? *Br J Sports Med.* 2001;35(5):291.

Cummings GS, Crutchfield CA, Barnes MR. *Orthopedic Physical Therapy Series: Soft Tissue Changes in Contractures.* Atlanta, GA: Stokesville Publishing Company; 1995.

Dalton E. Professional discovery through personal disaster. *Massage Magazine.* 2002;94.

Danto JB. Review of integrated neuromusculoskeletal release and the novel application of a segmental anterior/posterior approach in the thoracic, lumbar, and sacral regions. *JAOA: J Am Osteopath Assoc.* 2003;103(12): 583-596.

Davidson CJ, Ganion LR, Gehlsen GM, Verhoestra B, Roepke JE, Sevier TL. Rat tendon morphologic and functional changes resulting from soft tissue mobilization. *Med Sci Sports Exerc.* 1997;29(3):313.

Dicke E. *Meine Bindegewebsmassage.* Stuttgart, Germany: Hippokrates; 1953.

Dicke E, Shliack H, Wolff A. *A Manual of Reflexive Therapy of the Connective Tissue.* Scarsdale, NY: Simon; 1978.

Fung Y. Elasticity of soft tissues in simple elongation. *Am J Physiol—Legacy Content.* 1967;213(6):1532-1544.

Gallagher A. The integrated approach. *Massage Aust.* 2003:28-35.

Gläser O, Dalicho WA. *Segmentmassage; Massage reflektorischer Zonen, verl.* Leipzig, Germany: Georg Thieme; 1955.

Hammer WI. How does friction massage help tendinitis heal. *J Soft Tissue Manipulation.* 1999;7:20-21.

Hardy MA. The biology of scar formation. *Phys Ther.* 1989;69(12): 1014-1024.

Head H. On disturbances of sensation with especial reference to the pain of visceral disease. *Brain.* 1893;16(1-2):1-133.

Holey L, Lawler H. The effects of classical massage and connective tissue manipulation on bowel function. *Br J Ther Rehabil.* 1995;2(11):627-631.

Hunter G. Specific soft tissue mobilization in the treatment of soft-tissue lesions. *Physiotherapy.* 1994;30:15-21.

James N. Tendon and ligament healing: a new approach through manual therapy. *Massage Magazine.* 2001.

Jamison C, Marangoni R, Glaser A. Viscoelastic properties of soft tissue by discrete model characterization. *J Biomech.* 1968;1(1):33-46.

Khan KM, Cook JL, Taunton JE, Bonar F. Overuse tendinosis, not tendinitis. *Phys Sportsmed.* 2000;28(5):38-48.

King RK. Myofascial breathwork: a regenerative bodywork approach. *J Bodywork Movement Ther.* 2002;6(4): 224-225.

King RK. *Myofascial Massage Therapy: Towards Postural Balance.* Chicago, IL: Bobkat Productions; 1996.

LaBan MM. Collagen tissue: implications of its response to stress in vitro. *Arch Phys Med Rehabil*. 1962;43:461-466.

Latz J. Connective tissue massage. *Massage Bodywork*. 2011;16(12).

Latz J. Key elements of connective tissue massage. *Massage Ther J*. 2003;41: 46-53.

Leahy PM. Improved treatments for carpal tunnel and related syndromes. *Chiropr Sports Med*. 1995;9:6-9.

Leahy P, Mock L. Myofascial release technique and mechanical compromise as peripheral nerves of the upper extremity. *Chiropr Sports Med*. 1992;6: 139-150.

Lowther DA. The effect of compression and tension on the behavior of connective tissue. In: Glasgow EF, Twomey LT, Scull ER, Klenhans AM, Edczek RM, eds. *Aspects of Manipulative Therapy*. 2nd ed. London, UK: Churchill Livingstone; 1985:16-22.

Mackenzie SJ. *Symptoms and Their Interpretation*. London, UK: Shaw and Sons; 1909.

Myers T. Some thoughts on intra-nasal work. *J Bodywork Movement Ther*. 2001;5(3):149-159.

Myers TW. A structural approach. *J Bodywork Movement Ther*. 1998;2:14-20.

Nilsson N, Christensen HW, Hartvigsen J. The effect of spinal manipulation in the treatment of cervicogenic headache. *J Manipulative Physiol Ther*. 1997;20(5):326-330.

Oschman JL. What is healing energy? Part 5: gravity, structure, and emotions. *J Bodywork Movement Ther*. 1997;1(5): 297-305.

Oschman J. Structural integration (rolfing), osteopathic, chiropractic, feldenkrais alexander, myofascial release and related methods. *J Bodywork Movement Ther*. 1997;1:305-309.

Pellecchia GL, Hamel H, Behnke P. Treatment of infrapatellar tendinitis: a combination of modalities and transverse friction massage versus iontophoresis. *J Sport Rehabil*. 1994;3(2):135.

Rigby BJ, Hirai N, Spikes JD, Eyring H. The mechanical properties of rat tail tendon. *J Gen Physiol*. 1959;43(2):265-283.

Rigby B. The effect of mechanical extension upon the thermal stability of collagen. *Biochim Biophys Acta*. 1964;79:634-636.

Riggs A. Deep tissue massage: a visual guide to techniques. *Massage Bodywork*. 2005;20:38-49.

Robertson A, Gilmore K, Frith PA, Antic R. Effects of connective tissue massage in subacute asthma. *Med J Aust*. 1984;140(1):52-53.

Smith F. Causes of and treatment options for abnormal scar tissue. *J Wound Care*. 2005;14(2):49-52.

Stromberg D, Wiederhielm C. Viscoelastic description of a collagenous tissue in simple elongation. *J Appl Physiol*. 1969;26(6):857-862.

Turchaninov R, Prilutsky B. Massage therapy: a beneficial tool in treating fibromyalgia. *Massage Bodywork*. 2004;19:82.

Weinstock DC. Conscious bodywork. *Massage Bodywork*. 2000;15(24).

CHAPTER 11

References

*Randomized Controlled Trial
†Systematic Review

1. Benjamin PJ, Tappan FM. *Tappan's Handbook of Healing Massage Techniques*. 4th ed. Upper Saddle River, NJ: Pearson Prentice Hall; 2005.

2. Fritz S. *Fundamentals of Therapeutic Massage*. 3rd ed. St. Louis, MO: Mosby-Yearbook; 2004.

3. Fritz S. *Sports and Exercise Massage*. St. Louis, MO: Elsevier; 2005.

4. Salvo SG. *Massage Therapy: Principles and Practice*. 2nd ed. Philadelphia, PA: WB Saunders; 2003.

5. Yates J. *A Physician's Guide to Therapeutic Massage*. 3rd ed. Toronto, ON: Curties Overset; 2004.

6. Hollis M. *Massage for Therapists*. 2nd ed. Oxford, England: Blackwell Science; 1998.

7. Holey E, Cook E. *Evidence-Based Therapeutic Massage*. 2nd ed. Edinburgh, Scotland: Churchill Livingstone; 2003.

8. de Domenico G, Wood EC. *Beard's Massage*. 4th ed. Philadelphia, PA: WB Saunders; 1997.

9. Mense S, Simons DG, Russell IJ. *Muscle Pain: Understanding Its Nature, Diagnosis, and Treatment*. Baltimore, MD: Lippincott Williams & Wilkins; 2001.

10. Madenci E, Altindag O, Koca I, Yilmaz M, Gur A. Reliability and efficacy of the new massage technique on the treatment in the patients with carpal tunnel syndrome. *Rheumatol Int*. 2011; published online September 28:1-9.

11. Lederman E. *The Science and Practice of Manual Therapy*. Edinburgh, Scotland: Elsevier/Churchill Livingstone; 2005.

12. Pike G, Pike G. *Sports Massage for Peak Performance*. New York, NY: Harper Perennial; 1997.

13. Benjamin PJ, Lamp SP. *Understanding Sports Massage*. Champaign, IL: Human Kinetics; 1996.

14. Bob Karcy Productions. *A Soigneur's Sports Massage. The Massage Therapy Video Library: Sports Massage Series, Volume 4*. [Video]. New York, NY: View Video; 1988.

15. Smith LL, Keating MN, Holbert D, et al. The effects of athletic massage on delayed onset muscle soreness, creatine kinase, and neutrophil count: a preliminary report. *J Orthop Sports Phys Ther*. 1994;19(2):93.

16. Payne R. *Relaxation Techniques*. 3rd ed. Edinburgh, Scotland: Elsevier/Churchill Livingstone; 2005.

17. Trager M, Hammond C. *Trager Mentastics: Movement as a Way to Agelessness*. Barrytown, NY: Station Hill Press; 1987.

18. Nikola RJ. *Creatures of Water*. 3rd ed. Salt Lake City, UT: Europe Therapeutic; 1997.

19. Ramsey SM. Holistic manual therapy techniques. *Prim Care*. 1997;24(4):759-786.

20. Blackburn J. Trager psychophysical integration—an overview. *J Bodywork Mov Ther*. 2003;7(4):233-239.

21. Lederman E. *Harmonic Technique*. Edinburgh, Scotland: Churchill Livingstone; 2000.

22. Salter RB. The biologic concept of continuous passive motion of synovial joints. The first 18 years of basic research and its clinical application. *Clin Orthop*. 1989;242:12.

23. Akeson WH, Amiel D, Woo SY. Physiology and therapeutic value of passive motion. In: Helminien JH, Kivaranka I, Rammi M, eds. *Joint Loading—Biology and Health of Articular Structures*. Bristol: John Wright; 1987:375-394.

24. Levick JR. Synovial fluid and transsynovial flow in stationary and moving normal joints. In: Helminien JH, Kivaranka I, Rammi M, eds. *Joint Loading—Biology and Health of Articular Structures*. Bristol: John Wright; 1987:149-186.

25. Frank C, Akeson W, Amiel D, Coutts R. Physiology and therapeutic value of passive joint motion. *Clin Orthop*. 1984;185:113.

26. Korcok M. Motion, not immobility, advocated for healing synovial joints. *JAMA*. 1981;246(18):2005-2006.

27. Gelberman RH, Menon J, Gonsalves M, Akeson WH. The effects of mobilization on the vascularization of healing flexor tendons in dogs. *Clin Orthop*. 1980;153:283-289.

28. O'Sullivan SB. Strategies to improve motor control. In: O'Sullivan SB, Schmitz J, eds. *Physical Rehabilitation, Assessment and Treatment*. Philadelphia, PA: FA Davis; 1988.

29. Foster KA, Liskin J, Cen S, Abbott A, Armisen V, Globe D. The trager approach in the treatment of chronic headache: a pilot study. *Altern Ther Health Med*. 2004;10:40-46.

30. Dyson-Hudson TA, Shiflett SC, Kirshblum SC, Bowen J, Druin EL. Acupuncture and trager psychophysical integration in the treatment of wheelchair user's shoulder pain in individuals with spinal cord injury. *Arch Phys Med Rehabil*. 2001;82(8):1038-1046.

31. Whitt PL, MacKinnon J. Trager psychophysical integration: a method to improve chest mobility of patients with chronic lung disease. *Phys Ther*. 1986;66:214-217.

32. Hill PD, Humenick SS, Tieman B. Maternal activities used to soothe crying of 3-week-old breastfed infants. *J Perinat Educ*. 1997;6:13-20.

33. Bonnard M, Pailhous J. Contribution of proprioceptive information to preferred versus constrained space-time behavior in rhythmical movements. *Exp Brain Res*. 1999;128(4):568-572.

34. Benjamin BE, Piltch C. Ben Benjamin's corner. Massage therapists need to embrace research. *Massage Ther J*. 2005;44:32-35.

35. White-Traut RC, Goldman MBC. Pre-mature infant massage: is it safe? *Pediatr Nurs*. 1988;14:285-289.

36. White-Traut RC, Nelson MN. Maternally administered tactile, auditory, visual, and vestibular stimulation: relationship to later interactions between mothers and premature infants. *Res Nurs Health*. 1988;11(1):31-39.

37. Duval C, Lafontaine D, Hébert J, Leroux A, Panisset M, Boucher JP. The effect of trager therapy on the level of evoked stretch responses in patients with Parkinson's disease and rigidity. *J Manipulative Physiol Ther*. 2002;25(7): 455-464.

38. Upledger JE, Vredevoogd JD. *Craniosacral Ther*. Seattle, WA: Eastland Press; 1983.

Further Reading

Arabaci R. Acute effects of pre-event lower limb massage on explosive and high speed motor capacities and flexibility. *J Sports Sci Med*. 2008;7:549-555.

Bauer W, Short CL, Bennett GA. The manner of removal of proteins from normal joints. *J Exp Med*. 1933;57(3):419.

Blackburn J. Trager 2: hooking up: the power of presence in bodywork. *J Bodywork Mov Ther*. 2004;8(2):114-121.

Blackburn J. Trager: at the table—part 3. *J Bodywork Mov Ther*. 2004;8(3):178-188.

Blackburn J. Trager: mentastics-presence in motion—part 4. *J Bodywork Mov Ther*. 2004;8(4):265-277.

Haynes W. Rolling exercises designed to train the deep spinal muscles. *J Bodywork Mov Ther*. 2003;7(3):153-164.

Hendricks T. The effects of immobilization on connective tissue. *J Man Manipulative Ther*. 1995;3(3):98-103.

Hopper D, Deacon S, Das S, et al. Dynamic soft tissue mobilisation increases hamstring flexibility in healthy male subjects. *Br J Sports Med*. 2005;39(9):594-598.

Johnson SK, Frederick J, Kaufman M, Mountjoy B. A controlled investigation of bodywork in multiple sclerosis. *J Altern Complement Med*. 1999;5(3):237-243.

Korner AF, Guilleminault C, Van den Hoed J, Baldwin RB. Reduction of sleep apnea and bradycardia in preterm infants on oscillating water beds: a controlled polygraphic study. *Pediatrics*. 1978;61(4):528-533.

Pederson DR. The soothing effect of rocking as determined by the direction and frequency of movement. *Can J Behav Sci*. 1975;7(3):237.

Povareshchenkova YA, Petrov D. Modulation of the presynaptic inhibition of spinal α-motoneurons during mechanical stimulation of different types. *Hum Physiol*. 2008;34(1):97-102.

Rood M. The use of sensory receptors to activate, facilitate, and inhibit motor response, autonomic and somatic, in developmental sequence. In: Sattely C, ed. *Approaches to the Treatment of Patients with Neuromuscular Dysfunction*. Dubuque, IA: William C. Brown; 1962.

Solodkov A, Povareshchenkova YA. Dynamics of neuromuscular system recovery as a consequence of various massage techniques as determined from electroneuromyography parameters. *Hum Physiol*. 2006;32(5):599-608.

Tolle R. The trager approach. *Massage Ther*. 2005;44:60-67.

*Vermeulen HM, Rozing PM, Obermann WR, le Cessie S, Vlieland TPMV. Comparison of high-grade and low-grade mobilization techniques in the management of adhesive capsulitis of the shoulder: randomized controlled trial. *Phys Ther*. 2006;86(3):355-368.

Vrugt DT, Pederson DR. The effects of vertical rocking frequencies on the arousal level in two-month-old infants. *Child Dev*. 1973;44:205-209.

Wyke BD. Articular neurology and manipulative therapy. In: Glasgow EF, Twomey LT, Scull ER, eds. *Aspects of Manipulative Therapy*. Edinburgh, Scotland: Churchill Livingstone; 1987.

CHAPTER 12

References

*Randomized Controlled Trial

†Systematic Review

1. Frownfelter DL. *Chest Physical Therapy and Pulmonary Rehabilitation: An Interdisciplinary Approach*. Chicago, IL: Year Book Medical Pub; 1987.
2. Frownfelter DL, Dean E. *Principles and Practice of Cardiopulmonary Physical Therapy*. 3rd ed. St. Louis, MO: Mosby Inc.; 1996.
3. de Domenico G, Wood EC. *Beard's Massage*. 4th ed. Philadelphia, PA: WB Saunders; 1997.
4. Benjamin PJ, Tappan FM. *Tappan's Handbook of Healing Massage Techniques*. 4th ed. Upper Saddle River, NJ: Pearson Prentice Hall; 2005.
5. Holey E, Cook E. *Evidence-Based Therapeutic Massage*. 2nd ed. Edinburgh, Scotland: Churchill Livingstone; 2003.
6. Hollis M. *Massage for Therapists*. 2nd ed. Oxford, England: Blackwell Science; 1998.
7. American Physical Therapy Association. *Guide to Physical Therapist Practice*. 2nd ed. Alexandria, VA: American Physical Therapy Association; 1999.
8. Fritz S. *Fundamentals of Therapeutic Massage*. 3rd ed. St. Louis, MO: Mosby-Yearbook; 2004.
9. Loving J. *Massage Therapy*. Stamford, CT: Appleton & Lange; 1999.
10. Salvo SG. *Massage Therapy: Principles and Practice*. 2nd ed. Philadelphia, PA: WB Saunders; 2003.
11. Yates J. *A Physician's Guide to Therapeutic Massage*. 3rd ed. Toronto, ON: Curties Overset; 2004.
12. Ciesla ND. Chest physical therapy for patients in the intensive care unit. *Phys Ther*. 1996;76(6):609-625.
†13. Jones A, Rowe BH. Bronchopulmonary hygiene physical therapy in bronchiectasis and chronic obstructive pulmonary disease: a systematic review. *Heart Lung J Acute Crit Care*. 2000;29(2):125-135.
14. Ambrosino N, Callegari G, Galloni C, Brega S, Pinna G. Clinical evaluation of oscillating positive expiratory pressure for enhancing expectoration in diseases other than cystic fibrosis. *Monaldi Arch Chest Dis*. 1995;50(4):269-275.
15. Thomas J, Cook D, Brooks D. Chest physical therapy management of patients with cystic fibrosis. A meta-analysis. *Am J Respir Crit Care Med*. 1995;151(3):846-850.
16. Gallon A. Evaluation of chest percussion in the treatment of patients with copious sputum production. *Respir Med*. 1991;85(1):45-51.
17. Connors A Jr., Hammon W, Martin R, Rogers R. Chest physical therapy. The immediate effect on oxygenation in acutely ill patients. *Chest*. 1980;78(4):559-564.
18. Van der Schans C, Piers D, Postma D. Effect of manual percussion on tracheobronchial clearance in patients with chronic airflow obstruction and excessive tracheobronchial secretion. *Thorax*. 1986;41(6):448-452.
19. Davis K, Johannigman JA, Campbell RS, et al. The acute effects of body position strategies and respiratory therapy in paralyzed patients with acute lung injury. *Crit Care*. 2001;5(2):81-87.
20. Fink JB. Positioning versus postural drainage. *Respir Care*. 2002;47(7):769-777.
21. Jones A, Rowe B. Bronchopulmonary hygiene physical therapy for chronic obstructive pulmonary disease and bronchiectasis. *Cochrane Database Syst Rev*. 1998;4:CD000045.
22. Raoof S, Chowdhrey N, Raoof S, et al. Effect of combined kinetic therapy and percussion therapy on the resolution of atelectasis in critically ill patients*. *Chest*. 1999;115(6):1658-1666.
23. Hardy KA, Anderson BD. Noninvasive clearance of airway secretions. *Respir Care Clin N Am*. 1996;2(2):323-345.
24. McIlwaine MP, Davidson AG. Airway clearance techniques in the treatment of cystic fibrosis. *Curr Opin Pulm Med*. 1996;2(6):447-451.
25. Thomas J, DeHuek A, Kleiner M, Newton J, Crowe J, Mahler S. To vibrate or not to vibrate: usefulness of the mechanical vibrator for clearing bronchial secretions. *Physiother Can*. 1995;47(2):120-125.
26. Pryor J. Physiotherapy for airway clearance in adults. *Eur Respir J*. 1999;14(6):1418-1424.
27. McIlwaine PM, Wong LT, Peacock D, Davidson AGF. Long-term comparative trial of conventional postural drainage and percussion versus positive expiratory pressure physiotherapy in the treatment of cystic fibrosis. *J Pediatr*. 1997;131(4):570-574.
28. Oermann CM, Sockrider MM, Giles D, Sontag MK, Accurso FJ, Castile RG. Comparison of high-frequency chest wall oscillation and oscillating positive expiratory pressure in the home management of cystic fibrosis: a pilot study*. *Pediatr Pulmonol*. 2001;32(5):372-377.
29. Whitman J, Van Beusekom R, Olson S, Worm M, Indihar F. Preliminary evaluation of high-frequency chest compression for secretion clearance in mechanically ventilated patients. *Respir Care*. 1993;38(10):1081.
30. Dean E, Dean E. Oxygen transport: a physiologically-based conceptual framework for the practice of cardiopulmonary physiotherapy. *Physiotherapy*. 1994;80(6):347-354.
31. Hess DR. The evidence for secretion clearance techniques. *Respir Care*. 2001;46(11):1276-1293.
32. Dallimore K, Jenkins S, Tucker B. Respiratory and cardiovascular responses to manual chest percussion in normal subjects. *Aust J Physiother*. 1998;44:267-274.
33. Dall'Alba PT, Burns YR. The relationship between arterial blood gases and removal of airway secretions in neonates. *Physiother Theory Pract*. 1990;6(3):107-116.
34. Eales CJ, Barker M, Cubberley NJ. Evaluation of a single chest physiotherapy treatment to post-operative, mechanically ventilated cardiac surgery patients. *Physiother Theory Pract*. 1995;11(1):23-28.
35. Stiller K, Jenkins S, Grant R, Geake T, Taylor J, Hall B. Acute lobar atelectasis: a comparison of five physiotherapy regimens. *Physiother Theory Pract*. 1996;12(4):197-209.
36. Krause MF, Hoehn T. Chest physiotherapy in mechanically ventilated children: a review. *Crit Care Med*. 2000;28(5):1648.
37. Boyd S, Brooks D, Agnew-Coughlin J, Ashwell J. Evaluation of the literature on the effectiveness of physical therapy modalities in the management of children with cystic fibrosis. *Pediatr Phys Ther*. 1994;6(2):70.
38. Langenderfer B. Alternatives to percussion and postural drainage: a review of mucus clearance therapies: percussion and postural drainage, autogenic drainage, positive expiratory pressure, flutter valve, intrapulmonary percussive ventilation, and high-frequency chest compression with the ThAIRapy Vest. *J Cardiopulm Rehabil Prev*. 1998;18(4):283.
39. Hammon WE, McCaffree D, Cucchiara A. A comparison of manual to mechanical chest percussion for clearance of alveolar material in patients with pulmonary alveolar proteinosis (phospholipidosis). *Chest*. 1993;103(5):1409-1412.

40. Varekojis SM, HerbertDouce F, Flucke RL, et al. A comparison of the therapeutic effectiveness of and preference for postural drainage and percussion, intrapulmonary percussive ventilation, and high-frequency chest wall compression in hospitalized cystic fibrosis patients. *Respir Care*. 2003;48(1):24-28.

41. Fritz S, Chaitow L, Hymel G. *Clinical Massage in the Healthcare Setting*. St. Louis, MO: Mosby; 2007.

42. Griffin JW. Use of proprioceptive stimuli in therapeutic exercise. *Phys Ther*. 1974;54(10):1072-1079.

43. Lederman E. *Fundamentals of Manual Therapy*. New York, NY: Churchill Livingstone; 1997.

44. Belanger A, Morin S, Pepin P, Tremblay M, Vachon J. Manual muscle tapping decreases soleus H-reflex amplitude in control subjects. *Physiother Can*. 1989;41(4):192-196.

45. Cafarelli E, Sim J, Carolan B, Liebesman J. Vibratory massage and short-term recovery from muscular fatigue. *Int J Sports Med*. 1990;11(6):474-478.

46. Soh TS, Soh SC, Ng LL. Inter-rater reliability of percussion note as a respiratory assessment tool. *Physiother Singapore*. 1998;1:9-12.

47. Wood EC, Becker PD, eds. *Beard's Massage*. 3rd ed. Philadelphia, PA: WB Saunders; 1981.

48. Gameros Gardea RA. Inhalation therapy in asthma. *Rev Alerg Mex*. 1996;43(5):109-115.

49. Horiuchi K, Jordan D, Cohen D, Kemper MC, Weissman C. Insights into the increased oxygen demand during chest physiotherapy. *Crit Care Med*. 1997;25(8):1347.

50. Imle PC, Mars MP, Ciesla ND, Anderson PA, Delaney PA. The effect of chest physical therapy on intracranial pressure and cerebral perfusion pressure. *Physiother Can*. 1997;49(1):48-55.

51. Chen HC, Liu CY, Cheng HF, Ho SC, Chiang LL, Kuo HP. Chest physiotherapy does not exacerbate gastroesophageal reflux in patients with chronic bronchitis and bronchiectasis. *Changgeng Yi Xue Za Zhi*. 1998;21(4):409-414.

52. Travell JG, Simons DG. Myofascial pain and dysfunction. In: *The trigger point manual, volume 1*. Baltimore: Williams & Wilkins; 1983.

53. Morningstar MW, Strauchman MN. Manipulation under anesthesia for patients with failed back surgery: retrospective report of 3 cases with 1-year follow-up. *J Chiropr Med*. 2012;11:30-35.

54. Hoyle JA, Marras WS, Sheedy JE, Hart DE. Effects of postural and visual stressors on myofascial trigger point development and motor unit rotation during computer work. *J Electromyogr Kinesiol*. 2011;21(1):41-48.

55. Moor FB. *Manual of Hydrotherapy and Massage*. Nampa, ID: Pacific Press Publishing Association; 1964.

56. Colby LA, Kisner C. *Therapeutic Exercise: Foundations and Techniques*. 5th ed. Philadelphia, PA: FA Davis; 2007.

57. American Physical Therapy Association. *Guide to Physical Therapist Practice*. Alexandria, VA: American Physical Therapy Association; 2005.

58. Carr L, Pryor J, Hodson M. Self chest clapping: patients' views and the effects on oxygen saturation. *Physiotherapy*. 1995;81(12):753-757.

59. O'Sullivan SB. Strategies to improve motor control. In: O'Sullivan SB, Schmitz J, eds. *Physical Rehabilitation, Assessment and Treatment*. Philadelphia, PA: FA Davis; 1988.

Further Reading

Blazey S, Jenkins S, Smith R. Rate and force of application of manual chest percussion by physiotherapists. *Aust J Physiother*. 1998;44(4):257-264.

Chopra SK, Taplin GV, Simmons DH, Robinson GD Jr., Elam D, Coulson A. Effects of hydration and physical therapy on tracheal transport velocity. *Am Rev Respir Dis*. 1977;115(6):1009-1014.

Cochrane G, Webber B, Clarke S. Effects of sputum on pulmonary function. *Br Med J*. 1977;2(6096):1181-1183.

Comoss P, Hillegass EA, Sadowsky HS, Jewell DV. Essentials of cardiopulmonary physical therapy. *J Cardiopulm Rehabil Prev*. 1994;14(12):138.

Egbert LD, Battit GE, Welch CE, Bartlett MK. Reduction of postoperative pain by encouragement and instruction of patients. *N Engl J Med*. 1964;270(16):825-827.

Hussey J. Effects of chest physiotherapy for children in intensive care after surgery. *Physiotherapy*. 1992;78(2):109-113.

Irwin S, Tecklin JS. *Cardiopulmonary Physical Therapy*. St. Louis, MO: Mosby; 1990.

Kremer H. Continuing education in anesthesia and intensive care at the Limburg St. Vincenz Hospital. stimulating respiratory therapy—an alternative to the chemical club. Study of respiratory stimulating cutaneous administration in intensive care patients. *Krankenpfl J*. 2002;40(5-6):162-169.

La Grasse P. Still in favor of mechanical vibration ... "Mechanical massage at the Battle Creek Sanitarium." *Massage Ther*. 2005;43:20.

Mackenzie CF, Imle PC, Ciesla N. *Chest physiotherapy in the intensive care unit*. 2nd ed. Baltimore, MD: Williams and Wilkins; 1989:380.

Miller WF. Rehabilitation of patients with chronic obstructive lung disease. *Med Clin North Am*. 1967;51(2):349-361.

Nguyen HP, Le DL, Tran QM, Nguyen VT, Nguyen NO. Chromassi: a therapy advice system based on chrono-massage and acupression using the method of ZiWuLiuZhu. *Medinfo*. 1995;8(pt 2):998.

Oermann CM, Swank PR, Sockrider MM. Validation of an instrument measuring patient satisfaction with chest physiotherapy techniques in cystic fibrosis*. *Chest*. 2000;118(1):92-97.

Opdekamp C. Role of physical therapy in the infant. Role of assistive equipment in the physical therapy of patients with cystic fibrosis. *Rev Mal Respir*. 2003;20(2 pt 2):S177-S188.

Perrotta C, Ortiz Z, Roque M. Chest physiotherapy for acute bronchiolitis in paediatric patients between 0 and 24 months old. Cochrane Database Syst Rev. 2006;1:CD004873.

Pham QT, Peslin R, Puchelle E, Salmon D, Caraux G, Benis AM. Respiratory function and the rheological status of bronchial secretions collected by spontaneous expectoration and after physiotherapy (author's transl). *Bull Physiopathol Respir (Nancy)*. 1973;9(2):293-314.

Pryor JA, Webber BA. *Physiotherapy for Respiratory and Cardiac Problems*. Philadelphia, PA: Churchill Livingstone; 1998.

Watchie J. *Cardiopulmonary Physical Therapy: A Clinical Manual*. Philadelphia, PA: WB Saunders; 1995.

CHAPTER 13

References

*Randomized Controlled Trial
†Systematic Review

1. Fritz S. *Fundamentals of Therapeutic Massage*. 3rd ed. St. Louis, MO: Mosby-Yearbook; 2004.

2. Benjamin PJ, Tappan FM. *Tappan's Handbook of Healing Massage Techniques*. 4th ed. Upper Saddle River, NJ: Pearson Prentice Hall; 2005.

3. Salvo SG. *Massage Therapy: Principles and Practice*. 2nd ed. Philadelphia, PA: WB Saunders; 2003.

4. Quality Assurance Committee of the College of Massage Therapists of Ontario. *Code of Ethics and Standards of Practice*. Toronto, ON: College of Massage Therapists of Ontario; 2006.

5. de Domenico G, Wood EC. *Beard's Massage*. 4th ed. Philadelphia, PA: WB Saunders; 1997.

6. Holey E, Cook E. *Evidence-Based Therapeutic Massage*. 2nd ed. Edinburgh, Scotland: Churchill Livingstone; 2003.

7. Beck M. *Milady's Theory and Practice of Therapeutic Massage*. 3rd ed. Albany, NY: Milady; 1999.

8. Wood EC, Becker PD, eds. *Beard's Massage*. 3rd ed. Philadelphia, PA: WB Saunders; 1981.

9. Lederman E. *The Science and Practice of Manual Therapy*. Edinburgh, Scotland: Elsevier/Churchill Livingstone; 2005.

10. Mennell JB. Physical treatment by movement, manipulation and massage. *Am J Med Sci*. 1947;213(1):125.

11. Simons DG, Travell J, Simons LS. *Myofascial Pain and Dysfunction: The Trigger Point Manual: Upper Half of Body*. Vol 1. Baltimore, MD: Williams & Wilkins; 1999.

12. Michlovitz S. *Thermal Agents in Rehabilitation*. 3rd ed. Philadelphia, PA: FA Davis; 1996.

13. Cummings GS, Tillman LJ. Remodeling of dense connective tissue in normal adult tissues. In: Currier DP, Nelson RM, eds. *Dynamics of Human Biologic Tissues*. Philadelphia, PA: FA Davis; 1992:45-73.

14. O'Sullivan SB. Strategies to improve motor control. In: O'Sullivan SB, Schmitz J, eds. *Physical Rehabilitation, Assessment and Treatment*. Philadelphia, PA: FA Davis; 1988.

*15. Le Blanc-Louvry I, Costaglioli B, Boulon C, Leroi AM, Ducrotte P. Does mechanical massage of the abdominal wall after colectomy reduce postoperative pain and shorten the duration of ileus? Results of a randomized study. *J Gastrointest Sur*. 2002;6(1):43-49.

16. Fritz S, ed. *Fundamentals of Therapeutic Massage*. St. Louis, MO: Mosby-Lifeline; 1995.

17. Stillerman E. *The Encyclopedia of Bodywork*. New York, NY: Facts on File; 1996.

18. Hoehn-Saric R. Psychic and somatic anxiety: worries, somatic symptoms and physiological changes. *Acta Psychiatr Scand*. 1998;98:32-38.

19. Millenson JR. *Mind Matters: Psychological Medicine in Holistic Practice*. Seattle, WA: Eastland Press; 1995.

20. Hollis M. *Massage for Therapists*. 2nd ed. Oxford, England: Blackwell Science; 1998.

21. Kim MA, Sakong JK, Kim EJ, Kim EH. Effect of aromatherapy massage for the relief of constipation in the elderly. *Taehan Kanho Hakhoe Chi.* 2005;35(1):56-64.

22. Jeon SY, Jung HM. The effects of abdominal meridian massage on constipation among CVA patients. *Taehan Kanho Hakhoe Chi.* 2005;35(1):135.

23. Emly M, Wilson L, Darby J. Abdominal massage for adults with learning disabilities. *Nurs Times.* 2001;97(30):61-62.

24. Preece J. Introducing abdominal massage in palliative care for the relief of constipation. *Complement Ther Nurs Midwifery.* 2002;8(2):101-105.

25. Shirreffs CM. Aromatherapy massage for joint pain and constipation in a patient with Guillian Barré. *Complement Ther Nurs Midwifery.* 2001;7(2):78-83.

†26. Ernst E. Abdominal massage therapy for chronic constipation: a systematic review of controlled clinical trials. *Res Complement Med.* 1999;6(3):149-151.

27. Emly M. Abdominal massage. *Nurs Times.* 1993;89(3):34-36.

28. Resende TL, Brocklehurst JC, O'Neill PA. A pilot study on the effect of exercise and abdominal massage on bowel habit in continuing care patients. *Clin Rehabil.* 1993;7(3):204-209.

29. Klauser AG, Flaschentrager J, Gehrke A, Muller-Lissner SA. Abdominal wall massage; effect on colonic function in healthy volunteers and in patients with chronic constipation. *Z Gastroenterol.* 1992;30:246-251.

30. Burrows J. Tidy's massage and remedial exercises in medical and surgical conditions. *Br J Ind Med.* 1962;19(2):146.

Further Reading

American Physical Therapy Association. *Interactive Guide to Physical Therapist Practice.* Alexandria, VA: American Physical Therapy Association; 2003.

Arvedson JE. *Medical Gymnastics and Massage in General Practice.* London: JA Churchill; 1930.

Baumgartner AJ. *Massage in Athletics.* Minneapolis, MN: Burgess Publishers; 1947.

Beard G. History of massage technique. *Phys Ther Rev.* 1952;32:613.

Bohm M, Gould E. *Massage: Its Principles and Techniques.* Philadelphia, PA: JB Lippincott; 1913.

Claire T. *Bodywork: What Kind of Massage to Get-and How to Make the Most of It.* New York, NY: William Morrow; 2006.

Collinge W. *The American Holistic Health Association Complete Guide to Alternative Medicine.* New York, NY: Warner Books; 1996.

Cyriax J. Theory and practice of massage. In: Cyriax J, Coldham M, eds. *Textbook of orthopaedic medicine.* Vol 2;1984:267-274.

Cyriax JH, Cyriax P. *Cyriax's Illustrated Manual of Orthopaedic Medicine.* 2nd ed. Stoneham, MA: Butterworth-Heinemann; 1993.

Dorinson SM. Massage, manipulation, and traction. *Calif Med.* 1960;93(3):184.

Hoffa A. *Technik der Massage.* Stuttgart: Verlag von Ferdinand Enke; 1897.

Kellogg JH. *The Art of Massage: A Practical Manual for the Nurse, the Student and the Practitioner.* Battle Creek, MI: Modern Medicine Publishing; 1929.

Kellogg JH. *The Art of Massage.* Battle Creek, MI: Modern Medicine Publishing; 1923.

King RK. *Performance Massage.* Champaign, IL: Human Kinetics; 1993.

Loving J. *Massage Therapy.* Stamford, CT: Appleton & Lange; 1999.

Macías MML. Abdominal massage: therapy for the control of chronic constipation. *Rev Enfermer (Barcelona, Spain).* 1985;8(79-80):16.

McMillan M. *Massage and Therapeutic Exercise.* 2nd ed. Philadelphia, PA: WB Saunders; 1925.

Meagher J. *Sports Massage.* Barrytown, NY: Station Hill Press; 1990.

Prosser EM. *A manual of Massage and Movement.* 2nd ed. London: Faber & Faber; 1941.

Rattray F, Ludwig L. *Clinical Massage Therapy.* Toronto, ON: Talus Inc; 2000.

Selye H. History and present status of the stress concept. In: Goldberger L, Breznitz S, eds. *Handbook of Stress: Theoretical and Clinical Aspects.* New York, NY: Macmillan; 1982:7-17.

Seyle H. *The physiology and Pathology of Exposure to Stress.* Montreal: Acta; 1950.

Tappan FM. *Healing Massage Techniques: Holistic, Classic, and Emerging Methods.* Norwalk, CT: Appleton & Lange; 1988.

Tidy NM, Stevenson JL. Massage and remedial exercises. *Am J Nurs.* 1934;34(4):401.

Westland G. Massage as a therapeutic tool: I. *Br J Occup Ther.* 1993.

Yates J. *A Physician's Guide to Therapeutic Massage.* 3rd ed. Toronto, ON: Curties Overset; 2004.

Ylinen J, Cash M. *Sports Massage.* London: Stanley Paul; 1980.

Zhang Y, Zhang Y, Cheng Y. Clinical observation of constipation due to deficiency of vital energy treated by massage and finger pressure methods. *Chin J Nurs.* 1996;31(2):97.

CHAPTER 14

References

*Randomized Controlled Trial
†Systematic Review or Meta-Analysis

1. Wale JO. *Tidy's Massage and Remedial Exercises.* 11th ed. Bristol: John Wright and Sons; 1968.

2. Thomson A, Skinner A, Piercy J. *Tidy's Physiotherapy.* 12th ed. Oxford: Butterworth Heinemann; 1991.

3. Field TM. Massage therapy effects. *Am Psychol.* 1998;53(12): 1270.

4. Field T. Massage therapy. *Med Clin North Am.* 2002;86(1): 163-171.

5. Field T. *Massage Therapy Research.* 1st ed. Edinburgh: Churchill Livingstone Elsevier; 2006.

6. Moyer CA, Rounds J, Hannum JW. A meta-analysis of massage therapy research. *Psychol Bull.* 2004;130(1):3.

7. Rich GJ. *Massage Therapy: The Evidence for Practice.* 1st ed. Edinburgh: Mosby; 2002.

8. MacDonald G. *Massage for the Hospital Patient and Medically Frail Client.* 1st ed. Philadelphia, PA: Lippincott Williams & Wilkins; 2004.

9. Rattray F, Ludwig L. *Clinical Massage Therapy.* Toronto, ON: Talus; 2000.

10. American Physical Therapy Association. *Interactive Guide to Physical Therapist Practice.* Alexandria, VA: American Physical Therapy Association; 2003.

11. Goodman CC, Boissonnault WG, Fuller KS. *Pathology: Implications for the Physical Therapist.* 2nd ed. Philadelphia, PA: Saunders; 2003.

12. Lee A, Holdsworth M, Holland A, Button B. The immediate effect of musculoskeletal physiotherapy techniques and massage on pain and ease of breathing in adults with cystic fibrosis. *J Cyst Fibros.* 2009;8(1):79-81.

13. Batavia M. Contraindications for therapeutic massage: do sources agree? *J Bodywork Mov Ther.* 2004;8(1):48-57.

14. Whitehill W, Gustman B. Massage and skin conditions: indications and contraindications. *Athlet Ther Today.* 2002;7(3):24-28.

15. Walton T. Exploring contraindications to massage therapy. *J Soft Tissue Manipulation.* 1999;6:5-13.

16. Miesler D. Geriatric massage: assessment and contraindications for the geriatric client. *Massage Bodywork.* 1996;11(66).

17. Asdonk J. Effectiveness, indications and contraindications of manual lymph drainage therapy in painful edema. *Z Lymphol.* 1995;19(1):16-22.

18. Reader M, Young R, Connor JP. Massage therapy improves the management of alcohol withdrawal syndrome. *J Altern Complement Med.* 2005;11(2):311-313.

19. Post-White J, Kinney ME, Savik K, Gau JB, Wilcox C, Lerner I. Therapeutic massage and healing touch improve symptoms in cancer. *Integr Cancer Ther.* 2003;2(4):332.

20. Field T, Pickens J, Prodromidis M, et al. Targeting adolescent mothers with depressive symptoms for early intervention. *Adolescence.* 2000;35(138): 381-414.

21. Kerr CE, Wasserman RH, Moore CI. Cortical dynamics as a therapeutic mechanism for touch healing. *J Altern Complement Med.* 2007;13(1): 59-66.

*22. Billhult A, Lindholm C, Gunnarsson R, Stener-Victorin E. The effect of massage on cellular immunity, endocrine and psychological factors in women with breast cancer—a randomized controlled clinical trial. *Auton Neurosci.* 2008;140(1-2):88-95.

*23. Billhult A, Lindholm C, Gunnarsson R, Stener-Victorin E. The effect of massage on immune function and stress in women with breast cancer—a randomized controlled trial. *Auton Neurosci.* 2009;150(1-2):111-115.

*24. Beider S, Moyer CA. Randomized controlled trials of pediatric massage: a review. *Evid Based Complement Altern Med.* 2007;4(1):23-34.

25. Labrique-Walusis F, Keister KJ, Russell AC. Massage therapy for stress management: implications for nursing practice. *Orthop Nurs.* 2010;29(4):254.

26. Listing M, Krohn M, Liezmann C, et al. The efficacy of classical massage on stress perception and cortisol following primary treatment of breast cancer. *Arch Women Mental Health.* 2010;13(2):165-173.

27. Russell NC, Sumler SS, Beinhorn CM, Frenkel MA. Role of massage therapy in cancer care. *J Altern Complement Med.* 2008;14(2):209-214.

28. Moyer CA, Seefeldt L, Mann ES, Jackley LM. Does massage therapy reduce cortisol? A comprehensive quantitative review. *J Bodywork Mov Ther.* 2011;15(1):3-14.

*29. Mitchinson AR, Kim HM, Rosenberg JM, et al. Acute postoperative pain management using massage as an adjuvant therapy: a randomized trial. *Arch Surg.* 2007;142(12):1158.

30. Haraldsson K, Fridlund B, Baigi A, Marklund B. The self-reported health condition of women after their participation in a stress management programme: a pilot study. *Health Soc Care Community.* 2005;13(3):224-230.

31. Diego MA, Field T, Hernandez-Reif M, et al. Aggressive adolescents benefit from massage therapy. *Adolescence.* 2002;37:597-608.

32. Remington R. Calming music and hand massage with agitated elderly. *Nurs Res.* 2002;51(5):317.

33. Rowe M, Alfred D. The effectiveness of slow-stroke massage in diffusing agitated behaviors in individuals with Alzheimer's disease. *J Gerontol Nurs.* 1999;25(6):22.

34. Field T. Violence and touch deprivation in adolescents. *Adolescence.* 2002;37(148):735-749.

35. Field TM, Quintino O, Hernandez-Reif M, Koslovsky G. Adolescents with attention deficit hyperactivity disorder benefit from massage therapy. *Adolescence.* 1998;33:103-108.

36. Khilnani S, Field T, Hernandez-Reif M, Schanberg S. Massage therapy improves mood and behavior of students with attention-deficit/hyperactivity disorder. *Adolescence.* 2003;38(152):623-638.

37. Hernandez-Reif M, Field T, Ironson G, et al. Natural killer cells and lymphocytes increase in women with breast cancer following massage therapy. *Int J Neurosci.* 2005;115(4):495-510.

38. Hernandez-Reif M, Ironson G, Field T, et al. Breast cancer patients have improved immune and neuroendocrine functions following massage therapy. *J Psychosom Res.* 2004;57(1):45-52.

39. Hernandez-Reif M, Field T, Largie S, et al. Parkinson's disease symptoms are differentially affected by massage therapy vs. progressive muscle relaxation: a pilot study. *J Bodywork Mov Ther.* 2002;6(3):177-182.

40. Boylan M. Massage boosts immunity in breast cancer patients. *J Aust Tradit Med Soc.* 2005;11(2):59.

41. Diego MA, Field T, Hernandez-Reif M, Shaw K, Friedman L, Ironson G. HIV adolescents show improved immune function following massage therapy. *Int J Neurosci.* 2001;106(1-2):35-45.

42. Field T, Cullen C, Diego M, et al. Leukemia immune changes following massage therapy. *J Bodywork Mov Ther.* 2001;5(4):271-274.

43. Baskwill A, Kilty M, Hamilton A, Atkinson H. Massage therapy positively impacts quality of life for HIV+ individuals. *J Soft Tissue Manipulation.* 2003;11:4.

44. Lovas JM, Craig AR, Segal YD, Raison RL, Weston KM, Markus MR. The effects of massage therapy on the human immune response in healthy adults. *J Bodywork Mov Ther.* 2002;6(3):143-150.

45. Henrickson M. Clinical outcomes and patient perceptions of acupuncture and/or massage therapies in HIV-infected individuals. *AIDS Care.* 2001;13(6):743-748.

46. Shor-Posner G, Miguez MJ, Hernandez-Reif M, Perez-Then E, Fletcher M. Massage treatment in HIV-1 infected Dominican children: a preliminary report on the efficacy of massage therapy to preserve the immune system in children without antiretroviral medication. *J Altern Complement Med.* 2004;10(6):1093-1095.

47. Goodfellow LM. The effects of therapeutic back massage on psychophysiologic variables and immune function in spouses of patients with cancer. *Nurs Res.* 2003;52(5):318.

48. Birk TJ, McGrady A, MacArthur RD, Khuder S. The effects of massage therapy alone and in combination with other complementary therapies on immune system measures and quality of life in human immunodeficiency virus. *J Altern Complement Med.* 2000;6(5):405-414.

49. Victor W, Vieweg R, Pandurangi AK. The relation of stress and psychiatric illnesses to coronary heart disease. *Acta Psychiatr Scand.* 2006;113(4):241-244.

50. Brosschot JF, Pieper S, Thayer JF. Expanding stress theory: prolonged activation and perseverative cognition. *Psychoneuroendocrinology.* 2005;30(10):1043-1049.

51. Shepshelovich D, Shoenfeld Y. Prediction and prevention of autoimmune diseases: additional aspects of the mosaic of autoimmunity. *Lupus.* 2006;15(3):183-190.

52. Heller DP, Heller L. Somatic experiencing in the treatment of automobile accident trauma. *US Assoc Body Psychother J.* 2004;3(2):42-52.

53. Price C. Characteristics of women seeking body-oriented therapy as an adjunct to psychotherapy during recovery from childhood sexual abuse. *J Bodywork Mov Ther.* 2004;8(1):35-42.

54. Dryden T, Fitch P. Recovering body and soul from post-traumatic stress disorder. *Massage Ther J.* 2000;39:41-60.

55. Kline Leidy N. A physiologic analysis of stress and chronic illness. *J Adv Nurs.* 1989;14(10):868-876.

56. Selye H. Stress and the reduction of distress. *J S C Med Assoc.* 1979;75(11):562-566.

57. Selye H. Forty years of stress research: principal remaining problems and misconceptions. *Can Med Assoc J.* 1976;115(1):53.

58. McCaffrey R, Locsin RC. Music listening as a nursing intervention: a symphony of practice. *Holist Nurs Pract.* 2002;16(3):70.

59. Engebretson J, Wardell DW. Research: Reiki induces relaxation, liminal state of awareness. *Alternative Therapies in Health and Medicine.* 2002;8(2):48-53.

60. Brooks WW, Conrad CH, Nedder AP, Bing OHL, Slawsky MT. Thoracic massage permits use of echocardiography in unanesthetized rats. *Comp Med.* 2003;53(3):288-292.

61. Foeldi M, Strössenreuther RHK. *Foundations of Manual Lymph Drainage.* St. Louis, MO: Elsevier Mosby; 2005.

62. Lederman E. *Harmonic Technique.* Edinburgh: Churchill Livingstone; 2000.

63. Andrade CK, Clifford P, Andrade C. *Outcome-Based Massage.* Baltimore, MD: Lippincott Williams & Wilkins; 2001.

64. Hendrickson T. *Massage for Orthopedic Conditions.* Baltimore, MD: Lippincott Williams & Wilkins; 2003.

65. Diego MA, Field T, Sanders C, Hernandez-Reif M. Research: Moderate-pressure massage increases relaxation. *International Journal of Neuroscience.* 2004;114:31-45.

*66. Hattan J, King L, Griffiths P. The impact of foot massage and guided relaxation following cardiac surgery: a randomized controlled trial. *J Adv Nurs.* 2002;37(2):199-207.

67. Oh HJ, Park JS. Effects of hand massage and hand holding on the anxiety in patients with local infiltration anesthesia. *Taehan Kanho Hakhoe Chi.* 2004;34(6):924-933.

68. Kober A, Scheck T, Schubert B, et al. Auricular acupressure as a treatment for anxiety in prehospital transport settings. *Anesthesiology.* 2003;98(6):1328.

69. Jirayingmongkol P, Chantein S, Phengchomjan N, Bhanggananda N. The effect of foot massage with biofeedback: a pilot study to enhance health promotion. *Nurs Health Sci.* 2002;4(3):A4-A4.

70. Kim MS, Cho KS, Woo HM, Kim JH. Effects of hand massage on anxiety in cataract surgery using local anesthesia. *J Cataract Refract Surg.* 2001;27(6):884-890.

71. Stephenson N, Dalton JA, Carlson J. The effect of foot reflexology on pain in patients with metastatic cancer. *Appl Nurs Res.* 2003;16(4):284-286.

72. Pattillo MM. Therapeutic and healing foot care: a healthy feet clinic for older adults. *J Gerontol Nurs.* 2004;30(12):25-32; quiz 50-1.

73. Wang HL, Keck JF. Foot and hand massage as an intervention for postoperative pain. *Pain Manage Nurs.* 2004;5(2):59-65.

*74. Siev-Ner I, Gamus D, Lerner-Geva L, Zaidel S, Achiron A. Reflexology treatment relieves symptoms of multiple sclerosis: a randomized controlled study. *Mult Scler.* 2003;(9):356-361.

75. Kohara H, Miyauchi T, Suehiro Y, Ueoka H, Takeyama H, Morita T. Combined modality treatment of aromatherapy, footsoak, and reflexology relieves fatigue in patients with cancer. *J Palliat Med.* 2004;7(6):791-796.

76. Cottingham JT, Porges SW, Lyon T. Effects of soft tissue mobilization (rolfing pelvic lift) on parasympathetic tone in two age groups. *Phys Ther.* 1988;68(3):352-356.

77. Cottingham JT, Porges SW, Richmond K. Shifts in pelvic inclination angle and parasympathetic tone produced by rolfing soft tissue manipulation. *Phys Ther.* 1988;68(9):1364-1370.

78. Turchaninov R. *Therapeutic Massage: A Scientific Approach.* Phoenix, AZ: Aesculapius Books; 2000.

79. Turchaninov R. *Medical Massage.* 2nd ed. Phoenix, AZ: Aesculapius Books; 2006.

80. Okvat HA, Oz MC, Ting W, Namerow PB. Massage therapy for patients undergoing cardiac catheterization. *Altern Ther Health Med.* 2002;8(3):68-70, 72, 74-75.

81. Price S, Price L. *Aromatherapy for Health Professionals.* 2nd ed. Edinburgh, Scotland: Churchill Livingstone; 1999.

82. Fellowes D, Barnes K, Wilkinson S. Aromatherapy and massage for symptom relief in patients with cancer. *Cochrane Database Syst Rev.* 2004;2:CD002287.

83. Field T. Massage and aroma therapy. *Int J Cosmetic Sci.* 2004;26(3):169-170.

84. Field T, Hernandez-Reif M, Taylor S, Quintino O, Burman I. Labor pain is reduced by massage therapy. *J Psychosom Obstet Gynecol.* 1997;18(4):286-291.

85. Lee SY. The effect of lavender aromatherapy on cognitive function, emotion, and aggressive behavior of elderly with dementia. *Taehan Kanho Hakhoe Chi.* 2005;35(2):303.

86. Payne RA, Donaghy M. *Relaxation Techniques.* 3rd ed. Edinburgh: Elsevier Churchill Livingstone; 2005.

87. Hanley J, Stirling P, Brown C. Randomised controlled trial of therapeutic massage in the management of stress. *Br J Gen Pract.* 2003;53(486):20.

88. Bay E. *Empowered breathing* audiotape. *The Relaxation Response Ltd.*; audioptape (Toronto, Ontario).

89. Nikola RJ. *Creatures of Water.* 3rd ed. Salt Lake City, UT: Europa Therapeutic; 1997.

90. Fowlie L. *Heat and Cold as Therapy.* Toronto, ON: Curties-Overzet Publications; 2006.

91. Cullen LA, Barlow JH. A training and support programme for caregivers of children with disabilities: an exploratory study. *Patient Educ Couns.* 2004;55(2):203-209.

92. Smith MC, Kemp J, Hemphill L, Vojir CP. Outcomes of therapeutic massage for hospitalized cancer patients. *J Nurs Sch.* 2002;34(3):257-262.

93. Field T, Diego M, Cullen C, Hernandez-Reif M, Sunshine W, Douglas S. Fibromyalgia pain and substance P decrease and sleep improves after massage therapy. *J Clin Rheumatol.* 2002;8(2):72.

94. Tsay SL, Rong JR, Lin PF. Acupoints massage in improving the quality of sleep and quality of life in patients with end-stage renal disease. *J Adv Nurs.* 2003;42(2):134-142.

*95. Williams A, Vadgama A, Franks P, Mortimer PS. A randomized controlled crossover study of manual lymphatic drainage therapy in women with breast cancer-related lymphoedema. *Eur J Cancer Care.* 2002;11(4):254-261.

96. Field T, Hernandez-Reif M, Diego M, Feijo L, Vera Y, Gil K. Massage therapy by parents improves early growth and development. *Infant Behav Dev.* 2004;27(4):435-442.

97. Shen P. Two hundred cases of insomnia treated by otopoint pressure plus acupuncture. *J Tradit Chin Med.* 2004;24(3):168-169.

*98. Soden K, Vincent K, Craske S, Lucas C, Ashley S. A randomized controlled trial of aromatherapy massage in a hospice setting. *Palliat Med.* 2004;18(2):87-92.

99. Weze C, Leathard HL, Stevens G. Evaluation of healing by gentle touch for the treatment of musculoskeletal disorders. *Am J Public Health.* 2004;94(1):50.

100. Dieter JNI, Field T, Hernandez-Reif M, Emory EK, Redzepi M. Stable preterm infants gain more weight and sleep less after five days of massage therapy. *J Pediatr Psychol.* 2003;28(6):403.

101. Wang XH, Yuan YD, Wang BF. Clinical observation on effect of auricular acupoint pressing in treating sleep apnea syndrome. *Zhongguo Zhong Xi Yi Jie He Za Zhi.* 2003;23(10):747-749.

102. Barlow J, Cullen L. Increasing touch between parents and children with disabilities: preliminary results from a new programme. *J Fam Health Care.* 2002;12(1):7-9.

103. Ferber SG, Laudon M, Kuint J, Weller A, Zisapel N. Massage therapy by mothers enhances the adjustment of circadian rhythms to the nocturnal period in full-term infants. *J Dev Behav Pediatr.* 2002;23(6):410.

*104. Tsay SL, Chen ML. Acupressure and quality of sleep in patients with end-stage renal disease—a randomized controlled trial. *Int J Nurs Stud.* 2003;40(1):1-7.

105. Agarwal KN, Gupta A, Pushkarna R, Bhargava SK, Faridi MM, Prabhu MK. Effects of massage & use of oil on growth, blood flow & sleep pattern in infants. *Indian J Med Res.* 2000;112:212-217.

106. Cassar MP. The application of massage in psychogenic disorders. *Positive Health.* 2004;June(100):45.

107. Richards K, Nagel C, Markie M, Elwell J, Barone C. Use of complementary and alternative therapies to promote sleep in critically ill patients. *Crit Care Nurs Clin North Am.* 2003;15(3):329-340.

108. Cassar M. *Handbook of Clinical Massage.* 2nd ed. Edinburgh: Churchill Livingstone; 2004.

109. Mamtani R, Cimino A. A primer of complementary and alternative medicine and its relevance in the treatment of mental health problems. *Psychiatr Q.* 2002;73(4):367-381.

110. Field T, Diego M, Hernandez-Reif M, et al. Lavender fragrance cleansing gel effects on relaxation. *Int J Neurosci.* 2005;115(2):207-222.

111. Rexilius SJ, Mundt C, Erickson Megel M, Agrawal S. Therapeutic effects of massage therapy and handling touch on caregivers of patients undergoing autologous hematopoietic stem cell transplant. *Oncol Nurs Forum.* 2002;29(E35):E35.

112. Field T, Quintino O, Henteleff T, Wells-Keife L, Delvecchio-Feinberg G. Job stress reduction therapies. *Altern Ther Health Med.* 1997;3(4):54.

113. Cho YC, Tsay SL. The effect of acupressure with massage on fatigue and depression in patients with end-stage renal disease. *J Nurs Res: JNR.* 2004;12(1):51.

114. Yang JH. The effects of foot reflexology on nausea, vomiting and fatigue of breast cancer patients undergoing chemotherapy. *Taehan Kanho Hakhoe Chi.* 2005;35(1):177-185.

115. Cassileth BR, Vickers AJ. Massage therapy for symptom control: outcome study at a major cancer center. *J Pain Symptom Manage.* 2004;28(3):244-249.

116. Deng G, Cassileth BR, Yeung KS. Complementary therapies for cancer-related symptoms. *J Support Oncol.* 2004;2(5):419.

117. Stucki MOG. Physical therapy in the treatment of fibromyalgia. *Scand J Rheumatol.* 2000;29(113):78-85.

118. Cupido C. *Effects of Massage Therapy After Exhaustive Endurance Exercise in Young Healthy Males* [Masters]. McMaster University; 2010.

119. Archer P. *Therapeutic Massage in Athletics.* Philadelphia, PA: Lippincott Williams & Wilkins; 2006.

120. Thrash A, Thrash C. *Home Remedies.* Seale, AL: Thrash Publications, Rt; 1981.

121. Iwama H, Akama Y. Skin rubdown with a dry towel activates natural killer cells in bedridden old patients. *Med Sci Monit.* 2002;8(9):CR611-CR615.

122. Hart S, Field T, Hernandez-Reif M, et al. Anorexia nervosa symptoms are reduced by massage therapy. *Eat Disord.* 2001;9(4):289-299.

123. Hernandez-Reif M, Field T, Field T, Theakston H. Multiple sclerosis patients benefit from massage therapy. *J Bodywork Mov Ther.* 1998;2(3):168-174.

124. Bredin M. Mastectomy, body image and therapeutic massage: a qualitative study of women's experience. *J Adv Nurs.* 1999;29(5):1113-1120.

125. van der Riet P. Massaged embodiment of cancer patients. *Aust J Holist Nurs.* 1999;6:4.

126. Price C. Body-oriented therapy in recovery from child sexual abuse: an efficacy study. *Altern Ther Health Med.* 2005;11(5):46.

127. van der Riet P. Ethereal embodiment of cancer patients. *Aust J Holist Nurs.* 1999;6(2):20-27.

128. van der Riet P. The sexual embodiment of the cancer patient. *Nurs Inq.* 1998;5(4):248-257.

129. Mines S. Healing triumphs over domestic violence. *Massage Bodywork.* 2001;16(17).

130. Mattsson M, Wikman M, Dahlgren L, Mattasson B, Armelius K. Body awareness therapy with sexually abused women. Part 2: evaluation of body awareness in a group setting. *J Bodywork Mov Ther.* 1998;2(1):38-45.

131. Kim J, Jang S, Kim Y, Lee S, Song J. Developing CD-ROM based multimedia digital textbook of "San-yin-jiao (SP-6) pressure for reducing the labor pain and shortening the labor time." *Medinfo.* 2001;10(2):1038-1041.

132. Erickson S. How to understand tissue memory and its implications. *Massage Ther J.* 2003;42:70-77.

133. Wittink H, Michel TH. *Chronic Pain Management for Physical Therapists.* 2nd ed. Boston, MA: Butterworth-Heinemann; 2002.

134. Chu JJ. Managing cancer symptoms with massage therapy. *Am J Nurs.* 2005;105:72.

*135. Chang MY, Wang SY, Chen CH. Effects of massage on pain and anxiety during labour: a randomized controlled trial in Taiwan. *J Adv Nurs.* 2002;38(1):68-73.

136. Sola I, Thompson E, Subirana M, López C, Pascual A. Non-invasive interventions for improving well-being and quality of life in patients with lung cancer. *Cochrane Database Syst Rev.* 2004;Oct 18(4):CD004282.

137. Hernandez-Reif M, Field T, Krasnegor J, Theakston H. Lower back pain is reduced and range of motion increased after massage therapy. *Int J Neurosci.* 2001;106(3-4):131-145.

138. Hernandez-Reif M, Field T, Largie S, et al. Childrens' distress during burn treatment is reduced by massage therapy. *J Burn Care Res.* 2001;22(2):191.

*139. Fischer RL, Bianculli KW, Sehdev H, Hediger ML. Does light pressure effleurage reduce pain and anxiety associated with genetic amniocentesis? A randomized clinical trial. *J Matern Fetal Neonat Med.* 2000;9(5):294-297.

140. Hernandez-Reif M, Martinez A, Field T, Quintero O, Hart S, Burman I. Premenstrual symptoms are relieved by massage therapy. *J Psychosom Obstet Gynecol.* 2000;21(1):9-15.

141. Richards KC, Gibson R, Overton-McCoy AL. Effects of massage in acute and critical care. *AACN Adv Crit Care.* 2000;11(1):77.

142. Stephenson NN, Weinrich SP, Tavakoli AS. The effects of foot reflexology on anxiety and pain in patients with breast and lung cancer. *Oncol Nurs Forum.* 2000;27:67-72.

143. Field T, Diego M, Cullen C, et al. Carpal tunnel syndrome symptoms are lessened following massage therapy. *J Bodywork Mov Ther.* 2004;8(1):9-14.

144. Roy EA, Hollins M, Maixner W. Reduction of TMD pain by high-frequency vibration: a spatial and temporal analysis. *Pain.* 2003;101(3):267-274.

145. Van Den Dolder PA, Roberts DL. A trial into the effectiveness of soft tissue massage in the treatment of shoulder pain. *Aust J Physiother.* 2003;49(3):183-194.

146. Bag B, Karabulut N. Pain-relieving factors in migraine and tension-type headache. *Int J Clin Pract.* 2005;59(7):760-763.

*147. Cook C, Guerrerio J, Slater V. Healing touch and quality of life in women receiving radiation treatment for cancer: a randomized controlled trial. *Altern Ther Health Med.* 2004;10(3):34.

148. Bodhise PB, Dejoie M, Brandon Z, Simpkins S, Ballas SK. Non-pharmacologic management of sickle cell pain. *Hematology.* 2004;9(3):235-237.

†149. Huntley AL, Coon JT, Ernst E. Complementary and alternative medicine for labor pain: a systematic review. *Obstet Gynecol.* 2004;191(1):36-44.

150. Norrbrink Budh C, Lundeberg T. Non-pharmacological pain-relieving therapies in individuals with spinal cord injury: a patient perspective. *Complement Ther Med.* 2004;12(4):189-197.

151. Simkin P, Bolding A. Update on nonpharmacologic approaches to relieve labor pain and prevent suffering. *J Midwifery Womens Health.* 2004;49(6):489-504.

152. Yildirim G, Sahin NH. The effect of breathing and skin stimulation techniques on labour pain perception of Turkish women. *Pain Res Manage.* 2004;9(4):183-187.

153. Chung UL, Hung LC, Kuo SC, Huang CL. Effects of LI4 and BL 67 acupressure on labor pain and uterine contractions in the first stage of labor. *J Nurs Res.* 2003;11(4):251-260.

154. Dudley G, McGrath KN, Pheley AM. Length of stay and medication use in hysterectomy patients treated with a single massage treatment. *J Bodywork Mov Ther.* 2003;7(4):222-227.

155. Piotrowski MM, Paterson C, Mitchinson A, Kim HM, Kirsh M, Hinshaw DB. Massage as adjuvant therapy in the management of acute postoperative pain: a preliminary study in men. *J Am Coll Surg.* 2003;197(6):1037-1046.

156. Sakurai M, Suleman MI, Morioka N, Akça O, Sessler DI. Minute sphere acupressure does not reduce postoperative pain or morphine consumption. *Anesth Analg.* 2003;96(2):493.

157. Stephenson NLN, Dalton JA. Using reflexology for pain management. *J Holist Nurs.* 2003;21(2):179-191.

*158. Taylor AG, Galper DI, Taylor P, et al. Effects of adjunctive Swedish massage and vibration therapy on short-term postoperative outcomes: a randomized, controlled trial. *J Altern Complement Med.* 2003;9(1):77-89.

*159. Bellieni CV, Bagnoli F, Perrone S, Nenci A, Cordelli D, Fusi M. Effect of multisensory stimulation on analgesia in term neonates: a randomized controlled trial. *Pediatr Res.* 2002;51(4):460.

160. Dryden T, Menard MB, Hunter W. The effect of a single massage on pain sensation and pain unpleasantness. *J Soft Tissue Manipulation.* 2002;10:20.

*161. Le Blanc-Louvry I, Costaglioli B, Boulon C, Leroi AM, Ducrotte P. Does mechanical massage of the abdominal wall after colectomy reduce postoperative pain and shorten the duration of ileus? Results of a randomized study. *J Gastrointest Surg.* 2002;6(1):43-49.

*162. Lemstra M, Stewart B, Olszynski W. Effectiveness of multidisciplinary intervention in the treatment of migraine: a randomized clinical trial. *Headache.* 2002;42(9):845-854.

163. Akbayrak T, Citak I, Demirturk F, Akarcali I. Manual therapy and pain changes in patients with migraine: An open pilot study. *Adv Physiother.* 2001;3(2):49-54.

164. Billhult A, Dahlberg K. A meaningful relief from suffering: experiences of massage in cancer care. *Cancer Nurs.* 2001;24(3):180.

165. Gentz BA. Alternative therapies for the management of pain in labor and delivery. *Clin Obstet Gynecol.* 2001;44(4):704.

166. Kubsch SM, Neveau T, Vandertie K. Effect of cutaneous stimulation on pain reduction in emergency department patients. *Accid Emerg Nurs.* 2001;9(3):143-151.

167. Shirreffs CM. Aromatherapy massage for joint pain and constipation in a patient with Guillian Barré. *Complement Ther Nurs Midwifery.* 2001;7(2):78-83.

168. Field T, Peck M, Hernandez-Reif M, Krugman S, Burman I, Ozment-Schenck L. Postburn itching, pain, and psychological symptoms are reduced with massage therapy. *J Burn Care Rehabil.* 2000;21(3):189.

169. Gallagher G, Rae CP, Kinsella J. Treatment of pain in severe burns. *Am J Clin Dermatol.* 2000;1(6):329-335.

170. Grealish L, Lomasney A, Whiteman B. Foot massage: a nursing intervention to modify the distressing symptoms of pain and nausea in patients hospitalized with cancer. *Cancer Nurs.* 2000;23(3):237.

†171. Pan CX, Morrison RS, Ness J, Fugh-Berman A, Leipzig RM. Complementary and alternative medicine in the management of pain, dyspnea, and nausea and vomiting near the end of life: a systematic review. *J Pain Symptom Manage.* 2000;20(5):374-387.

*172. Uher EM, Vacariu G, Schneider B, Fialka V. Comparison of manual lymph drainage with physical therapy in complex regional pain syndrome, type I. A comparative randomized controlled therapy study. *Wien Klin Wochenschr.* 2000;112(3):133-137.

*173. Wilkie DJ, Kampbell J, Cutshall S, et al. Effects of massage on pain intensity, analgesics and quality of life in patients with cancer pain: A pilot study of a randomized clinical trial conducted within hospice care delivery. *Hosp J.* 2000;15(3):31-53.

174. Sellick SM, Zaza C. Critical review of 5 nonpharmacologic strategies for managing cancer pain. *Cancer Prev Control.* 1998;2(1):7-14.

175. Apostle-Mitchell M, MacDonald G. An innovative approach to pain management in critical care: therapeutic touch. *Off J Can Assoc Crit Care Nurs.* 1997;8(3):19-22.

176. Barnes J. Myofascial release in treatment of thoracic outlet syndrome. *J Bodywork Mov Ther.* 1996;1(1):53-57.

177. Goffaux-Dogniez C, Vanfraechem-Raway R, Verbanck P. Appraisal of treatment of the trigger points associated with relaxation to treat chronic headache in the adult. Relationship with anxiety and stress adaptation strategies. *Encephale.* 2003;29(5):377-390.

178. Tsao JCI. Effectiveness of massage therapy for chronic, non-malignant pain: a review. *Evid Based Complement Altern Med.* 2007;4(2):165-180.

*179. Jane SW, Chen SL, Wilkie DJ, et al. Effects of massage on pain, mood status, relaxation, and sleep in taiwanese patients with metastatic bone pain: A randomized clinical trial. *Pain.* 2011;152(10):2432-2442.

*180. Frey Law LA, Evans S, Knudtson J, Nus S, Scholl K, Sluka KA. Massage reduces pain perception and hyperalgesia in experimental muscle pain: a randomized, controlled trial. *J Pain.* 2008;9(8):714-721.

*181. Cherkin DC, Sherman KJ, Kahn J, et al. Effectiveness of focused structural massage and relaxation massage for chronic low back pain: protocol for a randomized controlled trial. *Trials.* 2009;10(1):96.

182. Seers K, Crichton N, Martin J, Coulson K, Carroll D. A randomised controlled trial to assess the effectiveness of a single session of nurse administered massage for short term relief of chronic non-malignant pain. *BMC Nurs.* 2008;7(1):10.

*183. Bauer BA, Cutshall SM, Wentworth LJ, et al. Effect of massage therapy on pain, anxiety, and tension after cardiac surgery: a randomized study. *Complement Ther Clin Pract.* 2010;16(2):70-75.

184. Listing M, Reißhauer A, Krohn M, et al. Massage therapy reduces physical discomfort and improves mood disturbances in women with breast cancer. *Psycho-Oncology.* 2009;18(12):1290-1299.

185. Kimber L, McNabb M, Haines A, Brocklehurst P. Massage or music for pain relief in labour: A pilot randomised placebo controlled trial. *Eur J Pain.* 2008;12(8):961-969.

186. Duygu A, Handan A, Gözüm S, Orbak Z, Karaca Çifçi E. Effectiveness of massage, sucrose solution, herbal tea or hydrolysed formula in the treatment of infantile colic. *J Clin Nurs.* 2008;17(13):1754-1761.

187. Wesa K, Cassileth B, Jain S. The effectiveness of biofield therapies for decreasing symptoms of pain and anxiety, and improving QoL. *Focus Altern Complement Ther.* 2011;16(1):62-65.

188. Jackson E, Kelley M, McNeil P, Meyer E, Schlegel L, Eaton M. Does therapeutic touch help reduce pain and anxiety in patients with cancer? *Clin J Oncol Nurs.* 2008;12(1):113-120.

†189. Ernst E. Massage therapy for cancer palliation and supportive care: a systematic review of randomised clinical trials. *Support Care Cancer.* 2009;17(4):333-337.

190. Rapaport MH, Schettler P, Bresee C. A preliminary study of the effects of a single session of Swedish massage on hypothalamic–pituitary–adrenal and immune function in normal individuals. *J Altern Complement Med.* 2010;16(10):1079-1088.

191. Wang AT, Sundt III TM, Cutshall SM, Bauer BA. Massage therapy after cardiac surgery. *Semin Thorac Cardiovasc Surg.* 2010;22(3):225-229.

192. Clifford P. Outcome based treatment planning for clients with cancer. *J Soft Tissue Manipulation.* 2003;11:3.

193. Crawford JS, Simpson J, Crawford P. Myofascial release provides symptomatic relief from chest wall tenderness occasionally seen following lumpectomy and radiation in breast cancer patients. *Int J Radiat Oncol Biol Phys.* 1996;34(5):1188-1189.

194. Gray RA. The use of massage therapy in palliative care. *Complement Ther Nurs Midwifery.* 2000;6(2):77-82.

*195. McNeely ML, Magee DJ, Lees AW, Bagnall KM, Haykowsky M, Hanson J. The addition of manual lymph drainage to compression therapy for breast cancer related lymphedema: a randomized controlled trial. *Breast Cancer Res Treat.* 2004;86(2):95-106.

196. Yates JS, Mustian KM, Morrow GR, et al. Prevalence of complementary and alternative medicine use in cancer patients during treatment. *Support Care Cancer.* 2005;13(10):806-811.

197. Roy L. Massage therapy for people with cancer: a practitioner's experience. *Posit Health.* 2004;96:48-50.

198. Klein J, Griffiths P. Acupressure for nausea and vomiting in cancer patients receiving chemotherapy. *Br J Community Nurs.* 2004;9(9):383-388.

*199. Szuba A. Research watch: the addition of manual lymph drainage to compression therapy for breast cancer related lymphedema: a randomized controlled trial. *Lymphat Res Biol.* 2005;3:36-41.

200. Shin YH, Kim TI, Shin MS, Juon HS. Effect of acupressure on nausea and vomiting during chemotherapy cycle for Korean postoperative stomach cancer patients. *Cancer Nurs.* 2004;27(4):267.

201. Wilcock A, Manderson CA, Weller R, et al. Does aromatherapy massage benefit patients with cancer attending a specialist palliative care day centre? *Palliat Med.* 2004;18(4):287-290.

202. Dunwoody L, Smyth A, Davidson R. Cancer patients' experiences and evaluations of aromatherapy massage in palliative care. *Int J Palliat Nurs.* 2002;8(10):497.

203. Gecsedi RA. Massage therapy for patients with cancer. *Clin J Oncol Nurs.* 2002;6(1):52-54.

204. Robin K. Pediatric cancer patients turn to alternative therapies. *HerbalGram.* 2002;Summer(55):13.

205. Kalauokalani D, Cherkin DC, Sherman KJ, Koepsell TD, Deyo RA. Lessons from a trial of acupuncture and massage for low back pain: patient expectations and treatment effects. *Spine.* 2001;26(13):1418.

*206. Hsieh LLC, Kuo CH, Yen MF, Chen THH. A randomized controlled clinical trial for low back pain treated by acupressure and physical therapy. *Prev Med.* 2004;39(1):168-176.

207. Quinn C, Chandler C, Moraska A. Massage therapy and frequency of chronic tension headaches. *Am J Public Health.* 2002;92(10):1657.

208. Main CJ, Spanswick CC. *Pain Management: An Interdisciplinary Approach.* Edinburgh: Elsevier Health Sciences; 2000.

209. Fitch P. Massage strategies for depressed clients. *Massage Ther J.* 2003;42:58-64.

210. Geisbrecht D. Third party series: credibility, accountability and third party payers. *Body Polit.* 2004;42:58.

†211. Khadilkar A, Milne S, Brosseau L, et al. Transcutaneous electrical nerve stimulation for the treatment of chronic low back pain: a systematic review. *Spine.* 2005;30(23):2657.

212. Barker R, Lang T, Steinlechner B, et al. Transcutaneous electrical nerve stimulation as prehospital emergency interventional care: treating acute pelvic pain in young women. *Neuromodulation.* 2006;9(2):136-142.

213. Brosseau L, Yonge K, Marchand S, et al. Efficacy of transcutaneous electrical nerve stimulation for osteoarthritis of the lower extremities: a meta-analysis. *Phys Ther Rev.* 2004;9(4):213-233.

214. King EW, Audette K, Athman GA, Nguyen HOX, Sluka KA, Fairbanks CA. Transcutaneous electrical nerve stimulation activates peripherally located alpha-2A adrenergic receptors. *Pain.* 2005;115(3):364-373.

215. Miller L, Mattison P, Paul L, Wood L. The effects of transcutaneous electrical nerve stimulation on spasticity. *Phys Ther Rev.* 2005;10(4):201-208.

216. Resende MA, Sabino GG, Candido CRM, Pereira LSM, Francischi JN. Local transcutaneous electrical stimulation (TENS) effects in experimental inflammatory edema and pain. *Eur J Pharmacol.* 2004;504(3):217-222.

217. Sarzi-Puttini P, Cimmino MA, Scarpa R, et al. Osteoarthritis: an overview of the disease and its treatment strategies. *Semin Arthritis Rheum.* 2005;35(1):1-10.

218. Brüggemann W, Uehleke B. *Kneipp vademecum pro medico.* 13th ed. Würzburg: Aufl. Sebastian Kneipp Gesundheitsmittel-Verlag; 1992.

219. Gwilt M, Athis J. Treating venous leg ulceration with complementary therapy. *Community Nurse.* 2000;6(9):51-53.

220. Felty CL, Rooke TW. Compression therapy for chronic venous insufficiency. *Semin Vasc Surg.* 2005;18(1):36-40.

221. Kessler T, de Bruin E, Brunner F, Vienne P, Kissling R. Effect of manual lymph drainage after hindfoot operations. *Physiother Res Int.* 2003;8(2):101-110.

*222. Andersen L, Højris I, Erlandsen M, Andersen J. Treatment of breast-cancer-related lymphedema with or without manual lymphatic drainage: a randomized study. *Acta Oncol.* 2000;39(3):399-405.

†223. Preston N, Seers K, Mortimer P. Physical therapies for reducing and controlling lymphoedema of the limbs. *Cochrane Database Syst Rev.* 2004;(4):CD003141.

224. Campisi C, Boccardo F, Casaccia M. Post-mastectomy lymphedema: surgical therapy. *Ann Ital Chir.* 2002;73(5):473.

225. Campisi C, Boccardo F, Zilli A, et al. Lymphedema secondary to breast cancer treatment: possibility of diagnostic and therapeutic prevention. *Ann Ital Chir.* 2002;73(5):493.

226. Casley-Smith JR. Changes in the microcirculation at the superficial and deeper levels in lymphoedema: the effects and results of massage, compression, exercise and benzopyrones on these levels during treatment. *Clin Hemorheol Microcirc.* 2000;23(2-4):335-343.

227. Kasseroller RG, Schrauzer GN. Treatment of secondary lymphedema of the arm with physical decongestive therapy and sodium selenite: a review. *Am J Ther.* 2000;7(4):273.

228. Kriederman B, Myloyde T, Bernas M, et al. Limb volume reduction after physical treatment by compression and/or massage in a rodent model of peripheral lymphedema. *Lymphology.* 2002;35(1):23-27.

229. Hertling D, Kessler RM. *Management of Common Musculoskeletal Disorders: Physical Therapy Principles and Methods.* 4th ed. Philadelphia, PA: Lippincott Williams & Wilkins; 2006.

230. Colby LA, Kisner C. *Therapeutic Exercise: Foundations and Techniques.* 5th ed. Philadelphia, PA: FA Davis; 2007.

231. Werner RA, Benjamin BE. *A Massage Therapist's Guide to Pathology.* Baltimore, MD: Lippincott Williams & Wilkins; 2002.

232. Dery M, Yonuschot G, Winterson B. The effects of manually applied intermittent pulsation pressure to rat ventral thorax on lymph transport. *Lymphology.* 2000;33(2):58.

233. Lederman E. *The Science and Practice of Manual Therapy.* Edinburgh: Elsevier/Churchill Livingstone; 2005.

234. Petermans J, Zicot M. Musculo-venous pump in the elderly. *J Mal Vasc.* 1994;19(2):115-118.

235. Kelly DG. *A Primer on Lymphedema.* Upper Saddle River, NJ: Prentice Hall; 2002.

†236. Preston N, Seers K, Mortimer PS. Physical therapies for reducing and controlling lymphoedema of the limbs. *Cochrane Database Syst Rev.* 2008;2008(3).

237. Harris S, Hugi M, Olivotto I, Levine M. Steering committee for clinical practice guidelines for the care and treatment of breast cancer. Clinical practice guidelines for the care and treatment of breast cancer: 11. Lymphedema. *CMAJ.* 2001;164(2):191-199.

238. Johansson K, Albertsson M, Ingvar C, Ekdahl C. Effects of compression bandaging with or without manual lymph drainage treatment in patients with postoperative arm lymphedema. *Lymphology.* 1999;32(3):103-110.

239. De Godoy J, Batigalia F. Preliminary evaluation of a new, more simplified physiotherapy technique for lymphatic drainage. *Lymphology.* 2002;35(2):91.

240. Sabir'ianov AR, Sabir'ianova ES, Epishev VV. Trends in variability of the central blood circulation in healthy individuals in response to massage of the collar cervical region. *Vopr Kurortol Fizioter Lech Fiz Kult.* 2004;Nov-Dec(6):13-15.

241. Liu Y, Xu S, Yan J, et al. Capillary blood flow with dynamical change of tissue pressure caused by exterior force. *Sheng Wu Yi Xue Gong Cheng Xue Za Zhi.* 2004;21(5):699-703.

242. Tsarev AI, Ezhova VA, Kunitsyna LA, Slovesnov SV, Chukreeva LN, Kolesnikova EI. Aromamassage of the cervical collar region in the combined treatment of patients with atherosclerotic dyscirculatory encephalopathy. *Vopr Kurortol Fizioter Lech Fiz Kult.* 2004;Sept-Oct(5):6-7.

243. Drust B, Atkinson G, Gregson W, French D, Binningsley D. The effects of massage on intra muscular temperature in the vastus lateralis in humans. *Int J Sports Med.* 2003;24(6):395-399.

244. Hinds T, McEwan I, Perkes J, Dawson E, Ball D, George K. Effects of massage on limb and skin blood flow after quadriceps exercise. *Med Sci Sports Exerc.* 2004;36(8):1308.

245. Mur E, Schmidseder J, Egger I, et al. Influence of reflex zone therapy of the feet on intestinal blood flow measured by color Doppler sonography. *Forsch Komplementarmed Klass Naturheilkd.* 2001;8(2):86-89.

246. Martin NA, Zoeller RF, Robertson RJ, Lephart SM. The comparative effects of sports massage, active recovery, and rest in promoting blood lactate clearance after supramaximal leg exercise. *J Athl Train.* 1998;33(1):30.

247. Perle SM. Effleurage massage, muscle blood flow and long-term post-exercise strength recovery. *J Sports Chiropract Rehabil.* 1996;10:102.

248. Robertson A, Watt J, Galloway S. Effects of leg massage on recovery from high intensity cycling exercise. *Br J Sports Med.* 2004;38(2):173-176.

249. Kniazeva TA, Minenkov AA, Kul'chitskaia DB, Apkhanova TV. Effect of physiotherapy on the microcirculation in patients with lymphedema of lower extremities. *Vopr Kurortol Fizioter Lech Fiz Kult.* 2003;(1):30-32.

250. Morhenn VB. Firm stroking of human skin leads to vasodilatation possibly due to the release of substance P. *J Dermatol Sci.* 2000;22(2):138-144.

251. Turchaninov R, Prilutsky B. Massage therapy: a beneficial tool in treating fibromyalgia. *Massage Bodywork.* 2004;19:82.

252. Michlovitz S. *Thermal Agents in Rehabilitation.* 3rd ed. Philadelphia, PA: FA Davis; 1996.

253. Varekojis SM, HerbertDouce F, Flucke RL, et al. A comparison of the therapeutic effectiveness of and preference for postural drainage and percussion, intrapulmonary percussive ventilation, and high-frequency chest wall compression in hospitalized cystic fibrosis patients. *Respir Care.* 2003;48(1):24-28.

254. Oermann CM, Sockrider MM, Giles D, Sontag MK, Accurso FJ, Castile RG. Comparison of high-frequency chest wall oscillation and oscillating positive expiratory pressure in the home management of cystic fibrosis: a pilot study*. *Pediatr Pulmonol.* 2001;32(5):372-377.

255. Fink JB. Positioning versus postural drainage. *Respir Care.* 2002;47(7):769-777.

256. Maa SH, Sun MF, Hsu KH, et al. Effect of acupuncture or acupressure on quality of life of patients with chronic obstructive asthma: a pilot study. *J Altern Complement Med.* 2003;9(5):659-670.

257. Persad R. *Massage Therapy and Medications*. Toronto, ON: Curties-Overzet Publications; 2001.

258. de Domenico G, Wood EC. *Beard's Massage*. 4th ed. Philadelphia, PA: WB Saunders; 1997.

259. Hess DR. The evidence for secretion clearance techniques. *Respir Care*. 2001;46(11):1276-1293.

260. Fritz S. *Fundamentals of Therapeutic Massage*. 3rd ed. St. Louis, MO: Mosby-Yearbook; 2004.

261. Clay JH, Pounds DM. *Basic Clinical Massage Therapy: Integrating Anatomy and Treatment*. Philadelphia, PA: Lippincott Williams & Wilkins; 2003.

262. Cantu RI, Grodin AJ. *Myofascial Manipulation: Theory and Clinical Application*. 2nd ed. Gaithersburg, MD: Aspen; 2001.

263. Stanborough M. *Direct Release Myofascial Technique*. Vol 4. Edinburgh: Churchill Livingstone; 2004.

264. Smith J. *Structural Bodywork*. Edinburgh: Elsevier Churchill Livingstone; 2005.

265. Travell JG, Simons DG. *Myofascial Pain and Dysfunction: The Trigger Point Manual*. Vol 2. Baltimore, MA: Lippincott Williams & Wilkins; 1992.

266. Alexander D. *Massage therapy self care manual*. Ottawa, Ontario: Sohnen-Moe Associates, Inc; 2005.

267. Lundberg U. Muscle tension. *J Soft Tissue Manipulation*. 2006;13:3.

268. Hernandez-Reif M, Field T, Largie S, et al. Cerebral palsy symptoms in children decreased following massage therapy. *Early Child Dev Care*. 1999;175(5):445-456.

269. Hou CR, Tsai LC, Cheng KF, Chung KC, Hong CZ. Immediate effects of various physical therapeutic modalities on cervical myofascial pain and trigger-point sensitivity. *Arch Phys Med Rehabil*. 2002;83(10):1406-1414.

270. Archer PA. Three clinical sports massage approaches for treating injured athletes. *Athlet Ther Today*. 2001;6(3):14-20.

271. Kostopoulos D, Rizopoulos K. *The manual of trigger point and myofascial therapy*. Thorofare, NJ: Slack; 2001.

272. Simons DG, Travell J, Simons LS. *Myofascial Pain and Dysfunction: The Trigger Point Manual: Upper Half of Body*. Vol 1. Baltimore, MD: Williams & Wilkins; 1999.

273. Lucas KR, Polus BI, Rich PA. Latent myofascial trigger points: their effects on muscle activation and movement efficiency. *J Bodywork Mov Ther*. 2004;8(3):160-166.

274. Weiss JM. Pelvic floor myofascial trigger points: manual therapy for interstitial cystitis and the urgency-frequency syndrome. *J Urol*. 2001;166(6): 2226-2231.

275. Delaney J, Leong KS, Watkins A, Brodie D. The short-term effects of myofascial trigger point massage therapy on cardiac autonomic tone in healthy subjects. *J Adv Nurs*. 2002;37(4):364-371.

276. Simons D, Mense S. Understanding and measurement of muscle tone as related to clinical muscle pain. *Pain*. 1998;75(1):1-17.

277. Michelotti A, Steenks M, Farella M, Parisini F. Short-term effects of physiotherapy versus counselling for the treatment of myofascial pain of the jaw muscles. *J Oral Rehabil*. 2002;29(9):874-874.

278. McPartland JM. Travell trigger points—molecular and osteopathic perspectives. *J Am Osteopath Assoc*. 2004;104(6):244-249.

279. Vaughn BF. Integrated strategies for treatment of spasmodic torticollis. *J Bodywork Mov Ther*. 2003;7(3):142-147.

280. Sefton J. Alternative and complementary concepts. Myofascial release for athletic trainers, part 3: specific techniques. *Athl Ther Today*. 2004;9(3):40-41.

281. Wheeler L. Advanced strain counterstrain. *Massage Ther J*. 2004;43(4).

282. O'Sullivan SB. Strategies to improve motor control. In: O'Sullivan SB, Schmitz J, eds. *Physical Rehabilitation, Assessment and Treatment*. Philadelphia, PA: FA Davis; 1988.

283. Bandy WD, Sanders B. *Therapeutic Exercise: Techniques for Intervention*. Baltimore, MD: Lippincott Williams & Wilkins; 2001.

284. Nyland J. *Clinical Decisions in Therapeutic Exercise: Planning and Implementation*. Upper Saddle River, NJ: Pearson Prentice Hall; 2006.

285. Rochet JM, Zaoui A. Burn scars: rehabilitation and skin care. *Rev Pract*. 2002;52(20):2258-2263.

286. Guler-Uysal F, Kozanoglu E. Comparison of the early response to two methods of rehabilitation in adhesive capsulitis. *Swiss Med Wkly*. 2004;134(23-24): 353-358.

287. Wies J. Treatment of eight patients with frozen shoulder: a case study series. *J Bodywork Mov Ther*. 2005;9(1):58-64.

288. Barnes JF. Myofascial release. In: Hammer WI, ed. *Functional Soft-Tissue Examination and Treatment by Manual Methods*. 2nd ed. Gaithersburg, MD: Jones & Bartlett Learning; 1999:533-548.

289. Smith F. Causes of and treatment options for abnormal scar tissue. *J Wound Care*. 2005;14(2):49-52.

290. Mannheim CJ. *The Myofascial Release Manual*. 3rd ed. Thorofare, NJ: Slack; 2001.

291. Sefton J. Myofascial release for athletic trainers, part 2: guidelines and techniques. *Athl Ther Today*. 2004;9:52-53.

292. Brosseau L, Casimiro L, Milne S, et al. Deep transverse friction massage for treating tendinitis. *Cochrane Database Syst Rev*. 2002;4:CD003528

293. Boisaubert B, Brousse C, Zaoui A, Montigny JP. Nonsurgical treatment of tennis elbow. *Ann Readapt Med Phys*. 2004;47(6):346-355.

294. Roques C. Massage applied to scars. *Wound Repair Regen*. 2002;10(2):126-128.

295. Davies C. Self-treatment of lateral epicondylitis (tennis elbow): trigger point therapy for triceps and extensor muscles. *J Bodywork Mov Ther*. 2003;7(3):165-172.

296. Gerwin RD. A review of myofascial pain and fibromyalgia–factors that promote their persistence. *Acupunct Med*. 2005;23(3):121-134.

297. Fredericson M GM. Quick solutions for iliotibial band syndrome. *Phys Sportsmed*. 2000;28(2):53-68.

298. Jurgel J, Rannama L, Gapeyeva H, Ereline1 J, Kolts I, Paasuke M. Shoulder function in patients with frozen shoulder before and after 4-week rehabilitation. *Medicina (Kaunas)*. 2005;41(1):30-38.

299. Lowe W. *Orthopedic Massage: Theory and Technique*. Edinburgh: Mosby; 2003.

300. Alexander D. Myofascial therapy response. *J Bodywork Mov Ther*. 1999;3(4):191-197.

301. Hawes MC, Brooks WJ. Reversal of the signs and symptoms of moderately severe idiopathic scoliosis in response to physical methods. *Stud Health Technol Inform*. 2002;91:365-368.

302. Myers TW. *Anatomy Trains*. Edinburgh: Churchill Livingstone; 2001.

303. Moore MK. Upper crossed syndrome and its relationship to cervicogenic headache. *J Manipulative Physiol Ther*. 2004;27(6):414-420.

304. Simons DG, Mense S. Diagnosis and therapy of myofascial trigger points. *Schmerz*. 2003;17(6):419-424.

305. Simons DG. Understanding effective treatments of myofascial trigger points. *J Bodywork Mov Ther*. 2002;6(2):81-88.

306. Gyllensten AL, Hansson L, Ekdahl C. Patient experiences of basic body awareness therapy and the relationship with the physiotherapist. *J Bodywork Mov Ther*. 2003;7(3):173-183.

307. Fitch P. Massage strategies for depressed clients. Massage *Ther J*. 2003;42:58-64.

308. Henriksen M, Højrup A, Lund H, Christensen L, Danneskiold-Samsøe B, Bliddal H. The effect of stimulating massage of thigh muscles on knee joint position sense. *Adv Physiother*. 2004;6(1):29-36.

309. Alexander D. Unravelling compensatory patterns. *J Soft Tissue Manipulation*. 2005;12:6.

310. Sefton JEM, Yarar C, Carpenter DM, Berry JW. Physiological and clinical changes after therapeutic massage of the neck and shoulders. *Man Ther*. 2011;16(5):487-494.

311. Lovas J, Craig A, Tran Y, Middleton J. The role of massage therapy in managing secondary conditions associated with spinal cord injury: an integrative model. *Top Spinal Cord Inj Rehabil*. 2008;14(1):61-75.

312. Manella C, Backus D. Gait characteristics, range of motion, and spasticity changes in response to massage in a person with incomplete spinal cord injury: case report. *Int J Ther Massage Bodywork*. 2011;4(1):28.

313. Zhou X, Zheng K. Treatment of 140 cerebral palsied children with a combined method based on traditional Chinese medicine (TCM) and western medicine. *J Zhejiang Univ Sci B*. 2005;6(1):57.

314. Wine ZK. Russian medical massage: massage for spasticity. *Massage Mag*. 1996;1:80.

315. Unknown. Tips for working with paralysis, other disabilities. *Massage Bodywork*. 2000;15:30.

316. Wang XH, Zhang LM, Han M, Zhang KQ, Jiang JJ. Treatment of Bell's palsy with combination of traditional Chinese medicine and western medicine. *Hua Xi Kou Qiang Yi Xue Za Zhi*. 2004;22(3):211-213.

317. American Physical Therapy Association. *Guide to Physical Therapist Practice*. Alexandria, VA: American Physical Therapy Association; 1999.

318. Porth C, Matfin G. *Pathophysiology: Concepts of Altered Health States*. 8th Ed. Baltimore, MD: Lippincott Williams & Wilkins. 2009.

319. Bucci C. Condition-Specific Massage Therapy. Baltimore, MD: Lippincott Williams & Wilkins. 2012.

320. Hendrickson T. *Massage for Orthopedic Conditions*. Baltimore, MD: Lippincott Williams & Wilkins. 2003.

321. US National Library of Medicine. Pubmed Health (online). 2012.

322. Page P, Frank C, Lardner R. *Assessment and Treatment of Muscle Imbalance: The Janda Approach*. Champaign, IL: Human Kinetics. 2009.

Abnormal connective tissue density: Irregular connective tissue remodeling that occurs during the consolidation and maturation stages of connective tissue healing.

Accessory joint motion: The range of motion within synovial and secondary cartilaginous joints that is not under voluntary control and can, therefore, only be obtained passively by the clinician. These motions, also known as joint play movements, are essential for full and pain-free active range of motion.

Active exercise: Exercise that is performed voluntarily without assistance.

Active listening: To restate a speaker's thoughts and feelings in the listener's own words; also known as paraphrasing. It is an effective way to clarify client desires or goals.

Active range of motion: The amount of joint motion that can be achieved by the client during the performance of unassisted voluntary joint motion.

Active Release®: A soft tissue system developed by chiropractor Michael Leahy for treatment of chronic and repetitive strain injuries. Active Release protocols for individual muscles combine simultaneous active or passive movement with application of specific and deep neuromuscular techniques.

Active trigger point: A trigger point that refers pain in a characteristic pattern whether the muscle in which it is located is working or at rest.

Activity or activity capacity: An individual's execution of a task or action in an ideal situation.

Acupoint: In Traditional Chinese Medicine and related systems, a point on a meridian that can be stimulated by various methods to achieve complex effects on physiological function that are usually manifested in areas that are remote to the point of application.

Acupressure: A type of massage that uses specific compression to stimulate acupoints and meridians to achieve complex effects on physiological function that are usually manifested in areas that are remote to the point of application.

Acupuncture: A technique for treating disease or pain or by inserting into the skin at specific points needles that are then twirled, heated, or subjected to weak electrical current.

In Traditional Chinese Medicine, acupuncture is used to treat a wide range of medical conditions, but its use in the West is usually confined to treatment of pain.

Acute pain: Pain provoked by noxious stimulation produced by injury and/or disease with unpleasant sensory and emotional experiences (see Pain).

Acute stage (of inflammation): The early response to tissue damage marked by local vasodilation and the influx of white blood cells. Acute inflammation is suggested in orthopedic practice when the client complains of diffuse pain that is felt at rest and made worse by movement.

Adherence: The extent to which clients follow the instructions for care that they negotiate with their health care providers.

Adhesions: A binding together with dense connective tissue of tissues that normally glide or move in relation to each other, with resultant loss of mobility. Like scars, adhesions may result from the replacement of normal tissue that has been destroyed by burn, wound, surgery, radiation, or disease with connective tissue.

Adhesive capsulitis: Inflammation and fibrosis of the shoulder joint capsule that causes painfully limited range of motion.

Aerosol therapy: The use of medicated mists to treat respiratory conditions.

Agonist/antagonist balance: The ability of opposing groups of muscles to reciprocally contract and lengthen through the full range of active movement.

AIDS: Acquired immunodeficiency syndrome; caused by infection with the human immunodeficiency virus (HIV).

Airway clearance: Ability to move pulmonary secretions effectively through the use of normal mechanisms of cough and the mucociliary escalator.

Alarm phase: The first phase of the general adaptation syndrome or nonspecific response to stress described by Hans Selye (1907–1982). It consists of nervous and endocrine responses to mobilize the organism for "flight or fight."

Alexander, F. Mathias: (1869–1955) An Australian actor who developed a system of movement training in response to difficulties he experienced in on-stage performance.

Alexander technique: A method of retraining movement that is taught by certified instructors in one-on-one guided sessions. Alexander technique emphasizes coordinated, easy, balanced movement performed with an aligned, elongated spine.

Algometer: A device that measures tissue sensitivity to pressure.

Aligned: Arranged in a line. A well-aligned spine tends towards shallow, even curves and bilateral symmetry.

Altered body image: A change in the way a person perceives his or her body, as happens in eating disorders or after disfiguring accidents.

Amplitude of technique: An indication of the size of the area that is covered by a technique.

Analgesia: Pain relief.

Anatomical barrier in soft tissue: The final resistance to normal tissue range of motion that is provided by bone, ligament, or soft tissue. Motion beyond the anatomical barrier results in tissue damage.

Anatomy Train: A continuous, connected, linear myofascial pathway that runs through the body. Eleven such pathways have been described in detail by Thomas Myers in the book, *Anatomy Trains*.

Antalgic: Literally, against pain. With an antalgic gait, the stance phase on the painful side is shortened.

Anxiety: A state of uneasiness, apprehension, or dread accompanied by physical symptoms such as restlessness, muscle tension, rapid heart rate, and difficulty breathing.

Anxiety disorders: A group of related mental illnesses that involve severe anxiety in response to stress.

Armoring: Myofascial hardness associated with chronically elevated muscle resting tension.

Aromatherapy: The use of essential oils distilled from plants to affect mood or to treat impairments or conditions. The fragrant oils are inhaled or diluted in carrier oil and applied during massage.

Arousal: The process of awaking or stimulating.

Arterial supply: The volume of oxygenated blood carried by arteries that reaches a given structure.

Attention: The clinician's capacity to focus on the sensory information that he or she receives primarily, but not exclusively, through his or her hands.

Automobilization: Joint mobilization performed by a client on him or herself.

Autonomic balance: Appropriate, healthy functioning of the sympathetic and parasympathetic branches of the autonomic nervous system.

Autonomic phenomena: Disturbances of the autonomic nervous system, such as vertigo, that may accompany myofascial trigger points in particular muscles.

Barnes, John F.: (1939–) American physical therapist who has contributed to the development of Myofascial Release and taught it extensively in workshops. Basic theory and technique related to this approach are presented in Chapter 10, Connective Tissue Techniques.

Barrier-release phenomenon: The therapist engages the tissue barrier at the point at which the therapist palpates a resistance to tissue motion. If the therapist sustains the pressure on the tissue barrier, a "release" may occur after a latency period that will vary with the nature and state of health of the tissue. This release results in a reduction of the resistance that will enable the therapist to move the tissue beyond the location of the original barrier without increasing the pressure of palpation.

Best research evidence: The best available clinical, client-centered research that examines the accuracy, safety, and efficacy of diagnostic and assessment tests, prognosis markers, and therapeutic interventions.

Biofeedback: A technique for training a person to influence autonomic body processes. Using information supplied from monitoring devices, the subject learns to control basic parameters, such as heart rate, and then to influence related activities such as blood pressure.

Biotensegrity system: A biological system in which the biomechanical forces allow both movement and the maintenance of static postures.

Body functions: The physiological functions of the anatomical systems of the body.

Body image: How a person mentally perceives his or her own body.

Body structures: The various anatomical structures and systems of the body.

Bodywork: A contemporary term that embraces massage and related approaches that contact or move the client's tissues to achieve educational or therapeutic effects.

Boundary violations: When the therapist crosses the ethical and interpersonal limits that have been established for the therapeutic relationship with the client.

Box kneading: A two-handed form of kneading in which the hands are positioned so that they are diametrically opposed on a limb, then compress toward each other, and then move proximally. This stroke is recommended to increase fluid return.

Broad-contact compression: A nongliding neuromuscular technique, delivered with a broad contact surface, that engages the client's muscle with the pressure and release of the stroke administered perpendicular to the surface of the client's body.

Broad-contact kneading: A gliding petrissage technique performed in circles or ellipses with a large contact surface such as the palm.

Burnout: A condition resulting from chronic stress that is characterized by physical and emotional exhaustion and is sometimes accompanied by clinical depression or illness.

Bursitis: Inflammation of a bursa.

Cadence: Rhythm.

Capsular laxity: Anatomical or pathological lengthening of the joint capsule.

Capsular restriction: Anatomical or pathological shortening of the joint capsule.

Capsulitis and synovitis: Inflammation of the joint capsule and associated internal ligaments and of the synovium.

Case-control study: A study in which researchers identify individuals who have similar outcomes and examine their history to determine if they received the same intervention.

Case report: A type of descriptive research that presents an accurate, brief, and clear narrative report of a single instance or event in a systematic format.

Case series: A summary of findings on a group of participants with similar characteristics or who received the same intervention without reference to findings on a control group.

Caution: A sign, symptom, evaluation, or diagnosis that directs the clinician to be prepared to modify a given procedure in order to reduce the risks associated with its application.

Center of gravity: The point in the center of an object, where the object's mass behaves as if it were concentrated. The center of gravity of the upright adult human is anterior to the S2.

Centrifugal: 1. Directed away from the heart or distally. 2. Opposed to the direction of venous and/or lymphatic return. 3. Directed away from an area of local pathology.

Centripetal: Directed towards the heart or proximally.

Chaitow, Leon: British osteopath and naturopath and editor of the *Journal of Bodywork and Movement Therapies* who has written extensively on manual therapy and natural healing.

Chest wall: All the structures in the thorax and outside the lungs that move during breathing, including the ribs, intercostal muscles, diaphragm, fascia, and skin.

Chest wall mobility: The ability of the chest wall and its component structures and tissues to move freely.

Chi (Qi): In Traditional Chinese Medicine, life force or energy. Chi circulates through the body in well-defined cycles through conduits or channels called meridians.

Chronic inflammation: See Chronic stage (of inflammation).

Chronic obstructive pulmonary disease: A pulmonary disorder that is characterized by the presence of increased airway resistance.

Chronic pain: Pain that persists beyond the usual course of healing of an acute disease or beyond the reasonable time in which the injury is expected to heal. Some authors define chronic pain in terms of duration of pain, with a lower limit of duration ranging from 6 weeks to 6 months; others define chronic pain in terms of an increasing dissociation from the physical etiology and increasing affective and cognitive dimensions of pain.

Chronic pain syndrome: A clinical syndrome in which clients present with high levels of pain that is chronic in duration, functional impairment, and depression.

Chronic restrictive pulmonary disease: A pulmonary disorder that is characterized by the restriction of lung expansion, such as interstitial fibrosis.

Chronic stage (of inflammation): The later response to tissue damage, marked by consolidation and maturation of collagen in scar tissue. Chronic inflammation is suggested in orthopedic practice when the client complains of localized pain that is felt only during specific movements, in a small part of the range or at the end range.

Chronic stress: A prolonged and heightened state of arousal that has negative physiological and psychological consequences.

Circulatory massage: The use of massage techniques, such as superficial effleurage and petrissage, to increase regional or systemic venous and lymphatic return or arterial supply.

Clapping: A form of percussion that is used to mechanically loosen secretions in the lungs and to facilitate airway clearance.

Classical massage, or classic massage: See Swedish massage.

Client-centered care: This approach to care looks beyond the mere delivery of services to the client to include advocacy, empowerment, respect for the client's autonomy, and the client's participation in decision making. When a therapist commits to client-centered care, the client and therapist share the decision-making about how the intervention will proceed.

Client examination: The systematic collection of information on the client's health status and clinical condition through history taking, a general systems review, and tests and measures.

Client values: The unique preferences, goals, and expectations that each client brings to the therapeutic relationship.

Clinical care: Therapists provide clinical care to their clients as they conduct their examinations and interventions.

Clinical competence to treat: The therapist's clinical training permits him or her to treat a given client's condition.

Clinical decision-making: The process by which clinicians synthesize and analyze information on their clients' conditions and use the results of their analysis to formulate and progress a therapeutic intervention for their clients. Also known as clinical reasoning and clinical problem-solving.

Clinical decision-making model: A framework that demonstrates a process by which therapists can synthesize and analyze information on their clients' conditions and use the results of their analysis to formulate and progress a therapeutic intervention for their clients.

Clinical depression: A mood disorder characterized by sadness, despair, or apathy that is severe enough to affect a person's ability to perform activities of daily living and to fulfill social roles.

Clinical experience: The experience that a therapist acquires by treating clients in clinical settings. Clinical experience (expertise), best research evidence, and patient values are the components of evidence-based practice.

Clinical expertise: The therapist's ability to use his or her clinical skills and past experience to identify each client's unique health status and the potential risks and benefits of interventions that he or she could use in each case.

Clinical findings: The results of tests and measures and the lists of impairments, body structures and functions, functional limitations, activity limitations, and limitations in participation with which the client presents.

Clinical hypothesis: The clinician's hypothesis about the client's key clinical problems.

Clinical indication: A sign, symptom, evaluation, or diagnosis that directs the clinician to apply a certain procedure.

Clinical problem: The client's presenting issues related to the impairments or functional limitations he or she is experiencing as a result of his or her medical condition.

Clinical problem list: A summary of the client's impairments and functional limitations that will be addressed within the plan of care.

Clinical stage of inflammation: The clinician's judgment of the stage of inflammation of an injury made by evaluating the severity of the client's symptoms and the results of tests such as range of motion.

Clonus: A cyclical, spasmodic hyperactivity of antagonistic muscles that occurs at a regular frequency in response to a quick stretch stimulus.

Coarse vibration: A form of vibration that has an amplitude of 1 cm or more and that intergrades with shaking.

Cochrane Database of Systematic Reviews: A collection of systematic reviews and meta-analyses that rigorously summarize and interpret the results of high-quality medical research, usually randomized controlled trials.

Cognitive Transactional Model of Stress: Lazarus and Folkman's model of stress as the condition that results when a person's interactions with his environment leads him to perceive a discrepancy between the demands of the situation and the resources of the person's biological, psychological, or social systems.

Cogwheel rigidity: A ratchet-like response to passive movement, alternating between giving way and resistance.

Coherence: Consistent order and structure of a massage sequence or intervention that results from clear and consistent intention(s) on the part of the therapist.

Cohort study: A study that follows the outcomes of a group of participants who researchers identify as having received the intervention and a group with similar characteristics who did not.

Cold mitten friction: An application of cold water with friction of a coarse towel or sponge that acts as a tonic. A full body application takes 20–30 minutes.

Cold pack: A container filled with cold water, frozen gel, or crushed ice that is applied locally to relieve pain or reduce edema.

Collagen: An important structural protein of connective tissue that combines into fibers whose great tensile strength reinforces ligaments, tendons, fascia, and cartilage.

Collagen cross-link: A chemical bond between adjacent fibers of collagen that reduces mobility of the fibers with respect to each other. Frequency of cross-links increases with age, injury, and immobility and can restrict mobility of the tissue as a whole.

Combines with: When one technique is said to "combine" with another, it means that the two techniques may be executed simultaneously.

Compartment syndrome: Elevation of fluid pressure within a closed fascial compartment that is caused by trauma or repetitive exercise such as running. Reduced perfusion can result in hypoxia, nerve damage, and muscle necrosis.

Compensatory changes: Changes in biomechanics that accumulate progressively throughout the body after an injury as a result of pain or the effects of scar tissue.

Compensatory strategy: A technique that is used as a means of compensating for an impairment that is not amenable to active treatment.

Complementary treatment techniques: Techniques that therapists use as an adjunct to the primary treatment techniques. In the case of massage treatments, the primary treatment technique would be massage techniques, and other techniques would be used in a complementary manner.

Complex decongestive therapy (also known as complex or complete decongestive physiotherapy, CDT, or CDP): A treatment regimen for lymphedema that includes massage, bandaging or compression garments, specific exercises, and education on hygiene.

Complex regional pain syndrome: A condition in which people present with persistent, severe pain and/or allodynia (painful response to non-painful stimulus), dystrophic changes, and vasomotor dysfunction as a result of an unstable sympathetic nervous system following an injury or surgery to an extremity.

Compression: Any force that is oriented in a manner so that its effect is to shorten or compact a tissue or structure.

Compression garment: An elastic sleeve or similar garment that is meant to cover a region and exert pressure on it to prevent or reduce the accumulation of edema.

Conceptual framework: A set of empirical generalizations that provides a means of organizing and integrating observations about a specific set of behaviors that one observes in a particular setting.

Conceptual model: A diagram that shows the proposed causal linkages among a set of concepts that the individual believes to be related to a particular health problem.

Congruency: The point at which a therapist and client are in agreement on process, action, and effect. It also may refer to the therapist's inward integrity being represented in outward action and word.

Connective tissue: Tissues that consist of several different types of cells, such as fibroblasts and fat cells, and elastin and collagen fibers embedded in a matrix of gelatinous material, the consistency of which varies in response to many factors. Nerves, blood vessels, lymph vessels, myofibrils, and organs are found within connective tissue.

Connective tissue disease (CTD): A group of diseases that affect connective tissues such as muscle, cartilage, tendon, or skin. They are often autoimmune and inflammatory in nature. Examples include systemic lupus erythematosus, rheumatoid arthritis, Sjögren's syndrome, scleroderma, and mixed connective tissue disease.

Connective tissue massage (CTM): A system of massage developed by Elizabeth Dicke and popular in Europe in which connective tissue techniques are applied in precise sequences to the skin and superficial fascial layers to elicit specific physiological reflex effects.

Connective tissue matrix: The intercellular portion of connective tissue that contains protein-based fibers and ground substance.

Connective tissue techniques: Massage techniques that palpate, lengthen, and promote remodeling of connective tissue.

Connective tissue zones: Specific areas of muscle and related fascia of the back that exhibit increased tone in response to visceral pathology. According to the theory of Connective Tissue Massage, manipulating a zone associated with an organ will reflexly improve the function of that organ.

Consent: See Informed consent.

Consolidated edema: Edema in the chronic stage, where inflammatory exudate has been replaced with dense fibrous connective tissue.

Consolidation: Combining or grouping into a single unit.

Contact surface: The portion of the clinician's hand or arm that is used to execute the stroke.

Context: A brief description of how a massage technique is conventionally sequenced in relation to other techniques.

Contextual factors: An individual's personal and environmental factors, which can have an effect on health.

Contractile tissue: Muscle, with its enveloping fascial layers, associated tendon(s), and periosteal attachments.

Contracture: A permanent muscular shortening due to a variety of physiological changes in muscle, such as fibrosis or loss of muscular balance.

Contraindication: A sign, symptom, evaluation, or diagnosis that directs the therapist to avoid applying a certain procedure.

Controlled lean posture: An inclined, aligned posture used to efficiently transfer the clinician's body weight to the client in a controlled manner.

Contusion: A bruise.

Cortisol: A hormone (hydrocortisone) produced by the adrenal cortex. It has multiple physiological effects that counteract the effects of stress.

Countertransference: Occurs when the therapist projects feelings onto a client that are unconscious, unprocessed, or unexpressed or idealizes the client in some way.

Cranial (craniosacral) rhythm: A subtle, palpable rhythm that occurs 6–14 times a minute and is caused by rhythmic flow of cerebrospinal fluid through the central nervous system.

Craniosacral Therapy: Involves assessing and adjusting the movement of the cerebrospinal fluid (CSF), which can become restricted by trauma and stress. Practitioners apply gentle and subtle manipulations to skull, spine, diaphragm, and fascia. Craniosacral therapy originated with osteopath William Sutherland and has been further developed by osteopath John Upledger.

Creep: Viscoelastic stretch of connective tissue that occurs when it is subjected to sustained tension and that is palpable.

Crepitus: A vibration of variable fineness that is associated with roughened gliding surfaces of a tendon or its sheath or of the articulating surfaces of a joint. Crepitus can sometimes be heard, as well as palpated.

Cross-link: See Collagen cross-link.

Cutaneous reflex: An involuntary response caused by stimulation of receptors in the skin.

Cyriax, James H.: (1904–1985) British orthopedic surgeon and author of an influential textbook of orthopedics that is still in print. Cyriax popularized range of motion testing to identify orthopedic conditions and the use of cross-fiber friction to treat many overuse conditions.

Decerebrate rigidity: Rigidity that occurs as a result of brainstem lesions. It presents clinically as sustained contraction and posturing of the trunk and lower limbs in extension.

Decorticate rigidity: Rigidity that occurs as a result of brainstem lesions. It presents clinically as sustained contraction and posturing of the trunk and lower limbs in extension and the upper limbs in flexion.

Deep effleurage: A general gliding manipulation performed with long strokes and moderate-to-heavy centripetal pressure that deforms superficial or deep layers of muscle.

Deep fascia: Connective tissue layer that lies immediately superficial to, or between, muscle fibers. The primary functions of the deep fascia are to allow muscles to move freely, to carry nerve and blood vessels, to fill the space between muscles, and to provide an origin for muscles.

Deep tissue massage: An imprecise term that suggests that connective tissue and/or neuromuscular techniques are being applied with enough force to deform myofascial tissue that lies beneath the investing layer of the deep fascia.

Deform: To change shape.

Deformation: The change in shape of a tissue or structure when it is subjected to pressure.

Delayed-onset muscle soreness (DOMS): Muscle soreness felt 24–72 hours after vigorous or unaccustomed exercise, probably caused by microtearing in the muscle fibers.

Dependent edema: An increase in extracellular fluid volume that is localized in a dependent area, such as a limb.

Depression: See Clinical depression.

DeQuervain's tenosynovitis: Overuse inflammation of the tendon and/or synovial sheath of the extensor pollicis brevis and abductor pollicis longus muscles.

Dermatomal pain: Pain in the pattern of a dermatome. Injury of a dorsal root may result in sensory loss in the skin or may be felt as a burning or electric pain.

Dermatome: An area of skin supplied by one dorsal nerve root.

Dermis: The first layer of connective tissue.

Diagnosis: The process and result of analyzing and organizing the findings from the client examination into clusters or syndromes.

Diaphragmatic breathing: An exercise that trains the client to consciously use the diaphragm during breathing.

Dicke, Elizabeth: German physiotherapist who developed connective tissue massage (Bindegewebsmassage) in the 1930s in response to personal illness.

Direct: In the context of connective tissue techniques, direct means that the therapist directs the force of the technique toward, and then through, the primary tissue restriction. This is in contrast to indirect techniques in which the therapist applies the force, or moves the client, away from the fascial barrier or restriction of motion.

Direct effect: A direct therapeutic effect

Direct fascial technique: A slow, gliding connective tissue technique that applies a moderate, sustained tensional force to the superficial fascia or to the deep fascia and associated muscle. It results in palpable viscoelastic lengthening and plastic deformation of the fascia.

Direct inhibitory pressure: Specific compression applied to a tendon as a means of inhibiting the tone of the related muscle for a short period of time.

Direction of technique: The direction of the applied force. The direction given in the description of techniques is the direction in which the greatest force is applied during the pressure phase of the stroke.

Disability: When an individual is unable to perform his or her socially defined tasks, activities, or roles to the expected level.

Disablement Model: An extension of the medical model that broadened the therapist's approach to examination, evaluation, and treatment to encompass the client's functional limitations and disability, as well as his or her presenting impairments.

Discharge: The transition of the client from the therapist's care to self-care or to treatment by another therapist.

Discharge Phase: The final phase of the clinical decision-making process that involves the transition of the client from the therapist's care to self-care or to treatment by another therapist.

Discrimination: The clinician's ability to distinguish fine gradations of sensory information.

Dislocation (luxation): The displacement of a bone from its normal position in a joint.

Dissociation: An impaired perception of reality often accompanied by a numbing of emotions or a disconnecting from the present. A client who is dissociated may appear to exhibit a profound apathy or inability to make decisions or initiate movements or actions. The client may be unaware of the present, of sounds and activities around them, or of the perception of pain.

Distraction: See Traction.

Drag: 1. Tensile force, stretching force, or traction force exerted along a single tissue layer. 2. Inherent tissue resistance to such force.

Drainage technique: Any massage technique or related technique, such as elevation of a limb, that increases the return flow of lymph or venous blood.

Draping: The process by which the clinician covers and uncovers portions of the client's body during treatment, while maintaining modesty and respecting appropriate client–clinician boundaries.

Dry brushing: Systematic brushing of the skin with a (natural) bristle brush, administered as a tonic, to exfoliate, and to stimulate skin metabolism.

Dual relationships: When the professional and social roles and interactions between two people overlap. This may occur when therapists treat family members, friends, or colleagues. Dual relationships are not necessarily wrong or unethical, but they can present uncomfortable situations or conflicts of interest for the therapist and client.

Duration of technique: An estimate of a reasonable length of time for which a single technique may have to be applied by a competent clinician to begin to achieve the specified outcomes.

Dyspnea: Shortness of breath, labored or difficult breathing, or uncomfortable awareness of one's breathing.

Ease of movement: Movement that is comfortable and that requires minimal effort.

Eastern-influenced massage systems: Massage systems originating in Asia that are based on radically different conceptual models of body processes than those used in Western medicine, such as energy (Chi) and meridians. Examples of Eastern approaches are Shiatsu, Amma, Thai massage, acupressure, and Jin Shin Do.

Ectomorph: A person with a build that is lean, slender, and sparsely muscled.

Edema: An accumulation of fluid in cells, tissues, or serous cavities. Edema has four main causes: increased permeability of capillaries, decreased plasma protein osmotic pressure, increased pressure in capillaries and venules, and lymphatic flow obstruction.

Effleurage: A group of general gliding manipulations performed with centripetal pressure and varying pressures.

Effusion: Excessive fluid in the joint capsule, indicating irritation or inflammation of the synovium.

Elastic: Capable of returning to original size and shape after being stretched or deformed.

Elastic barrier in soft tissue: The resistance that the clinician feels at the end of the passive range of motion of the tissue when she is taking the "slack" out of the tissue.

Elastic deformation: Deformation in response to applied force that disappears after the force is removed; spring-like behavior.

Elastic recoil: The return towards original size and shape demonstrated by elastic substances.

Elastic stretch: Stretch that disappears after the tensile force is removed.

Electromyography (EMG): A technique for recording the electrical (physiological) activity of muscles at rest and while contracting.

Electronic muscle stimulation (EMS): A modality where electric impulses are applied externally to muscle to make it contract.

Elevated resting tension: Increase in firmness to palpation of muscles at rest.

Endangerment sites: Areas of the human body over which the use of direct or sustained pressure is contraindicated.

End feel: (1) The qualities of motion or resistance to motion that the clinician palpates in the joint at the end of passive range of motion. (2) For massage techniques, end feel is the quality of resistance to further movement that is perceived by the practitioner at the end of the massage stroke. End feel is related to tissue constituents such as fat, connective tissue (scar tissue), muscle, etc.

Endomorph: A person with a build where the trunk is ample and rounded, with a high percentage of body fat.

Endorphins: A group of peptide neurotransmitters produced in the brain that act to reduce pain by binding to opiate receptor sites.

Energetic approaches: Approaches, such as Therapeutic Touch or Reiki, that use the simple forms of touch to manipulate the energy field or magnetic field of the client's body. See also Eastern approaches to massage.

Engage: To enter into contact with. In this text, a tissue is said to be "engaged" during a technique if it is significantly deformed during the technique's application.

Entrainment: The alteration of a biological rhythm in response to an external stimulus.

Entrapment neuropathy: Nerve compression that can result from bony deformity or muscle and connective tissue shortening and inflammation associated with trigger point activity, fascial restrictions, overuse syndromes, and other clinical conditions.

Environmental factors: Aspects of an individual's environment that can act as facilitators or barriers to the individual's health or wellness.

Episode of care: A series of interventions from initial visit to discharge within a single period that a client receives for a specific condition.

Epithelium: A layer of closely packed columnar or squamous cells that have little intercellular material between them.

Ergonomic: Related to the design and use of workplace equipment that enhances worker wellness.

Evaluation: The synthesis of the information from the client examination.

Evaluative Phase: The steps in the Evaluative Phase revolve around formulating and confirming a clinical hypothesis about the client's clinical problem or wellness goals.

Evidence: Information on clinical care that researchers and therapists collect in a systematic manner.

Evidence-based medicine (EBM): The integration of best research evidence with clinical expertise and client values.

Evidence-based practice: The integration of best research evidence with clinical expertise and client values to treat individual clients.

Evidence house: An approach proposed by Jonas that includes many kinds of rigorous research methods, rather than Sackett's hierarchical model. Jonas suggests that including a variety of research methodologies, such as qualitative research methods, can provide a more balanced and complete picture of what constitutes massage and how it works.

Examination: The collection of information on the client's health status and clinical condition through history taking, a general systems review, and tests and measures.

Exercise tolerance: The ability to perform cardiopulmonary work.

Exhaustion phase: The third and final phase of the general adaptation syndrome or nonspecific response to stress described by Hans Selye (1907–1982). It is characterized by physical and emotional exhaustion and is sometimes accompanied by illness.

Explicit memory: The verbal, narrative memory that derives from the hippocampus and that is evoked when a person relates a story.

Extensibility: Ability to extend or lengthen.

Facilitated segment: A spinal segment whose joints are dysfunctional as a result of visceral imbalance or pathology. Muscles adjacent to the facilitated segment show elevated resting tension and may be edematous or fibrotic. See also Connective tissue zone and Viscerosomatic reflex.

Fascia: A tough fibrous membrane composed of dense connective tissue. Superficial fascia contains fat, nerves, and blood vessels and joins the skin to the underlying layer. Deep fascia supports and separates the muscles. Subserous fascia lies between the deep fascia and the body cavities.

Fascial binding: See Fascial restrictions.

Fascial restrictions: The loss of mobility of one fascial layer with respect to another because of the loss of fluid consistency of ground substance and development of collagenous cross-links. Fascial restrictions can result from repair of tissue damage and from prolonged immobility.

Fascial sheath: An envelope of fascia that surrounds another structure, for example a muscle.

Fascial splinting: Regional thickening and hardening of fascia in response to increased biomechanical load.

Fasciculations: Localized, subconscious muscle contractions that result from the contraction of the muscle cells innervated by a single motor axon and thus do not involve the entire muscle.

Fasciitis: Inflammation of fascia.

Fatigue: Extreme tiredness or exhaustion; decreased capacity for physical or mental work.

Feldenkrais Method: A system, developed by Moshe Feldenkrais (1904–1984), that teaches mindful movement and efficient patterns for functional activities. Instruction by certified practitioners occurs in individual or group settings.

Fibromyalgia: A chronic rheumatic syndrome characterized by widespread musculoskeletal pain, the presence of specific tender points, severe fatigue, and sleep disturbances.

Fibroplasia: The phase of wound repair when fibroblasts grow and form new extracellular matrix and collagen. Fibroplasia occurs after the inflammatory phase and before the remodeling phase.

Fibrosed edema: See Consolidated edema.

Fibrosis: Formation of (excess) fibrous connective tissue during the process repair.

Fibrositic deposit or nodule: An outdated term used to describe hard pea-sized deposits in muscle and connective tissue that would now probably be recognized as myofascial trigger points.

Fine vibration: A superficial reflex technique in which a fast, oscillating or trembling movement is produced on the client's skin that results in minimal deformation of subcutaneous tissues.

Flexibility: The ability to bend without breaking.

Fluidotherapy: The application of warmed cellulose particles suspended in forced dry air to heat an injured body part prior to exercise.

Force of palpation: The direction and manner in which manual strength is applied to tissues during palpation that results in tissues being compressed, stretched, sheared, bent, and twisted.

Fracture: Interruption in the continuity of a bone.

Framework: The manner in which the intervention is delivered including timing, location, appointment setting, common responses, payment, and issues of confidentiality. It also describes the ethical foundations for decision-making to which the therapist commits. When a therapist's framework is clear to a client, then the client may appreciate the client roles and expectations as well as what the therapist is able to do.

Framing general massage technique: A general massage technique that is repeated at intervals during the course of a massage sequence. A framing technique serves as the principal palpation tool, connects the other techniques used, and imparts a sense of structure to the sequence.

Fremitus: A pulmonary vibration that a clinician can palpate over the rib cage as the client speaks or vocalizes.

Friction: 1. A repetitive, specific, nongliding, connective tissue technique that produces movement between the fibers of dense connective tissue, increasing tissue extensibility. 2. Historically, the term "friction" has a broad, ambiguous usage that has embraced virtually any manner of rubbing between two surfaces.

Fulling: A form of broad-contact kneading in which the hands compress down and away from each other to spread or broaden the muscle belly and then lift the muscle up on the return stroke.

Functional instability: Instability of a joint under load.

Functional limitation: A restriction of the individual's ability to execute a task or action in an ideal situation.

Functional outcome: The outcome that is related to the client's functional limitation.

Galvanic stimulation: See Electronic muscle stimulation.

Gate theory of pain: The widely quoted theory, first proposed by Melzack and Wall in the 1960s, that proposes that perception of painful stimuli in higher brain centers can be inhibited by stimulation of large fiber afferents.

General adaptation syndrome: The nonspecific response to stress first described by Austro-Canadian endocrinologist Hans Selye (1907–1982). It consists of three sequential psychoneuroimmulogical phases termed alarm, resistance, and exhaustion.

General massage (general full-body massage): Massage that includes all regions of the body. General massage commonly takes 60–90 minutes to perform but can be completed in as little as 15 minutes.

General technique: A technique that is applied to an entire region or a larger portion of the body or applied using a broad surface such as the palm, or both.

Glide: Movement of the clinician's hand across the client's skin.

Grade of injury: Severity of injury. An orthopedic injury may be assigned a numerical grade of 1, 2, or 3 to represent a mild, moderate, or severe injury.

Grounding: A practitioner's awareness of his or her contact and connection with the earth. The posture and alignment exercises described in Chapter 6 increase this awareness.

Ground substance: See Matrix.

Guided awareness: A technique where the therapist guides the client to focus his or her awareness on a body part or process.

Hatha yoga: As practiced in the West, Hatha yoga is usually the exercise of performing various postures, called asanas. Traditional Indian Hatha yoga is a comprehensive discipline that includes moral guidelines, asanas, breathing exercises, and meditation.

Healing Touch: An energetic approach similar to Therapeutic Touch and Reiki. Practitioners use the simplest form of touch to manipulate the energy field or magnetic field of the client's body.

Health: A dynamic process that encompasses multiple domains, including the individual's physical, emotional, social, and intellectual dimensions. In addition, some definitions of health address the individual's ability to fulfill his or her social roles and respond to environmental stressors.

Health-related quality of life: The objective and subjective dimensions of an individual's ability to function in, and derive satisfaction from, a variety of social roles in the presence of impaired health status.

Holding: See Unnecessary muscle tension.

Homeostasis: The state of internal stable equilibrium that is maintained by healthy living organisms in response to external and internal changes.

Hospice: A facility or organization that provides palliative care and physical, spiritual, emotional, and economic support for the terminally ill and their families.

Hot pack: A container filled with hot water, gel, or clay that is applied locally to increase circulation and produce analgesia.

H-reflex: A measure of spinal reflex (motoneuron) excitability that is based on the time required for a stimulus applied to a sensory nerve to travel to the spinal cord and return down the motor nerve. The H-reflex is increased in conditions of spastic paralysis.

Hyaluronic acid: A glycosaminoglycan found in the extracellular matrix of connective tissues that contributes to the lubricating qualities of synovial fluid and cartilage.

Hydration: The bonding of water molecules to another compound.

Hyperarousal: An abnormally heightened state of arousal.

Hyperemia: An increase in the amount of blood flowing through a body part, indicated by redness. Hyperemia can be caused by massage and by applications of heat or cold.

Hyperreflexia: Exaggerated deep tendon reflexes.

Hypersensitivity: This is the sudden painful, jolting, ticklish, or uncomfortable reaction that a client has when touched by the therapist. Hypersensitivity may be caused by an old, unresolved injury or trauma or as a result of chronic protection, overuse, or postural dysfunction.

Hyperstimulation analgesia: Pain relief that occurs as a result solely of somatic sensory stimulation in the form of heat, cold, touch, vibration, or movement. See Gate Theory of Pain.

Hypertonia: A general term used to refer to muscle tone that is above normal resting levels, regardless of the mechanism for the increase in tone.

Hypertrophy: Increase in the size of an organ or structure, usually due to growth of individual cells rather than an increased number of cells.

Hypotonia: A general term used to refer to muscle tone that is below normal resting levels, regardless of the mechanism for the decrease in tone.

Ice massage (cryomassage): Superficial massage with ice, a cold pack, or an instrument performed locally to reduce pain and inflammation.

Identification: The clinician's ability to distinguish between healthy and dysfunctional tissue states and to identify tissues and structures and their responses to applied force.

Impairment: A loss or abnormality of the affected individual's body structures or functions that occurs as a result of the initial or subsequent pathophysiology.

Impairment-related outcome: The outcome that is related to the impairment of the client's body structure or function.

Implicit memory (tissue memory): The nonnarrative, nonverbal, and sensory-motor memory that is typically recorded in the amygdala. When implicit memory is evoked, a client will feel as if the memory is happening in the present.

Indication: A sign, symptom, evaluation, or diagnosis that directs the therapist to apply a certain procedure.

Indirect: Techniques in which the therapist applies the force, or moves the client, away from the fascial barrier or restriction of motion.

Indurated: Hardened.

Inertial resistance: The resistance of an object to applied force that depends on its mass.

Inert tissues: Tissues that do not contract, for example, ligament, capsule, and nerve.

Infant massage: A modified form of classical massage designed for infants. Infant massage improves infant development and parent–child bonding and can be used to treat colic.

Informed consent: Obtaining clear and informed consent for treatment from a client involves ensuring that the client understands the intent and direction of therapy. This process requires that the therapist explain exactly what he or she is going to do and how he or she will achieve the specified outcomes. It also requires that the client hears and understands the therapist's explanation, since clients who do not hear the explanation may agree without understanding what the therapist means.

Inquiring touch: Intelligent Touch is inquiring touch. A good clinician is constantly asking questions, and the use of massage is no exception to this requirement. The use of inquiring touch does not imply that the clinician's touch feels tentative to the client or that it lack firmness when required.

Intelligent Touch: The learned skills essential for successful clinical use of massage: attention and concentration, discrimination, identification, inquiry, and intention.

Interferential current: The crossing of two independent medium frequency electrical currents to create a different frequency current at the point of intersection of the two currents. This is used to stimulate large impulse fibers and interferes with the transmission of pain messages at the spinal cord level.

Intergrades with: To merge gradually one into another. When one technique is said to "intergrade" with another, the two techniques can be performed consecutively and will merge gradually one into another since there are intermediate hybrid forms of the technique that lie between and resemble both techniques.

International Classification of Functioning, Disability and Health: A model that presents human function, health, and disability as an interaction between the individual, the disease process, and the environment in which the individual lives.

Interstitial fluid pressure: Pressure that is caused by the amount of fluid in the interstitium or intercellular spaces. The interstitial fluid pressure reflects the degree of hydration of the tissue, and the forces that govern it are described in Starling's Law.

Intervention: 1. A single instance during which a clinician delivers care to the client. 2. A technique or series of techniques that are used to address a client's impairments or wellness goals.

Intractable: Unresponsive to treatment.

Investing layer of the deep fascia: Dense connective tissue layer that lies between the superficial fascia and muscle.

Ischemic compression: See Specific compression and Trigger point pressure release.

Joint integrity: The extent to which a joint conforms to the expected anatomical and biomechanical norms.

Joint manipulation: A high-grade joint mobilization.

Joint mobilization: A technique in which therapists apply controlled, graded force to produce accessory joint motions (joint play) in order to restore altered biomechanics (i.e., to restore normal joint play) of the target joint to reduce pain and improve range of motion.

Joint play: Small movements that occur between synovial joint surfaces that are necessary for normal joint functioning during range of motion. These motions can be produced by the therapist in a passive client, but they are not under voluntary control and cannot be performed actively by the client.

Joint position sense: Ability to accurately locate a joint in space using only proprioceptive information (i.e., when blindfolded).

Joint range of motion: The capacity of the joint to move within the anatomical or physiological range of motion that is available at that joint based on its arthrokinematics and the ability of the periarticular connective tissue to deform. Range of motion reflects the function of the contractile, nervous, inert, and bony tissues and the client's willingness to perform a movement.

Jump sign: Pain behavior, such as wincing and attempted withdrawal, that a client shows when a trigger point is compressed.

Kellogg, J. H.: (1852–1943) American medical doctor who ran the Battle Creek Sanitarium, a health resort that emphasized vegetarian meals, enemas, and exercise. Kellogg wrote well-known texts on massage and hydrotherapy and started a company to market whole-grain cereals.

Key signs: The results of tests and measures that are characteristic for any given orthopedic condition.

Key trigger point: A trigger point that is responsible for activating one or more satellite trigger points. Inactivation of a key trigger point will inactivate its associated satellites.

Kinetic chain: The series of joints that connect the bones of the upper limb or the lower limb.

Kneading: A gliding neuromuscular technique, performed in circles or ellipses, that repeatedly compresses superficial tissues and muscle against underlying structures and releases them. See also Petrissage.

Lactate: The byproduct of anaerobic glycolysis that accumulates in muscles during intense exercise. Accumulation of lactate is no longer believed to be responsible for delayed-onset muscle soreness.

Latent trigger points: Trigger points that are not painful in and of themselves unless they are being palpated.

Lead pipe rigidity: Constant resistance to passive movement.

Lederman, Eyal: British osteopath and author of several books and articles on manual therapy.

Legal right to treat: The therapist's scope of practice permits him or her to treat a given client's condition.

Level of arousal: Level of alertness.

Levels of evidence: A hierarchy of research designs created by Sackett et al. that ranks several different types of studies. Studies at the top of the hierarchy provide the strongest evidence of a cause-and-effect relationship between the intervention and the outcome and vice versa.

Life Events Model of Stress: Holmes and Rahe's model of stress that examined the nature and consequences of negative life events and proposed that interpersonal stressors are predictive of increases in disease activity.

Lifelong learning: The philosophy that learning is required throughout the lifespan of a professional career.

Lifestyle: The way a person (or a group) lives, including attitudes, values, worldview, patterns of social relations, consumption, entertainment, and dress.

Lift/lifting: Lifting of the tissues perpendicularly off the surface of the body, as occurs with some forms of petrissage like picking-up.

Ligament insufficiency: Anatomical or pathological shortening of the capsular ligament.

Ligament laxity: Anatomic or pathologic lengthening of the capsular ligament.

Lipoma: A benign fatty tumor.

Local reflex signs: An effect observed in a particular region that is mediated by the nervous system. Examples are discoloration of the skin (blanching or flushing) or more general autonomic responses such as sweating and nausea.

Lomilomi: A traditional shamanic massage form from Hawaii that is done to heal and to mark life passages. Lomilomi uses repetitive centripetal elongated gliding strokes, and sessions last for 2 hours or longer.

Long-axis traction: Traction in which force is applied parallel to the length of a limb.

Lubricant: A substance, such as oil, that a therapist uses to control the amount of glide, friction, and drag that occurs between his or her moving hands and the client's skin.

Lunge: A movement used during massage, in which the therapist slowly shifts her body weight onto her forward leg by bending that knee and straightening the back leg, while keeping her torso perfectly poised and upright.

Lunge and lean: A movement used during massage in which the therapist inclines her body forward (leans) as she shifts her weight onto her forward leg during a lunge.

Lunge and reach: A movement used during massage in which the therapist extends both arms straight ahead at navel level as she shifts weight onto her forward leg during a lunge.

Lymphatic return: The volume of lymph returned to the venous system through the lymphatic vessels.

Lymph drainage techniques: See Drainage techniques.

Lymphedema: Accumulation of abnormal amounts of lymph fluid and associated swelling of subcutaneous tissues that result from the obstruction, destruction, or hypoplasia of lymph vessels.

Manual lymph drainage (MLD): Comprehensive massage systems designed to enhance lymphatic return (e.g., Vodder, Leduc). These systems may incorporate various massage techniques but often rely extensively on what is termed in this text as superficial lymph drainage technique. MLD also uses other massage techniques, such as petrissage and direct fascial technique, to address consolidated edema associated with chronic conditions.

Matrix (extracellular matrix): The portion of connective tissue found between the cells. It includes proteoglycans, matrix proteins, and water, but not protein fibers such as collagen.

Maturation (of connective tissue): The last period of the chronic stage of inflammation (from the 2nd month to a year after injury), when collagen turnover declines and the scar tissue becomes mostly fibrous.

Mechanical effects of massage: Effects that are caused by physically moving the tissues by compression, tension (stretch), shearing, bending, or twisting.

Mechanical techniques: Massage techniques that compress, stretch, shear, bend, or twist the tissues.

Mechanoreceptor: A receptor for information about movement, tension, pressure, or touch.

Medical massage: The use of massage to help clients with medical conditions return to an optimal state of health.

Medical Model: Clinical model that focused on measuring and treating the client's presenting impairments without a specific consideration of the client's other personal factors.

Mennell, James Beaver: (1880–1957) A British doctor who taught medical massage at St. Thomas's Hospital in London from 1912 to 1935 and wrote an influential textbook on the subject. Mennell's experiences treating the wounded of

World War I convinced him first hand of the efficacy of medical massage.

Meridian: In Traditional Chinese Medicine, a conduit or channel through which energy (qi, chi, ch'i) circulates through the body in well-defined cycles.

Mesomorph: A person with a build that is well-muscled.

Meta-analysis: A form of research in which the results of different, similar studies are pooled and analyzed.

Mobilization: See Joint mobilization.

Modality: Any therapeutic technique. Some examples of physical modalities include hot packs, cryotherapy, ultraviolet radiation, TENS, traction, acupuncture, massage, joint mobilization, and therapeutic exercise.

Model: 1. A framework or system of ideas used to explain the workings of the world. 2. A diagram that represents an idea, phenomena, or relationship between variables.

Moist heat: Superficial heat that is accompanied by a small amount of steam, such as is obtained from a hydrocollator hot pack or thermophore.

Motoneuron (motor neuron) excitability: See H-reflex.

Motor point: The place where a motor neuron enters a muscle.

Muscle endurance: A muscle's ability to contract, or maintain torque, over a number of contractions or a period of time. Conversely, fatigue is inability to maintain torque, or the loss of power, over time.

Muscle energy techniques: Osteopathic techniques in which the patient contracts a muscle in one of a number of ways to promote its relaxation. The patient's position and the duration, direction, and force of the contraction are controlled and gently resisted by the practitioner.

Muscle extensibility: The ability of a muscle and its associated fascia to undergo lengthening deformation during the movement of a joint through its anatomic range.

Muscle integrity: The extent to which a muscle conforms to the expected anatomical and biomechanical norms.

Muscle performance: A muscle's capacity to do work based on its length, tension, and velocity. Neurological stimulus, fuel storage, fuel delivery, and balance, timing, and sequencing of muscle contraction influence integrated muscle performance.

Muscle power: Work produced by a muscle per unit of time (strength × speed).

Muscle resting tension: The firmness to palpation at rest observed in muscles with normal innervation. Traditionally, muscle resting tension has been described as resulting from the physiological properties of muscle, such as viscosity, elasticity, and plasticity, rather than from motor unit firing.

Muscle spasm: Involuntary contraction of a muscle that results in increased muscular tension and shortness that cannot be released voluntarily.

Muscle squeezing: A petrissage technique in which one or both hands are used to grasp, lift, and squeeze a muscle, muscle group, or body segment without glide.

Muscle strain or tear: Lesion or inflammation of muscle fibers that can occur in response to trauma.

Muscle strength: The force or torque produced by a muscle or group of muscles to overcome a resistance during a maximum voluntary contraction.

Muscle tone: Resting tension and responsiveness of muscles to passive elongation or stretch.

Myofascial balance: Appropriate distribution of tension throughout the connective tissues of the myofascial network. Good myofascial balance promotes upright posture and efficiency and ease of movement.

Myofascial network: The muscles and associated connective tissues (tendons, aponeuroses, and fascia) of the locomotor system. This network forms part of a greater system that includes all the structural connective tissues of the body.

Myofascial pain syndrome: The sensory, motor, and autonomic symptoms caused by myofascial trigger points.

Myofascial release: 1. A connective tissue technique that combines nongliding fascial traction with varying amounts of orthopedic stretch and that results in palpable viscoelastic lengthening and plastic deformation of the fascia. 2. A system of treatment that uses the myofascial release technique in conjunction with craniosacral, osteopathic, and other soft tissue techniques.

Myofascial trigger point: A hyperirritable spot in skeletal muscle that is associated with a hypersensitive palpable nodule in a taut band. The area is painful on compression and can give rise to a variety of symptoms, such as referred pain, referred tenderness, motor dysfunction, and autonomic phenomena.

Myofascial unit: One muscle and its associated tendons, aponeuroses, and fascial wrappings.

Myotatic unit: A functional unit of an agonist and its antagonist muscles.

Myotherapy: A method of treating myofascial trigger points, popularized by Bonnie Prudden, that uses specific compression and active exercise to restore full, pain-free movement to muscles.

Myotomal pain: Pain in a myotome, or a group of muscles that are supplied by one nerve root.

Nerve entrapment: Compression of a peripheral nerve or nerve root.

Neurapraxia: Loss of nerve conduction due to compression, without structural change in the axon.

Neurogenic pain: Pain that results from noninflammatory dysfunction of the peripheral or central nervous system that does not involve nociceptor stimulation or trauma.

Neuromuscular facilitation: The application of techniques, such as tapping and quick stretch, to strengthen the contraction of a muscle. These techniques are often applied immediately prior to exercise for clients who have CNS disorders.

Neuromuscular inhibition: The application of massage techniques, such as static contact, or other techniques, such as prolonged cold, to reduce the strength of contraction or tone of a muscle. These techniques are often applied immediately prior to exercise for clients who have CNS disorders.

Neuromuscular Technique (NMT): As defined by Chaitow and others, a complex massage system that includes specific finger and thumb techniques that resemble stripping and direct fascial technique.

Neuromuscular techniques: Massage techniques that palpate muscle, affect the level of resting tension of muscles, and have additional psychoneuroimmunological effects.

Neuromuscular tone: Muscle resting tension and responsiveness of muscles to passive elongation or stretch.

Nociception: The stimulus of pain receptors and the resulting transmission of information about pain to the central nervous system (CNS). Nociceptive information can be modulated in the CNS so that the resulting perception of pain is heightened or reduced.

Nociceptive pain: Sensitization of peripheral nociceptors as a result of injury to a muscle or a joint that causes increased release of neurotransmitters in the dorsal horn of the spinal cord. The sensitized dorsal horn neurons demonstrate increased background activity, increased receptive field size, and increased responses to peripherally applied stimuli.

Nongliding: A technique in which no movement occurs of the hand relative to the skin.

Nonmyofascial trigger point: A hyperirritable spot in scar tissue, fascia, periosteum, ligament, or joint capsule that is associated with a hypersensitive palpable nodule in a taut band.

Nonspecific (treatment) effects: Positive treatment effects that are not caused by the specific action of the intervention, but rather are due to a subject's expectations of benefit. Placebo response.

Numeric rating scale: A numeric scale that clients use to rate the intensity of pain or other subjective symptoms. Zero represents no pain, and 10 represents the worst pain imaginable or previously experienced. The client makes the rating verbally or using a visual scale such as the Visual Analog Scale.

Object of palpation: The chosen portion of the sensory field on which the clinician focuses attention during palpation. The object being palpated is not necessarily a physical object; instead, it may be a characteristic, such as temperature, or a phenomenon, such as resistance to movement.

OBM clinical decision-making: A structured process in which the therapist and client work together to (a) identify the client's impairments and the desired outcomes based on those impairments and (b) develop and implement a treatment plan to achieve those outcomes.

Osteopathy: 1. A branch of medicine that uses manual therapy, in addition to other treatment techniques such as medication and surgery, to treat the full range of conditions. A central tenet of osteopathy is that good structural relationships will positively influence function. 2. A form of alternative therapy that uses a variety of manual techniques, such as craniosacral technique, to treat the musculoskeletal system.

Outcome-Based Massage (OBM): A systematic treatment approach in which therapists provide massage interventions with the goal of achieving specified outcomes that are tailored to address each client's unique needs, presenting issues, and preferences.

Outcome for body structure and function: The outcome that is related to the impairment of the client's body structure or function.

Outcome measure: A variable that is measured in order to gauge the client's progress towards an outcome.

Outcome or Outcome of care: The result of a single intervention or of all of the interventions in the plan of care as a whole.

Overpressure: With respect to massage techniques, an increase of manual pressure applied to a particular structure, such as a group of lymph nodes, often at the end of a stroke.

Overtreatment: Application of techniques for too long a time or with too much force, so that undesirable consequences occur.

Oxytocin: A neurotransmitter hormone that stimulates uterine contractions during labor and the production of milk.

Pain: An unpleasant sensation associated with actual or potential tissue damage that is mediated by specific nerve fibers to the brain where its conscious appreciation may be modified by various factors.

Pain scale: A verbal or visual analog scale that rates a client's experience of pain with numbers from 0 (no pain) to 10 (worst pain ever experienced).

Palliative care: Any form of medical care or treatment that aims to alleviate symptoms without curing.

Palpation: A method of examination in which the therapist uses the hands and fingers to gather information about the location, size, shape, firmness, temperature, and sensitivity of tissues and structures.

Parasympathetic: The branch of the autonomic nervous system with efferent fibers that exit through several cranial nerves and the 2nd to 4th sacral nerves. It slows the heart rate, increases intestinal secretion and peristalsis, constricts bronchioles, and is associated with a general relaxation response of the organism—"rest and digest."

Parasympathetic response: See Parasympathetic.

Parkinsonian rigidity: Rigidity that occurs as a result of basal ganglia lesions. It presents clinically as a tight contraction of both agonist and antagonist muscles throughout the movement (lead pipe rigidity).

Participation or participation capacity: An individual's involvement in a life situation or ability to execute a task within his or her environment.

Passive movement techniques: Massage techniques that primarily palpate the movement of tissues and structures and result in the repetitive movement of soft tissue masses over the underlying structure(s) with varying degrees of joint motion.

Passive range of motion: The amount of joint motion available when an examiner moves a joint through its anatomical or physiological range, without assistance from the client, while the client is relaxed.

Passive relaxed movements: See Passive range of motion.

Pathophysiology: Physiological changes that occur as a result of a medical condition.

Peer supervisor: When therapists are confused by some aspect of the therapeutic process, it is recommended that they consult an experienced peer or supervisor who may assist them in sorting out the problem. This approach to self-care helps therapists to avoid ethical dilemmas and to ensure that they have sufficient resources to help them provide appropriate care.

Percussion, or percussive techniques: Massage techniques that deform and release tissues quickly through controlled, repeated, rhythmic, light striking.

Perfusion: Local circulation of blood through a specific tissue or organ.

Personal factors: Personal characteristics that can have an impact on an individual's health or wellness.

Petrissage: A group of related neuromuscular techniques that repetitively compress, shear, and release muscle tissue with varying amounts of drag, lift, and glide.

Physiological barrier in soft tissue: The resistance that determines the range of motion of soft tissue that is available under normal conditions. In other words, the range of motion of the tissue lies between the two physiological barriers, with the least amount of resistance being apparent at the midrange.

Physiological Model of Stress: Hans Selye's model of stress that is based on the interaction of the adrenal cortex and the neuroendocrine and immune systems during stress. Stress in this model is defined as the body's automatic response ("fight or flight") to a demand that is placed on it.

Picking-up: A one-handed or two-handed gliding petrissage technique in which muscle is lifted and squeezed between the fingers and the abducted thumb.

Piriformis syndrome: A syndrome of posterolateral hip and leg pain caused by a tight piriformis. This may in turn cause sacroiliac joint dysfunction and sciatic nerve entrapment.

Pitting edema: Edema that retains the indentation produced by the pressure of palpation.

Placebo: An intervention that is known not to actively cause specific treatment effects and that is used to replace a specified intervention. It is often used in research.

Plan of care: The systematic set of therapeutic techniques selected by the clinician to achieve the identified outcomes or wellness goals for a client.

Plastic deformation: Deformation in response to applied force that remains after the force is removed; putty-like behavior.

Pliability: The inherent quality of tissue that refers to the ease with which it is bent, twisted, sheared, elongated, or compressed.

Polarity therapy: An energetic approach developed by Randolph Stone, D.O., D.C., N.D. (1890–1981), that uses static contact to treat blockages in the biomagnetic field of the body.

Positional release: A group of related osteopathic techniques that relieve tension and pain in muscles through positioning and gentle sustained pressure.

Positioning: The alignment and support of the client's body by the clinician in preparation for the application of massage.

Post-event massage or post-event sport massage: Massage that is delivered following an event, often a sports event to help the athlete cool down while maintaining high levels of oxygen to help with the oxygen debt.

Postintervention pain/soreness: Pain that arises after an intervention. When due to massage, it may be due to mild inflammation caused by work that is done too quickly, activation of a latent trigger point, or a shift in tension related to postural rebalancing.

Postisometric relaxation (PIR): A technique developed by Karel Lewit, M.D., where the client contracts a tense muscle isometrically against resistance and then relaxes completely as the therapist takes up the slack.

Posttraumatic stress disorder: Severe psychological distress that develops after events in which a person is a witness to or exposed to the threat of death or serious injury. Disabling symptoms may include recurrent memories, fears, feelings of helplessness, rage, and avoidance behavior.

Postural awareness: See Posture.

Postural condition: Any condition of impaired or deficient posture, such as hyperlordosis, hyperkyphosis, scoliosis, and upper and lower cross syndromes. Postural conditions involve (at least) the impairments of adaptive shortening, adaptive lengthening, and impaired postural awareness.

Postural drainage: The use of positioning to promote the movement of bronchial secretions through the lungs; conventionally used in conjunction with percussion.

Postural drainage and percussion (PDP): The use of postural drainage and clapping (cupping) to mechanically loosen secretions in the lungs and facilitate airway clearance. Clapping is followed by, or alternated with, rapid compression and release of the rib cage.

Postural exercise: Any exercise (e.g., stretching, strengthening, or awareness) that is designed to improve posture.

Postural imbalance: Lack of balanced length and strength that is seen between agonist and antagonist groups of muscles in postural conditions.

Postural malalignment: Abnormal joint alignment caused by soft tissue imbalance or deformity within a bone.

Postural scan: A test in which the therapist observes the client's body structure for alignment, symmetry, and muscular balance. A postural scan is performed with the client standing and viewed from the front, back, and both sides.

Postural tone: The development of muscular tension in skeletal muscles that participate in maintaining the positions of different parts of the skeleton. The cerebellum regulates postural tone. Unlike muscle resting tension, constant muscle activation is required for the maintenance of postural tone, and the self-sustained firing of motor neurons

may reduce the need for prolonged synaptic input in this situation.

Postural weakness: Weakness that is seen in muscles that show adaptive lengthening in postural conditions.

Posture: The positioning and alignment of the skeleton and associated soft tissues in relation to gravity, the center of mass, and the base of support of the body.

Power: See Muscle power.

Power differential: A difference in the perceived or actual power between individuals in a relationship.

Power stroke: That portion of a circular or elliptical massage technique where pressure is applied to the client's tissues, usually by pushing the hand away from the body and adding some amount of body weight; contrasted with return stroke.

Practice guidelines: Broad guidelines for the treatment of medical conditions that provide therapists with a general framework for planning and progressing interventions. These condition-specific practice guidelines and professional practice guidelines outline a general guide to prognoses, expected numbers of visits per episode of care, outcome measures, and relevant types of intervention for a range of medical conditions.

Precompetition sports massage: Sports massage performed up to 24-hours before competition, which seeks to enhance arousal and awareness, while promoting relaxation of skeletal muscle.

Pressure of technique: The amount of force per unit area of contact surface that the clinician applies.

Pressure stroke: See Power stroke.

Pretest–posttest design: An experimental research design in which subjects are tested before and after the intervention period.

Prevention: A clinical approach that focuses on impeding the development of impairments and medical conditions, rather than treating them after they occur.

Primary impairment: Any loss or abnormality of the client's body structures or functions that occurs as a result of the pathophysiology of a medical condition.

Primary research: The original research conducted by therapists or researchers. Types of primary research include: clinical trials, surveys, ethnographies, and a variety of other research designs.

Primary source: A source that directly documents the primary research, which is the original research conducted by therapists or researchers. Primary sources are typically professional journals, conference presentations, and, occasionally, text books.

Principles of (sequence) design: Principles for selecting and ordering massage techniques to achieve specific clinical outcomes.

Process of care: The manner in which care is delivered, and the activities that take place within and between the clinician and the client. This encompasses the interpersonal aspects of the client–clinician interaction and the technical aspects of how the clinician provides care.

Prognosis: The process of predicting the client's level and timing of improvement.

Progression: Incremental changes in the techniques used to treat a client's clinical condition or address the client's wellness goals. Stages of progression reflect the clinical course and prognosis for a given condition and client. Therapists can use information from several sources to guide treatment progression. These sources include practice guidelines, findings from the client examination, and clinical experience.

Progressive relaxation: A method to reduce stress and train muscular relaxation developed by Edmund Jacobsen in the 1920s. The client alternately tenses and relaxes groups of muscles sequentially throughout the body.

Proprioception: Awareness of position, weight, and movement of the body as a whole and of its parts in relation to each other.

Proprioceptive neuromuscular facilitation (PNF): Developed in the 1940s by Dr. Kabat and physical therapists Margaret Knott and Dorothy Voss, is a method of increasing range of motion, strength, endurance, joint stability, and motor control through the stimulation of proprioceptors. Techniques include Hold-Relax, Rhythmic Initiation, Slow Reversal, and Rhythmic Stabilization.

Proprioceptive palpation: A form of palpation in which the clinician uses proprioceptive sense to gauge how the client's compressed tissues are deforming under the application of the clinician's body weight.

Proprioceptive stimulation techniques: The application of massage techniques, such as tapping, or other techniques, such as quick stretch, to strengthen the contraction of muscle; often done immediately prior to exercise for clients who have CNS disorders.

Psychoneuroimmunology: The science that studies the relationships between the nervous, endocrine, and immune systems and how these relationships affect behavior.

Pulse: Periodic, regular expansion and contraction of arterial walls in response to the fluid wave caused by contraction of the heart.

Qi: See Chi.

Qualitative research: Research that uses the collection and analysis of word-based experiential and observational data, rather than numbers. Qualitative research assumes that people define reality.

Quality of life: The objective and subjective dimensions of an individual's ability to function in, and derive satisfaction from, a variety of social roles.

Quantitative research: Research that uses the collection and analysis of numerical data. The underlying assumption in quantitative research is that there is a reality that exists independently of people.

Radicular pain: Pain that is felt in a dermatome, myotome, or sclerotome because of direct involvement of a spinal nerve or nerve root. Also known as nerve root pain.

Radiculopathy: Pathology of a nerve root that commonly produces radicular pain.

Randomized clinical trial (RCT): A clinical trial whose participants have been randomly allocated to treatment and control groups. RCTs are highly ranked in the hierarchy of quantitative research methods. Sometimes called a randomized controlled trial.

Rate of technique: An indication of how fast the force is applied. The rate may describe the speed of the movement of the clinician's hand over the client's skin (distance per second), the frequency of repetitions of a described technique (repetitions per second), or both.

Reactive cramping/tightening: The undesirable elevation of resting tension in a massaged muscle group or its antagonist that may appear shortly after treatment. It indicates activation of a latent trigger point or a shift in tension related to postural rebalancing.

Reactive hyperemia: Hyperemia that is caused by short applications of cold.

Recovery: The improvement in the client's impairments that are the result of a medical condition.

Red flag: A sign or symptom that indicates the presence of a condition requiring immediate medical attention.

Re-examination: Ongoing repetition of the examination process to determine the client's progress towards his or her clinical or wellness goals.

Referred pain: Pain that is felt at another part of the body that is at a distance from the tissues that have caused it because the referred site is supplied by the same or adjacent neural segments.

Referred tenderness: Tenderness to palpation that is felt at another part of the body that is at a distance from the tissues that have caused it because the referred site is supplied by the same or adjacent neural segments.

Reflex effect: An effect where functional change is mediated by the nervous system (as opposed to a mechanical effect).

Reflex sympathetic dystrophy (RSD): See Complex regional pain syndrome.

Reflex technique: A massage technique whose effects are largely or solely reflex effects.

Reflexology: A system of manual treatment that applies specific compression to reflex points in the foot or hand to normalize function in distant body segments or organs.

Reiki: An energetic approach similar to Therapeutic Touch and Healing Touch. Practitioners use the simplest form of touch to manipulate the energy field or magnetic field of the client's body.

Relaxation: 1. The process of releasing mental or physical tension. 2. A state of low mental or physical tension. See Parasympathetic.

Repetitive strain injury (repetitive motion trauma, cumulative trauma syndrome): Damage to muscles, tendons, or nerves in the upper body that is caused by the sustained postures and repetitive movements such as keyboarding.

Research competency: The ability to conduct research.

Research literacy: The ability to find, understand, and critically evaluate research evidence for application in professional practice.

Resilience: The inherent quality of tissue that restores original form after deformation by applied force.

Resistance: The inherent quality of tissue that counteracts the tendency of applied force to produce movement of the tissue.

Respiratory rhythm: Periodic, regular movement of the chest wall that occurs during breathing.

Resting muscle tension: The firmness to palpation at rest observed in muscles with normal innervation or the perceived texture of muscle during palpation.

Restorative sleep: Restful sleep that is conducive to health. Sleep disturbances from various causes may alter sleep architecture, so that sleep occurs but does not have its normal restorative effects.

Restrictive, or pathological barriers, in soft tissue: Barriers that are observed when soft tissue dysfunction is present. They can be located anywhere between the normal physiological barriers, can limit the available range of motion within the tissues, and can alter the position of the midrange. A restrictive barrier will change the quality of the movement and the "feel" at the

end of the tissue range of motion. This is analogous to the abnormal end feels observed in joints.

Retrograde: Proceeding backwards from the endpoint. In the case of abdominal massage, if a technique is applied in a retrograde order, it means that the technique is applied first over the sigmoid colon, then the descending colon, then the transverse colon, and lastly over the ascending colon.

Retrostasis: Pushing of excess fluid away from an area of the body due to vasoconstriction caused by local application of cold for more than 10 minutes.

Return stroke: The portion of a circular or elliptical massage technique where the hand glides to its original position with little or no pressure.

Rhythmic mobilization: A technique in which entire structures are repetitively moved, resulting in the movement of soft tissue over bone and the movement of related joints and internal organs.

Rib cage mobility: The capacity of the rib cage to move within the available anatomical range of motion during respiration, based on the arthrokinematics of the joints of the rib cage and the thoracic spine, and the ability of the periarticular connective tissue to deform.

Rigidity: Increased muscular tone that results from brainstem or basal ganglia lesions. Rigidity involves a uniformly increased resistance in both agonist and antagonist muscles, resulting in stiff, immovable body parts, independent of the velocity of the stretch stimulus.

Rocking: A technique in which gentle, repetitive oscillation of the body is produced by repeatedly pushing the pelvis or torso from a midline resting position into lateral deviation and then allowing it to return.

Rolf, Ida P.: (1896–1979) American biochemist, originator of Structural Integration and Rolfing, and author of the text *On the Integration of Human Structures*. Dr. Rolf was an influential innovator; for example, she likely introduced both the use of the elbow and forearm as a contact surface and the simultaneous use of massage and active movement.

Rolfing (The Rolf Method of Structural Integration): The massage-related approach developed by Ida Rolf combines the following features: the aim of lengthening and balancing the myofascial network to improve posture and movement, an emphasis on connective tissue techniques, a series of 10 sessions, and the use of movement and postural awareness exercises.

Salt glow: An application of wet salt to the client's skin with rubbing. A full-body application takes 20–30 minutes, acts as a tonic, and strongly stimulates peripheral circulation.

Satellite trigger point: A trigger point that is activated by a key trigger point by being in its area of referral or by being its antagonist or synergist.

Scanning, or stroking, palpation: Palpation that moves relatively quickly over a large area. Therapists use this when they want to collect information from a wide area.

Scapulohumeral rhythm: The ratio between glenohumeral motion and scapulothoracic motion during shoulder abduction. The normal ratio is 2 degrees of glenohumeral motion for 1 degree of scapulothoracic motion, after 20 degrees.

Scar: The fibrous tissue that replaces normal tissues that have been destroyed by a burn, wound, surgery, radiation, or disease.

Sclerotomal pain: Pain in a sclerotome, an area of bone or fascia innervated by one segmental nerve root.

Seated aligned posture: A posture used during massage, in which the therapist sits upright in a relaxed manner, while requiring his or her awareness of his or her pelvis contacting the chair.

Secondary effect: An indirect therapeutic effect.

Secondary impairments: Any loss or abnormality of the client's body structures or functions that occurs as a result of the primary impairments.

Secondary research: Studies that summarize and draw conclusions from primary research studies. Examples are nonsystematic literature reviews, systematic literature reviews, and meta-analyses.

Secondary source: A summary of the information presented in a primary source. Secondary sources can include secondary research studies, such as literature reviews and meta-analyses. Other secondary sources are textbooks, the popular media, the Internet, professional courses, and professional journals.

Sedation: The process of calming or allaying nervous excitement. See Relaxation.

Segmental vertebral dysfunction: Abnormal movement of the joints in a contiguous section of the spine that often involves adjacent areas of hyper- and hypomobility.

Self-care activities: Any actions that clients perform on their own behalf to promote wellness or treat impairments.

Self-mobilization: See Automobilization.

Shoulder separation: An injury in which the acromioclavicular and coracoclavicular ligaments are torn.

Sequence: A structured, outcome-based series or succession of massage techniques that comprise an intervention or a part of an intervention.

Serotonin: A widely spread neurotransmitter, 5-hydroxytryptamine, that is involved in depression, appetite, nausea, intestinal motility, sleep cycles, and obsessive compulsive disorders.

Shaking: A passive movement technique in which soft tissue, primarily muscle, is repetitively moved back and forth over the underlying bone, with minimal joint movement.

Sham: A type of placebo treatment that mimics the form of the actual treatment without actively causing specific treatment effects.

Shear/shearing: Deformation that involves sliding of adjacent layers over each other.

Shiatsu: A complex Japanese system of massage, based on the meridian system, that makes extensive use of specific compression.

Simons, Dr. David: American medical doctor and coauthor with Dr. Janet Travell of both volumes of *Myofascial Pain and Dysfunction,* the first and most authoritative text reference about trigger points.

Skin: A layer of epithelium, the epidermis, and the dermis.

Skin rolling: A gliding connective tissue technique in which tissue superficial to the investing layer of deep fascia is grasped, continuously lifted, and rolled over underlying tissues in a wave-like motion.

Slow-stroke back rub: A light massage of short duration, often performed by nursing staff in hospitals, and the subject of numerous clinical trials.

Societal limitations: Those limitations to an individual's level of function that can be attributed to physical or attitudinal barriers in society.

Soft tissue: Pliable tissue such as muscle, tendon, fascia, ligament, synovial capsule, cartilage, and nerve.

Soft tissue dysfunction: Abnormal function of soft tissues, such as muscle, tendon, fascia, ligament, synovial capsule, cartilage, and nerve, due to impairment or pathophysiology.

Soft tissue range of motion: Available range of motion of soft tissue that is analogous to the range of motion available in joints. Within this range of motion, normal soft tissue has three barriers or resistances that can limit movement.

Solid edema: See Consolidated edema.

Somatoemotional release: 1. The phenomenon of emotional release that occurs in response to a touch therapy and manifests as sighs, crying, laughing, muscle twitches, or anger. 2. A service-marked method of the Upledger Institute that teaches the techniques and skills required to deal with this phenomenon.

Somatovisceral reflex: A reflex in which touch, pressure, or thermal stimulation applied to musculoskeletal tissues affects visceral function.

Spasm: A sudden, involuntary contraction of skeletal or smooth muscle that causes increased tension in the muscle and often pain. Spasms of skeletal muscle are accompanied by motor neuron firing.

Spasticity: Increased muscular tone that results from an upper motor neuron lesion that may or may not be associated with reflex hyperexcitability. Spastic muscle exhibits velocity-dependent increase in tonic stretch reflexes. The quicker the stretch is, the more pronounced the resistance of the spastic muscle.

Specific compression: A nongliding neuromuscular technique in which pressure is applied to the target tissue with a specific contact surface in a direction that is perpendicular to the target tissue.

Specific kneading: A gliding petrissage technique performed in circles or ellipses and delivered with a small contact surface such as the thumb.

Specific technique: A technique that is applied to a localized area, applied with a small contact surface, or both.

Sports massage: Massage performed on athletes performed before, between, or after events, for the purpose of preparation, recovery, maintenance, or rehabilitation.

Sprain: Overstretching, partial tearing, or complete tearing of a ligament due to trauma.

Spray and stretch: A method of inactivating trigger points in which skin overlying the muscle and area of referral is cooled with vapocoolant spray while the muscle is simultaneously stretched. The alternative ice and stretch method has a similar effect but avoids the use of chemicals that damage the ozone layer.

Standard (Universal) Precautions: A set of procedures designed to prevent the spread of infectious diseases that describes how to handle blood, serous fluids, and any material that has come in contact with them. These precautions include handwashing and wearing protective equipment such as gloves, masks, and gowns.

Standing aligned posture: A posture used during massage in which the therapist stands upright in a relaxed manner while refining her awareness of her feet contacting the ground.

Standing controlled lean: A movement used during massage in which the therapist leans forward from the lunge position to contact the client and transfers some of his or her weight to the client in a controlled manner.

Standing upright posture: See Standing aligned posture.

State anxiety: A measure that represents a person's experience of anxiety at a given moment in time. It is opposed to trait anxiety, which measures anxiety as a more enduring character trait.

Static contact: A superficial reflex technique in which the clinician's hands contact the client's body without motion and with minimal force.

Static palpation: Palpation that involves no movement of the palpating hand and is best suited for palpating moving phenomena such as pulse or respiratory rhythm.

Stiffness: Resistance to applied forces; rigidity.

Stimulating massage: Massage that is quick paced and performed to decrease fatigue, increase arousal, or prepare for activity.

Stimulation: Sensory input.

Strain: Trauma to a muscle and/or its tendon from overstretching or violent contraction. There may be tearing of fibers with a palpable depression in the muscle.

Strain-counterstrain: See Positional release.

Strength: The maximum force that a muscle or muscle group can produce against resistance.

Stress: Any physical, physiological, or psychological stimulus that disrupts homeostasis.

Stress response: The individual's cognitive, physiological, affective, or behavioral response to the stressor or stress-causing agent.

Stripping: A slow, specific, gliding, neuromuscular technique that is applied from the origin of a muscle to its insertion for the purpose of reducing the activity of trigger points.

Stroke volume (cardiac stroke volume): The amount of blood pumped by the left ventricle of the heart in one contraction.

Structural Integration: A generic term for the massage systems descended from the work of Ida Rolf, whose practitioners use connective tissue techniques and education to realign clients' bodies in a series of 10 or more interventions.

Structure of care: The human, physical, and financial resources that are available for the delivery of care.

Substance P: A peptide neurotransmitter that is involved in the regulation of depression, anxiety, and pain and in the body's response to stress and noxious stimuli.

Superficial effleurage: A gliding manipulation performed with light centripetal pressure that deforms subcutaneous tissue down to the investing layer of the deep fascia.

Superficial fascia: Connective tissue layer that is deep to the skin that houses fat and water; that provides a path for nerves and vessels; and that may contain, in certain areas of the body, striated muscle that controls the movement of the skin, such as the platysma muscle.

Superficial fluid techniques: Massage techniques that are applied to tissues superficial to muscle that increase the return flow of lymph and possibly venous blood.

Superficial lymph drainage technique: A nongliding technique performed in the direction of lymphatic flow using short, rhythmical strokes with light pressure that deforms subcutaneous tissue without engaging muscle.

Superficial reflex techniques: Massage techniques that palpate the skin and primarily affect level of arousal, autonomic balance, and the perception of pain.

Superficial stroking: A superficial reflex technique that involves unidirectional pressureless gliding over the client's skin with minimal deformation of subcutaneous tissues; usually applied over large areas.

Supports: Objects such as pillows and bolsters that are used to make the client more comfortable, stable, or accessible during massage.

Swedish massage: A system of massage, consolidated by Per Henrik Ling (1776–1839), that includes effleurage, petrissage, friction, tapotement, and shaking (or vibration). It is one of the technical foundations for Outcome-Based Massage.

Swelling: An abnormal enlargement of a segment of the body.

Sympathetic response: A response caused by activating the sympathetic division of the autonomic nervous system, whose efferent fibers exit through the thoracolumbar spinal nerves. Effects include increased heart rate, vasoconstriction in the skin and viscera, vasodilation in skeletal muscle, dilation of bronchioles, and secretion of epinephrine and norepinephrine.

Systematic review: A type of secondary research that evaluates findings from individual studies and combines these findings using statistical techniques.

Systemic connective tissue disorders: See Connective tissue disease.

Tai Chi: An oriental movement discipline, which is related to martial arts, in which choreographed sequences of slow dance-like movements are practiced to develop awareness, flexibility, strength, and poise.

Tapotement: See Percussion.

Taut band: A group of tense muscle fibers that extend from a trigger point to the muscle's attachments and that will twitch when the trigger point is palpated.

Taxonomy: System of classification.

T-bar: A T-shaped instrument that is gripped in the hand and used to perform massage techniques to reduce hand strain.

Tendinitis: Inflammation of the peritendinous tissues that can occur in response to repetitive mechanical trauma.

Tendinopathy: Pathology of a tendon.

Tendinosis: Unlike tendinitis, which is an inflammatory condition, tendinosis refers to common overuse conditions of a tendon with a histopathology that is consistent with a noninflammatory, degenerative process of unclear etiology.

TENS (transcutaneous electrical nerve stimulation): The application of mild electrical stimulation to electrodes attached to the skin for analgesia.

Tension, or tensile force: Any force that is so oriented that its effect is to lengthen a tissue or structure.

Terminus stroke (MLD): A stroke applied just above the clavicle that milks the junctions of the right lymphatic and thoracic ducts with the subclavian veins. This stroke begins a drainage sequence for any region of the body.

Thai massage: An Eastern massage approach performed with the client clothed and lying on the floor that makes extensive use of specific compression along meridians and passive stretching.

Theory: An organized set of facts that explains the relationships between a group of observed phenomena.

Therapeutic contract: The agreement between therapist and client as to what goals are to be addressed, how the therapy will proceed, and what is expected of each person.

Therapeutic effects: The effects produced by a technique that are used to achieve clinical outcomes. A massage technique can produce multiple therapeutic effects. These may occur locally, only on the site of manipulation, or generally throughout the client's body. The therapeutic effects of massage techniques fall into six categories: mechanical, physiological, psychological, reflex, psychoneuroimmunological, and "energetic."

Therapeutic rapport: A relationship of mutual trust and sympathy between a therapist and client.

Therapeutic relationship: The therapeutic relationship is the trust relationship that forms between a client and a therapist where the needs of the client, the ethical considerations of the therapist, and the boundaries of what is possible contain and frame the outcomes of care.

Therapeutic Touch: An energetic approach developed by Delores Kreiger, RN, in the 1970s. Practitioners use the simplest form of touch and may also move their hands above the surface of the body to manipulate the energy field or magnetic field of the client's body.

Therapeutic ultrasound: A treatment modality in which high-frequency sound waves are used to treat musculoskeletal injuries. Effects may be due to warming of tissues, increased blood flow, and stimulation of healing.

Thixotropy: The property of some colloids by which they become more fluid when subjected to movement or heat and less fluid when subjected to stasis or cold.

Thoracic outlet (compression) syndrome (TOS): A group of conditions caused by compression of the subclavian vessels and trunks of the brachial plexus in the region(s) of the clavicle, the first rib, and the anterior scalene and pectoralis minor muscles. Symptoms may include pain, swelling, and neurological symptoms in the upper limb.

Tissue memory: This occurs when a client is touched by a therapist in a way that reminds the client of another earlier and often significant life experience. A cascade of emotional and biochemical responses occur within the client that may cause concern, fear, or bewilderment for the client.

Tissues engaged by technique: The target tissues or layers of tissue to which the clinician directs the pressure of the stroke and that are mechanically deformed by application of the technique.

Tone: See Muscle tone.

Torticollis: A condition in which the head is tilted toward one side and rotated towards the opposite side. It may be congenital or caused by unilateral spasm or trigger points in the sternocleidomastoid.

Touch Research Institute (University of Miami): The Touch Research Institute was formally established in 1992 by Tiffany Field, Ph.D., at the University of Miami School of Medicine. Since that time, numerous researchers there have published dozens of articles investigating the effects of massage on a variety of population groups and clinical conditions.

Touch-triggered memory: A memory that is triggered by touch. See implicit memory and somato-emotional release.

Traction: A sustained pulling force. Manual traction is commonly applied to separate joint surfaces or oriented parallel to the long axis of a limb.

Traditional Chinese Medicine (TCM): An ancient, vast, and sophisticated system of philosophy, clinical theory, and practice that has come to the attention of the West in recent decades primarily because of the evidence for the analgesic effects of acupuncture. Fundamental to the system of Chinese medicine are several interrelated concepts that have no parallel concepts in Western medicine. In Chinese medicine, energy (chi) circulates through the body in well-defined cycles through conduits or channels called meridians.

Trager Method of Psychophysical Integration: A method of passive rocking and rhythmic mobilization that teaches awareness of relaxation, ease, lightness, and freedom of movement developed by Dr. Milton Trager. Table work is supplemented with dance-like active movements taught to clients for home use to achieve the same ends.

Trait anxiety: A measure of anxiety as an enduring character trait. It is opposed to state anxiety, which measures a person's experience of anxiety at a given moment in time.

Transcutaneous electrical nerve stimulation: See TENS.

Transference: Occurs when a client idealizes and projects feelings onto the therapist that are unconscious, unprocessed, or unexpressed. When unresolved feelings or childhood issues are "transferred" onto the therapist, then a client is said to be experiencing transference.

Transitional stroke: A massage stroke that is used between regions or between techniques that take more time. Superficial effleurage and superficial stroking are commonly used transitional strokes.

Traumatic edema: Edema that results from trauma.

Travell, Dr. Janet: (1901–1997) American medical doctor, and senior coauthor with Dr. David Simons of both volumes of *Myofascial Pain and Dysfunction,* the first and most authoritative text reference about trigger points.

Treatment: 1. A clinical intervention that is directed to an impairment in the client's body structure or function. 2. A series of interventions that make up an episode of care.

Treatment of impairments: Treatment when the aim is to reduce the impairments associated with medical conditions.

Treatment Phase: The Treatment Phase is an ongoing cycle of treatment, re-examination, and treatment progression that begins after the therapist completes the plan of care.

Treatment Planning Phase: The steps in the Treatment Planning Phase involve identifying body structures and functions that are appropriate for treatment and selecting treatment techniques that will produce improvements in the client's impairments in body structures and functions, functional limitations, or overall wellness.

Tremors: Rhythmic movements of a joint that result from involuntary contractions of antagonist and agonist muscle groups.

Trigger point: See Myofascial trigger point.

Trigger point pain: Referred pain that arises in a trigger point but is felt at a distance that is often entirely remote from its source. The pattern of referred pain is diagnostic of the site of origin. The distribution of referred trigger point pain rarely coincides entirely with the distribution of a peripheral nerve or dermatomal segment.

Trigger point pressure release: A specialized application of specific compression for reducing the activity and symptoms of myofascial trigger points.

Trigger point syndrome: See Myofascial pain syndrome.

Trophic changes: Changes in local tissue health usually due to interruption of peripheral nerve supply to an area.

Twitch response: A transient reflex contraction of the muscles fibers in the taut band that contains a trigger point, caused by palpation of the trigger point.

Ultrasound: See Therapeutic ultrasound.

Unnecessary muscle tension: Unwitting muscular contraction or muscle tension that is under voluntary control.

Upledger, John: American osteopathic physician and author of numerous texts on craniosacral and related therapies. He is the founder of the Upledger Institute in Florida, which offers training in a wide variety of manual therapies.

Upper-cross syndrome: A postural syndrome in which the pectorals, upper trapezius, and levator scapulae tighten and shorten, while the rhomboids, serratus anterior, middle and lower trapezius, and deep neck flexors weaken.

Varicosities: Enlarged twisted veins that are commonly found on the legs.

VAS (visual analog scale): A scale that clients use to rate the intensity of pain or other subjective symptoms. The client marks the rating on a 10-cm line with descriptors at each end.

Venous insufficiency (venous stasis): Reduced return flow of venous blood usually from the lower limb that is caused by incompetent valves and venous hypertension.

Venous return: The volume of blood returned to the heart through the veins.

Venous ulcer: A slow-healing ulcer associated with impaired venous return that is usually located above the medial malleolus.

Vestibular reflex: A reflex that depends on sensory information from the labyrinth of the ear.

Visceral pain: Pain in areas of the viscera that are supplied by a nerve root.

Viscerosomatic reflex: A reflex in which visceral dysfunction affects the function of musculoskeletal tissues. See Connective tissue zone.

Viscoelastic: Showing both viscous/plastic and elastic behavior. For a viscoelastic stretch, some of the length that the tissue gains during the stretch will remain when one releases the tensile force.

Viscoelastic deformation: Deformation in response to applied force that partially remains after the force is removed; viscoelastic deformation combines spring-like and putty-like behavior.

Viscosity, or fluid viscosity: The property of fluids and semifluids that offers resistance to flow, i.e., stickiness.

Vodder, Emil: Originator in the 1920s and 1930s of what later became the Vodder method of Manual Lymph Drainage. There are now numerous lymphatic drainage schools that have been influenced to some degree by the Vodder method.

Wellness: The state of an individual that encompasses both a balance of mind, body, and spirit and individuals' self-perception of their well-being, which is distinct from his or her state of "health."

Wellness behavior: Personal factors that play a central role in wellness, such as self-nurturance, healthy lifestyles, readiness for change, and perceived health.

Wellness goals: Clinical goals for optimizing clients' body structures and functions to enhance their levels of wellness.

Wellness Interactions Model: A model that shows an ongoing interaction between a person, wellness, and the person's environment. In this model, an individual's level of wellness can affect any aspect of his or her person at any point in life, and vice versa. At the same time, that individual exists within an environment in which the barriers and facilitators to wellness will influence his or her level of wellness.

Wellness intervention: A systematic application of therapeutic techniques to achieve a client's wellness goals, rather than the improvement of impairments.

Wellness massage: Massage to achieve a client's wellness goals for body structures and functions that are free of impairments.

Whole Systems massage: The Whole Systems approach takes a broader view of the client within the therapeutic environment and therapist-client relationship, rather than focusing on the client's medical condition or wellness goals alone. Looking at outcomes from this perspective will consider the client's experiences of massage, psychosocial effects of the therapeutic environment, a client's expectations of the therapist, and even the therapist's perspective.

Whole systems research: An approach for examining the complex interrelationship between the specific and nonspecific effects of a massage intervention or a massage practice as a whole.

Wide-stance knee bend: A posture and movement used during massage in which the therapist stands with widely placed feet and then flexes and extends the knees to lower and raise the upright torso in relation to the floor.

Wringing: A petrissage technique in which muscle is lifted and sheared between contact surfaces that are moving in opposite directions.

Yin and yang: In Traditional Chinese Medicine, the two basic qualities of energy. Yin energy, metaphorically described as "female" and "negative," is ascending and is associated with hollow organs such as the stomach. Yang energy, metaphorically characterized as "male" and "positive," is descending and is associated with solid organs such as the liver. Health is conceptualized as a dynamic balance between yin and yang energy flowing in precise diurnal patterns through the various meridians.